A World Geography of Human Diseases

A World Geography of Human Diseases

Edited by

G. Melvyn Howe

*Department of Geography,
University of Strathclyde,
Glasgow, Scotland*

1977

ACADEMIC PRESS
London New York San Francisco
A Subsidiary of Harcourt Brace Jovanovich, Publishers

ACADEMIC PRESS INC. (LONDON) LTD.
24/28 Oval Road,
London NW1

United States Edition published by
ACADEMIC PRESS INC.
111 Fifth Avenue
New York, New York 10003

Illustrations in Chapter 9 by R. Willcox

Library of Congress Catalog Card Number: 77 71825
ISBN: 0 12 357150 2

Printed in Great Britain by
Willmer Brothers Limited, Birkenhead

Contributors

A. P. Ball, B.Sc., M.B., M.R.C.P.(U.K.). *Senior Registrar, Department of Medicine (Sub-department of Communicable and Tropical Diseases), East Birmingham Hospital, Birmingham, England*

A. W. A. Brown, Ph.D. *Emeritus Professor, Michigan State University (Department of Entomology), East Lansing, Michigan, U.S.A.*

L. Burgess, B.A. *Lecturer, Division of Earth and Biological Sciences, Derby College of Art and Technology, Derby, England,* formerly *Research Student, Department of Geography, University of Strathclyde, Glasgow, Scotland*

A. B. Christie, M.A., M.D., F.R.C.P., F.F.C.M., D.Ph., D.Ch. *Professor of Infectious Diseases, University of Benghazi, Libya,* formerly *Honorary Physician, Fazakerley Hospital, Liverpool, England*

R. Elsdon-Dew, M.D., D.Sc., F.R.S.(S.Af.). Formerly *Director, Amoebiasis Research Institute for Parasitology, Durban, S. Africa*

J. A. Forbes, A.M., M.B., B.S., F.R.A.C.P., F.A.C.M.A. *Medical Superintendent, Fairfield Hospital, Fairfield, Victoria, Australia*

G. Ffrench, M.A., M.D., M.R.C.P. *Department of Industrial Medicine, Central Middlesex Hospital, London, England*

P. Gatenby, B.A. *Research Student, Department of Geography, University of Strathclyde, Glasgow, Scotland*

J. Giggs, B.A., Ph.D. *Lecturer, Department of Geography, University of Nottingham, Nottingham, England*

C. R. Gillis, M.B., Ch.B., M.D. *Director, West of Scotland Cancer Intelligence Unit, Ruchill Hospital, Glasgow, Scotland*

G. Melvyn Howe, M.Sc., Ph.D., D.Sc. *Professor of Geography, University of Strathclyde, Glasgow, Scotland*

H. Jusatz, Dr. Med. *Professor and Director, Geomedical Research Unit, Heidelberg Academy of Sciences, Heidelberg, W. Germany*

W. E. Kershaw, C.M.G., V.R.D., M.D., D.Sc. *Professor of Biol-*

ogy, University of Salford, lately *Walter Myers and Everett Dutton Professor of Parasitology and Entomology, Liverpool School of Tropical Medicine and University of Liverpool, England*

A. Learmonth, M.A., Ph.D. *Professor of Geography, The Open University, Walton, Buckinghamshire, England*

J. May, M.D.† *Consultant to the Tunisian National Institute of Nutrition and Food Technology, Agency for International Development and the United Nations Development Programme.*

G. H. Rée, M.B., B.Chir., M.R.C.P., D.C.M.T. *Senior Lecturer, Department of Clinical Tropical Medicine, Hospital for Tropical Diseases, London, England*

J. L. Reed, M.B., B.Chir., F.R.C.P., F.R.C.Psych. *Senior Lecturer, Department of Psychological Medicine, St. Bartholomew's Hospital, London, England*

G. Sangster, M.D., F.R.C.P.(Ed.). *Consultant Physician, Infectious Diseases Unit, City Hospital, Edinburgh,* and *Hon. Senior Lecturer, University of Edinburgh, Scotland*

G. C. Schild, B.Sc., Ph.D., F.I.Biol. *Head of Division of Virology, National Institute for Biological Standards and Control, Hampstead, London, England*

I. Sutherland, M.A., D.Phil. *Director, Statistical Research and Services Unit, Medical Research Council, University College Hospital Medical School, London, England*

R. R. Willcox, M.D., F.R.C.P. *Consultant Venereologist, St. Mary's Hospital, London* and *King Edward VII Hospital, London, England. Member of W.H.O. Expert Panel on Venereal Infections and Treponematoses*

J. C. Young, B.Sc. Ph.D. *Warden of Clare Hall and Lecturer in Geography, University of Leicester, England*

†deceased

Foreword

Gordon T. Stewart
Mechan Professor of Community Medicine in the University of Glasgow, Scotland

In a world in which the word International is more likely to raise suspicious than wise thoughts, it is a relief as well as a privilege to introduce a book written with sanity and benevolence. Professor Melvyn Howe has harnessed the study of geography to the service of human needs in several ways but in none more so than in expanding the base of medical knowledge. In the present volume he deals with the main diseases of mankind on a global basis, bringing together a group of well-known experts for the purpose.

In the context of health, geography has to be viewed both regionally and nationally. Disease does not usually respect frontiers though it can be stopped at a frontier by resolute action, as in the case of some of the major communicable diseases. This is where detailed knowledge of geography becomes not just helpful but indispensable. The control of smallpox, for instance, required knowledge in the first place of its prevalence within and between countries; of its spread along routes of commerce and migration; of the acceptability of vaccines and health education by backward peoples; and of the continuing need for surveillance and evaluation of intervention. In the case of smallpox, from all accounts, the story is successful as well as interesting. However there are many other diseases which are still communicated across wide areas of land and sea whose control requires still more understanding of what is going on in various parts of the world. This is where differences in social environment, culture and administration may be as important or more important than purely physical differences between countries and regions: control of cholera, malaria, trachoma and schistosomiasis becomes practicable only when policies and programmes are based on an understanding of these aspects of geography.

The same considerations apply to non-communicable diseases. Coronary heart disease is prevalent in developed Western countries and much less prevalent in less developed Asiatic and tropical countries; where the Western pattern of living has been modified to apply some of the lessons of the East, there is evidence of benefit. In these matters we stand on the threshold of some very friendly doorways to knowledge. Through these doorways, communities can see and exchange knowledge of each others' health hazards; they can observe also the trials and errors pointing, by accident or design, to possible solutions of difficulties which, in the light of knowledge, are seen to be illusory. We already know this from successes in overcoming deficiency diseases arising from malnutrition. It seems likely that the same might soon apply to degenerative diseases, cancer and mental disorders.

In this book, Professor Howe and his contributors are not prophesying or presuming. They are stating what is known about a selected range of important diseases in terms of pattern, distribution and trend. This tells us where we stand, what we have accomplished and what still confronts us. More than that, it tells us how much we have to learn and gain by sharing and applying such knowledge.

Preface

Just over a hundred years ago, in 1860 and 1864 respectively, August Hirsch, one time Professor of Medicine in the University of Berlin, published the first edition of his two-volume monumental "Handbuch der historisch-geographischen Pathologie". Between 1881 and 1886 the second edition was published and translated into English as "Handbook of Geographical and Historical Pathology". The book was written at a time when ill-balanced humours in the individual, "constitutions", divine vengeance from wrong doings, putrefaction (especially of unburied human corpses), miasmatic emanations, smelly drains, etc. were still being invoked in the causation, breeding and transmitting of disease. Hirsch's classic, and seminal medical geography, is concerned essentially with geographical distributions of acute infective diseases (Vol. 1), chronic infective, toxic, parasitic, septic and constitutional diseases (Vol. 2) and diseases of organs and parts (Vol. 3). Though lacking illustrative maps this major work attempts to relate spatial patterns of incidence of disease with differences in local environments in the various parts of the world.

New concepts concerning man's relationships with his total environment, exciting advances in bacteriology, virology and biochemistry, new knowledge relating to nutrition, pollutants, drugs and a whole host of other environmental stimuli, combined with great strides in genetics and improved statistical data and statistical techniques prompted this present volume as possibly a 20th century version of the "Handbook". As in the Hirsch work, the purpose is to demonstrate the global variability and spatial patterns of disease. Spatial relationships and inter-relationships of environmental and aetiological factors have been adopted as its theme. Twenty-two authors have contributed expert knowledge to the study. The diseases selected were the personal choice of the editor; they in no way represent a comprehensive list. Not all of the main killing or debilitating diseases are included, though those which receive attention together most certainly account for the major share of the 60 million or more who die annually and of the millions more who survive to suffer pain and distress. The omission of any one particular disease, as for example trypanosomiases or plague, in no way detracts from its significance or seriousness in terms of human health.

The book is global in its approach and inter-disciplinary in character, with contributors drawn from a variety of academic disciplines. Treatment of the subject matter tends to differ in practically every case and no attempt has been made to produce uniformity of view or literary style. A short glossary of scientific terms used is given at the end of the book (p. 577). In the difficult and sometimes contentious issues relating to the aetiology of disease it seemed important to draw on experience and wisdom from different quarters and to attempt an objective judgement.

The introductory chapter expands on the concept that disease represents maladjustment or a lack of harmony in the environment. This is followed in Part One by a consideration of those diseases for which the aetiology is largely known (cholera, smallpox, malaria, tuberculosis, etc.). Such diseases could be greatly reduced in frequency and virtually eliminated, as with smallpox (Chapter 11), if only sufficient finance could be devoted to raising levels of sanitation and nutrition and to implementing necessary programmes of vaccination and control of insect vectors. This obviously presupposes a stable political scene, an incorruptible administration, competent workers and a dedication to detail.

Part Two deals with industrial lung diseases, illnesses associated with drug abuse, deficiency diseases, mental illnesses, cardiovascular diseases and cancer. The latter diseases are thought of as being chronic "degenerative" diseases but the marked geographical variation in frequency which they display suggests that—as with infectious diseases—some environmental risk factors or stimuli are involved in their development.

The aim has been to produce a much shorter book than that published by Hirsch. Consequently all contributors have had to accept the necessity of compressing their work into a relatively small number of words, with the high degree of selection and generalization which this process involves. I record with real pleasure my thanks to all the experts who have contributed to this book, not least to their considerable patience and forebearance during the delays which inevitably accompany a multi-authored work. An obvious debt is due to authors, editors and publishers who have given permission to reproduce published material. All acknowledgements are listed separately. I extend particular thanks to Mrs J. Holme and Mrs J. MacIver of the Cartographic Staff of the Department of Geography in the University of Strathclyde who prepared most of the maps and diagrams in a form suitable for publication, and Miss A. Laing and Mrs J. Simpson for the preparation of the final manuscript.

As this book was about to be printed, the sad news was received of the death of one of its contributors, Dr. Jacques May, author of "Deficiency Diseases" (Chapter 20). He and his wife were killed in a motor car accident in Tunisia on 30th June 1975. One-time director of the Medical Geography Department of the American Geographical Society, his maps of the global distribution of infectious diseases have become common tools in teaching medicine throughout the world. While engaged in this kind of work he became increasingly convinced that food and nutrition were the most fundamental health problems of mankind and between 1960 and 1973 he wrote a 12-volume series, "The Ecology of Malnutrition". It is in recognition of his efforts on behalf of medical geography and with all respect and affection this book is now dedicated to him.

July 1977 *G. M. Howe*

Acknowledgements

The editor wishes to acknowledge the following with thanks for permission to reprint certain chapters, excerpts of chapters and figures which were first published in books and in journals. Wm Heinemann Medical Books (Introduction); Prof. L. J. Bruce Chwatt, *Entomological Society of America*, *American Geographical Society*, W.H.O., University, Milton Keynes, U.K. (Chapter 3); Dr M. A. Bhatty (Chapter 5); Controller, H.M.S.O., London (Chapter 6); U.S. Dept. Health, Education and Welfare, W.H.O. (Chapter 9); W.H.O. (Chapter 11); W.H.O., Dr Paul Boes, Dr (Col.) Philip K. Russell (Chapter 12); W.H.O., *Royal Geographical Society*, Dr G. F. Pyle, Prof. G. Melvyn Howe, Dr N. McGlashan, Prof. A. T. A. Learmonth, Dr R. Grau (Chapter 17); Dr R. Lynn (Chapter 18); Sir R. Doll, Mr D. S. MacLean (Chapter 19); *Amer. Geog. Soc.*, *Nat. Geog. Soc.* (Chapter 20).

Contents

List of Figures

List of Tables

To the Memory of
Jacques M. May

Introduction

The Environment, Its Influences and Hazards to Health*

G. Melvyn Howe

The term "environment" suggests different things to different people. To the meteorologist and climatologist, for instance, it means the atmosphere, but to the environmental engineer it usually means the atmosphere in an enclosed space. "Environment" to the ecologist is synonymous with the term "habitat" within which plants and animals live. Historically environment has been frequently equated with sanitation. Such views on what constitutes environment are rather restricted. In the present context the term "environment" is assumed to have a broader connotation and to refer to the totality of the external influences—natural and man-made—which impinge on man and affect his well-being. It thus embraces the life support systems and also the multiplicity of stimuli and hazards, direct and indirect, which man experiences. This, the *external* environment (nurture) stands in contrast with man's *internal* environment (nature) which relates to an individual's biological system, i.e. his genetic make-up.

LIFE SUPPORT SYSTEMS

Life support systems are those environmental conditions which are necessary for human life. They include air, water, food and shelter.

* Reprinted from *Environmental Medicine* (edited by G. Melvyn Howe and John A. Loraine) by kind permission of the publishers William Heinemann Medical Books, London.

For instance, a supply of free oxygen is essential for respiration. This is obtained from the atmosphere. A man deprived of oxygen dies in a few minutes. It is fortunate that oxygen is abundant almost everywhere in the atmosphere and is uniformly distributed over the globe. Where oxygen does run short, as in very high mountains, then man cannot live at all, though he may pass through such regions in the pressurized cabins of modern aircraft or struggle up into them for a few hours or days—at the cost of great difficulty and exhaustion. In the lower part of the atmosphere (i.e. the troposphere) where man normally lives, pure dry air is a mixture of at least nine gases. By volume two of these, oxygen and nitrogen, make up over 99%, 21% consisting of oxygen and 78% of nitrogen. Should the percentage of oxygen fall below 16% anoxia develops. This affects bodily functions and brain centres. Life cannot be sustained if the oxygen concentration is below 6%.

Water is another integral part of the life support systems. The need for water is as universal as the need for oxygen. However, in contrast to oxygen, water has a variable spatial distribution in that some regions have an excess of water, either annually or seasonally, and others a deficiency, either annually or seasonally. Furthermore, much of the water is too salty for man. *Homo sapiens* can live at most for about a week without drinking water, but in individual cases survival may be measured in days.

Food nutrients, in certain minimum amounts and proportions, are required to ensure active life and successful procreation of the species. Carbohydrates, fats and proteins form the major portion of man's diet while minerals and vitamins are present in smaller quantities. That man is closely dependent upon his environment for the provision of these requirements is all too obvious.

An equally close man–environment relationship exists in the case of shelter or housing. Shelter is necessary to provide protection from environmental extremes of heat, cold, moisture, aridity, sunshine or wind. Life or settlement would be impossible in several parts of the world were it not for adequate shelter. At the same time shelter provides the place where people care for most of their bodily needs, rear their children and keep their possessions. Important too is the fact that shelter provides a retreat where the individual may enjoy quietude and privacy, particularly where there are large numbers of people living in close proximity to one another.

HAZARDS AND INFLUENCES OF THE ENVIRONMENT

The environment provides man with the essential life support systems but it also presents him with a variety of hazards which may prejudice his health. If health is "a state of complete physical, mental and social well-being and not merely the absence of disease or infirmity" (W.H.O.), it represents a balanced relationship of the body and mind and complete adjustment to the total environment. Disease, on the other hand, is maladjustment or maladaptation in an environment, a reaction for the worse between man and hazards or adverse influences in his *external* environment. The response of the individual to these influences is conditioned by his genetic make-up or *internal* environment. Environmental influences or hazards may be categorized as (*a*) physical, (*b*) biological and (*c*) human.

Physical environment

Ever since the time of Hippocrates the weather and climate have been postulated as influencing, either favourably or unfavourably, man's well-being. The main problem is to isolate those components—solar radiation (including heat, measured in terms of temperature), air movement (wind), precipitation (rain, mist, snow, sleet, hail), moisture (humidity, fog, dew, frost), etc.—which have a direct and/or specific influence on man.

Solar radiation includes cosmic rays, gamma rays, X-rays, ultraviolet rays, luminous rays and infrared rays. Prolonged exposure to radiations may induce skin burns, cancers, genetic mutations and other biological changes.

Whilst water is essential to support life it can, nevertheless, provide a range of health hazards. Many pathogens responsible for disease are essentially water-borne (Table 1.1).

In addition to the water-borne pathogens there are often impurities in water which may have adverse effects on health. These include pesticides, herbicides, lead, zinc, mercury, arsenic, nitrates, fluorides, selenium, molybdenum, cadmium and sodium.

Differences in the trace element contents of soils, vegetables and atmosphere, in the character of the water supply, and in background radiation can be related to differences in the basic rock structure of countries and localities, in rock type, and in the general relief of the

Pathogen	Disease
Algae	Gastro-enteritis
Bacteria	Cholera, dysentery, paratyphoid, typhoid
Parasites	Malaria, tapeworm, yellow fever, schistosomiasis
Protozoa	Dysentery
Viruses	Infectious hepatitis, poliomyelitis

Table 1.1 Diseases associated with water-borne pathogens

land. For instance, sedimentary rocks have a lower content of the radioactive elements uranium and thorium and provide less gamma-ray background than igneous rocks. Rocks, together with their overlying soils, may have anomalous trace element or micro-nutrient contents. The essential trace elements are more important in the nutrition of man than their organic micro-nutrient counterparts, the vitamins. The former cannot be synthesized as can the vitamins, but must be present in the environment within a relatively narrow range of concentration. Both trace-element deficiencies and excesses kill. Soils derive their trace elements from the soil, parent rock material, applied fertilizers, and agricultural dusts and sprays, and pass in their trace-element characteristics to vegetable matter growing on them. Vegetable matter used as food may thus repeat the trace element peculiarities of the soil and of the parent geological material. An excess of mercury, lead, cadmium and selenium, whether eaten in vegetable matter or animal foods, can seriously affect health. Deficiencies of, for example, copper, iron, manganese, zinc, iodine, flourine, cobalt and molybdenum may give rise to nutritional problems.

Biological environment

Man's body provides a rich ground for parasites. Several parasites live in or within man permanently, without causing any structural change or functional disturbance. On the skin there are staphylococci, in the mouth non-pathogenic strains of streptococci and in the colon the organism, *Escherichia coli*. In the atmosphere there are pathogenic bacteria and pathogenic viruses which are responsible for many human diseases. One of the intriguing features of the micro-organisms which attack man is their natural history and the ways in which they, the disease agents, are transmitted from person to person. It is here that relationships between disease agents, the diseases they cause, and the physical and human environment, are particularly evident. For example, cholera, has a two-factor complex—causative organism and host. The causative organism, *Vibrio cholerae*, is introduced into the human body directly and, as far as is known, only man can be infected by it. Physical environmental factors thought to correlate with, and possibly to govern, cholera endemicity are high temperatures, low-lying lands, ponds and lakes and other bodies of water rich in organic matter and salts, and sheltered from the rays of the sun and from the rain. On the other hand, typhoid, caused by the bacterium *Salmonella typhosa*, usually enters the body through the mouth in contaminated food, milk or water. Water contaminated by infected sewage provides a major means of spread. There are other infectious diseases which are vector-borne. Bubonic plague, for instance, is primarily an infectious disease of certain species of rodent. The pandemics of this disease in the past were the result of fortuitous invasions of the human body by internal pathogens of these rodents. In the Great Pestilence or Black Death of the fourteenth century the pathogen was the bacillus *Pasteurella pestis* which produced endemic infection in rats. It was transmitted from plague-infected rats to man through the bite of infected rat fleas (*Xenopsylla cheopis*). Rodents acted as host to the plague bacillus and the flea was the carrier or vector. The malaria parasites (*Plasmodia*) are transmitted by female *Anopheles* mosquitoes. Yellow fever, a viral disease, is transmitted by the mosquito *Aedes aegypti*. This same vector also carries dengue. Mosquitoes are either known or suspected vectors for a group of viruses thought to cause encephalitis.

In each case disease is the result of a complicated natural history. Different hosts and vectors of several pathogenic viruses, pathogenic bacteria and parasitic organisms, are differently affected by geographical conditions and controls. Furthermore, disease agents may be carried by different vectors in different parts of their range, as in the case of malaria.

Whether it be causative organism (virus, bacterium, spirochaete, rickettsia), intermediate host or vector, each element in the disease complex has its own specific environmental requirements. Each element, including man himself, is inescapably bound up with the geographical environment. Disease in any given locality is the result of a combination of geographical circumstances which bring together disease agent, vector, intermediate host, reservoir and man at the most auspicious time. Knowledge of these relationships and of each element in the complex is a prerequisite to a true understanding of infectious disease, its distribution and control. But relationships are rarely simple or static, on the contrary, they are complicated and undergo continuous change. Despite this, man's ability to modify certain environmental conditions, his use of pesticides and his ever-increasing technology, have succeeded in bringing a new perspective to the control of vector-borne diseases. Several of the viral and microbial diseases are effectively inhibited by antibiotics such as chloramphenicol and the synthetic penicillins. In consequence smallpox, plague, typhus and cholera are now virtually banished from the West and the incidence of scarlet fever, diphtheria and poliomyelitis is very low. Serious infectious disease is now absent from most of the developed countries of the world as are the environmental conditions likely to bring about their return. However, in the present era of rapid air travel, a person may acquire a serious infectious disease and travel thousands of miles in a fraction of the incubation period of the disease. Thus, he may enter a country such as Britain in the silent stage of an infection in the absence of any clinical symptoms. Such a situation, whereby a person may be at home for a week or more before becoming ill and where the diagnosis of the illness may be delayed or missed, is likely to be exacerbated with the increasing speed, size and frequency of air travel.

Human environment

The human, or socio-cultural environment, is essentially man made and relates to the density, geographical distribution and mobility of populations, to occupations, to socio-economic status, to housing, to diets, to habits, customs and general life-styles.

The size of a country's population is obviously important in that the larger the number of people the more there are at risk of exposure to disease. If the population is too large in proportion to its natural resources, the availability of capital, etc., then, accordingly, living standards will be much lower than they might be under different circumstances.

Overpopulation does not depend merely upon the total number living in a country or on the density of the population. A population density of 60 persons to the square kilometre may mean overpopulation in one area but underpopulation in another. Much depends upon the available resources and the degree of cultural development. A country is not necessarily overpopulated simply because it is incapable of providing sufficient food to support its people; such a country may be able to employ its labour force more effectively in manufacturing industry, exporting its surplus of manufactured goods in exchange for food-stuffs. Where this is not possible and a country becomes overpopulated, as is evident in, for example, mainland China, India, Bangladesh, Indonesia and parts of the Mediterranean and the West Indies, the evils of overcrowding—slums, mass unemployment, poverty and disease—are all too evident.

Population density and population distribution vary within countries. Patterns of settlement are the outcome of physical, historical and economic factors. In Egypt, for instance, there is a striking contrast between a large area of desert which is virtually uninhabited and the Nile valley and delta which have a huge concentration of people. In places there is a rural density of over 400 persons per square kilometre, and, including towns and cities, there is an overall density of 960 per square kilometre. The average figure of 25 persons per square kilometre for the whole of Egypt is thus totally misleading.

Bangladesh, with an overall population density of 433 persons per square kilometre, is the most densely populated country in the world. Taiwan comes second with 384 persons per square kilometre followed by Belgium and South Korea, each with 316 persons per square kilometre. The United Kingdom is the ninth most densely populated country in the world; England and Wales together are second after Bangladesh and Taiwan. Over 80% of the population of the United Kingdom lives in towns and 7.4 million out of a total population of 55.34 million (1971), i.e. 13%, live in Greater London. If the optimal population for a country is taken as "the maximum which can be maintained indefinitely without detriment to the health of individuals from pollution or from social or nutritional stress", then clearly Britain is overpopulated.

People today are mobile to a remarkable degree, and in countries like Britain there is a slackening of close family ties and social relationships. Many urban dwellers have moved further away from centres of towns and their places of work and have taken up residence in suburbs, in nearby market towns and in so-called "new towns". Change of place of residence involves not only physical disturbance but also a social disturbance since people are obliged to create entirely new social environments for themselves. There is at the same time the inevitable journey to work. This may be long or short, but it involves extra energy and takes toll of physical and mental reserves.

Pilgrimages of people to places such as Mecca, Jerusalem or Lourdes, seasonal movement of labour, as in the U.S.S.R., Switzerland or Bolivia, the movement of traders along ancient caravan routes, or roads and railways or by sea present hazards to health. The paths of infection by such diseases as cholera or plague have been traced along ancient trade routes by land and sea. Ships carry people who may be contaminated; ships also carry rats which may alight at ports of call. Seaports have thus become, quite naturally, secondary sources of disease diffusion. The role of air travel in the modern spread of disease has already been mentioned.

Occupation is one way of measuring "socio-economic" status, with its implications in respect of family income, living standards and life-styles. Furthermore, many occupations carry with them hazards to health. As early as 1775 Percival Pott drew attention to soot as a cause of scrotal cancer in chimney sweeps. Silicosis is a risk in quarrying and glass manufacture and there is an above-average incidence of pneumoconiosis among coal miners. Lead, mercury, arsenic, fluoride, asbestos, chromium and benzene are among the recognized poisonous materials used in modern industry. These and hundreds more new chemicals are being introduced into the environment each year. Man's reaction to such chemicals depend on the toxicity of the chemical, the duration of exposure, the concentration of the chemical and the genetic susceptibility of the individual. Diseases or disorders commonly associated with atmospheric pollutants and thought to be aggravated by them, include chronic bronchitis, pneumonia, lung cancer, emphysema and asbestosis.

Housing in the West has improved considerably. In medieval Britain, for instance, the common folk lived in dark, verminous, unventilated, wattle and daub, thatched-roofed dwellings which harboured plague. Densely packed, back-to-back dwellings lacking drains, water closets or other basic facilities characterized nineteenth-century Liverpool, Glasgow, Manchester, Birmingham, Leeds, Sheffield, Bradford, Nottingham, Newcastle and other industrial towns, all of which had bad records for tuberculosis. Housing in twentieth-century Britain is of stone, brick or concrete, supplied with clean, running water and flush toilets, usually with baths and showers; the houses are now often centrally heated and/or air conditioned. The artificial interior climates of many of these houses, offices and public buildings are often quite different from the climate out of doors. Whether such artificial climates are optimal for a person's physical or mental functioning is not known. It is thought, however, that air conditioning provides relative freedom from infection for the occupants of buildings in which it is installed due both to the withdrawal of infected air and to the filtration of incoming air.

Food constitutes yet another important factor of the human environment worthy of the closest of attention in the context of human health. Man needs food as a source of energy for undertaking work, and as a source of raw material with which to perform the process of tissue building and the perpetuation of the species, *homo sapiens*. Diets in most of the densely populated developing countries of the world are defective both in quantity and quality. Among the most serious deficiency states now prevailing in such areas are kwashiorkor, beri-beri, pellagra, rickets and goitre. At the same time poor nutrition predisposes to infections, particularly to tuberculosis and to infestations such as hookworm. In the West there has been a profound change in food and dietary habits. In particular this has involved a reduction in the amount of protein consumed and an increase in carbohydrate intake. It has been suggested that, compared with man's total evolutionary history, the relatively short time since he changed from a protein-rich to a carbohydrate-rich diet has not permitted adaptation. Sugar, in particular, is used in ever-increasing quantities, and chemicals are added to food and drink ostensibly to improve palatability and appearance. High blood lipid levels (lipid being the general term which includes fats and fat-like compounds) are thought to be of aetiological importance in coronary arterial disease.

The unrestricted use of powerful chemical pesticides based on organo-phosphorus compounds and chlorinated hydrocarbons, while revolutionizing the chemical attack against harmful insects and pests, upsets the balance of soil ecosystems and may well prove a serious source of contamination of food supplies. Dichloro-diphenyl-trichlorethane (DDT), dieldrin, aldrin and related substances persist in soils and accumulate in animal and body fat.

The modern town, the social habitat of industrialized man, is characterized by high density living, overcrowding, a polluted atmosphere and noise. Air pollution is a major social problem. Sources include motor vehicles, railway trains, aircraft, domestic heating, chemical plant, fuel-burning factories and offices, refuse disposal and thermo-electric generating stations. Studies have shown that atmospheric pollution is associated with the occurrence and worsening of many respiratory diseases including chronic bronchitis, lung cancer, emphysema and asthma. As distinct from man-made atmospheric pollution there is the atmosphere pollution from natural sources such as pollens and dust which, either singly or possibly in association with certain kinds of food or emotional stress, cause asthma.

Cigarette smoking, a social habit of long standing, has also been associated epidemiologically with respiratory and heart diseases. Carcinogenic hydrocarbons, notably 3,4-benzpyrene, have been isolated from tars of cigarette smoke and from the soot of polluted atmosphere.

Other social habits likely to prejudice health and promote disease include gluttony leading to obesity, chronic alcoholism leading to physical disease (gastritis and cirrhosis of the liver) and mental deterioration, and promiscuity leading to venereal disease. Several countries now appear to be experiencing an epidemic of drug dependence among teenagers in which opiates, cocaine, amphetamine and cannabis have pride of place.

In contrast to the rather more tranquil life of past generations the tempo and tensions of contemporary westernized urban societies are such as to lead to "stress", believed by some to be a factor in producing coronary heart-disease, cerebro-vascular disease and some forms of cancer. How much mental illness is due to the stresses of modern life, to genetic causes, or to influences in youth in the Freudian sense, remains to be established. Certainly cacophonous noises from motor vehicles, railway trains, jet aircraft, building-site machinery, pneumatic drills and a multiplicity of other man-made sources, provide a contributory environmental hazard. For example, it is thought that the acoustic discomfort associated with winds blowing against high-rise and tower blocks of flats results in nervous strain among the occupants, largely due to fear of actual physical harm.

MAN'S INTERNAL ENVIRONMENT

External environmental influences and hazards act on man, but the response in almost every case is thought to be conditioned by the genetic make-up of the individual. There appears to be a hereditary predisposition on the part of some individuals to certain diseases. Illness attributable solely to inherited characteristics, such as haemophilia, is rare. On the other hand some associations between the ABO blood groups and disease have been proved beyond reasonable doubt. Thus the incidence of peptic ulcer is 40% higher in persons of blood group O than in those belonging to blood groups A, B or AB. The increased risk attaching to blood group O is about 25% more common in gastric ulcer. Again, it has been established that cancer of the stomach is about 25% more common in persons of blood group A than in those of other groups. Pernicious anaemia is similarly associated with group A. In addition, there appears to be an association between group A and diabetes mellitus, bubonic plague, and carcinoma of the cervix, pancreas, prostate and stomach. Smallpox and pituitary adenomata have an O group association; broncho-pneumonia, infantile diarrhoea, salivary gland tumours and tumours of the ovary appear to have an A group association.

It is open to question whether the associations are truly causal in the sense that a person of blood group O is intrinsically more liable to peptic ulcer, or whether persons of other blood groups are protected against the disease. Similarly it is possible that blood group A does not carry a liability to cancer of the stomach but that other blood groups have a special protection against the disease. At present views on this subject are conflicting.

FURTHER READING

Arthur, D. R. (1969). "Survival: Man and his Environment". English Universities Press, London.

Arvill, R. (1969). "Man and Environment". Penguin Books, London.
Bach, W. (1972). "Atmospheric Pollution". McGraw-Hill, New York.
Barr, J. (1970). "The Assaults on our Senses". Methuen, London.
Black, J. D. (1968). "The Management and Conservation of Biological Resources". Philadelphia.
Bresler, J. B. (Ed.) (1968). "Environments of Man". Addison-Wesley, Reading, Mass.
Burton, I. (1968). The quality of the environment: a review. *American Geographical Review* **58**, 472.
Carr, D. E. (1965). "The Breath of Life". W. W. Norton, New York.
Clements, F. W. and Rogers, J. F. (1960). "Diet in Health and Disease". Sydney.
Economic Commission to Europe (1971). Symposium on problems relating to the environment. United Nations, New York.
Erlich, P. R. and Erlich, A. (1970). "Population Resources and Environment". W. H. Freeman, San Fransisco.
Holdren, J. P. and Ehrlich, P. R. (Eds) (1971). "Global Ecology". Harcourt Brace Jovanovich, New York.
Howe, G. M. (1972). "Man, Environment and Disease". Barnes and Noble, New York and David and Charles, Newton Abbot. Penguin Books, Harmondsworth (1976).
Loraine, J. A. (1972). "The Death of Tomorrow". Heinemann, London.
Medical Research Council (1956). "The Hazards to Man of Nuclear and Allied Radiations". Cmnd. 9780, H.M.S.O., London.
Mellanby, K. (1969). "Pesticides and Pollution". Fontana, London.
Perloff, H. S. (Ed.) (1969). "The Quality of the Urban Environment". John's Hopkins Press, Baltimore.
Powles, J. (1972). The medicine of industrial man. *The Ecologist* **2**, 10, 24.
Purdom, P. Walton (Ed.) (1971). "Environmental Health". Academic Press, New York.
Rodda, M. (1967). "Noise and Society". Oliver and Boyd, London.
Royal College of Physicians (1970). "Air Pollution and Health". Pitman, London.
Royal Commission on Environmental Pollution (1971). First Report, Cmnd. 4585, London, H.M.S.O.
Royal Commission on Environmental Pollution (1972). Second Report. Cmnd. 4894, London, H.M.S.O.
Ward, M. A. (Ed.) (1970). "Man and his Environment", Proceedings of the first Banff conference on pollution (May 16–17, 1968). Penguin Press, London.

Part One

1. Schistosomiasis

G. H. Rée

Schistosomiasis is a disease of countries with warm climates. It is estimated that it affects nearly 200 million people. Early Egyptian records refer to haematuria—a symptom of one form of the disease—and ova of schistosomes have been detected in an Egyptian mummy of the 20th dynasty (B.C. 1250–1000). Though the cause of schistosomiasis was discovered in 1851, the life cycle of the parasite elucidated in 1915 and effective treatment introduced in 1918, it remains one of the few communicable diseases of man which is increasing in prevalence throughout the tropical and subtropical world.

AETIOLOGY

Schistosomiasis is caused by digenetic trematodes of the super family Schistosomatoidiae. The three species commonly affecting man, *Schistosoma haematobium*, *S. mansoni* and *S. japonicum*, have similar life cycles involving a sexual stage in man, and an asexual stage in various species of mollusc which are the intermediate hosts. Other species, such as *S. intercalatum*, may infect man, particularly in equatorial Africa, but are of lesser significance.

Life cycle of schistosoma

The mature adult *S. haematobium* are found in the veins of the vesical plexus, and ova are excreted in the urine. *S. mansoni* and *S.*

japonicum inhabit the veins of the mesenteric plexus and ova are excreted in the faeces. When ova come into contact with fresh water, a free swimming miracidium emerges, which penetrates an appropriate snail. Within the snail, numerous cercariae are produced; these are periodically shed into water, penetrate the skin of a vertebrate host and after migration through the tissues, mature in the appropriate venous plexus.

Geographical distribution

Schistosomiasis is necessarily limited by the distribution of the molluscan intermediate host. Though not all areas of suitable snail distribution are foci of transmission they constitute the potential foci. The main geographical distributions of the three important human forms of the disease are shown in Fig. 1.1.

Within endemic areas, the distribution is not uniform. Instead there are focal patterns in which prevalence and intensity of infection vary greatly from area to area. This is due not only to the presence or absence of suitable snails, but also to such topographical and social variants as water supplies, water usage and population densities in relation to natural water contact and usage. The chances of acquiring the infection are smaller when a small population uses a large body of water than when a large population uses a small area of water. In some localities of low prevalence and intensity of infection, usually where adults particularly are infected, the disease may not be being transmitted or the transmission may proceed only at a very low level after being introduced into the area. Paucity of medical facilities, particularly in the rural areas of the developing world, may also contribute to an underestimation of the degree of endemicity.

Ecological relationships

Ecology is the study of the relationship between living organisms and their surroundings. In the case of schistosomiasis, it involves a study of the complex relationships between man and his internal and external environment, the snails and their environment and the parasites and their surroundings in man, water and snails.

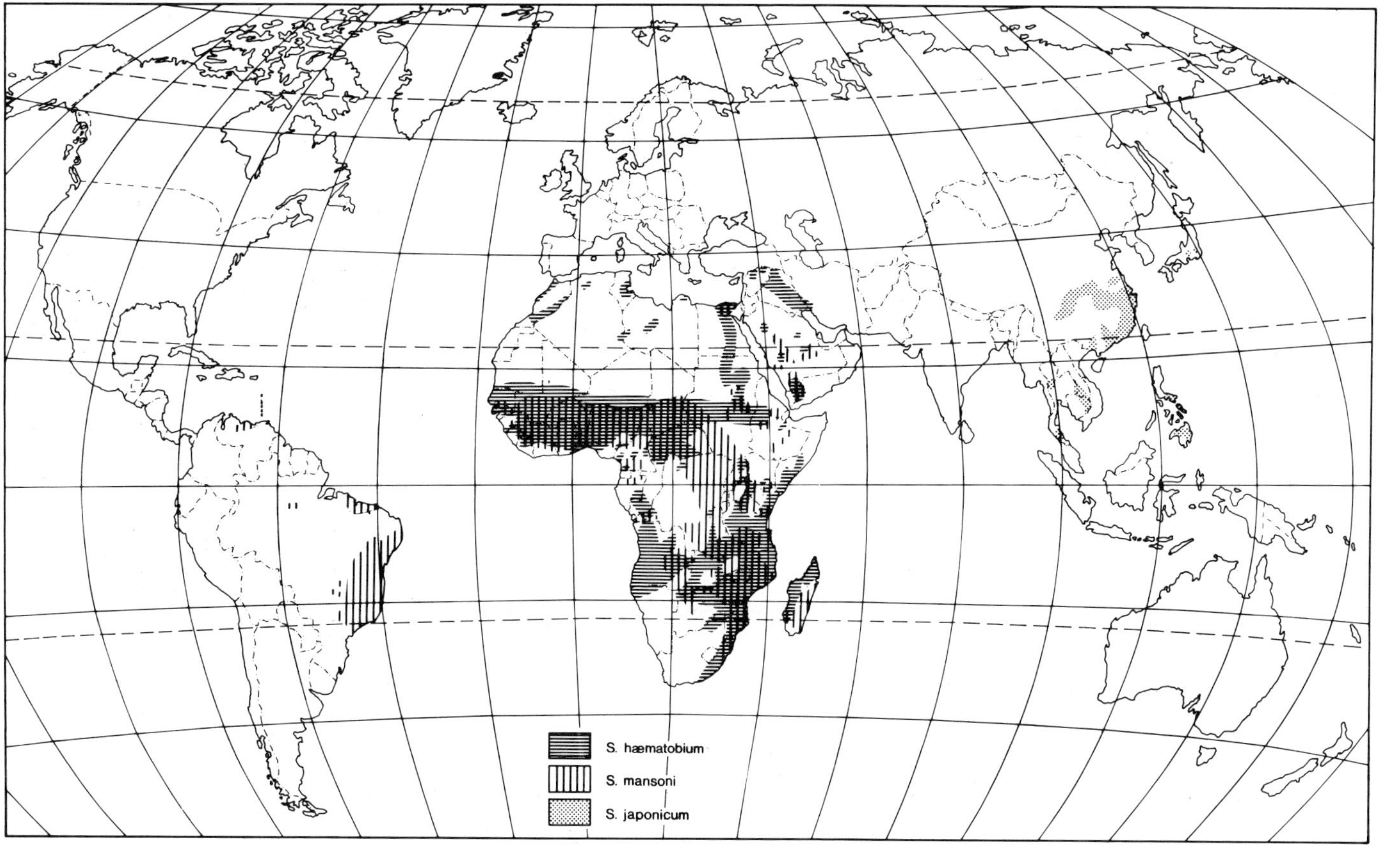

Fig. 1.1 Global distribution of the three important forms of schistosomiasis.

Molluscan intermediate hosts

The intermediate hosts of *S. haematobium* belong to the family *Planorbidae* and are in the genus *Bulinus*: of *S. mansoni* in the genus *Biomphalaria*. The intermediate hosts of *S. japonicum* belong to the family *Hydrobiidae* in the genus *Oncomelania*.

Bulinids are not found in the New World; they extend over most of Africa, the Middle East, Mauritius, the Cape Verde Islands and some areas of Portugal. These snails are ovate and sinistral. Biomphalaria species are found in both the Old and New Worlds. There is a wide distribution in sub-Saharan Africa, usually at intermediate altitudes but at sea level in parts of west and south Africa. Their small numbers in the coastal plains of east Africa is thought to be due to thermolability. Though found in Egypt, they are absent from most of the North African coast. The snails exist in Israel and parts of the Arabian peninsula. In the New World, they extend from the southern United States to Chile with irregular occurrences in the Caribbean Islands. It is probable that the New World species developed from a common ancestral root and are not of recent introduction from the Old World. Biomphalaria are discoid snails. Both Bulinus and Biomphalaria are non-operculate, aquatic and hermaphroditic.

By contrast Oncomelania are operculate, amphibious and dioecious. This species is limited to the Far East, China, Japan, Formosa, Philippines and some areas of South-East Asia. The snails are dextral, conical or sub-conical.

Snail ecology

Though acquatic, Planorbids are capable of withstanding dessication for relatively long periods of time. Seasonal transmission of schistosomiasis may occur in pools which dry out completely during the dry season, the snails aestivating in the mud until the pool fills. Infection with schistosomes may render snails more susceptible to dessication.

Planorbid snails may be found in a wide variety of habitats ranging from swamps and pools—seasonal or perennial—to large bodies of water such as Lake Victoria. Though not found in swiftly moving waters, such waters nevertheless have areas of stagnant shallows which may support numerous colonies of snails. Molluscs are not found in sea water, nor in swamps irrigated by tidal river water. They can, however, withstand wide ranges of chemical and physical conditions of water, though low levels of dissolved electrolytes are not well tolerated. This is presumably owing to inability to maintain their own electrolyte balance. Snails feed on algae and diatoms present in the water, though distribution of species is not related to a particular microflora. Sewage was at one time, but not now, thought to be advantageous to snail colonization. The snails generally show a wide ecological tolerance, and it is considered difficult to separate the ecological requirements of the various species.

Miracidia

Miracidia emerge from viable ova when these come into contact with fresh water. Their emergence results partly from osmotic action, and partly from their own movements. They are free swimming organisms which do not feed and have a life of about 24 hours. The three human species differ in size, but are morphologically and behaviourally similar.

Miracidia are small ciliated organisms, which swim by ciliary motion and by irregular contractions of the body. Though the swimming pattern is apparently random, marked, but non-specific, chemotactic responses to snail hosts occur. They are positively phototropic and negatively geotropic and are found just below the surface of the water, where the majority of molluscs are located.

Miracidia can penetrate many species of snails, but if the host is inappropriate a rapid tissue reaction occurs and the miracidium is walled off and destroyed by amoebocytes. A further reaction of the mollusc has been termed hypersensitivity. Snails which are normally susceptible to one strain of parasite are rapidly killed when exposed to another strain. Strain differences are also of importance in terms of infectivity to the snail. A strain of *S. mansoni* from one area may fail to infect a snail from another area, even though that snail is a good host for its own local strain of *S. mansoni*.

The miracidium develops into a first stage sporocyst, usually close to the area of penetration within an appropriate host. The mature sporocyst contains germinal cells, and from these second stage sporocysts bud off. These migrate to other parts of the snail's body—usually the liver and ovotestis. Further germination occurs and within a period of 4–7 weeks cercariae are developed. By this means several thousand cercariae emerge from a single miracidium, each of the same sex as the original miracidium. Under field conditions, snails are rarely infected by more than a single miracidium; there is some evidence that the development of sporocysts inhibits the further penetration of miracidia.

The effect of the larval parasitism on the snails is variable. On rare occasions self cure after an initial production of cercariae has been noted. However, mortality, increased by a factor of 1.3–3.5 among infected snails, is usual. In addition, eggs laid by infected snails are more commonly sterile than eggs of uninfected species.

Cercariae

Cercariae emerge from the snails over a period of time, rising rapidly to a peak, and declining gradually over a period of weeks. Cercariae of *S. mansoni* and *S. haematobium* generally leave the snail host under the influence of heat and light, and the time of emergence tends to remain fairly constant. By contrast, long periods of light are required to stimulate the emergence of *S. japonicum* and maximal numbers are found in the early evening.

After leaving the host, cercariae have a life in water of about 48 hours though their infectivity to the final host decreases after about 24 hours. They do not feed but possess large glycogen reserves. Factors, such as increasing temperature, which stimulate the use of these reserves, reduce the life span of the cercariae.

Cercariae are usually found just below the surface of the water. Swimming activity tends to be intermittent and when it ceases they slowly sink. The stimulus to location of the vertebrate host is unknown, but is not chemotactic. The ability of cercariae to infect the host is affected by their age, water temperature, water turbulence and flow rate. Not all cercariae which contact the host necessarily penetrate the skin. The time taken for *S. mansoni* to achieve complete penetration is about 5 minutes. Should the skin dry before penetration is complete the cercariae are destroyed.

Each cercaria as it penetrates human skin, and particularly after repeated exposures, gives rise to an element of a papular rash, known as swimmers itch or cercarial dermatitis. This appears to be more common following repeated exposure to non-human, particularly avian, schistosome cercariae.

Following penetration of the skin, the cercariae lose their tails and are termed schistosomulae. These migrate, either through the lymphatic or venous systems to the right side of the heart and thence to the lungs where some destruction occurs. From the lungs the survivors migrate either via the circulation or directly through the diaphragm to the liver where further destruction may occur. The survivors grow in the liver and when sexually mature, migrate to the appropiate venous plexus. As a result of destruction of schistosomulae in lungs and liver, the number of mature worms which finally develop is always much less than the number of cercariae which successfully penetrated the skin. Human infections may consist of only 10 or less adult worms. Since the worms are dioecious, unisexual infections are necessarily sterile and do not give rise to clinical disease. The stimulus to conjugation is unknown, but when this occurs the female is held in the gynaecophoric canal of the male and egg laying commences. The prepatent period, i.e. from cercarial penetration to appearance of eggs in excreta, is about 6 weeks, but may be considerably longer. The life expectancy of the mature worms, evidenced by continued egg laying in persons removed from endemic areas, may be up to 20 years. It is probably usually significantly less and may be as short as 2 years.

Clinical disease is associated with the presence of schistosome ova in the tissues; the adult worms, for reasons which will be considered later, are involved in more occult pathological processes. The maximal daily egg production by the worms varies with the species; for *S. mansoni* it is about 200 a day and *S. japonicum* about 1000 a day. These figures are not absolute, strain differences being associated with different egg production.

The human disease

For ova deposited by the female in the veins of the appropriate plexus there are three possible modes of disposal. They may be (a) extruded through the viscus wall and excreted in urine (*S. haematobium*) or faeces (*S. mansoni*, *S. japonicum*), (b) retained in the wall of the viscus or (c) carried embolically to the liver or other sites.

Ova in excreta maintain continued transmission and are of considerable diagnostic value. In the tissues, ova induce the formation of foreign body granulomata which, with the passage of time, give rise to dense fibrosis. The clinical effects of schistosomiasis are largely determined by the granuloma and the subsequent fibrosis. Apart from haematuria, symptoms of schistosomiasis are usually due to the complications, such as portal hypertension, pyelonephritis and hydronephrosis. In areas of heavy infection with urinary schistosomiasis an association has been found between the disease and the subsequent development of bladder cancers.

EPIDEMIOLOGY

Schistosomiasis caused by *S. haematobium* is a disease of man only: some animals, particularly baboons and monkeys, are found infected with *S. mansoni* but this probably represents reverse zoonotic transmission from man to animals. *S. japonicum* is a true zoonosis and animals ranging from cows to small rodents are found naturally infected and are of great epidemiological importance. It is of interest that the species of *S. japonicum* found in Taiwan, apparently morphologically identical to other forms of *S. japonicum*, is wholly zoophilic and not transmissible to man.

Schistosomiasis is largely a disease of rural areas, though transmission occurs in some urban situations. Within endemic areas, a focal distribution is evident.

In infected populations both maximal prevalence and intensity of infection occur in children and young adults and diminish with increasing age. This diminution is less evident in *S. japonicum* infections. The morbidity and mortality of the disease are highest in areas of high endemicity and the results of clinical studies suggest that those with heavy infections are more liable to potentially fatal complications than those with light infections. Studies of patients suffering from *S. haematobium* infections have shown that resolution of urinary tract abnormalities may occur, either spontaneously or after parasitological cure and such resolution is more likely with light infections.

The morbidity of the disease is difficult to assess owing to the many nutritional and parasitic diseases which affect patients from the tropics. The numerous symptoms complained of by malnourished Puerto Ricans with *S. mansoni* subsided when they were fed on an improved diet despite the withholding of specific parasitological treatment. Detailed life statistics are not usually available in those countries where schistosomiasis is endemic. It is known, however, that the disease is of social and economic importance. Though the proportionate mortality is low the large number of persons infected leads to a numerically large number of deaths which are directly attributable to the disease. No genetic or racial resistance or predisposition to the disease has been demonstrated.

It is assumed that the decreasing prevalence of schistosomiasis with age is attributable to the slow but steady development of immunity. It has long been known that humoral antibodies to different stages of the parasite arise during the course of the infection and this fact is fully exploited in sero-diagnostic procedures. However protection by these antibodies has not been proved. Passive transfer of gamma globulin from infected persons has not changed the parasitological status of recently infected persons. It has been shown in experimental animals that during their period of maturation, schistosomes incorporate host material into their tegument derived from either red cells or blood group substances which renders them non-antigenic and protects them against antibody attack. A "lethal antibody" to newly-invading schistosomulae has been detected in the experimental animals, which prevents superinfection (concomitant immunity). It is, however, the adult worm (shown by transfer experiments) which provides the main stimulus to the development of immunity against cercarial challenge. It is not known whether a similar situation arises in man.

The falling prevalence rates in adult life may also be explained in terms of decreasing exposure. The inability of the worms to multiply within the definitive host, coupled with a finite life span, must lead to spontaneous parasitological (though not necessarily pathological) cure if further exposure to cercarial infected water does not occur. This requires an assessment of how and why infection is acquired. Exposure in childhood is readily evident in the contact children have with water when playing. As age increases, such play exposure diminishes and subsequent contact with water is either occupational or accidental. Occupational exposure for men includes agriculture, fish farming and boating. For women it would include agriculture and the washing of clothes and utensils. Accidental exposure might follow from the traversing of infected water courses or ritual washings. Unlike bathing and swimming, both types of exposure are usually associated with only partial immersion of the body. The provision of piped water supplies in many urban areas may, partially, explain the absence of the diseases in urban areas.

In many tropical areas, agricultural irrigation is seasonal, and is dependent upon seasonal rains. Rain temporarily increases the area of habitat suitable for the molluscs. It also increases water flow rates in rivers and irrigation ditches, often sufficiently to remove snails or to prevent cercariae from attaching themselves to the vertebrate host. The development of perennial irrigation in Egypt from the old basin irrigation has meant a greater and more constant contact with infected water. This has led to a rapid and marked increase in the prevalence of schistosomiasis among the agriculture population. If contaminated faeces are deposited on the banks of water courses, rain will wash the excreta into the water and permit miracidia to continue the cycle. In dry areas miracidia are unable to reach water and the cycle terminates. This factor is less marked with *S. haematobium* because indiscriminate micturition into water courses is common.

Since the daily cercarial output from the snails is of limited duration—usually it is maximal about midday—and since the infectivity of cercariae diminishes with age, an assessment is required of the time of day at which exposure to contact occurs. It is evident that exposure to water shortly before the period of cercarial shedding will result in less infection than later. If, for example, washing of clothes is a morning occupation, then the risk for infection is decreased. In this context the effect, if any, of soap on cercariae is as yet unknown.

Religious practices may be involved in the epidemiology of schistosomiasis. Male Muslims indulge in ritual washing (*Wadu*) and prevalence rates are often higher in Muslims than in Christians. Again, children who attend school may have lower rates than those not attending school, through both diminished exposure resulting from time spent in classrooms and, it is hoped, education of the dangers from contact with infected water.

Economic effects of schistosomiasis

The economic losses due to schistosomiasis are difficult to assess, particularly in areas of subsistence farming. In Brazil, endemic areas are often areas of poor socio-economic status. Whether there is a cause-effect relationship between the disease and socio-economic status is uncertain. A known effect, however, is migration of infected populations to wealthier areas where, given the presence of suitable molluscs, extension of the disease is liable to occur.

CONTROL OF SCHISTOSOMIASIS

If it is accepted that schistosomiasis is a disease with significant morbidity, albeit a small mortality, then control becomes a necessity. The costs of control are at the moment high, and an assessment of the probable benefits to be expected from control are required before starting a long and costly scheme. Control of schistosomiasis has as its objectives eradication, prevention of spread of the disease, and elimination of morbidity and mortality.

Methods of control include mass therapy of infected individuals, environmental sanitation, control of human–water contact and snail control. In practice, combinations of all these have been used.

In 1918, tartar emetic was introduced into clinical medicine as an effective schistosomicidal drug. Though used occasionally on a mass scale unpleasant side effects, occasional fatalities (from cardiotoxity) and the need to give the drug by intravenous injection led most therapists to abandon this treatment as a form of control. Further research into trivalent antimonial compounds led to the production of a number of drugs which could be given by intramuscular injections. Though generally effective, all drugs showed side effects which correlated with retention of antimony in the body; none are ideal for mass use. Neither have newer non-antimonial drugs, such as niridazole (Ambilhar) and hycanthone, found acceptance on a mass scale. This is because of unpleasant and sometimes dangerous side effects, particularly in persons with liver damage. Though the requirements of an ideal drug are known, no such drug has yet been produced.

Environmental sanitation is primarily concerned with excreta disposal, a subject fraught with cultural taboos. Prolonged educational efforts, directed mainly at children, are required to overcome such taboos. In rural communities, the building, maintenance and use of latrines in the domestic situation is obviously desirable as part of general health policy; it is unlikely that provision of latrines in agricultural areas where people are working can be considered seriously as a preventative method. Likewise indiscriminate micturition, particularly while bathing, will continue despite the presence of latrines. Environmental sanitation is unlikely to affect the transmission of *S. haematobium*. The zoonotic nature of *S. japonicum* renders this method of control (by itself) inadequate.

Control of human contact with water presents logistic, economic, and cultural problems. Piped water supplies, footbridges over streams, fencing off of infected pools, adequate washing facilities for women and mechanization of farming techniques have all been advocated and, where implemented, have met with varying degrees of success. Urbanization has been beneficial in Japan; it is unlikely to be of great value in Africa in the immediate future. Control of snails has been the most widely advocated and practical method of control. This has been effected by three means, environmental control, biological control and chemical control, singly or in combination. Detailed knowledge of the ecology and biology of the molluscs is essential before any attempt can be made at snail control.

Environmental control of snails involves drainage of water. Where this is not practical other measures such as increasing water flow rates, removal of vegetation, the construction of ditches and irrigation canals are all of value. Should such measures not totally remove the snails, they may nevertheless render them more susceptible to molluscicides.

The development of industrial and civil engineering programmes has led to the formation of numerous quarries, pits and ditches, in many of which transmission of schistosomiasis now occurs. It is essential that authorities concerned with such programmes insist upon the proper control of these sites.

Biological control is defined as the control of pests and parasites by the use of other organisms. Control may be through predation, parasitism, direct or indirect competition, habitat modification or a combination of these. A number of laboratory studies have suggested practical methods of snail control but, in general, these have not proved satisfactory in the field, owing to the abnormal ecological conditions existing under laboratory conditions. With snail predators it is essential to use species which are not exclusively dependent on the snail for their food, otherwise control of the snail will lead to elimination of the predator and prepare the water for re-infection. Direct competition and predation are combined in the snail *Marisa cornuarietis*, which feeds on the aquatic plants favoured by Biomphalaria and also preys on them. The effect is not complete and, in addition, Marisa could become an important pest of wet cultivated crops.

Certain shrubs and trees contain saponins in their leaves and fruit which are toxic to snails. While the industrial extraction of these is not justified, planting of these near important sites of local transmission might be reasonable.

Chemical control or the application of chemical molluscicides has a number of advantages over other methods of control in that a rapid interruption of transmission occurs. Some molluscicides are also herbicidal thereby reducing the need for weed clearance. The active participation of the local population, often difficult to obtain, may not be required for this method of control. Disadvantages include relatively high cost, coupled with the need for repeated re-applications of the molluscicide over a period of time, the development of technical expertise in the application of the compounds and their potential to cause ill health in man.

The technical aspects of molluscicide application involve a knowledge of the quantity of chemical to put into the water, the type of water involved, the dispersability of the chemical and the likelihood of its reaching the lacustrine habitats of the snails, the dilution of chemical which occurs as it moves downstream and finally, the effect of organic compounds in the water on the chemical and physical stability of the molluscicide. Three molluscicides are in common use today. Copper sulphate which is very cheap is not very effective and is greatly affected by dissolved–solid content of water. Niclosamide (bayluscide), effective against both snails and their eggs, is of low toxicity to mammals, and physical and chemical factors in water cause only minimal inactivation of the chemical. Sodium pentachlorphenate (NaPCP) is an effective molluscicide but more difficult to handle than Niclosamide. It is an irritant to snails in low concentrations and may cause them to leave water (in the case of *S. japonicum*) and escape its lethal action. However, in very low concentrations, a lethal effect on snails eggs is present, which could be of value particularly in seasonal ponds. When snail populations become small repeated applications of NaPCP at low concentrations could be used to prevent re-establishment of the colony following the subsequent period of rains.

EXTENSION OF SCHISTOSOMIASIS

Despite the large body of knowledge which has been accumulated, schistosomiasis is increasing in prevalence. Numerous factors are involved, which can be briefly summarized. Due to the control of endemic diseases of high mortality the population in endemic areas is increasing. This increase in population has led to a need for improved agricultural techniques. Lack of irrigation water has been the chief factor in limiting agricultural development and the construction of large dams to overcome this has led to the creation of numerous artificial reservoirs. These reservoirs, in their turn, have become rapidly contaminated with snails. The creation of large artificial lakes has caused displaced populations to change their occupations and way of life. There has been a change from agriculture to fishing and boating, a change to occupations with increased risks of infection.

Endemic areas of schistosomiasis cut across political boundaries and the political co-operation necessary to ensure control of the disease is not always available. Migration and nomadism, still very common in Africa, offer a ready method of increasing prevalence since the snail hosts are generally more widespread than the disease. Infected populations may not be fully aware of their ill health and the co-operation and understanding of the population in control schemes may be achieved only with the greatest difficulty.

The economic losses from the disease, particularly in areas of subsistence farming, are difficult to estimate. Under such circumstances government interest and financial support is often hard to find. Finally, control schemes are expensive and have often proved to be failures. This has been due largely to inadequate pre-control study and preparation, and failure of long-term follow-up of the programme.

FURTHER READING

Bruijning, C. F. A. (1971). Water, health and economic progress. *Trans. Roy. Soc. Trop. Med. Hyg.* **65** (Suppl.), 47–52.

Forsyth, D. M. and Bradley, D. J. (1966). The consequences of bilharziasis. *Bull. W.H.O.* **34**, 715–735.

Jordan, P. and Webbe, G. (1969). "Human Schistosomiasis". Heinemann, London.

Smithers, S. R. (1972). Recent advances in the immunology of schistosomiasis. *Brit. Med. Bull.* **28**, 49–54.

Warren, K. S. (1973). Regulation of the prevalence and intensity of schistosomiasis in man: immunology or ecology. *J. Infec. Dis.* **127**, 595–609.

Wright, C. A. (1966). Relationships between schistosomes and their molluscan hosts in Africa. *J. Helminth.* **40**, 403–412.

Wright, C. A. (1968). Some views on biological control of trematode diseases. *Trans. Roy. Soc. Trop. Med. Hyg.* **62**, 320–324.

Woodruff, A. W. (Ed.) (1974). "Medicine in the Tropics". Churchill Livingstone, Edinburgh and London.

2. Filariasis

W. E. Kershaw

GENERAL

It is tempting for the uninitiated to regard the distribution of the filarial infections, particularly those which have achieved notoriety, such as river blindness and elephantiasis, as having a geographical dependence since the boundaries of their distribution on the widest scale are well defined.

There are some 600 or more species of filarial parasites of vertebrates, of which some half a dozen affecting man are important. These parasites, both male and female, are thin, thread-like nematodes, usually a few inches long. They live in the connective tissues of the vertebrate host where they produce the first of the four stages in the nematode life cycle. These are then so distributed that they can be ingested by the appropriate blood-sucking or fluid-imbibing insects for the next stage of their development. For example, the filariae which are responsible for elephantiasis occur in the blood and those for river blindness in the upper layers of the skin, where they are accessible to blood-sucking insects of the appropriate kind. The corresponding stages in some animals are excreted in the tears where other fluid-imbibing insects may act as the intermediate host.

The first-stage larva develops in the vector to a second stage and then to a third stage which is infective to the vertebrate host on biting. The vector may take other blood meals during the development of the parasite.

The parasite has no free-living form and therefore must live either in the vertebrate host or, for a short interval, in the insect vector. The vector has quite separate and distinct natural environments or ecological niches within the same general environment. It is necessary for the insect to be able to find its host and to decide that it is the appropriate one, then successfully to take a blood meal from it. This whole process occurs usually within a matter of minutes or even seconds. The vertebrate host and the insect vector share the same environment for a very short time. The so-called specific location of a disease therefore involves at least two quite separate components within that specific location. For example, man does not live under water as do the larval stages of the filaria-transmitting mosquito, nor does he live in the sand in the bottom of a freshwater swamp, as do the larval stages of *Chrysops* which transmits *Loa loa*. In many respects, therefore, the parasitologist is much less interested in the geographical distribution of filarial man than in the minutiae of the distribution of the vector. The so-called geographical distribution of the disease is meaningless unless it is understood as a mosaic made up of very well defined pieces of scientific information concerning the behaviour of the parasite, the host and the vector, and the interrelation of their separate environments.

This chapter will describe the filarial infections affecting man and how their make-up is relevant to their geographical distribution. Consideration will be given to: infection with *Loa loa*, which causes fugitive, irritating swellings in man and monkeys in the Guinea rain forests of Africa; Bancroftian filariasis and its relations which cause elephantiasis throughout the tropics; infections with *Onchocerca volvulus* which, in Africa, are associated with river blindness; and two other filarial infections, *Acanthocheilonema perstans* and *A. streptocerca* which, because they have a distribution common to some of the other filarial infections, may be confused with them. All these infections show great differences in their clinical manifestations and in the details of their life cycles; their vectors are widely divergent in habitat and in taxonomy. It is pertinent, therefore, to consider laboratory filarial infections by way of illustration of such general principles as may be applied.

The study of filariasis was impeded for many years because of the lack of an easily manipulable laboratory infection. In connection with the production of scrub typhus vaccine at the end of the Second

World War, wild cotton rats were imported into the United Kingdom from North America and were found to be infected naturally with their own filarial worm, *Litomosoides carinii*. This is no place to describe the efforts made to understand the infection and to establish it in the laboratory. The female worms are thread-like and about 10 cm (4 inches) long; the males are half this length and have a characteristically corkscrew-like tail. Both sexes live in the pleural cavities of the rat and sometimes in the peritoneal cavity. Their first-stage larvae (microfilariae) are found in the blood at all times during the day and night, the number of larvae there being proportional in single infections to the number of adult worms. Microfilariae live for weeks and the tropical rat mite, taking a blood meal, supports development of the parasite within its fat bodies to produce within a fortnight second and then third-stage infective forms 1 mm long. The mite takes two intermediate blood meals and then, on the infective meal, the third-stage infective larvae make their way into the tissues of another cotton rat. Within days these larvae establish themselves in its pleural cavity. The intensity of the infection as judged by either the number of adult worms or by the number of microfilariae in the peripheral blood, is dependent upon the number of infective forms to which the animal has been exposed. In this respect, the filariae differ completely from such infections as malaria or sleeping sickness, both of which, by the asexual development of the parasite within the host, are capable of saturating that host. In theory, one infective form can, by its potential for asexual multiplication and from one blood meal, produce just as heavy an infection as 1000 or more infective forms. In human filariasis this is not possible since asexual multiplication does not occur. One infective form means one adult worm and no more. To achieve intense infection (a matter of importance in considering river blindness) intense exposure over a long time is necessary since it is unusual in nature for large numbers of infective forms to be introduced into the host at one blood meal.

One infection may suppress in part the development of a subsequent infection. If the mammalian host is exposed constantly to small infections this suppression is well developed and continuously effective. If on the other hand the host is exposed to infections which, though heavy, are well separated and which allow immunity to decline, then suppression is less marked and the heavy infections are better established.

The host reacts to the presence of the parasite. In the cotton rat, reproductive activity of the female worm increases for weeks and the numbers of microfilariae in the peripheral blood increase, reaching a plateau after one or two months. The pleural cavities contain eosinophils and macrophages. Fibrin is deposited around the female worms which later become sclerosed. The male worms are later included in the same reaction. These eosinophilic granulomata become organized and fibrosed and form small white nodules in which the cuticle of the degenerating worms can still be recognized. The number of microfilariae in the peripheral circulation falls until they finally disappear. In the cotton rat this has no clinical effect on the host. These general pathological processes occur in all filarial infections but in man they differ in the details of their manifestations.

In the evolution of parasitism the ultimate trend is towards symbiosis or commensalism or perhaps beyond (when the host is better for having his parasites). This should not be regarded as a simple accidental enterprise on the part of the parasite only, but as an accidental enterprise of the whole parasite-host-vector-environment complex. None of the human filariae may be regarded as comparable to malaria or trypanosomiasis (sleeping sickness) or to some of the insect-borne viruses where infection can be lethal in a matter of hours. The filarial complexes have evolved in a balanced way and such clinically disabling results as may occur amongst those infected are comparatively rare. More harbour the parasite than suffer from disease. This may be due in part to the fact that the complex, as made up, contains mechanisms which tend to establish the infection at a level of equilibrium. Such mechanisms may combine to raise a low level of infection; alternatively they may tend to reduce a high level of infection.

The effect of the infection on vectors varies with the particular kind of vector and the type of infection. In some instances there appears to be little evidence to suggest that the vector is harmed by the development of the parasite within it. For example, up to half the body weight of *Chrysops* may consist of parasites and yet it can fly and feed with no disabilities except for an accident which is unique in vector-borne diseases and which will be described later. The tropical rat mite and the filarial mosquito may, however, have their powers of movement, flight and feeding interfered with; therefore heavily infected vectors which would otherwise be most likely to transmit the infection may not be capable of doing so because of their inability to find their host or to take a blood meal.

INFECTION WITH *LOA LOA*

Loa loa occurs in man and monkeys within the rain forest of West and Central Africa. The infection is found among inhabitants of small rain forest villages located within the patches of residual forest which lie west of the Niger in Nigeria and possibly also in similar situations in Ghana. Infection in man (it certainly occurs in monkeys) is thought to occur also in Uganda, the Congo and Angola. It does not occur in the rain forests of Amazonia in Latin America nor in those of India or Malaysia. The adult worms are about the same size as those in the cotton rat; they live in the subcutaneous tissues and in some of the deeper intermuscular planes of the host and migrate throughout those tissues, causing little trouble. Disturbance of the worms by trauma and by movement provokes local anaphylactic reactions which cause fugitive swellings (Calabar swellings) lasting several days. It is disfiguring for a lady to have a swollen orbit and disturbing if the worm crosses the conjunctiva. A swelling in the wrist of a man who has to drive a car over rough roads, or a swelling in the knee of someone who has to get about, may be very inconvenient. The infection lasts for many years. The microfilariae, if they are found in the blood of the host, are there during the day only. Most of those infected fail to show microfilariae in the peripheral blood, the maximum rate being 40% in adults of 40 years of age or over. These middle-aged people provide the effective reservoir of infection for the fly. This is therefore an infection with a 40-year time scale.

The vectors of the human infection are *Chrysops silacia* and *C. dimidiata* which bite man on the floor of the forest. Only the females take blood meals; males live on fruit or vegetable juice and are often found, together with females, amongst their prey in a nest of bambara bees. The females bite during the day; the microfilariae taken up with the blood meal migrate to the fat bodies in the abdomen of the fly. They develop here within five days and migrate to the muscles of the thorax whence, after a further five days, they are liberated into the general body cavity of the fly. During this time there is no real evidence of any pathological effect and the fly takes one or two intermediate blood meals. When the fly takes its final and infecting blood meal, and final it is, the membranes which join the mouthparts to the head rupture and the infective larvae stream down the mouthparts to lie on the skin of the host and penetrate the wound. In this manner, as many as a thousand larvae may have the opportunity of gaining entry. Having transmitted the infection in this way, the fly dies. In no other vector-borne infection does this occur.

The vectors of the monkey infection are *Chrysops langi* and *C. centurionis*. The infection in monkeys occurs in several species of *Cercopithicae*—in particular the Mona monkey and the putty nosed—and in the short-tailed drill, all of which live in the canopy of the forest. In the drill the worms are longer than in the human infection and the microfilariae occur in the blood during the night. The two vectors spend their entire adult life in the forest canopy 30–45 m (100–150 feet) above the ground; adults are never caught on the forest floor. They bite only at dusk and in the early hours of darkness when the monkeys congregate in the canopy to sleep. Man is rarely bitten by these two species (unless he happens to be a parasitologist engaged in research in the canopy of the forest at night). The infections in man and in monkeys are therefore quite distinct, even though they have the same general geographical distribution.*

*A historical note may be of interest here. Before the discovery of the two canopy-dwelling species of *Chrysops*, the only adult species which had been caught on the floor of the rain forest were adult female *C. silacia* and *C. dimidiata* which are man-biting. No males of any species had been caught on the forest floor. The presence of the two canopy-dwelling species was only revealed when it was necessary to produce, for laboratory experiments, *Chrysops* known to be free of infection. A random collection of larvae and pupae of *Chrysops* and other tabanids was taken from the bottom of freshwater swamps in flat country and from the sandy bottoms of clean rivers and streams in the mountainous parts of the Guinea rain forest. The larvae and pupae so gathered were reared in pots of wet sand. Surprisingly, there emerged, in roughly equal proportions, females *and* males, not only of the forest-floor-feeding *C. silacia* and *C. dimidiata* but also of *C. langi*, *C. centurionis* and *C. longicornis*. All larvae and pupae of these five species had been taken from similar habitats and yet only one adult male of any of the five species had been caught previously by man, and only one female adult of *C. langi*, *C. centurionis* or *C. longicornis* had been caught on the forest floor coming in to take blood meals from man or animals. Where were these adults living in nature and on what creatures did they feed? By the use of scaling ladders two species, *C. langi* and *C. centurionis*, were found living in the canopy of the forest and biting monkeys (and man if he happened to be there) only during the night. Adult female *C. silacia* and *C. dimidiata* were also present in the canopy but were biting there during day. Such adult females were already known to bite man and other animals on the forest floor during the day. On what *C. longicornis* feeds remains a mystery.

Although the rain forest may be regarded as one vast, uniform habitat, each separate host-parasite-vector complex is a local affair. The dispersal range of *Chrysops* is limited to about 1 mile, particularly if blood meals are readily available. The extensive distribution of *L. loa* in the Guinea rain forests in West and Central Africa may itself be regarded as a mosaic or patchwork comprising small, contiguous fragments, each self-maintaining and contributing little to its neighbours. The two important factors which prevent this infection from being labile are the limited dispersal of the fly and the fact that most people who are infected are not infective.

Rubber estates provide an interesting example of man's interference with the natural equilibrium of an infection. Rubber trees are no more than 20 m (70 feet) high and in this specialized vegetation there are no monkeys to provide blood meals for the two canopy-dwelling species of *Chrysops*. But the rubber estate is surrounded by swamps, the breeding places of *Chrysops* which are provided with a regular and plentiful source of human blood meals by the rubber tappers moving from tree to tree during the day. *C. silacia* and *C. dimidiata* abound, with the result that the rate of transmission of the infection in communities living in a rubber estate is higher than in the small and scattered villages of the forest, more people having microfilariae in their peripheral blood and at an earlier age. However, the clearing of a quarter of a mile of forest around an expanding village to provide farm land may be sufficient to bring about a substantial reduction in the rate of transmission, since the adult *Chrysops* is a shade-loving fly.

The distribution of *L. loa* in man and monkeys is dependent upon the four relevant species of *Chrysops* having suitable fresh water for breeding and rain forest with its canopy for their adult life. It seems likely that the forest *Chrysops* first evolved in the scattered trees and grasslands of the savanna and only later in its evolutionary adventure did it invade the rain forest (regarded by some as "savanna on stilts"). Nothing is known of the previous history of *L. loa* since it has no close relatives. Whether it was transmitted from the savanna by *Chrysops* or whether it evolved in the rain forest is not clear, nor is it clear whether those *Chrysops* which are now vectors of *L. loa* in man and monkeys diverged before they came into the forest or after they entered the forest. Two species remained in the canopy for the whole of their adult lives, both during the day and the night, getting their blood meals from whatever creatures happened to be there; and two, those transmitting human *L. loa*, developed the ability to take their meals during the day on the forest floor. The present distribution of infection with *L. loa* is thus a manifestation of the evolutionary adventures of *Chrysops*.

L. loa does not occur in the rain forests of the Amazon nor in those of India and Malaysia although *Chrysops* occurs in all these places. One assumes, therefore, that either it has evolved in Africa after the supposed separation of the continents or that it evolved before the separation and has subsequently died out elsewhere. It seems probable that it had the opportunity of establishing itself relatively recently in Central and South America by the importation of slaves from West Africa; however, since most of the slaves imported would have been young, they would not have had the microfilariae of *L. loa* in their peripheral blood to serve as a reservoir. An illustration by Pigafetta, dated 1598 in a *Journal of the Voyages of Magellan*, showing a man removing a guinea worm from his leg and another having a worm, presumably *L. loa*, removed from his eye, would seem to indicate that the worm has been recognized as early as the 16th century.

Some parasitic infections like Bancroftian filariasis which have several alternative vectors can adapt themselves to new circumstances. Bancroftian filariasis can be transmitted by *Culex fatigans* and by several species of anopheline mosquitoes; similar infections may be transmitted by *Aedes* and *Mansonia* species. This does not apply to *L. loa* which has no alternative set of vectors. Transmission of human *L. loa* is limited to two species of *Chrysops*, and limited not because other species cannot transmit it (all African species from the rain forest will do so in the laboratory) but because of their particular biting habits. For this reason *L. loa* has not the potential of Bancroftian filariasis for wider spread.

Human *L. loa* may be regarded as having long-term resilience since the present transmission is based on infections laid down 30 or 40 years ago. A person once infected by the fly remains infected, probably for the rest of his life; accordingly, the fly turn-over is slow. On the other hand, the infection is sensitive, in the short term, to local conditions affecting *Chrysops*, since the dispersal of *Chrysops* is limited and it will not cross unshaded clearings. In order to maintain transmission, there must be enough people in a community, and sufficient flies, to maintain transmission at a level which will produce the reservoir decades hence. A community, therefore, must be of a certain size: too small a community may allow transmission to die out, too large a community will reduce transmission by dint of the clearing by farming and other activities round an organized community. It follows that the infection is one associated with small villages in the forest rather than with towns.

Throughout the tropics botanists are concerned for the survival of the rain forests which are in places being wantonly destroyed. It is interesting to speculate on how the destruction of the forest or its management will affect. *L. loa*. If it is turned into rubber estates, human *L. loa* will increase if turned into farms, it will diminish. If forestry management is instituted, this would affect all the components of the infection, since the drainage of swamps and canalization of small rivers would destroy the breeding places of the fly, a thinner forest canopy might not provide sufficient shade for *Chrysops*, while human populations in a managed forest would be regulated if not removed, thus removing both the reservoir of infection and the blood meals for the fly.

INFECTION WITH *ACANTHOCHEILONEMA PERSTANS*

It is convenient to consider here one of the parasitic curiosities, *Acanthocheilonema perstans*, since many people in the Cameroon and eastern Nigeria who are infected with *L. loa* are also infected with this filaria. The adult filariae live in the connective tissues near the spine of a mammalian host; the microfilariae occur in the blood during the day and night and are very commonly found.

In the western Cameroon, where there are large banana plantations, infection with *Acanthocheilonema perstans* is universal, so much so that it is a badge of sojourn. It is also found in Uganda, Rhodesia and Zambia. The infection is transmitted by the biting midge, *Culicoides milnei* (*C. austeni*) which has adapted itself to spending its larval and pupal stages in the pinhead-sized pools of water left in the cut stems of banana plants. Banana cultivation involves the cutting of these stems at regular intervals. They are about 30 cm (1 foot) in diameter; each stem must contain many thousands of exuberantly moving larvae and pupae and there are millions of banana plants in a few square miles.

At the turn of the century *A. perstans* was suspected of being responsible for "negro lethargy" (later known as sleeping sickness) since it was very common in proximity to the plantations near the shores of Lake Victoria where sleeping sickness was rife. The distribution of the two conditions differed slightly and subsequently sleeping sickness was shown to be due to a trypanosome. The microfilariae of *A. perstans* are easily distinguished from those of *L. loa*. In the Cameroun, it is common to find people with Calabar swellings and adult *L. loa* worms crossing the eye but with the microfilariae of the concomitant infection *A. perstans* in their peripheral blood and not those of *L. loa*. There are several other species of man-biting *Culicoides* in the forest, mangrove swamps and grasslands but infection with *A. perstans* of such prevalence as occurs in the Cameroon reflects the presence of plantations of bananas or of the domestic plantain.

Culicoides milnei bites only at night in very dim light such as occurs when the moon is obscured by clouds. Even a temporary clearing of the moon will cause the midges to desist from biting. They do not bite when the night sky is clear nor where there are artificial lights brighter than a glimmer.

BANCROFTIAN FILARIASIS

Bancroftian filariasis occurs in man in the tropics and, in its later stages, is associated with the gross swellings of the limbs and genitalia known as elephantiasis. It is caused by several closely related parasites of which the most common is *Wuchereria bancrofti*. This particular parasite occurs only in man but several others may occur in animals such as cats. All are transmitted by mosquitoes, most commonly by *Culex fatigans* (which breeds in stagnant, polluted water) and by species of *Anopheles* and *Aedes*. Other related parasites are carried by *Mansonia* mosquitoes.

The principles of the infection are common to those of the other filariae but its course differs in detail. The infective forms, the third stage larvae, are transmitted by the infective mosquito at the time of biting and probably make their way direct from the insect's mouthparts into the wound. During their development to adults, it seems likely that the larvae remain in the same area in which they are implanted but are then usually held up in the first local lymph glands. Bites on the hand produce swellings in the lymph glands of the elbow while those occurring on the lower leg involve the lymph glands of the groin. During this time, which may be months, the host is in a state of developing sensitivity and allergy and may well develop asthma, eosinophilia and urticarial rashes.* The presence of these adult parasites in the lymph glands may produce, from time to time, allergic flares lasting days, weeks or even longer, with allergic cellulitis of the leg or arm accompanied by fever—"lymphangetic fever". These attacks may occur at intervals for several years.

Some 10–15 years after infection, microfilariae, the first-stage larvae, begin to appear in the peripheral blood. They are usually periodic and, in the case of *Wuchereria bancrofti* infections, may be present during the night. Some of the other infections are non-periodic or semi-periodic. After being present for perhaps 10 years, the microfilariae decline and gradually disappear from the peripheral blood.

About 10 years after the initial infection, the first of many, the attacks of lymphangetic fever begin to subside, leaving residual swellings. This condition may progress until a permanent swelling of the superficial tissues of the scrotum, leg, arm or breast develops. The swelling may be gross. A leg becomes perhaps 60 cm (2 feet) in diameter with heavily thickened skin and perhaps with large warts over the feet. This makes the gait ponderous, swinging and slow and the general appearance is ugly. The enlargement of the scrotum may be such as to require a small wheelbarrow to enable the man to get about. How far these unsightly deformities are disabling depends upon the mode of life of those infected. Lesions deep in the lymph glands of the abdomen may produce blockage of the lymphatic connections of the genito-urinary tract and allow the escape of chyle in the urine. The prevalence of deformities in a community is related to the intensity of infection over many years. Many of those individuals who are only lightly infected may be transmitting the infection to mosquitoes. They may have no overt symptoms themselves; indeed such symptoms may never develop.

*Some of the filariae which occur normally in animals may be implanted in man. Their development may be arrested in this abnormal host. Even so the parasites may continue to live in arrested development and be associated with such syndromes as pulmonary eosinophilia.

The present distribution of Bancroftian filariasis is dependent upon man's environment and is a measure of urbanization. Before the Second World War, the disease was considered to be merely an interesting vector-borne infection which occurred in the tropics. It did not excite public health interest, although there was a great deal of sympathy, particularly in the Pacific Islands, for individuals with elephantiasis. After the Second World War, however, with the increase in population in the tropics and increasing urbanization, the infection began to spread at an alarming rate which has now attracted universal concern. Examples of this increase in Sri Lanka, Burma and a small part of India will be given later; in the meantime consider the case of filariasis in a population which is in harmony with its environment and in equilibrium with its parasites. Such a community could be found in 1942 in Addu Atoll (which includes the island of Gan), the southernmost atoll of the Maldives. This atoll, some 32 km (20 miles) across in some 2000 fathoms of Indian Ocean, comprises several islands, the highest point being nowhere more than 1–1½ m (4–5 feet) above the sea. There were coconut trees and much mangrove. Until the Second World War the population was static. People lived in well-constructed houses built of coral blocks and had wells of clean water, probably derived from the rains. Anopheline mosquitoes bred in the wells and *Culex fatigans* bred in domestic utensils such as coconut shells. The islanders produced little copra since the area of the islands was small. Their main diet consisted of fish. Much sun-dried fish (Bombay duck) was bartered in Ceylon for rice; they had no currency.

The inhabitants of Addu Atoll lived with their infections: malaria; scrub typhus; filariasis and bony tuberculosis. The malaria was associated with a high infant mortality which kept the population in balance. There was of course no urbanization and no increase of population and the disease could not explode. The islanders accepted filariasis as a part of life and, perhaps unusually, believed it to be contagious. Anyone showing permanent swellings was transferred to an island used especially for this purpose where all the adults had elephantiasis.

Similar foci of filariasis could be found all over South East Asia and in the islands of the Pacific. Populations were controlled by malaria. There was little movement of rural populations to the cities and travel was slow, difficult and expensive. Sri Lanka at that time was a stable island. The population was static, the towns were small and the tea, rubber and copra plantations, together with trading in gems, provided a stable economy. Malaria was contained by surveillance. The malaria control campaign was designed to prevent the spread of malaria from the hyper-immune dry areas of the north-east of the island, through the intermediate zone, to the non-immune wet zone in the south-west. With the advent of DDT, the policy was changed and an attempt was made to eradicate malaria. This resulted in a marked lowering of the infant mortality and a consequent rapid increase in the population. There was concomitant urbanization. The villages in the south-west became towns and Colombo, the capital, developed satellite suburbs.

The suburbs of Colombo expanded but the provision of sanitary services in both the suburbs and in the coastal towns and villages failed to keep pace with that expansion. An individual septic tank for each house was provided in some towns but not in others since the expense of the installations was formidable. In consequence the established, old latrines tended to overflow during the rains, producing pools of polluted water in which the *Culex fatigans* mosquito bred readily and rapidly. Water supplies were given greater priority than sanitary services and the resulting easily accessible water in turn gave rise to more stagnant pools. The increasing popularity of the motor car ensured an increasing number of discarded motor tyres for use as convenient seats or as constituents of litter, which together with the ubiquitous tins, provided further breeding places. The breeding places of mosquitoes are therefore domestic; *C. fatigans* bite at night and the families in their nearby houses are available as a source of blood meals.

Coconuts are grown widely in Sri Lanka but the coconut industry is concentrated in the south-west of the country, particularly at Matara and in the intermediate zone near Karunegala. In Matara, the coconut trees are grown in rows, separated by long trenches of water which are used for retting. The nuts are harvested, the copra is removed and the husks put into the trenches, covered with palm leaves and heavy stones and are thus submerged. After some weeks the coconut fibres in the husks are separated and can then be milled for fibre and rope making. By this time the water in the retting pits is evil-smelling and allows an enormous population of *C. fatigans* to thrive, with the result that the naturally white coral side of the pits is black with a mat of adult mosquitoes. To remain in a plantation at night is not possible unless one is completely covered by a net. The intensity of transmission of infection in these plantations is extremely high.

Near Karunegala the palms are grown without retting pits between the rows of trees. Instead there is a large central retting pit built of concrete. The husks are put into the pit at one end and taken out at the other and it can take weeks or even months for a batch of husks to move along. The water is not so evil-smelling as in the small retting pits near Matara; it does not support the growth of mosquitoes nor of any other living creature.

This difference in retting procedures between the two areas would repay investigation. The implications in control are obvious. The retting pits at Matara are shaded by the palms; those at Karunegala are open to the direct rays of the sun.

In Burma the infection is a manifestation of faecal disposal. Rangoon is a city built on flat, reclaimed land in the delta of the Rangoon river; the magnificent Shwedagon Pagoda surmounts the one and only hill. Rangoon is a modern city and it has two sets of drains. The sewage, which is carried in deep drains, is dependent upon a series of pumps which give the sewage an artificial head of about a metre at intervals in its course to the sea. The superficial street and roof drains which take the rains have a separate course. The pumps, which were fitted in 1860 and were mining pumps made in Ruabon, North Wales, were designed to have a 30-year life. During the Second World War, some of the pumps broke down through lack of maintenance. As a result, many of the deep drains of Rangoon became clogged and ceased to function. Householders in much of Rangoon had to break the pipes at the point where the sewage pipes ran outside the houses into the deep drains. The superficial drainage system was thereby polluted and, with the general accumulation of debris following the degradation of a district, pools of polluted water became permanent. (This did not occur in those districts where the pumps were still working.) Filariasis, which had been a curiosity in Rangoon before the Second World War and was believed to occur only in migrants to that city from India, thus became widespread. Although many people had microfilariae in their blood at night, few had elephantiasis, except Indian migrants, but as a result of radio appeals made in 1961, people with elephantiasis, which they had only just begun to notice, came forward. The epidemic of filariasis in

Rangoon, which is continuing, began with the break-up of the drainage system. Noone used a mosquito net in Rangoon before the Second World War; 20 years later a net had become a necessity.

At the end of the Second World War, Burma was plagued with roving bands of dacoits and the population of Rangoon rose to two or three times its normal size as refugees from the north moved in to live in shanties in the streets. The authorities made a determined effort to re-house these refugees in three satellite towns on reclaimed land in the delta, with houses, stand-piped water and their own dry, deep privies. The water was constantly pumped out of this reclaimed land which was often below sea level. During the dry season the privies did not overflow, nor did the water accumulate; but during the rains, many privies did overflow and the nearby water, although eventually pumped out, stood long enough to permit the breeding of *C. fatigans*.

Elsewhere in Burma, filariasis exists but patchily. There is little in the Imlay lakes in the mountainous regions of the Shan States. The long main lake and the other smaller ones have clear water in which *C. fatigans* does not breed, nor does it breed in the fast-running mountain streams. In Taunji, the capital of the Shan States in the mountainous areas near China, there is no filariasis. Sewage disposal presents no difficulty, nor does storm water accumulate, since the run-off is so rapid. Again in the small coastal fishing villages of Tenasserim, there is no filariasis. Houses are built on stilts over the sea and each house has its own direct sewage disposal system based on the movements of the tides. In Mergui, on the other hand, an old established town on the maritime trade route to the Far East, filariasis does occur. Here, in the narrow strip of flat land between the hills and the sea, storm water can be held up in uncompleted drains where households are responsible for their own superficial drains. To this may be added water from flooded privies.

Mandalay has filariasis occurring in strips within the city. Much of the city has fast running rivers or streams which flow towards the Irrawaddy. Many of the houses have their own privies erected on the ends of gang-planks over the streams. The compounds are well drained and there is no accumulation of polluted water. These rivers run into man-made ditches which are slow-flowing and the houses on the banks of these ditches (which are perhaps 9–10 m wide) have privies in the gardens which are protected by small bunds. During the rains, as in the corresponding situation in the satellite towns in

Rangoon, the privies become water-logged, the accumulated water is held up by the bund and mosquitoes breed.

Near Delhi, infection is transmitted by *C. fatigans* which breeds not only in the usual domestic stagnant pools but also in wells used for irrigating the rice fields. Here the water is sufficiently polluted by decaying vegetation and dead birds to support the larvae and pupae of the mosquito.

The examples given above may be regarded as isolated problems arising from the wide differences in the nature of the breeding places of the mosquito. All could be effectively dealt with were it not for the high cost of, for example, providing adequate sanitary arrangements or reorganizing procedures in the coconut industry. Such measures would provide a more or less permanent solution by eradicating vector populations. However, in the event of a breakdown of environmental engineering, the flight range of *C. fatigans* would probably enable the species to re-establish itself. Near Delhi, where it is not possible to eliminate the breeding places by environmental engineering because the wells must be there for irrigation, attempts have been made to eradicate the mosquitoes by insecticides and by the manipulation of mosquito genetics; but temporary success has been followed by the re-establishment of a vector population from outside the area.

Filariasis is increasing at an alarming rate. Since it takes 30 or more years for microfilariae to appear in the peripheral circulation this dramatic explosion of filariasis can be regarded as an epidemic on a 30-year time scale. Thirty years from now the reservoir of infection will be enormous. How far this can be arrested is open to doubt unless by the application of costly sanitary engineering measures.

It is difficult to establish satisfactory control systems for many reasons. Not the least of the problems lies in the difficulty of obtaining accurate information from a survey of the human population. The microfilariae are present in the blood only during the night and householders do not take kindly to having blood films taken at 2 o'clock in the mornings. Furthermore, it has been well said that if a man has malaria and is ill, one gives him medicine and he is better; if he has filariasis and is well, one gives him medicine and he is ill. The treatment of filariasis by the piperazines invokes an immediate reaction by anaphylaxis—the Herxheimer reaction—and for several days, the man so treated has headache, a temperature, itching and malaise and will be off work. It is difficult, therefore, to persuade people to accept the treatment which would remove the reservoir of infection within a community.

Insecticides invoke resistance. A series of insecticides can be used, one being used after mosquitoes have developed resistance to another. Careful monitoring of mosquito populations for insecticide resistance is necessary and this requires sophisticated equipment and knowledge. It is difficult sometimes to ensure that the insecticide is applied in the correct place and in the correct manner since some insecticides have such an unpleasant residual smell that the operator may find himself a domestic outcast. Moreover, insecticides are made from petro-chemicals whose availability in the future may be called into question. The expense of the large-scale application of insecticides is beyond the pockets of many communities.

It is not easy to produce and maintain a reliable organization to attempt to control filariasis. It requires political stability, a reliable bureaucracy and a large number of dedicated operators who can be trusted to work without supervision and who must be recruited from the intelligent; they require much training. No country can contemplate the institution of control measures on a nationwide scale. Nevertheless, given determination and a sense of civic responsibility, each local infection could be tackled individually.

ONCHOCERCIASIS

Onchocerciasis in man occurs in West, Central and East Africa; reputedly in the Yemen; in Central America; and in the north part of Latin America. The parasite, *Onchocerca*, is transmitted by several species of *Simulium* (the buffalo gnat) which breeds in fast-running streams with turbulent and well-oxygenated water.

The life cycle of the infection in the host is similar in principle to that of the other filariae. Third-stage larvae are implanted when the infective fly takes a blood meal and they grow through the fourth stage to the adult form. Although they may migrate a little locally they probably remain relatively static compared with the body-wide migrations of *Loa loa*. Males and females congregate and produce local reactions which some years later produce fibrous nodules. Microfilariae (first-stage larvae) are found in the skin and are not found in the blood. The microfilariae are taken in by the biting

Simulium accidentally when it is taking a blood meal and they make their way within hours to the thoracic muscles of the insect, where they develop to the third larval stage. During this time the fly may well take in two or three blood meals. Having reached the infective form, microfilariae move to the haemocele and the head and are released by the fly in taking a further blood meal.

The clinical manifestations of infection in man differ according to the site of biting of the vector. In the African form, transmitted by *S. damnosum* and *S. neavei*, fibrous nodules occur on the legs and the lower part of the body, particularly on the knees, the iliac crests and the great trochanter; skin lesions are predominantly in these areas. The density of microfilariae in the skin is greatest in the quarters near the nodules, and when there are several, the highest counts are in the buttocks and in the calves. In persons standing up, *S. damnosum* and *S. neavei* bite mostly on the ankles and the lower legs, but they may bite elsewhere on the dependent parts in those sitting or lying down. The flies also bite on a forearm resting on a table top.

In Guatemala, Mexico and parts of South America, where transmission is by *S. ochraceum*, the nodules are found mostly on the head, as are the early skin changes. There is also an associated demonstrable soft tissue swelling which is not so noticeable in the legs in Africa. *S. ochraceum* bites on the head and neck and not on the ankles. The reasons for the difference in behaviour between these two related flies is not clear. In Venezuela, however, where *S. metallicum* transmits the infection, a pattern more like that of the African form occurs, corresponding to the biting behaviour of the vector. The Central American form has long been associated with eye changes, hence the old name of the parasite *Onchocerca cercutiens* or the blinding filaria. Even in the 1920s, the African form was thought to be unimportant but since then its association with river blindness has been realized.

In Africa, in a mild infection, i.e. in someone young who has not been repeatedly exposed to infection over a very long period or in an adult who has had a mild infection occasionally, the infection may remain localized to the leg or in the lower part of the trunk; there may be few or no microfilariae found in the shoulders and the head and neck; and there will be no eye changes. With oft-repeated infections, intensity of infection builds up; very large numbers of microfilariae occur in the lower limbs and buttocks and in the lower part of the trunk; they appear in the shoulders, in the skin of the head, in the conjunctiva and some in the anterior segment of the eye. Correspondingly, the skin changes become more extreme in the lower parts of the body and extend, in a less marked way, upwards.

Eye changes begin to appear in the anterior chamber after long exposure to intense infection and produce opacities of the cornea, a keratitis and deformity of the iris. These anterior segment changes are related to the intensity of the infection and occur in adults usually over the age of 35 years and are gradual in onset. They do not produce economic blindness in their early stages. There are, however, other eye changes in the posterior segment of the eye which occur in areas where onchocerciasis occurs, but also in other areas where it does not. These include atrophy of the optic nerve and a dissolution of the retina in which the remnants of the retina are seen as blotches of pigment against the intact coroid. Optic atrophy can occur from other causes and similar genetic abiotrophies occur in people who have never been in the tropics; these eye changes in areas where onchocerciasis occurs are not related to intensity of infection. They must be due to another mechanism in the infection, or to other causes not connected with it. Vitamin deficiency has been suggested. It is difficult to see how this problem can be answered. With the rapid interchange of modern African communities, it is no longer possible to analyse the genetic and infective background of small static groups.

The skin changes fall into a clear pattern. In the early stage of infection, there may be an allergic urticarial or oedematous rash and this is commonly complained of by adult Europeans exposed for the first time but, of course, is not noteworthy in the infant African. Similar reactions occur in infections with *L. loa* and Bancroftian filariasis. In these early stages the microfilariae occur immediately under the uppermost layer of the skin (*stratum corneum*) with few histological changes, but as the intensity of infection increases, the elastic tissues in that site become fewer and the skin takes on a rather smooth appearance; with increasing intensity of infection the elastin normal to the skin disappears, down to perhaps a millimetre or more. This process continues; the elastin is replaced by fibrous tissue and the normal structure of the skin becomes a thin layer of epithelium supported by fibrous tissue and all the special structures, such as capillary processes, disappear. The skin then looks like lizard skin. It is thin, inelastic and wrinkled. It has been described as senile skin, but the histological changes are quite different from those of ageing. The changes are specific to the infection.

Finally, in an intense infection the skin on the legs may be thickened due to the enormous increase of fibrous tissue, giving a woody feel, and the histological disturbance may produce large unpigmented patches. In these so-called "burned out" cases, microfilariae counts in the superficial layers of the skin are low.

The disposition of the microfilariae in the different layers of the skin is important in relation to transmission and, therefore, to the epidemiology of the infection. *Simulium*, unlike most other biting creatures, bites by "open-cast mining", by producing a tunnel until it tears apart the blood vessels of the papilla of the skin. It has not the mouthparts to seek a capillary as does the mosquito. It feeds only from the superficial layer and takes in the microfilariae with the tissue fluid which it has liberated, mixed with the blood. In an early infection, the microfilariae may be few but they are available to the fly. In a later infection, one of middle intensity, with no marked skin changes, the number of microfilariae available is much higher. When the skin changes become more extreme, numbers of microfilariae in the skin are enormous but, because they are mostly beneath the fibrous layers which have begun to replace the elastin, they are denied to the fly. Similarly, of course, any superficial skin snip will disclose only small numbers.

The most effective reservoirs available to the fly are thus the early mild and the middle cases, and not the late, extreme cases. The obvious cases of onchocerciasis are not the reservoir of infection and thus contrast with the transmission of *L. loa* in which the old cases of infection are the reservoir.

When the fly takes in a blood meal, the wall of the stomach secretes round the meal a membrane which for the most part seals it off. Before the membrane is fully formed some of the microfilariae in the blood meal are able to escape and make their way to the thoracic muscles by a route which is, as yet, undefined. The other microfilariae perish with the blood on digestion. The majority of those ingested cannot therefore proceed to development. It seems likely, however, that most of the microfilariae which establish themselves in the thorax may become infective. This cutting down of the population of the parasite ingested by the fly does not occur in *Chrysops* infected with *L. loa*. The infection with *Onchocerca* does not affect the behaviour of *Simulium*.

The distribution of *Simulium* is almost world wide. It breeds exclusively in fast-running water, in rivers and streams, in waterfalls and even in the cooling towers of electricity stations. In temperate zones and in the tundra it is a biting nuisance of enormous proportions. For example, during the building of the Alaskan Highway in North America, drastic measures had to be taken to control the fly in order to protect the work force. Similarly in eastern Canada, it was a severe biting nuisance during the building of a hydro-electric station at Churchill Falls. In both of these places the work force provided an abundant source of blood meals when other sources were scarce. This represents a regulating factor of the *Simulium* population. The biting nuisance arises when man invades an area which contains *Simulium* which have been feeding on other creatures. In such circumstances, *Simulium* may be acting as a vector for parasites of the creatures from which they obtain their normal blood meals; but these parasites are not transmissible to man. The *Onchocerca* parasite infecting man does not occur outside the tropics. It has been said that the commonest biting fly in England may be *Simulium* but the many species of *Simulium* rarely bite man. The parasites which it transmits are related to riverine creatures such as water birds and animals such as cattle and horses. Most cattle and horses in Britain are infected with their own kind of onchocerciasis.

Generally speaking, man is not a riverine creature in Britain. Those few men who spend much of their time in or near rivers are usually well protected against biting flies and the cold. In Africa, however, where human *Onchocerca* does occur, man is very often riverine, either perhaps as a ferryman or fisherman, or because the river is the sole source of water for his villages. He wears little clothing. As in Britain, a form of onchocerciasis occurs in cattle.

Simulium damnosum and many other species occur in the rain forest, in the savanna and in semi-arid areas of most of West and Central Africa. The fast-flowing and perennial streams and rivers in the mountainous rain forests are either boulder strewn or have pebbly bottoms. These rocks and stones, together with aquatic vegetation, support the larvae and pupae of *Simulium*. Transmission of the infection can occur therefore throughout the whole year. Most villages are near small streams and the intensity of infection may be high.

Breeding of *Simulium* in the savanna and in the drier parts of Africa is intermittent. Many water courses are without water during the dry season and there is no breeding. With the onset of the local rains, however, the rivers flow. The speedier parts, which have rocks and gravelly stones in their beds, will support the aquatic stages of *Simulium damnosum* as will the grass at the edge of the river bank. So too, will the grass in the stream bed when it becomes submerged as the river rises. In rivers such as the Niger, which at each flood receives waters from its local tributaries and also from the previous year's rainfall on the Atlantic coast of West Africa via the swamps of Timbuctu, there is a characteristic distribution of *Simulium*. Few *Simulium* larvae occur in the river itself, which for the most part has a sandy or muddy bottom, but they are plentiful along its banks near the confluence of the many small tributaries. A village may be on the banks of the Niger from which the villagers obtain their fish, but their infection is acquired from the small tributaries several hundred metres away.

In the Upper Volta and Sissili river basins, the general lack of water causes people to live near the rivers and infection here may be intense locally. It may be sufficient, because of the skin lesions and itching in the early infections, the nuisance of biting, and the eye changes, to depopulate considerable areas. While infection may be present over large areas, it seems likely that it is really a composite of many small local foci.

Much has been made of the flight range of individual flies. But flight range is a different concept from dispersal and, if blood meals are available, the fly population does not wander much. For example, in the villages of the southern edge of the Bauchi Plateau in Nigeria, the intensity of infection falls off very markedly within 3 or 4 km of the breeding places. A change in altitude in grassland areas, even between villages 2 miles apart, makes an even greater difference: one village may be free from infection while the other is heavily infected. This localization of infection, which is a reflection of limited dispersal, is different from flight range. When *Simulium* has been "controlled" in a stretch of river, it has no difficulty in restoring its population, either by the movement of larvae down river from established habitats upstream or perhaps by lateral invasion. In these circumstances there is no doubt that *Simulium* has a long flight range.

If eradication is the aim, it is difficult to see how any attempt to control *Simulium* over a very large area could be effective. Theoretically, however, it should be possible to reduce the transmission, and therefore the intensity, of infection to a level below which serious pathological results would not arise. Wherever there is a large work force, it may be necessary for psychological reasons to remove *Simulium* because of its known association with river blindness. For example, the work force engaged on the construction of the Kainji dam in North-West Nigeria was protected by the repeated use of DDT in some of the nearby tributaries. Similarly, in plantations sited in mountainous rain forest, it is possible markedly to reduce fly populations in the small streams near plantation villages. The building of dams for hydro-electric energy in localities in Africa where onchocerciasis occurs affects the distribution of *Simulium*. The raising of water levels in the old river bed and its tributaries often submerges the rocky outcrops which, with their vegetation, provide numerous opportunities for the breeding of *Simulium*. The human population which lived near the now submerged breeding places may well move their villages to the banks of unaffected tributaries where *Simulium* will still be breeding and transmission of the infection will therefore continue.

Attempts at controlling *Simulium* by soluble and non-selective insecticides have produced results which should have been anticipated. Being non-selective the insecticide has affected many other creatures in the river including the predators which feed on *Simulium* larvae. It takes many months to restore predator populations by upstream seeding but *Simulium* can restore itself in a matter of weeks, giving rise to an unrestrained population explosion.

The use of soluble insecticides, even at low, discreet dilutions, must therefore be a continuous process. Their use in some of the waterfalls in the Upper Nile has changed the biological character of the falls and of the river below.

Simulium feeds on particles of the same order of size as a red blood cell. It is possible, therefore, to use particulate insecticides which affect *Simulium* selectively but leave other creatures in the river undisturbed. The use of residual insecticides whose activity is maintained for a long time is not necessary. Less damage results from the use of insecticides which are hydrolized into inert substances within a few days, during which time they would have been effective on a few miles of river.

Insecticides are now becoming very expensive and it is a matter of administrative discretion whether a community can afford the cost of insecticides in its public health budget. Furthermore, the detailed ecological studies which are carried out in small temperate* rivers are virtually impossible in rivers like the Niger.

If it is desired to follow up any changes in the other creatures in the river as a result of the use of insecticides, difficulties arise due to the enormous differences in the ecology of aquatic creatures during the floods and during the dry season; for these reasons also it is difficult, if not impossible, to establish a biological baseline. The cost in skilled manpower, in transport and above all in time is astronomical. It might be much cheaper in the long run to remove the community away from the river and supply a piped water supply.†

S. damnosum has been described as the vector of human onchocerciasis in West and Central Africa. There are, however, many other species of *Simulium* in the rivers of these parts which feed not on man but on other creatures and which do not transmit onchocerciasis. In East Africa, human onchocerciasis is transmitted by *S. damnosum* and *S. neavei*. There are separate genetic strains of *S. damnosum*, distinguished by their chromosome patterns, within the

*Temperate rivers require management to take account of the water demands for industry, domestic water supplies, the disposal of sewage and industrial effluent; and of leisure pursuits such as game and coarse fishing, canoeing and sailing. The water is often re-used several times before it reaches the sea. This re-use of water is possible because rivers are self-cleaning. In tropical Africa, the great bodies of water are used for transport, irrigation and fish-hunting, as they always have been, and, in recent years, for the generation of hydro-electric energy. The water supplies to the few large cities require, of course, the same management as those in temperate zones.

†The control measures described have been those directed against the aquatic stages of the fly. Shortly after the Second World War, and in one special circumstance, *Simulium* was controlled by residual insecticides used against the adult fly. A few kilometres below the town of Kinshasa, the River Zaire, a deep, swift-flowing river several kilometres wide, becomes a series of turbulent rapids dotted with a large number of islands which are inaccessible by boat. On the south bank opposite these islands was a fishing village which had a very high incidence of onchocerciasis. It was assumed that the breeding places of the fly were on the margins of the islands and that the vegetation on these islands would act as resting places of emergent flies. Because of the enormous volume of the river, the use of DDT against the larval stages was out of the question. Accordingly, the assumed resting places were sprayed with DDT by means of a fixed wing aircraft. The population of *Simulium* in the village diminished markedly as a result of this operation.

general population of *S. damnosum*, which feed on other creatures. It is likely that the same phenomenon occurs in Central Africa. This presents a further complication in the interpretation of the epidemiology.

S. neavei is a special case. The larval and pupal stages of *S. damnosum* are found on sticks, stones and aquatic vegetation; *S. neavei* is supported in the water only on the backs and limbs of freshwater crabs in East Africa. There is no particular taxonomic relation between the type of crab and *S. neavei*. The relation is ecological and is determined by the behaviour of the crab at the altitude (1200–1600 m, 3800–5200 feet) at which *S. neavei* lives. It is one of some 15 or so species of *Simulidae* living within or just above this zone.

The *S. neavei* complex is associated with nine species of the freshwater crab *Potamonautes* belonging to five species groups. The low-country crab, *P. niloticus*, is found up to a limit of 1400 m (4600 feet) in the lower reaches of rivers in Uganda and Kenya. It lives in many habitats and in turbulent water. It is associated in its higher distribution with *S. neavei*. *P. berardi* occurs between 1100 and 3000m (3000 and 10 000 feet)—the greatest height at which collections were made on Mount Elgon; it lives under stones in the river beds and in burrows in the river banks, particularly in the forest. It supports *S. neavei* from the lower levels of its distribution up to the highest level of the distribution of *S. neavei* (i.e. 1600 m, 5200 feet). Similar closely related crabs occur in the upper reaches of the rivers in the mountains in Uganda and Kenya and support *S. neavei*. *S. neavei* is thus supported by the low-country crabs in their higher distribution and the separate groups of mountain crabs in their lower reaches, provided that they spend all their time in the water.

Another kind of crab occurs in Mount Kenya at altitudes of 1130–2070 m (3700–6800 feet) wherever loose, damp soil is present. This is commonly in the splash zone of waterfalls and among the tree ferns in the forest. It is rarely seen in the water and is never associated with *S. neavei*. Similar crabs occur in Kenya and Tanzania. The distribution of the freshwater crabs is wider than the distribution of *S. neavei*. There is a close correlation between the occurrence of the *S. neavei* complex and the distribution of uncleared forest which provides the shelter essential for the survival of the adult fly. Another complication arises from the introduction of trout in the Mount

Kenya and Aberdare mountains region. The *S. neavei* complex here is at present confined to the north-east Nyambeni forest, although formerly it was wide-spread in these highlands. It would appear that, following the introduction of trout, the number of crabs has been reduced to less than the number necessary for the maintenance of the population of the insect. There are few, if any, indigenous fish in the highland rivers of East Africa and little predation of the crabs by other aquatic animals.

S. neavei is restricted to a well-defined altitudinal range which overlaps that of both *P. niloticus* and *P. leveni* (one of the up-country crabs), except where this is modified by the presence or absence of forest and, in one restricted area, by the introduction of trout. Any crab which spends the whole of its time in the water at the altitude appropriate for *S. neavei* will support it. There is thus no evidence to suggest any specific taxonomic relation between any particular crab species and *S. neavei*.

INFECTION WITH *ACANTHOCHEILONEMA STREPTOCERCA*

In parts of West Africa, and particularly in the Cameroon, infection with *Acanthocheilonema streptocerca* occurs in man. It is probable* that the adult worms live near the spinal column in the chest. The microfilariae occur in the skin and are limited to the skin of the trunk; they do not occur in the limbs or in the extremities. Infection is often symptomless but some people have a mild rash which has the same distribution and appearance as mild seborrhoea in temperate climates, i.e. on the centre of the chest and between the shoulders. The vector is *Culicoides grahami*. It bites during the day but more particularly just before sunset. The larvae and pupae of this fly occur in wet soil and humus from decaying vegetation. The bites of the vector become conspicuous in Europeans exposed either for the first time or intermittently. The bites pass unnoticed for several weeks but with what must be a sensitization to the bites of this midge, red spots begin to appear about a quarter of an inch across. The spots are rarely attributed to the midge since it is so small. It is invisible to the

* The exact site is not known, for the infection is of no clinical importance and the inconspicuous worms are very difficult to find at *post mortem* examination.

inexpert eye until it has taken its full meal. The midge is commonly called "no-see-um". After a month or more, the subject becomes desensitized and the spots cease to appear. The infection is a parasitological curiosity. It may be confused with onchocerciasis if those examining skin snips are unaware of the infection.

Since several of these filariae may overlap in their distribution multiple infections are common. A person may well have infections with *L. loa*, *A. perstans*, *A. streptocerca* and *O. volvulus* and yet appear to be none the worse for it.

FURTHER READING

Loa loa and *Alanthocheilonema perstans*

Christie, C. (1903). The distribution of sleeping sickness, *filaria perstans* etc. in East Equatorial Africa. *Repts Sleep. Sickn. Comm. Roy. Soc.* **2**, 2.

Duke, B. O. L. (1972). Behaviour aspects of the life cycle of *Loa*. "Behaviour Aspects of Parasite Transmission" (Eds E. U. Canning and C. A. Wright). Linnean Soc., Academic Press, London and New York.

Gordon, R. M., Kershaw, W. E., Crewe, W. and Oldroyd, H. (1950). The problem of loiasis in West Africa with special reference to recent investigations at Kumba in the British Cameroons and at Sapele in Southern Nigeria. *Trans. Roy. Soc. Trop. Med. Hyg.* **44**, 11.

Kershaw, W. E. (1953). Studies on the epidemiology of filariasis in West Africa with special reference to the British Cameroons and the Niger Delta. II. The influence of town and village evolution and development on the incidence of infections with *Loa loa* and *Acanthocheilonema perstans*. *Ann. Trop. Med. Parasit.* **45**, 261.

Nicholas, W. L., Kershaw, W. E., Keay, R. W. J. and Zahra, A. (1953). Studies on the epidemiology of filariasis in West Africa with special reference to the British Cameroons and the Niger Delta. III. The distribution of *Culicoides* spp. biting man in the rain forest, the forest fringe and the mountain grasslands of the British Cameroons. *Ann. Trop. Med. Parasit.* **47**, 95.

Oldroyd, H. (1957). "The Horseflies of the Ethiopian Region", Vol. III. The Trustees of the British Museum.

Bancroftian Filariasis

Kershaw, W. E. (1962). A report on a visit to the filarial endemic areas in Ceylon in 1961 (report to the Government of Ceylon through the W.H.O.). W.H.O. Regional Office for S.E. Asia. SEA/Fil/2. 9.2.62.

Kershaw, W. E. (1962). A report on filariasis in the City of Rangoon and in Burma in 1961 (report to the Government of Burma through the W.H.O.). W.H.O. Regional Office for S.E. Asia. SEA/Fil/1. 9.2.62.

Kershaw, W. E. (1975). Filariasis in children due to infection with *Wucheria bancrofti*, *W. pacifica*, *B. malayi* and related filariae. *In* "Diseases of Children in the Sub-Tropics and Tropics" (Eds D. B. Jelliffe and Dr. J. P. Stanfield), (3rd edn). Edward Arnold, London.

Onchocerciasis

Duke, B. O. L. (1971). The ecology of onchocerciasis in man and animals. *In* "Ecology and Physiology of Parasites" (Ed. A. M. Fallis), pp. 213–222. Adam Hilger, London.

Hynes, H. B. N., Williams, T. R. and Kershaw, W. E. (1961). Freshwater crabs and *Simulium naevei* in East Africa. I. Preliminary observations made on the slopes of Mount Elgon in December 1960 and January 1961. *Ann. Trop. Med. Parasit.* **55**, 197.

Hynes, H. B. N., Williams, T. R. and Kershaw, W. E. (1964). Freshwater crabs and *Simulium naevei* in East Africa. II. Further observations made during a second visit in February–April, 1962, dry season. *Ann. Trop. Med. Parasit.* **58**, 159.

Kershaw, W. E., Duke, B. O. L. and Budden, F. H. (1954). The distribution of the microfilariae of *Onchocerca volvulus* in the skin of man and its relation to the skin changes and to eye lesions and blindness. *Brit. Med. J.* **2**, 724.

Kershaw, W. E. (1958). The population dynamics of infection with *Onchocerca volvulus* in the vector, *Simulium damnosum*. Proc. 10th Int. Congr. Entomology, Canada, 1956. III, 1958. *Trans. Roy. Soc. Trop. Med. Hyg.* **51**, 4.

Kershaw, W. E., Williams, T. R., Frost, S., Matchett, R. E., Mills, M. L., and Johnson, R. D. (1968). The selective control of *Simulium* larvae by particulate insecticides and its signicance in river management. *Trans. Roy. Soc. Trop. Med. Hyg.* **62**, 35–40.

Williams, T. R. (1968). The taxonomy of the East African river-crabs and their association with the *Simulium naevei* complex. *Trans. Roy. Soc. Trop. Med. Hyg.* **62**, 29–34.

3. Malaria

A. T. A. Learmonth

INTRODUCTION

Medical geography or nosogeography—the geography of disease— is often criticized as merely descriptive. If it is merely descriptive, of course, it may still be rendering a service, not least as one channel of communication for alerting general practitioners about risks to which their patients may have been exposed during holiday and business travel, etc. (Maegraith, 1965). It may appear at first sight that this essay, devoted to aspects of the geography of malaria, is predestined to fall into the merely descriptive category, since it is almost a century since Laveran first described the malaria parasite and 1897 when Ross and Grassi established the fundamentals of the malaria cycle. The cycle and vector mosquito (*Anopheles*—more strictly an alternate host), linking man and *Plasmodium*, the protozoal parasite, are widely known among laymen. The essential link is between infected and susceptible man, though transmission of *Plasmodium* from monkeys to man is now known to occur, while birds, rodents and other animals are also known to have their own malaria cycles. Figure 3.1 is the simplest possible view of the cycle. Granting the practical usefulness of straightforward description of the geography of malaria, and the now long-established understanding of the malaria cycle, is there a further and analytical function for geography? Surely it is possible that geographical analysis may complement other approaches in elucidating problems that still remain of both academic and practical importance. This is because the malaria cycle involves complexities concealed by the first simple

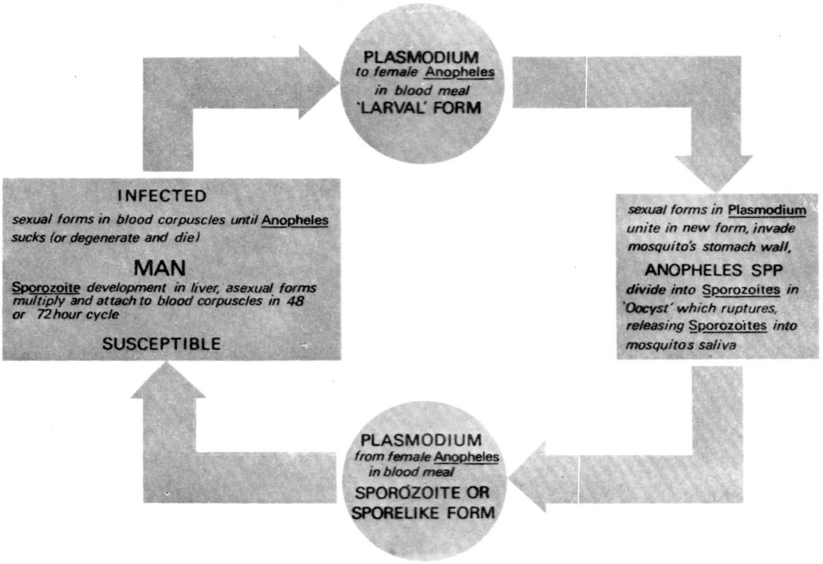

Fig. 3.1 The malaria cycle—a first diagrammatic representation.

cycle diagram (Fig. 3.1). Since malaria is a three-factor disease, a full study of it involves three ecologies (May, 1950); there are three sets of interacting relationships of each individual factor with its total environment, including of course the other two factors. A medical geography closely linked with ecological insight may give one essential approach to understanding the historical patterns of advance, retreat and persistence of the disease, of success or failure of eradication campaigns, and the areal or spatial distribution patterns of today.

A more complex flow diagram of the malaria cycle may be constructed (Fig. 3.2); but even this is a gross oversimplification of the complexities of the real world situation. There are the slightly differing ecologies and substantially differing, and changing, geographies of the several species of *Plasmodium* parasitic on man; there are the many vector species of *Anopheles*, with individual but at times rapidly evolving and changing preferences in feeding times and habits, resting places, sites for egg-laying and the like; ultimately even more difficult to represent diagrammatically, though somewhat easier to perceive, are the endless variations in the patterns of man's activities at work, at rest and at play, which may crucially affect man-mosquito contact and his risk of exposure to the malaria cycle.

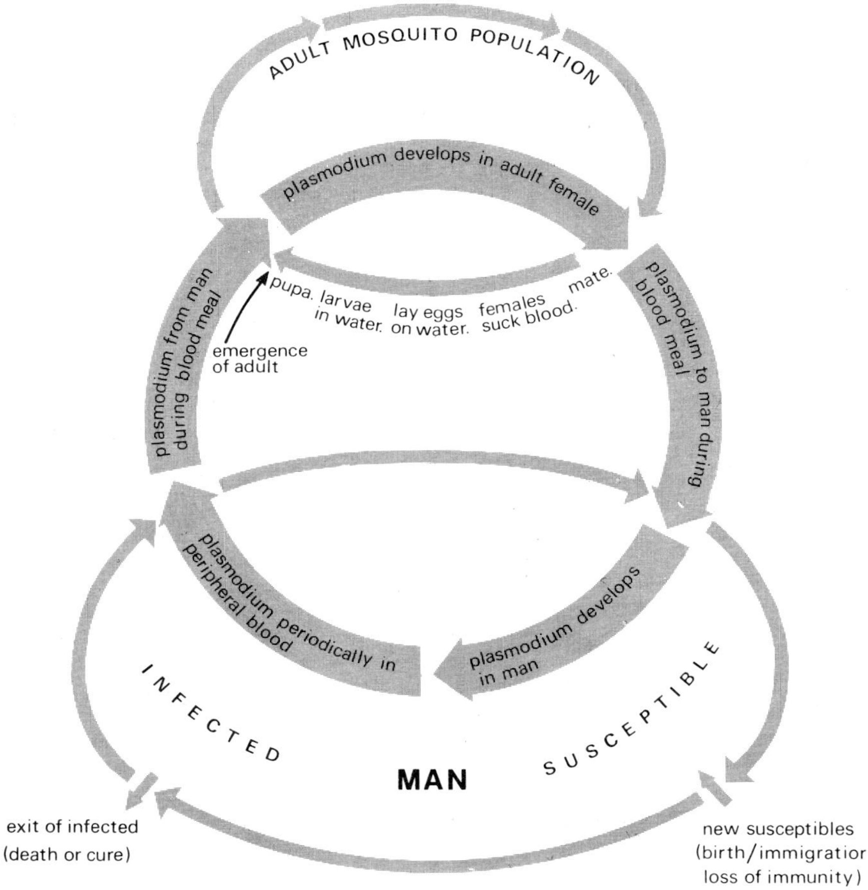

Fig. 3.2 The malaria cycle—a more complex diagram (Open University).

In this necessarily selective essay, there follow sections on the geography of species of *Plasmodium* affecting man, malaria as a community health problem, the world map of malaria in 1967, Bruce-Chwatt's regional analysis of 1970, case studies of the breaking of the malaria cycle at various points in different ecological circumstances and some conclusions.

THE CHANGING GEOGRAPHY OF SPECIES OF *PLASMODIUM* AFFECTING MAN

Figure 3.3 was compiled about 1950, before the campaigns to control

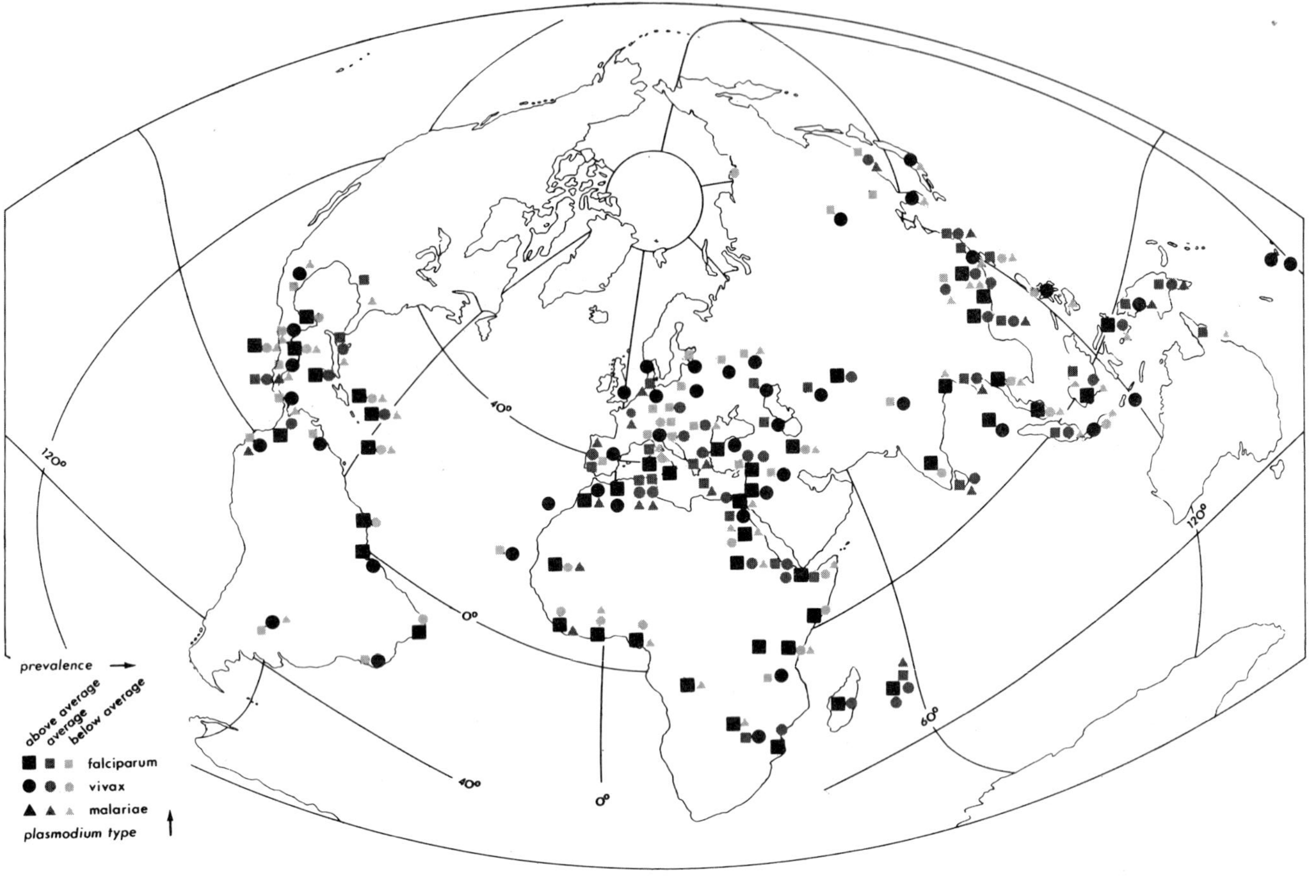

Fig. 3.3 Plasmodium species affecting man (May, 1951).

malaria had altered the distribution patterns of the main species of *Plasmodium* affecting man. It shows *Plasmodium falciparum* as the malaria parasite with widespread distribution in the tropics especially in Africa and the Americas. It causes the classical malignant tertian or sub-tertian fever.

Plasmodium vivax coexisted with *P. falciparum* over much of the tropics but with important areas of dominance, particularly in Asia. It extended into extra-tropical areas and polewards to the temperate regions. *Plasmodium malariae*, causing quartan fever, played a comparatively minor role, generally to *P. falciparum* and *P. vivax*, though it was important locally. *Plasmodium ovale*, generally causing a relatively mild and self-limiting form of tertian fever, occurred mainly in the forested lowlands of West Africa and in parts of East Africa.

The distributions shown in Fig. 3.3 have been considerably altered, mainly as a result of the differential impact of eradication programmes on the different species of *Plasmodium*. *P. vivax* has been virtually eliminated from temperate regions and from parts of Asia, notably India, so that its domain has contracted to approximate that of *P. falciparum*. There are, however, occasional recrudescences, as in India in 1976. *P. falciparum* in turn has contracted in the Americas, though it may remain important there in areas which are resistant to anti-plasmodial drug campaigns. In some areas, including temperate countries such as Rumania, *P. malariae* has tended to survive through its long life in the human host, though its disappearance along with *P. vivax* after eradication programmes is reported from U.S.S.R. Elsewhere, including parts of tropical Asia, *P. malariae* seems to have increased in both absolute and relative terms. In contrast, *P. ovale* seems to have been relatively little affected, remaining in its tropical forest environments and with a close, if possibly fortuitous, association with the areal distribution of *Anopheles melas* and *A. gambiae* form A. It has been reported from the Philippines and probably from New Guinea but the nature of the ecological links has yet to be established (W.H.O., 1968; Lysenko and Beljaev, 1969).

HISTORICAL DEVELOPMENT OF *PLASMODIUM*

The historic and pre-historic evidence concerning the origins and dispersal of *Plasmodium*, especially the species parasitic on man, have

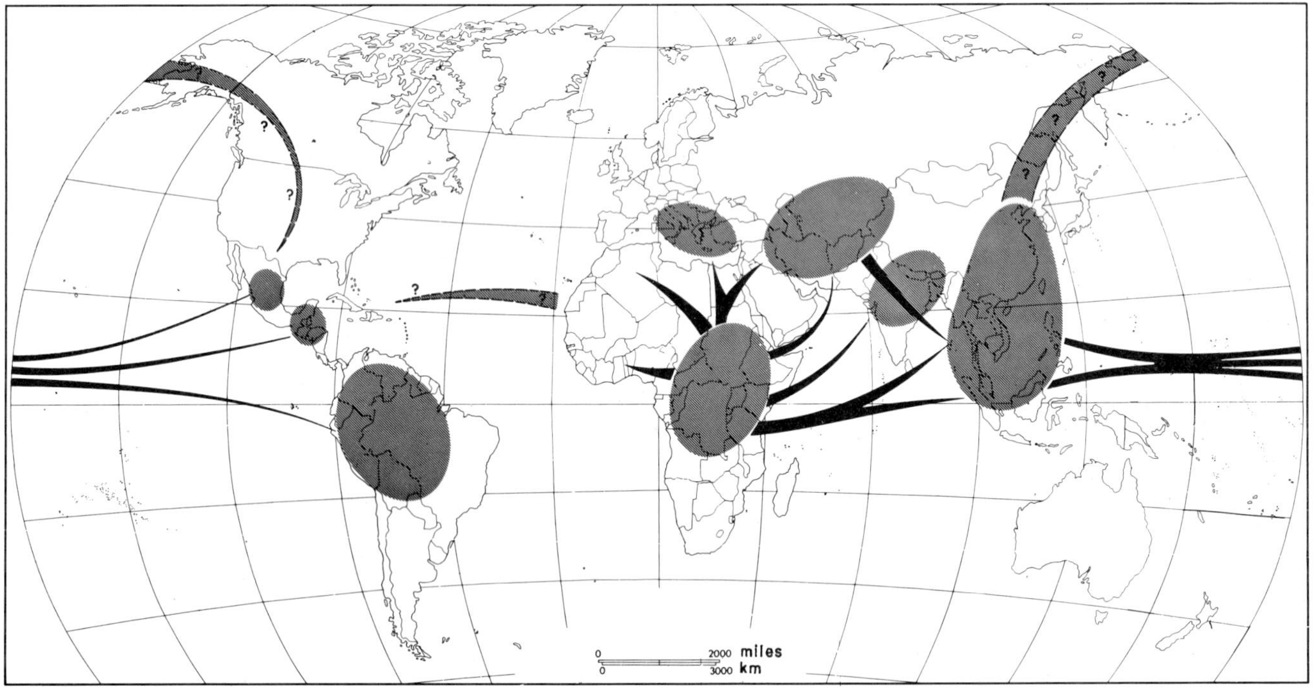

Fig. 3.4 Probable routes of spread of malaria in prehistoric and early historic times (Bruce–Chwatt, 1965).

recently been reviewed (Bruce–Chwatt, 1965). While the evidence is of necessity patchy, it seems likely that malaria originated in Africa. It maintained itself in small foci during Palaeolithic and Mesolithic times then dispersed with the agricultural revolution of Neolithic times to become established in the great riverine civilizations of the Indus valley, Mesopotamia, southern China and the Nile valley from where it reached the Mediterranean basin (Fig. 3.4). From these major foci it spread across most of the tropical world and much of the temperate world. In the Americas, the evidence is particularly difficult to interpret. Some workers support the view that there was a patchy distribution of malaria in pre–Columbian times, others say that it was one of the imports from Africa which accompanied the navigators and the slave trade. The evidence does not lend itself to linking the suggested dispersal pattern with the order of evolution of the several species of *Plasmodium* affecting man but the morphological and physiological evidence is interpreted as suggesting that *P. malariae* was evolved early to be followed by *P. vivax* and *P. ovale*. Its long life in man, suggesting a degree of commensality, might be regarded as compatible with this hypothesis.

Plasmodium falciparum is one of a small group which is comparatively less dependent than other species on the pre-erythrocytic phase of development in the mammalian host, i.e. the phase spent in the liver rather than in the blood (Shortt *et al.*, 1951). It is partly for this reason that *P. falciparum* is thought to be more recently evolved. However, *Plasmodium falciparum* may be associated with a lesser degree of pathogenicity among adults in holoendemic areas (see below) when compared with say *P. vivax*. This may be related to very close and comparatively closed interrelationships between particular communities of men, mosquitoes and *Plasmodium* during recent generations and up to the present with its rapid and widespread movement of people (in particular) over large areas of the globe.

MALARIA AS A COMMUNITY HEALTH PROBLEM

Malaria is a disease in which the blood and tissues of man are invaded by certain species of *Plasmodium*. The vector species of *Anopheles*, i.e. the adult females, are true alternate hosts. Both *Anopheles* and man are essential for particular stages of development of *Plasmodium*. At the same time blood-sucking is essential for ovulation in the fertilized female *Anopheles*. Other animals such as monkeys and birds have their own particular *Plasmodia* and malarial cycles. Simian malaria has been reported under natural conditions, as distinct from laboratory conditions, as being transmitted to man. It must now be regarded as possible, though so far unlikely, that malaria is really a zoonosis similar to plague or yellow fever rather than a purely human disease with several species of the pathogen (Bruce–Chwatt, 1968; Coatney, 1968).

THE GEOGRAPHY OF *ANOPHELES*

Apart from the cold deserts and much of the hot deserts, anopheline mosquitoes have a widespread distribution throughout the world. Their efficiency as vectors varies in the different species, but malaria as such has the potential of being almost a world-wide disease. Indeed it approached this status some 30 years ago. Paradoxically, however, malaria is also a local disease. Over considerable periods of time, it may depend on the maintenance of the malaria cycle between local communities of man, local populations of *Anopheles* and local strains of one or more of the species of *Plasmodium* parasitic on man. Many vector species are normally found overwhelmingly within a short flight range of those water bodies used by the gravid females for egg-laying. This flight range may be no more than 1–2 km, though recent records have shown that some strongly flying species or wind-blown *Anopheles* may reach distances of 10 or more km.

Such comparatively local relationships may be both close and almost closed. Moreover they may be perennial, as in equatorial rainforest conditions, or seasonal as in tropical summer rainfall or Mediterranean winter rainfall regions. Elsewhere they may be only occasional years in which transmission is possible or at least significant as a public health problem, i.e. in particularly wet years along the margins of the hot deserts, or sometimes in dry years in hot-wet areas as in Sri Lanka in 1935. Given a reservoir of infection the perennial transmission is likely to equate with endemic malaria. Tropical summer rainfall areas tend to have seasonal epidemics during and after the rains, winter rainfall areas have autumn and spring epidemics and areas with the odd favourable year for transmission have occasional though usually more catastrophic epidemics. Given the development of even partial individual immunity as a norm, including some though fairly short-lived congenital immunity in endemic areas, highly endemic areas are likely to include communities with comparatively high community immunity in adults. This immunity consists quite commonly of lesser degree of illness and lower mortality rates among adults and, in theory, might even reach perfect host-parasite adjustment. There is, however, some variation according to species of *Plasmodium; falciparum* seems to be associated with higher pathogenicity in general.

In contrast the areas of seasonal epidemics tend to have intermediate conditions. The areas subject to occasional years of catastrophic epidemics tend to have low immunity. They experience many severe illnesses and high mortality among all age groups of the population, but with a tendency to some concentration among the young and old. The economic and demographic effects of this epidemic incidence contrast with the high pathogenicity and mortality in highly endemic areas among older infants and children and, to a lesser extent in old people. Adults, as already noted, tend to suffer less illness and have lower death rates.

ENDEMICITY

W.H.O. have classified degrees of endemicity along the following lines, where the crude and equivocal spleen index is the best indicator for which data are available:

1. *Hypo-endemic:* childhood spleen-rate below 10% (children of 2–10 years)
2. *Meso-endemic:* childhood spleen-rate 10–24%
3. *Highly endemic:* childhood spleen-rate 25–49%
4. *Hyper-endemic:* childhood spleen-rate 50–74%
5. *Holo-endemic:* childhood spleen-rate 75% and over, associated with *high* adult spleen-rate
6. *Hyper-endemic:* childhood spleen-rate 75% and over, associated with almost complete freedom from adult sickness and low adult spleen-rates where the cycle has been maintained over long periods.

MACROGEOGRAPHY OF MALARIA

Malaria is, in some respects, a local disease. It is a consequence of local combinations of variables: several species of *Plasmodium* are concerned, scores of vector species of *Anopheles* with distinctive ecological preferences are involved with some tendency to change in habits, while man devises almost infinite variations in detail in his mode of life, patterns of activity and settlement forms, etc. A lifetime may thus be spent studying the microgeography of malaria without reaching an end. Even so there is a macrogeography within which medium and small areas of study may be fitted. One way of seeking some understanding of this macrogeography, on either a continental or world scale, is by means of a model or schematic map of a hypothetical malarial continent. The utility of the model approach is that the inquiry may begin with certain very broad simplifying assumptions. The model is then modified to remove these assumptions and, at the same time, varied to demonstrate the impact of particular variables. This use of a model is for teaching and demonstration purposes; it is not a research tool.

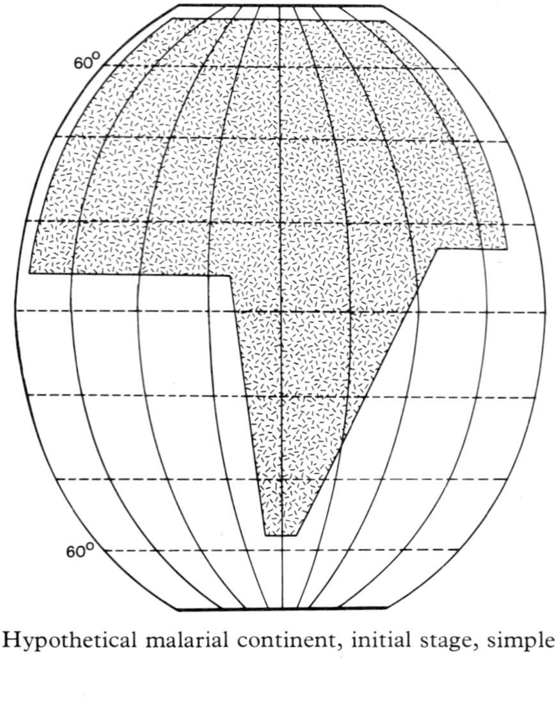

Fig. 3.5.1 Hypothetical malarial continent, initial stage, simple and massive.

Fig. 3.5.1 assumes a simple, massive continent. It stretches from about latitude 75°N to latitude 55°S and is a very rough generalization of the broad northern-hemisphere landmasses extending in relatively peninsular form towards or into the southern hemisphere. Temperature and rain-belts are assumed much as in the real world and will be discussed below in relation to malaria. At this stage only low to undulating relief is assumed together with a variety of water-bodies and hydrological conditions on land, e.g. still water, running water subject to spates, brackish water, etc. The latter represent the range of egg-laying conditions preferred by gravid female *Anopheles*. A uniform distribution of human population and of *Plasmodium* are assumed, both of a density sufficient for the malaria cycle to be effectively maintained as a public health problem. Finally the initial assumptions within the model include general economic underdevelopment, so that the malaria cycle is not inhibited, directly or indirectly, by man's technology.

The main climatic zones of the hypothetical continent are set out boldly in Fig. 3.5.2 very much as they appear in textbooks of climatology. Moving from the arctic circles towards the equator the

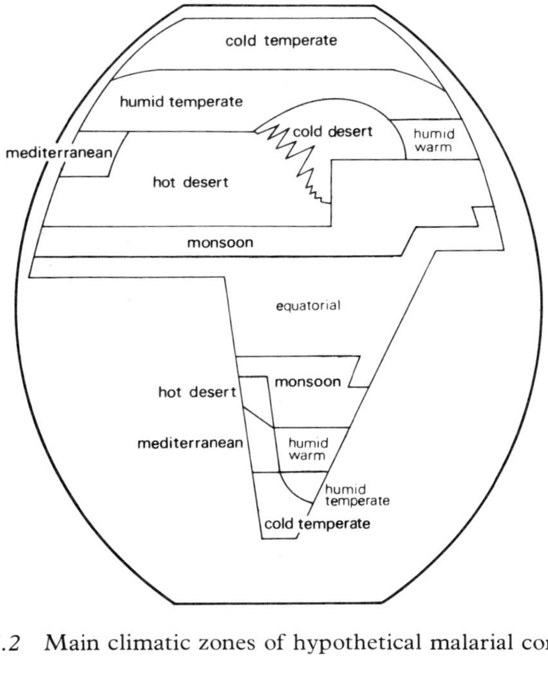

Fig. 3.5.2 Main climatic zones of hypothetical malarial continent.

climate sequence is polar, cold temperate, cold desert, warm humid temperate, mediterranean, hot desert, tropical summer rainfall and, finally, the equatorial hot, perennially wet zone. The influence of these climates on anopheline breeding are tabulated in Fig. 3.5.3

			winter	summer
1	cold temperate	temperature	O	O
		water	w	w
2	humid temperate	temperature	O	T
		water	w	w
3	cold desert	temperature	O	T
		water	o	o
4	mediterranean	temperature	T	T
		water	w	o
5	hot desert	temperature	T	T
		water	o	o
6	monsoon	temperature	T	T
		water	o	w
7	humid warm	temperature	T	T
		water	w	w
8	equatorial	temperature	T	T
		water	w	w

Fig. 3.5.3 Influence of warm and coldest months and of rainfall conditions on Anopheline activity in each climatic zone.

taking for purposes of simplicity only the temperature and rainfall conditions of the warmest and coolest months. As a very crude generalization anopheline breeding and activity generally may be related to temperatures above 16°C while average relative humidity of about 60% will provide conditions congenial to the mosquitoes for large parts of the day. Temperatures in excess of about 35°C and average relative humidities less than 25% mean that large parts of most days will prove uncongenial to *Anopheles*; they will tend to die off or aestivate. (These generalizations are presented as model-building assumptions, not as being in any way definitive.) Rainfall amounts may not be directly related to anopheline activities but a rainy season of three of more months is taken as being likely to provide some of the infinite variety of water bodies used by the different species of *Anopheles*. Fig. 3.5.4 links these tabulated effects on *Anopheles* back to the climatic zones of Fig. 3.5.2, which are now represented in relation to malarial conditions. As already suggested epidemic zones will have severe morbidity and mortality in all age

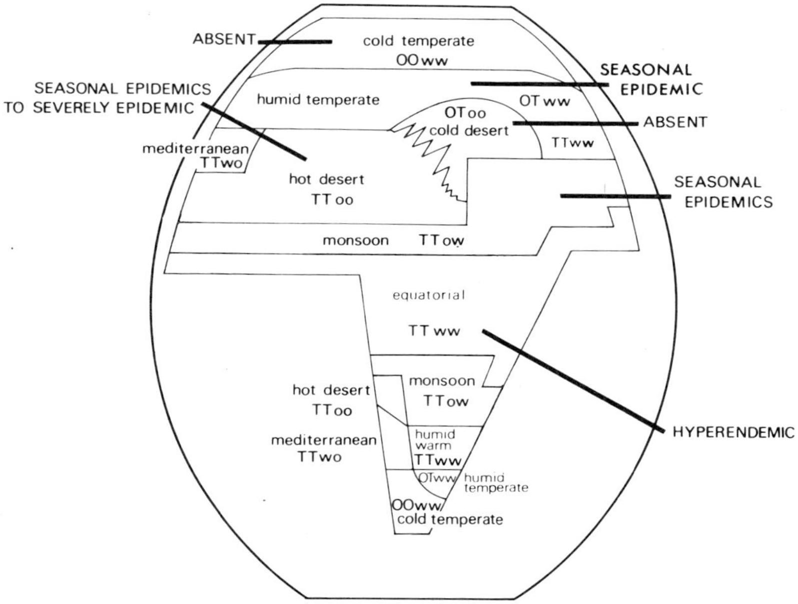

Fig. 3.5.4 Malarial conditions in the climatic zones.

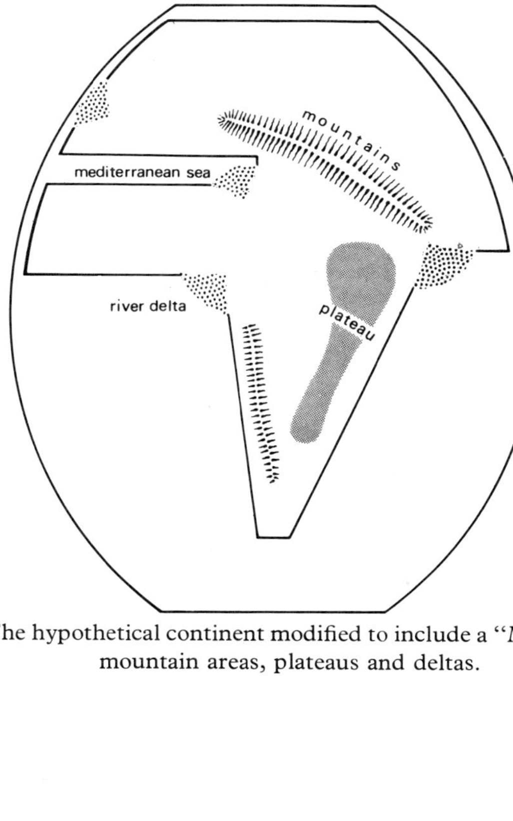

Fig. 3.5.5 The hypothetical continent modified to include a "Mediterranean" sea, mountain areas, plateaus and deltas.

groups, though with a tendency to concentrate among children and the aged. During epidemic seasons there will be a temporary increase in abortions, a reduction in conceptions and a consequential reduction in birth rates. Birth rates will recover between epidemics, probably quite rapidly, while community immunity will fall. In contrast will be the high child morbidity and mortality of hyper-endemic zones, with high immunity among adults, high abortion rates and low birth rates.

The hypothetical continent is modified in Fig. 3.5.5 to bring it nearer to real-world conditions. (This type of manipulation of the theoretical model—for pedagogic purposes rather than research—is one justification for its use.) A "mediterranean-type sea", mountain arcs of Alpine-Himalayan type, plateau blocks as in East Africa, and deltas analogous to those of the Rhine, Nile, Niger, Ganga–Brahmaputra and Mekong are inserted. Fig. 3.5.6 is a further elaboration of the model with perennial malaria extended into warm or hot climate deltas and the cold deserts of the high ridges represented as being free of malaria.

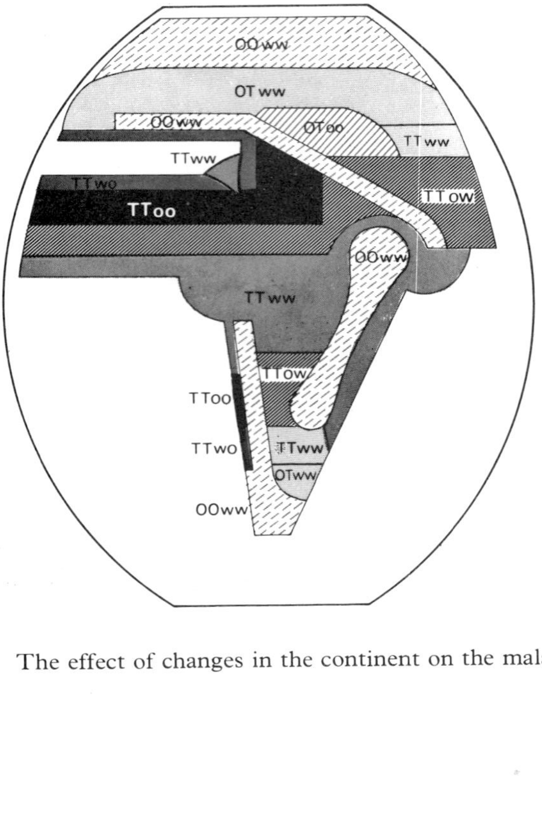

Fig. 3.5.6 The effect of changes in the continent on the malaria zones.

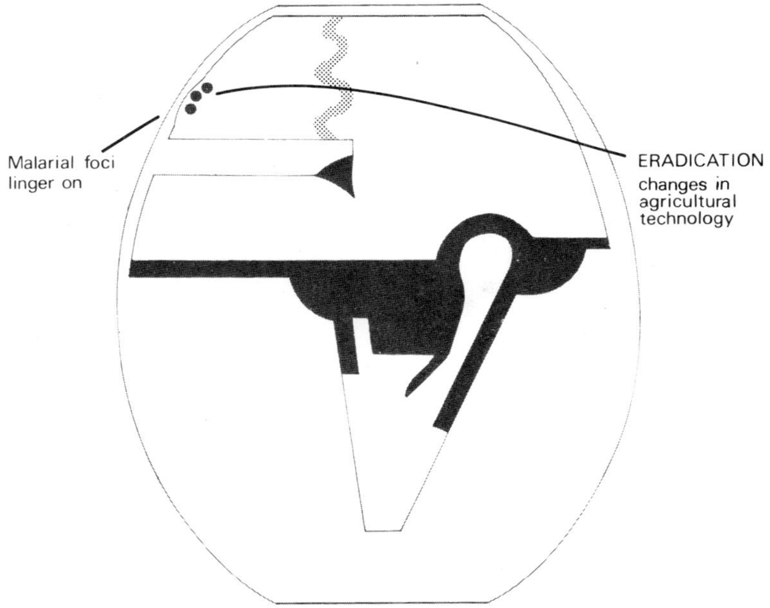

Fig. 3.5.7 Malaria eradicated in temperate zones by changes in agricultural technology, etc.

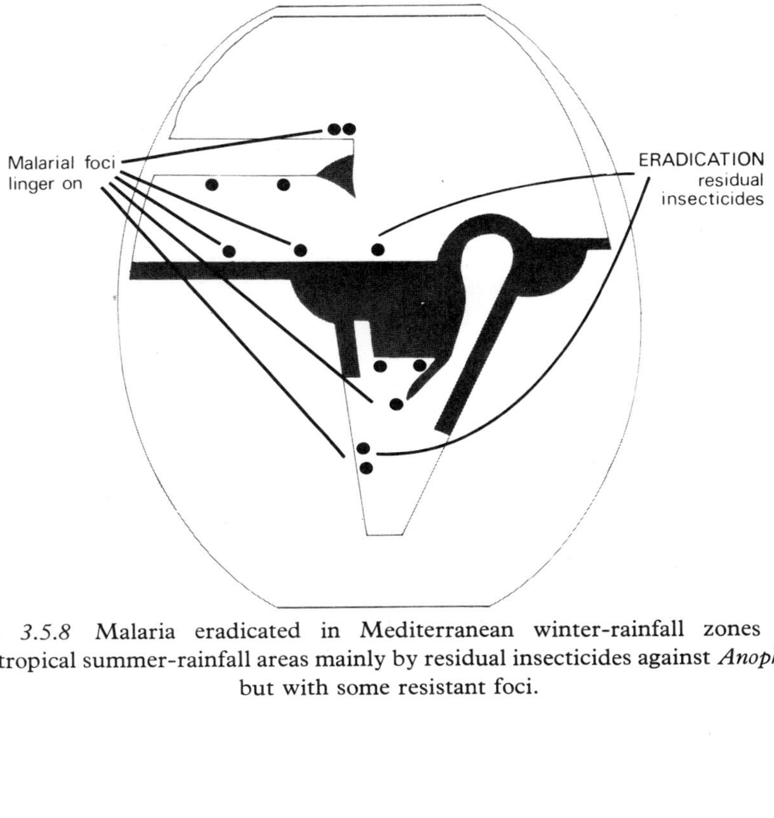

Fig. 3.5.8 Malaria eradicated in Mediterranean winter-rainfall zones and subtropical summer-rainfall areas mainly by residual insecticides against *Anopheles* but with some resistant foci.

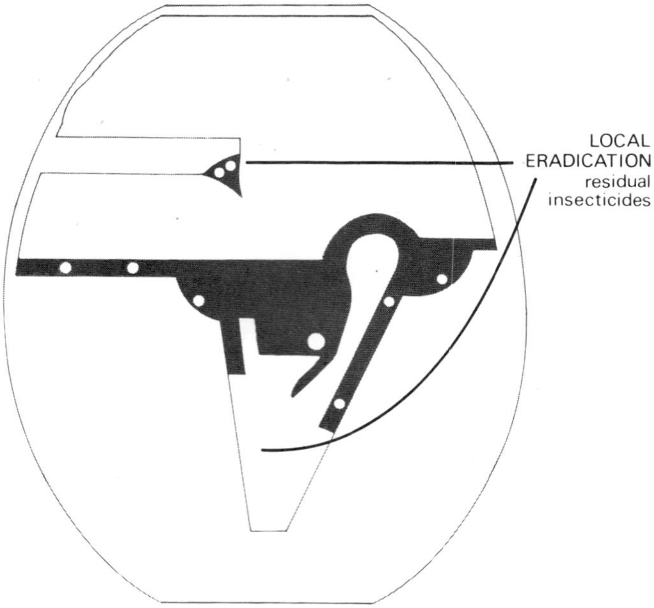

Fig. 3.5.9 Malaria resistant in main zone of perennial malaria, but with eradication in local areas.

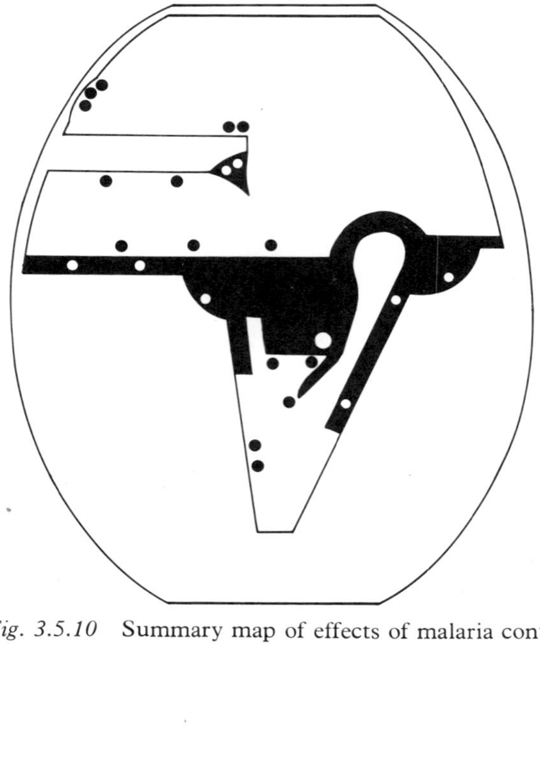

Fig. 3.5.10 Summary map of effects of malaria control.

Figs 3.5.7 to 3.5.10 represent manipulations of the model to show the impact of malaria eradication in different zones. Fig. 3.5.7 shows a temperate zone as largely cleared of malaria through changes in agricultural technology, better housing, etc. though retaining some resistent foci in deltaic areas. This sequence of eradication occurred in parts of western Europe as noted later. Figure 3.5.8 represents deliberate malaria eradication, mainly through the use of residual insecticides against adult *Anopheles*, though anti-larval measures, prophylactic and curative drugs may be assumed to have played a part in response to local variations in man-mosquito-*Plasmodium* relationships. Local areas resistant to eradication campaigns occur. Figure 3.5.9 represents the contrasted picture in the hyper-endemic areas of perennial malaria. Here only local areas have been cleared of malaria with large tracts proving too difficult for eradication campaigns. Reasons for this would include the low use of houses compared with forest sites as anopheline resting places, and the advance of "wilder" species or strains of *Anopheles* if a house-haunting species is eliminated. Figure 3.5.10 summarizes the eradication situation in the hypothetical continent.

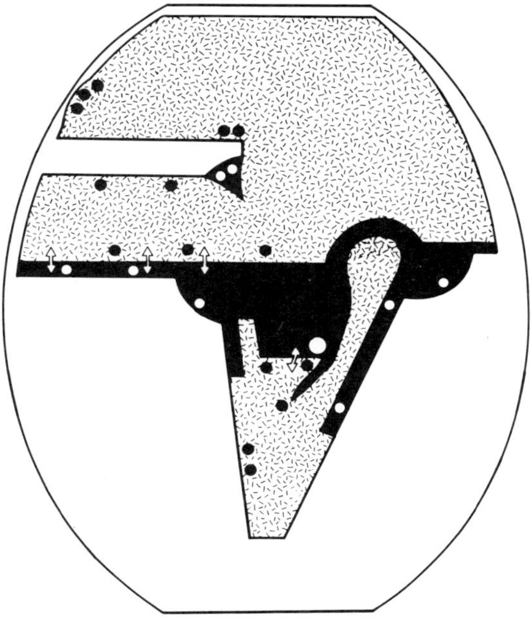

Fig. 3.5.11 Effects on malaria control of human migration across border between controlled and uncontrolled areas.

Two further manipulations of the model remain. Figure 3.5.11 is a reminder of the way that eradication campaigns may be disrupted by human migrations across the border between controlled and

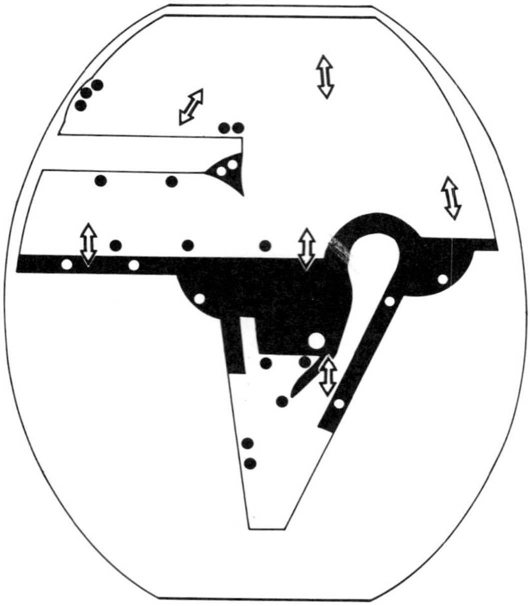

Fig. 3.5.12 Effects on malaria control of shift of climatic belts.

uncontrolled areas (Prothero, 1965). Figure 3.5.12 returns to the interplay between physiogeographic and biogeographical variables. It sketches the impact on malarial zones of shifts of the major climatic belts like the southward movement of the Saharan climate responsible for widespread drought in 1975, or the drought that brought dry-zone malaria vectors in force to the wet-zone of Sri Lanka (Ceylon) in the catastrophic epidemic of 1935. The advance of wetter climates northward can bring major regional epidemics, like that of Punjab in 1912.

The model having been used to present generalizations and manipulated to demonstrate the removal of simplifying assumptions, it is opportune to consider the W.H.O. world map of malaria for 1972 on the progress of malaria eradication in the main malaria regions of the world made by a leading malariologist (Bruce–Chwatt, 1970).

WORLD GEOGRAPHY OF MALARIA, 1972

The white areas of the map between the "past limits" line and the grey or black areas (Fig. 3.6) represent the very large areas of mainly seasonal but locally severe malaria from which the malaria cycle has retreated. In some areas, like much of western Europe, malaria retreated without specific campaigns against it. Instead the retreat came as a result of improvement in agricultural technology, housing and general standards of hygiene. Incidentally rather than advisedly, they broke the malaria cycle. In England, for instance, the main malaria vectors were *Anopheles messeae*, breeding in lowland rivers and freshwater swamps and *A. atroparvus* breeding in brackish water swamps; these included parts of coastal saltmarshes like those of the Thames estuary. The separation of cattlesheds from houses—the vectors being zoophilic—and the general improvement in house construction and surroundings were sufficient to break the malaria cycle, though with occasional recrudescence (Hackett, 1949; Smith, 1956; Shute, 1963). Elsewhere, however, the white areas on the map represent areas freed from malaria by carefully mounted campaigns during the last 30 years or so. These campaigns mainly involved some use of the so-called residual (long-lasting) insecticides such as DDT. The main attack has been directed against the adult mosquito, though anti-larval measures against water-bodies used for breeding and also therapeutic and prophylactic drugs have also played a part.

The grey areas of Fig. 3.6 show tracts—made up of countries or groups of countries—which have been virtually freed from malaria as a result of eradication programmes. They are in the final stages (called "consolidation") before the ceasing of the campaign, i.e. apart from surveillance measures to guard against the return of the active malaria cycle on a scale sufficient to constitute a public health problem. The black areas of Fig. 3.6 represent the areas from which the malaria cycle has not yet been removed. Some combination of circumstances, biological, economic and/or technological, has so far prevented the undertaking of eradication campaigns or their successful completion.

It is possible to generalize from an examination of such a small-scale map of the world (Fig. 3.6). The white and grey areas are generally towards the margin of the former extent of the world malaria belt, and towards the margins lie those where changes in

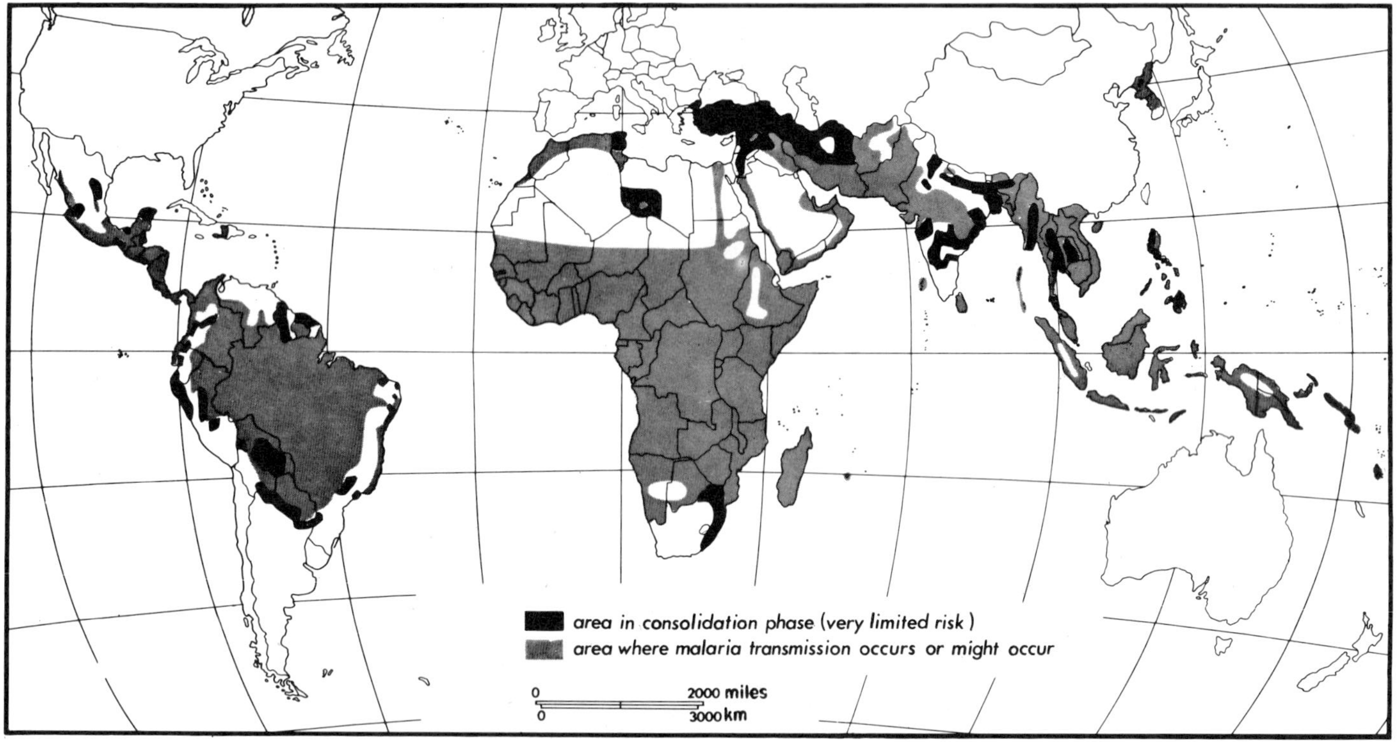

Fig. 3.6 Epidemiological assessment of world status of malaria, 1972 (W.H.O., 1974).

(Source: W.H.O. 16A5 Report on Malaria. Geneva, 1974.)

agricultural technique and such like (as noted for England) were crucial. Elsewhere the malaria was generally seasonal, since *Anopheles* vector species tended to be house-haunting for at least part of the year. This would be in the less congenial season for mosquitoes either when it was a hot dry summer stimulating aestivation or during a very cool or cold winter prompting hibernation. Since the vectors were house-haunting, residual insecticides campaigns against the adult mosquitoes were the more likely to be successful. The black areas, in contrast, are generally in the constantly wet and warm rainforest areas; there the norm is towards hyper-endemic or holo-endemic conditions (even super-endemic in little-disturbed tribal areas) and towards dominance of much less house-haunting species of *Anopheles*. The vector species tend to have resting places and aestivation sites scattered through jungles and forests and so are difficult to attack with residual insecticides, either against adults or against larvae, in their innumerable breeding places. Even if house-haunting species or strains are eradicated, their ecological niche tends to be reoccupied by an invading forest mosquito, which is often as efficient a vector as the supplanted species.

RESULTS OF MALARIA ERADICATION THROUGH THE ATTACK ON THE VECTOR

The following regional account by Prof. L. J. Bruce–Chwatt (1970) is reproduced by kind permission of The Entomological Society of America.

The results of the various malaria-eradication programmes in relation to the main vectors can be given in the broadest lines for the 12 epidemiological zones of the world according to the classification of Macdonald (1957) and Russell *et al.* (1963) (Fig. 3.7). The area extending from the countries on the western shore of the Pacific eastward to the New Hebrides (with the exclusion of Australia and islands of Indonesia) has been divided by Colbourne (1962a) into seven zones with very distinct characteristics. In the present review this large area falls within four epidemiological zones.

In the "Eurasian Northern Zone" malaria eradication has been achieved within 10 years after the start of the respective country programmes. *A.*

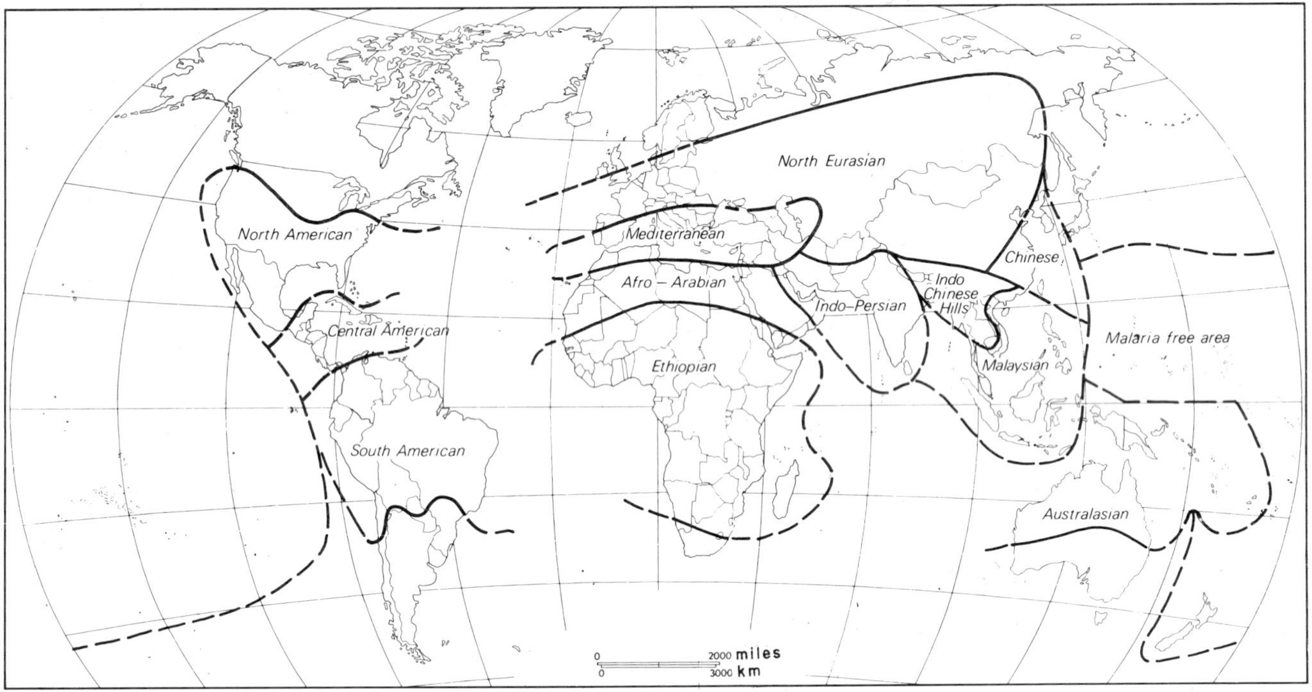

Fig. 3.7 Epidemiological malaria zones of the world (Bruce-Chwatt, 1970).

atroparvus Van Thiel and *A. messeae* Falleroni are the main vectors in this zone. They have easily responded to control measures by residual insecticides, mainly DDT; over most of this zone combined antimalaria methods were used extensively. In this large zone, anopheline species of the *maculipennis* group have maintained normal or slightly decreased susceptibility to DDT in spite of several years of residual spraying. An increased irritability to this insecticide did not interfere with the success of spraying operations. The outstanding early achievements of malaria eradication in the U.S.S.R. has been outlined (Bruce–Chwatt, 1959), but fuller information will be found in Sergiev *et al.* (1961) and Sergeiv (1968). In North China, malaria in the hills was carried by *A. pattoni* Christophers, while *A. sacharovi* Favre was the vector in the high plateau of the northwest; in the plains of North China as in the south, *A. sinensis* Weidemann was the main vector.

The "Chinese Zone" of the continent of Asia includes the coastal and southeast part of mainland China, Korea and the southern islands of Japan: the main vector in the plains is *A. sinensis*. In the foothills of South China *A. minimus* Theobald is an important vector, with *A. jeyporiensis candidiensis* Koizumi as a subsidiary. Little is known about malaria eradication in mainland China or North Korea, which are not included in the annual reports of the W.H.O. although it is believed that mosquito control by orthodox methods has greatly decreased the incidence of malaria. In South Korea, the eradication programme shows much progress. In Japan and the Ryukyu Islands, malaria has been eradicated, although DDT resistance in *A. sinensis* was reported in 1967 from Okinawa.

In the "Mediterranean Zone", where malaria eradication showed early and spectacular successes, the range of *A. atroparvus* extended over the whole coastal area of southwest Europe; *A. sacharovi* was the main vector of the southeastern coast, while *A. labranchiae* Falleroni extended over the western part of the North African shore and shared the central part of the Mediterranean Zone with *A. sacharovi*.

In Spain, Portugal, southern France, Romania, Yugoslavia and Italy, malaria eradication has been completed without any major obstacles. The relationship between resistance and irritability of *Anopheles*, their ecological zones and epidemiology of malaria, was particularly well studied in Italy (Mariani, 1956; Raffaele and Coluzzi, 1957; Coluzzi, 1965).

In Romania, *A. atroparvus*, *A. messeae* and *A. maculipennis* Meigen have shown a degree of resistance to dieldrin-benzene hexachloride (HCH) within four years after spraying, and by 1965 this resistance was found over the whole territory. It is likely that this was due to the widespread use of various insecticides in agriculture. There was a slow and small rise of tolerance to DDT but without any adverse effect on the programme. No resistance of *A. sacharovi* to dieldrin or DDT was observed, and since 1962 this mosquito has been almost completely absent from the coastal areas of the country (Lupasco and Duport 1968).

In Greece, *A. sacharovi* and *A. superpictus* Grassi were the main vectors of malaria. The zoophilic members of *A. maculipennis* complex were of little importance. The malaria-control campaign that began in 1946 had an immediate impact on the two main vectors. The cessation of DDT spraying in Crete and the Peloponnesus created the conditions of "anophelism without malaria" and paved the way to malaria eradication. The subsequent DDT resistance of *A. sacharovi* observed in 1951 had little influence on the outcome of the campaign. Even when dual resistance to insecticides was recognized in Greece in 1953, it was possible to cope with the operational problems by alternating insecticides, since resistance to DDT was not of a high order. In the southern provinces of Turkey, DDT resistance of *A. sacharovi* was recorded in 1959, and the use of dieldrin was indicated. Over the rest of the country DDT continued to be of value. However, in two localities in the consolidation phase of the programme double resistance of this species was found in 1967. There are areas of Turkey and Yugoslavia with foci of transmission ascribed to outdoor biting and exophily of *A. superpictus*; in a few localities of Turkey, the same phenomenon was reported in *A. claviger* (Meigen), a secondary vector.

In Lebanon and Israel, malaria eradication has been virtually accomplished. In Israel, a progressive disappearance of *A. sacharovi* was observed, leaving *A. sergentii* (Theobald) and perhaps *A. claviger*, as secondary vectors in some localities.

In Algeria and Morocco, full-scale malaria-eradication programmes have not yet started because of operational and other reasons, but there is little doubt that when properly carried out they will be successful. The fact that in Morocco *A. labranchiae* was found to be resistant to dieldrin in 1959 excludes the use of this insecticide. The malaria-eradication programme in Tunisia offers excellent prospects, as this country is at the periphery of the eastward distribution of *A. labranchiae*.

The "Afro-Arabian Desert Zone" shares the mosquitoes of three zoogeographical regions, and it is evident that the malaria-eradication programmes were more successful where palaearctic *Anopheles* were the main vectors. In Jordan, *A. sergentii* was responsible for some local transmission, but this did not interfere with the satisfactory progress of eradication, since the main vector was *A. sacharovi*. Recently in one isolated area of Jordan, *A. sergentii*, already known to be dieldrin-resistant since 1958, showed resistance also to DDT, and larvicidal methods were introduced.

In Egypt, a considerable degree of malaria control has been achieved; *A.*

pharoensis was found resistant to dieldrin in 1959, and more recently it has been found resistant to DDT in some areas of Egypt and in the Sudan; this resistance may be a technical obstacle to malaria eradication. Localized malarious areas (oases), where seasonal outbreaks are related to the presence of *A. sergentii*, *A. multicolor* Cambouliu, *A. hispaniola* (Theobald), and perhaps *A. dthali*, should not present any major problems. The presence of *A. gambiae* on the southern border of this zone should be watched carefully, especially as dieldrin/HCH resistance of this species has been reported from the Sudan.

In Saudi Arabia, malaria-control activities were affected in 1953 by the discovery of DDT resistance in *A. stephensi* Liston, five years after the start of the campaign. A change to dieldrin improved the situation, but in 1962 this species was found to be resistant to dieldrin in the oasis of Qatif, and further observations confirmed the double resistance of *A. stephensi* on both shores of the Persian Gulf. The operational importance of this finding is obvious, although alternative insecticides, such as malathion, are still of considerable value and are extensively used. The appearance of *A. stephensi* on the western shore of the Red Sea (Gad, 1967) is viewed with concern, and it is hoped that this invasion of the African continent by the Asian mosquito will be of transient character. This species showed double resistance in Saudi Arabia in 1967. DDT resistance in *A. fluviatilis* has been reported also from that country, where malaria eradication has not yet started. Saudi Arabia seems to be the source of imported malaria in Jordan.

The "Ethiopian Zone" covers the whole of sub-Saharan Africa and represents the greatest challenge to malaria eradication. The programme in South Africa and Swaziland, where *A. gambiae* and *A. funestus* Giles are the main vectors, are well advanced, and the prevalence of malaria is very low. Mauritius is now at the end of its most successful eradication programme; *A. funestus* has almost disappeared within two years following DDT spraying that started in 1949, and the density of *A. gambiae* showed a striking decrease. The annual number of cases of malaria on the island is less than 10, and most of them are imported. *A. gambiae* exhibits zoophilic trends in both Mauritius and South Africa, and its contact with man is tenuous.

In the three pilot projects on the mainland of Africa (Liberia, South Cameroon, Uganda) situated either in the forest area or in the highlands, the transmission of malaria has been interrupted. In these projects, *A. funestus* has virtually disappeared and *A. gambiae* showed a spectacular decrease. In the South Cameroon project, *A. moucheti* and *A. nili* (Theobald) have followed this trend; after the termination of these pilot projects *A. gambiae* density returned to its previous levels. and this return was followed by a resurgence of malaria, though no spectacular epidemic was observed.

In the remaining 20 pilot projects in tropical Africa carried out during the past 15 years and extending from Senegal in the north to Rhodesia in the south, interruption of transmission has not been achieved, though in most of them there was a considerable degree of control. Four of these projects deserve separate mention. In Zanzibar (Tanzania), the eradication programme based on the use of DDT resulted, after 10 years, in a striking reduction of malaria, but the persistent low-level transmission has been attributed to incomplete coverage, because of a large number of temporary shelters, and to the mobility of the human population. The irritant effect of DDT on the partially exophilic *A. gambiae* species B may also have played a part in this situation.

In northern Nigeria, a large-scale project in western Sokoto has been operating since 1954. Use of dieldrin was followed by a rapid emergence of highly resistant strains of *A. gambiae* species A and B in 1956; the subsequent use of DDT produced a good measure of control over several years, but not an interruption of transmission. The same was true in a more recent smaller project in northern Nigeria, in which insecticides and drugs were used (Foll *et al.*, 1965; Foll and Pant, 1966).

In the Taveta–Pare project in Tanzania, dieldrin resistance in *A. gambiae* species A and B has not appeared after six years of its use; the impact of the insecticide spraying on the amount of malaria was considerable. *A. funestus* was eliminated and failed to re-establish itself three years after the cessation of spraying, while *A. gambiae* slowly returned to its previous density but appears to have undergone some selection toward greater exophily. The first significant increase of cases following the termination of the project was observed after one year, but two years later the degree of transmission was still lower than before the start of the programme (Pringle, 1969).

Problems related specifically to malaria control and eradication by residual insecticides in tropical Africa have been outlined before (Bruce–Chwatt, 1954; W.H.O., 1962). Hamon *et al.* (1963), who reviewed the projects of malaria eradication in Africa, ascribe the failure of most of the projects to entomological factors: (a) resistance of *A. gambiae* to insecticides and particularly to the dieldrin/HCH group, (b) irritant effect of DDT, and (c) zoophilic and exophilic behaviour pattern of some populations of *A. gambiae*. Other factors such as imperfect coverage, duration of residual effect on mud walls and operational difficulties (e.g. population movements) play at least an equally important part.

No evidence of DDT resistance was found in *A. gambiae* s.l. before 1966, although isolated reports from northern Nigeria, Somalia and the Ivory Coast indicated a lower degree of susceptibility in some field trials. Recent reports of DDT resistance in species A and B from Upper Volta, Togo and Senegal in populations already resistant to dieldrin are now causing some concern. Resistance of *A. funestus* to dieldrin was reported in 1967 from

Ghana, Nigeria and Upper Volta; the same finding in *A. nili* was signaled from Ghana.

In the "Indo-Iranian Zone", good results have been achieved within a few years in Afghanistan and in northern Iraq and Iran, where *A. sacharovi* and *A. superpictus* are the main vectors of endemic malaria. However, in the southern parts of those countries where *A. stephensi* exists far inland from the coast, the malaria-eradication programme has encountered a major obstacle in the form of resistance of *A. stephensi*, first to DDT (1957) then to dieldrin/HCH (1959). In parts of this zone (especially in Iraq) more complete coverage with DDT spraying had a temporary effect but led to a higher degree of resistance; elsewhere malathion, propoxur and larvicidal treatment improved the situation.

However, one must not underrate the seriousness of the situation in this area where double resistance of *A. stephensi* has been confirmed (Zulueta *et al.*, 1968). The fact that all the "strains" of this species from India, Iran and Iraq are interfertile suggests the absence of an *A. stephensi* species complex.

The double resistance of *A. stephensi* has recently spread into Saudi Arabia, Iran, Iraq and to southern Pakistan, and the presence of this vector in the urban area of Karachi has created a difficult problem (U.S.P.H.S., 1968). The role played by *A. stephensi* in urban malaria is not new; it was investigated 40 years ago by Covell (1928) in Bombay, Calcutta, Bangalore and recently recorded in Gujerat State.

The tremendous malaria-eradication programme of India has been very successful, as in 1968 well over half the population of this country of more than 500 million was in areas in the maintenance phase and 150 million in the consolidation phase. Some difficulties have recently slowed the hitherto impressive progress of this campaign. The DDT resistance of *A. culicifacies* Giles first reported in 1960 from Baroda, has now spread to several Indian states and parts of Pakistan. Nevertheless, this does not seem to constitute a major problem, and renewal of transmission in some localities in the attack phase is probably due to incomplete insecticidal coverage. Perhaps more significant are a few limited urban areas of transmission owing to the DDT-resistant *A. stephensi*; this species has shown double resistance in Madras and in a few other areas.

There are small areas of DDT resistance in *A. fluviatilis* James in hill forest areas of Maharashtra and Mysore. Resistance to this insecticide was reported also in 1966 in *A. annularis* Van der Wulp, in Bangladesh (Rangpur) and in Baroda, where this species is of limited importance as a vector. Although in some parts of India foci of transmission have spread to previously cleared areas, those reverses are not due to entomological causes but rather to operational difficulties.

The recent widespread epidemic of vivax malaria in Ceylon is a serious setback to the impressive malaria eradication programme on this island, inhabited by 12 million people, where malaria eradication started in 1948 and where in 1966 only 308 cases of malaria were reported. Although some decrease of susceptibility to DDT of *A. culicifacies* was observed in 1964, there was no evidence of a wide-spread insecticide resistance of this species in Sri Lanka. The reasons for the present outbreak are complex, and are due to shortcomings of surveillance activity, unusual climatic conditions, unexpected population movements and perhaps importation of cases.

As pointed out by Hamon and Garret–Jones (1963), the fact that DDT resistance in *A. culicifacies* has only limited effect on the trend of transmission is rather unusual. It may be due to the instability of malaria association with this vector, but the possible impact of this phenomenon on the operational problems of eradication must not be under-estimated.

The "Zone of Indo-Chinese Hills" extends from northeastern India to southern China and southward to Burma, Thailand, Cambodia, Laos and Vietnam. Although in these countries malaria-eradication programmes encountered many difficulties of administrative, operational and other natures, it appears that in lowland areas, where *A. minimus* is the main vector, the interruption of transmission is feasible by residual spraying alone.

The recent reappearance of transmission in a few areas of Assam is due to operational problems not related to the resistance or behaviour pattern of the vector. Until recently, *A. minimus* was believed to be the only important vector of malaria in Thailand and adjacent countries. In Thailand, in areas where *A. minimus* was the main vector, the amount of malaria decreases spectacularly, and the vector has practically disappeared. We now know that *A. balabacensis* Baisas is the major vector in forested foothills of these countries. The species is greatly attracted to man, higher exophilic, and may easily evade insecticide-treated surfaces. For these and other reasons, eradication of malaria in areas where *A. balabacensis* is the main vector faces great obstacles (Scanlon and Sandhinand, 1965). In hilly and densely forested areas of Thailand, Cambodia and Vietnam, where *A. balabacensis* is the main or additional vector, residual spraying has not been effective. Lately DDT resistance in *A. culicifacies* has been reported from northern Thailand, but this should not affect the operational aspects of the present programme. In Vietnam, the vectorial role of *A. minimus* and *A. jeyporiensis* James has been confirmed, though *A. maculatus*, *leucophyrus* Dönitz, *subpictus* Grassi, and *sinensis* may transmit at a low level. *A. sundaicus* (Rodenwaldt) is an additional vector in coastal areas (Hien, 1968). In these countries it is virtually impossible to separate technical problems from operational obstacles (such as houses without real walls) or administrative shortcomings.

The "Malaysian Zone" includes the outstandingly successful programme in Taiwan where *A. m. minimus* was the vector in foothills and *A. sinensis* in the plains. In Taiwan, malaria eradication was achieved in 1965 without any major obstacles. The island inhabited by 13 million people had the advantage of well-developed administrative and rural health services and the programme was tailored to suit local conditions.

In Hong Kong and Singapore—two large urban areas of this zone—there is no local transmission of malaria. Elsewhere programmes are in varying stages of progress. In the Phillipines, *A. minimus flavirostris* Ludlow developed resistance to dieldrin/HCH and a reversion to DDT became necessary. The programme had many setbacks because of operational and administrative problems, and most of it is still in the attack phase.

In Malaya (West Malaysia), a pilot project was completed in 1964 in an area of Selangor where *A. campestris* Reid, *A. sundaicus* and *A. maculatus* were the main vectors, and *A. letifer* Sandosham was a subsidiary vector. Twice-yearly spraying of houses with DDT was combined with mass drug distribution and some larvicidal treatment of *A. maculatus* breeding places. *A. campestris* disappeared rapidly, but the density of other species was little affected. However, the transmission of malaria was interrupted, indicating the possibilities of malaria eradication in that area, especially as *A. letifer* and some other species were found to be of little importance as vectors in Selangor.

Malaria carried by the *A. leucosphyrus* group presents a serious challenge to eradication, since two of the important vectors of human malaria have prominent outdoor habits. *A. balabacensis* ranges as a vector through Assam, Burma, Thailand, North West Malaya and Borneo; *A. leucosphyrus* is a vector in Sarawak, North Borneo and Sumatra, and it was doubtful if it could be affected by residual insecticides. However, it was shown that it rested for some time on internal surfaces in Sarawak and Brunei, and that good coverage may result in interruption of transmission in many parts of the country. In North Borneo, an intensive campaign achieved equally good results, although in some pockets low level transmission by one of the species of the *barbirostris* group (perhaps *A. donaldi* Reid) persisted.

In Indonesia, the malaria-eradication programme is confined to Java, Bali and South Sumatra. It has shown considerable progress in the early period in spite of the fact that *A. sundaicus* developed dieldrin/HCH resistance on the south coast of Java and to DDT on the north coast. The replacement of dieldrin by DDT in the south has greatly improved the situation and the same was seen when DDT was substituted for dieldrin in the north. Neverthelsss, it appears that the DDT-susceptible strain of *A. sundaicus* has a high degree of irritability to this insecticide, and this characteristic may have an adverse effect on further results of spraying operations.

Dieldrin resistance in *A. minimus flavirostris* in eastern Java was of limited significance, as this species is not an important vector in this area. Double resistance in *A. aconitus* Dönitz, previously reported in only a few peripheral localities, has spread to central Java. Although the eradication programme has slowed down for various reasons, well over half of the densely populated area of Java remains in the consolidation phase.

In the "Australasian Zone", malaria eradication has been achieved in the Australian north-west, where *A. farauti* Laveran is the main vector with *A. bancrofti* Giles as its auxiliary. New Guinea is one of the most malarious parts of the West Pacific: transmission there is of the same order as that found in tropical Africa. The main vectors belong to the *A. punctulatus* group (*A. punctulatus* Dönitz, *A. farauti* and *A. koliensis* Owen). High levels of endemicity are seen in most coastal areas of New Guinea, where the *A. punctulatus* complex is prevalent, while a high degree of transmission is related to the presence of *A. farauti* alone. However, the greater exophily of the latter species, together with its adaptability to breeding in various waters, makes *A. farauti* difficult to control. In spite of serious operational difficulties, two pilot projects have reduced transmission to a very low level, though this does not necessarily indicate rapid eradication of malaria from New Guinea.

In the "North-American Zone" malaria eradication has been achieved in the United States, where nearly one quarter of the total population of the country resides in the previously malarious area.

The National Malaria Eradication Programme of the Unites States resulted 20 years ago in a dramatic decrease of malaria (Andrews, 1951), and over the following decade there persisted only a few minor foci of malaria with less than 20 indigenous cases. In 1963 there were only 3 locally transmitted cases of malaria in the United States. Although resistance of the common malaria mosquito, *A. quadrimaculatus* Say, to dieldrin/HCH was reported from Mississippi as early as 1956 and to DDT from Georgia and Maryland in 1960, this presented no problem. There have been no reports of insecticide resistance in *A. freeborni* Aitken from the western United States (Hinman, 1966).

In Mexico, the attack phase of malaria eradication was initiated in 1957, and five years later the incidence of malaria decreased spectacularly over three quarters of the whole malarious area. In the remaining one quarter of the country transmission persisted at a low level. The main zone of continuing transmission is the Pacific coastal area of Mexico with *A. albimanus* Wiedemann the main vector; several small zones with persisting transmission exist inland where *A. pseudopunctipennis* Theobald is the vector. Both species show a degree of outdoor biting. *A. aztecus* Hoffmann plays only a minor role in the highlands. The reasons for persistent transmission are complex as usual, *A. albimanus* has shown since 1959 a high degree of resistance to dieldrin. DDT resistance was found in 1961 but excitorepellency of this insecticide may be the main cause of its lack of effect, together with some aspects of human ecology. The same lack of response to dieldrin was noted in *A. pseudopunctipennis* in 1960, together with incipient resistance to DDT. In a small area of northern Mexico, *A. quadrimaculatus* has developed double resistance. At the present time, the final success of the programme hinges on the improvement of surveillance operations in the consolidation areas and the use of alternative mosquito-control methods in those parts of the country where the attack phase continues.

The "Central-American Zone" shows a peculiar mixture of failure and success as far as malaria eradication is concerned. The countries of Guatemala, El Salvador, Honduras, Nicaragua and Panama have been notoriously malarious, particularly on their coasts. The eradication programmes, started at the end of the 1950s, produced excellent control of disease, but during the past few years the progress has been slowed down in areas with about one fifth the population at risk. One of the main causes of this situation is the high degree of resistance of *A. albimanus* to both DDT and dieldrin/HCH reported in 1959–61. In some parts of this zone, the excitorepellancy and exophily of the main vector are also important obstacles to control by the use of usual insecticides. Most of these areas are on the Pacific coast, where there has been an extensive application of various insecticides for control of agricultural pest insects. Malathion has been used with some effect, though recently resistance to this insecticide was reported from Guatemala and Nicaragua.

In contrast to the situation in Central America, malaria eradication has made great strides in many Caribbean islands. It has been achieved and certified in Dominica, Grenada and Carriacou, Jamaica, St. Lucia and Trinidad and Tobago. In Barbados, Dominican Republic, Cuba, Puerto Rico, Martinique and Guadeloupe, the programme is in the consolidation or maintenance phase, this is in spite of the fact that *A. albimanus* developed dieldrin/HCH resistance in several of these islands. It is likely that success has been achieved by a judicious integration of DDT spraying and by well-conducted surveillance activities. In Trinidad, the presence of bromeliad-breeding and outdoor-biting *A.* (*Kerteszia*) *bellator* Dyar and Knab, incriminated as a secondary vector on the island and not easily controlled by DDT, created no difficulties for the interruption of transmission or achievement of eradication.

In Haiti, the eradication programme, carried out since 1962, had a major upset from hurricane "Flora" in 1963. The intensified control measures have decreased quite strikingly the amount of malaria during the past four years, but have not interrupted the continuing low-level transmission, in spite of large-scale chemotherapy. *A. albimanus* of Haiti, while resistant to dieldrin, has remained susceptible to DDT; its exophilic habits may be partly responsible for the continuation of transmission, but other, chiefly operational, difficulties are relevant to the present situation.

In the "South-American Zone" the outstanding and early success of the Venezuelan programme is well known: the major part of the country is certified malaria-free. Insecticidal spraying had a rapid effect on transmission by *A. albimanus* and *A. darlingi* Root in local association with *A. pseudopunctipennis*. *A. albitarsis* Lynch Arribálzaga, *A. albimanus* and occasionally *Kerteszia* are minor vectors. Local resistance to dieldrin has been reported in *A. albitarsis*, *A. aquasalis* Curry and some other secondary vectors, but the virtual disappearance of *A. darlingi* following the early DDT spraying was sufficient to interrupt transmission.

A continuing low-level transmission continues along the Venezuela-Colombia border where *A. nuneztovari* is the main transmitter; this is due partly to the exophily of the vector, partly to its decrease of susceptibility to DDT, and to a large extent to the movement of populations across the frontier.

In an equally successful malaria-eradication programme in Guiana the same virtual disappearance of *A. darlingi* from the coastal area took place; low-level transmission by nondomestic species such as *A. aquasalis* and *A. albitarsis* did not greatly interfere with the programme, but in the interior additional measures were necessary.

In Colombia and Equador, much of the malarious area is still in the attack phase for various operational reasons. The local resistance to dieldrin of *A. albimanus* cannot be incriminated as the cause of the slow progress of the campaign. No problems were encountered in areas of higher altitude where *A. pseudopunctipennis* is the vector.

Brazil is the largest country of South America, and its malaria-eradication programme that began more than 10 years ago has made much progress in the São Paulo area; the coastal strip from Espirito Santo to Rio Grande do Norte is still in the attack phase, while in the Amazon region little can be done at the present time. The pace of this huge campaign has been uneven for several reasons. *A. darlingi*, the main vector, is much less endophilic and anthropophilic in Brazil than in Venezuela or Guiana. Other vectors are *A. tarsimaculatus* Goeldi (= *albimanus*), *A. albitarsis* and *Kerteszia* in the south of the country. It is possible that the behaviour of *A. darlingi* is different at the centre of its geographical distribution and that this difference affects the response to the insecticidal spraying. Local resistance of *A. aquasalis* or *A. albitarsis* is of little importance; fortunately no resistance has been observed in *A. darlingi*.

In Argentina, Bolivia, Peru, Paraguay and other countries of South

America, programmes are in various stages, and the lack of uniformity of progress is mainly due to operational difficulties. No major entomological problems have been reported for *A. pseudopunctipennis* (although in Peru this species shows resistance to dieldrin), *A. albimanus* and *A. punctimacula* Dyar and Knab. *A. albitarsis*, *A. aquasalis* and *A. darlingi* are other vectors adapted to ecological conditions in this part of the world.

MALARIA CONTROL: CASE STUDIES

The aim of this section is to pursue the more complex diagram of the malaria cycle—viz. Fig. 3.2. The basic elements of Fig. 3.2 are repeated in each of Figs 3.5.8 to 3.5.12 and Fig. 6 in relation to six case study areas. They present the inter-related life cycles of vector species of *Anopheles* and of the species of *Plasmodium* parasitic on man and *Anopheles* as alternate hosts, together with the more complex and varied movements and activities of man. Some details of the local particularities of the malaria cycle gleaned from the literature are added. These include the species of *Plasmodium* and of *Anopheles* involved, the points of attack of malaria control campaigns—whether directed to the adult or the larval forms of *Anopheles*, or on *Plasmodium* by prophylactic or curative drugs. Where it seems appropriate or useful, changes in the local ecology of malaria after the campaign have been indicated.

Cameroon provides a good example of the difficulties presented to eradication campaigns by much of the equatorial and wet tropical forest lands of Africa and elsewhere. The two great vector *Anopheles* of Africa, *A. gambiae* and *A. funestus*, were present in their complementary roles: *A. funestus* the more closely associated with permanent water bodies, swamps and marshes; *A. gambiae* the vector thought of as the great opportunist species. *A. gambiae* adapts quickly to temporary water bodies of all kinds and invades relatively dry sites soon after temporary pools of all shapes and sizes have been provided by the rains. Early attempts to use curative drugs were partially successful, at least in the limited context of the timber industry. House-spraying with residual insecticides like DDT appeared in the 1950s and early 1960s as a possible *deus ex machina*. Considerable successes were attained. *A. funestus* was almost eradicated, along with the two forest species *A. moucheti* and *A. nili*. Even *A. gambiae* was

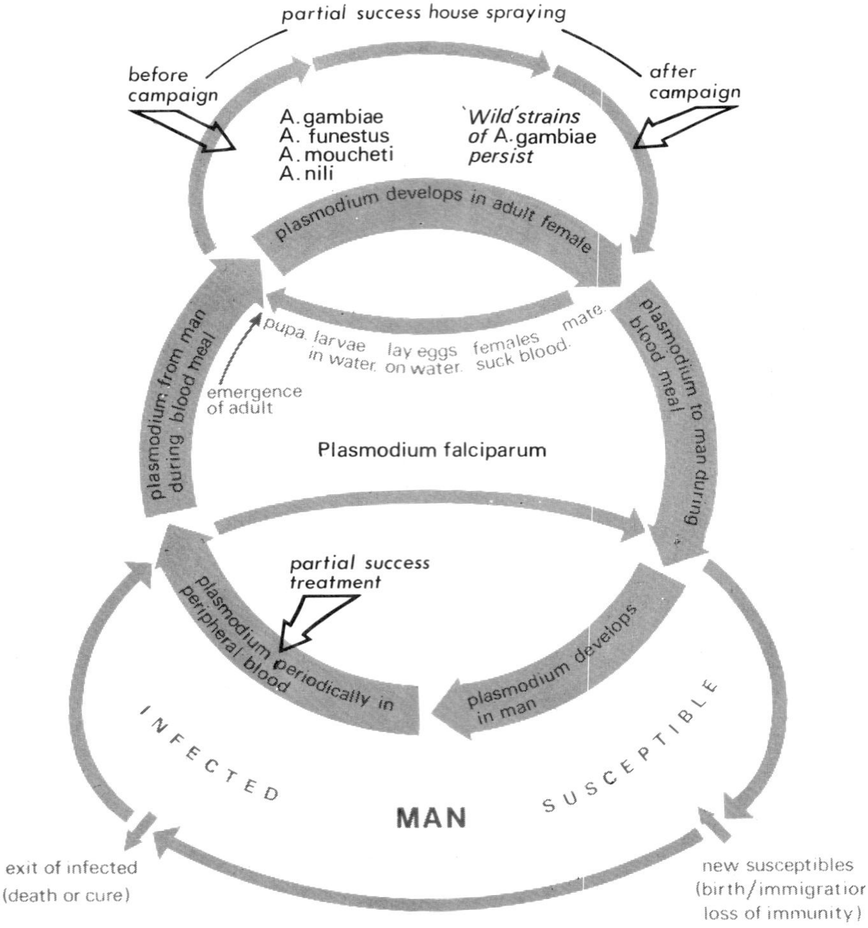

Fig. 3.8 Malaria control campaigns and the malaria cycle: Cameroon (Languillon *et al.*, 1956; Open University, 1971).

much reduced in and around dwellings and workplaces, but it became clear here, as elsewhere, that *A. gambiae* includes many strains of different preferences in places and times of feeding, breeding and resting. House-haunting strains were wiped out, but others remained, notably those which preferred resting after a blood meal in forest rather than domestic sites. Strains which act in this fashion but which also feed predominantly on animals are of less importance to human malaria than as a problem in social medicine, though individual cases of malaria in lumbermen and hunters may well be due to those mosquitoes. Limited and local malaria control in the economically important urban areas was clearly practicable, but would need constant surveillance and a changing armoury of control weapons. Early optimistic thought of complete eradication by the use of residual insecticides against the adult mosquitoes were soon dispelled. Well-populated plains enjoyed a reduced incidence, but flood-liable riverine flats remained meso-endemic. Given the exophilous strains of *Anopheles gambiae* and the extreme adaptibility of the species, the malariologists' early optimism became sharply qualified.

How representative is this case study from the Cameroon? A diagrammatic case is chosen but other areas described in the literature conform reasonably well, though with peculiarities related to a locally-varying disease ecology and disease cycle. Kpain in central Liberia, for instance, showed problems of accessibility, of missed houses, of missed roof-spaces in steep-roofed huts and of the use of temporary shelters away from permanent villages (Prothero, 1965, p. 109). Ruanda-Urundi has areas free from malaria at altitudes above 2000 m and with temperatures normally below those at which malaria transmission takes place. Above 1500 m, *Plasmodium* can develop in the mosquito only inside huts, so house spraying is effective; below this altitude, spraying is ineffective without reinforcement by drugs. There is now popular pressure for the use of anti-larval measures, because these reduce the incidence not only of *Anopheles* but also of non-malarious culicine mosquitoes which have a high nuisance value (Jadin *et al.*, 1952; Meyus *et al.*, 1962).

Figure 3.9 illustrates a tropical summer rainfall case, from the Udi plateau area in Nigeria. Much of the more humid of the tropical rainfall tracts have conditions broadly comparable with those described for the equatorial rainforest zone, and with the same two main vectors, *Anopheles funestus* and *A. gambiae*. The powers of adaptability of the vectors, however, are demonstrated by their dominance in the Udi plateau, a comparatively high and dry tract where water storage is a problem and large pots are used. A study in 1957, established that of the 2 million pots within the 100 square miles under survey, over a quarter contained larvae. Because the villagers were opposed to covering their pots, the use of dieldrin larvicidal pellets were advocated.

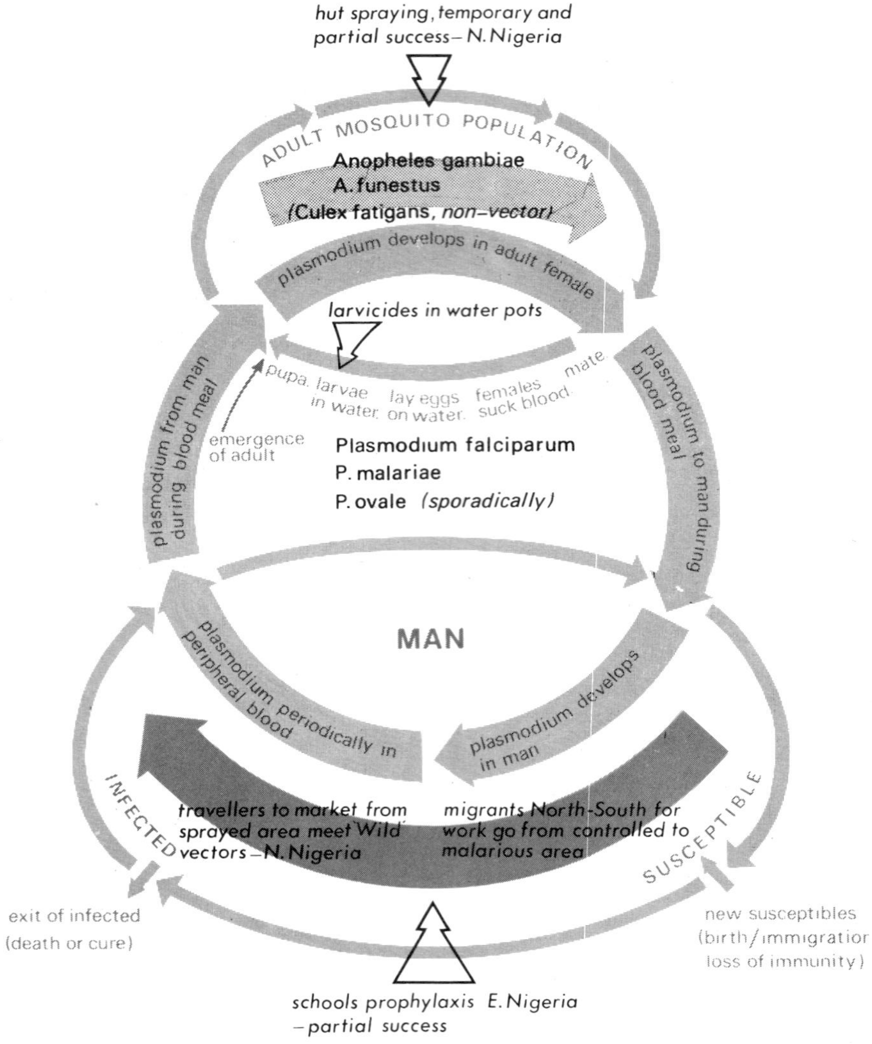

Fig. 3.9 Malaria control campaigns and the malaria cycle: Nigeria (Prothero, 1965; Bruce-Chwatt *et al.*, 1955–56; Arthur, 1965; Bruce-Chwatt, 1957; Dodge, 1966).

This was a special case. Over most of the summer rainfall area of northern Nigeria, the source of vectors was not so localized, and the vectors were judged sufficiently house-haunting for the more conventional spraying of hut walls to be used. However, a study conducted in 1966 showed how the increasing numbers of people going to local markets, often over distances of 15–25 km are exposed to vectors which have not been near their huts and so exposed to the insecticide sprays. A programme of prophylaxis in schools was tried

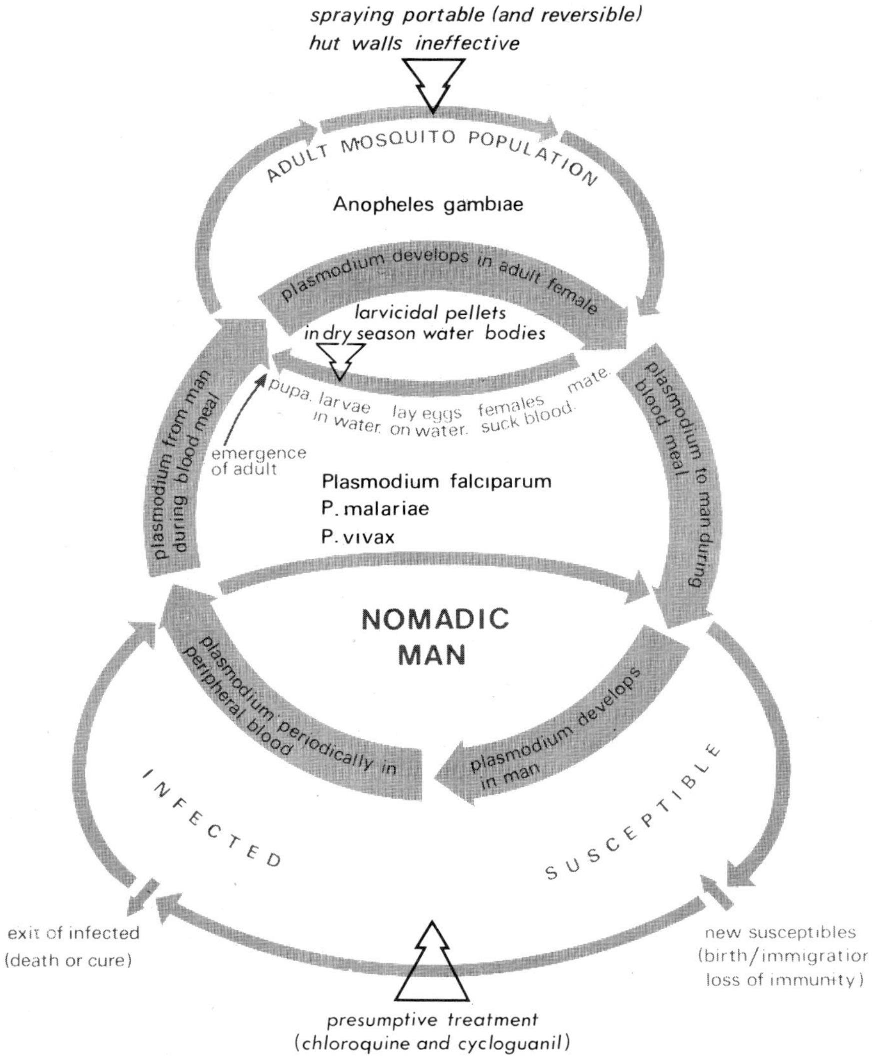

Fig. 3.10 Malaria control campaigns and the malaria cycle: Somalia (W.H.O., 1965).

(Source: W.H.O. Chronicle 1976 June, 1965).

E

in eastern Nigeria with the usual difficulties presented by irregular supplies, holidays, absenteeism, and children not swallowing tablets (Dodge, 1966). Fulani migration from north to south in search of harvest and other employment was studied by Prothero primarily as an example of dynamic human geography. This was subsequently established by Bruce–Chwatt to link up with difficulties which had been encountered in a malaria control campaign being conducted in western Sokoto (Prothero, 1965).

Figure 3.10 illustrates the malaria problem in a more extreme case of migratory movement, among truly nomadic people, 5 million strong, in fairly constant movement across the Horn of Africa. Their main dwellings are portable matting huts which lose insecticide very quickly, and whose sides may, in addition, be reversed when the hut is next taken down and reassembled. The people are most widely dispersed during the rainy season when transmission is most probable, and *Anopheles gambiae*, the main vector, has been shown to travel with the knocked down hut walls. Up to 1965, presumptive treatment with chloroquin was tried, but dieldrin pellets in residual breeding places, i.e. the limited number of breeding places in the dry season, has been recommended. In the same season, the population tends to be at its most concentrated round the wells, and it may be possible to administer a repository drug like cycloguanil (CI–501).

One of two case studies from the Mediterranean world is illustrated in Fig. 3.11. In Israel, the malaria cycle is attacked at almost every possible point where it might be broken. Movements of people appear in a different guise from the seasonal migration of the Fulani or the nomadic movements of Somalia. Instead the stream of immigrants and of foreign students, many of whom come from malarious countries, has made presumptive treatment an important weapon of control. Anti-larval and imagocidal spraying played their part in initial establishment of malaria control. They are continued now more in an effort to reduce the nuisance value of mosquitoes and free passenger and freight movements from restrictions than as part of the eradication campaign. Israel is one of the areas in which a change in the main vector and in its seasonal incidence has been recorded. The peak incidence has changed from July and November to October as *Anopheles sacharovi* along the coastlands and *A. superpictus* in the hills have been replaced as main vectors by *A. sergenti* which is associated with the increase in irrigation. Another

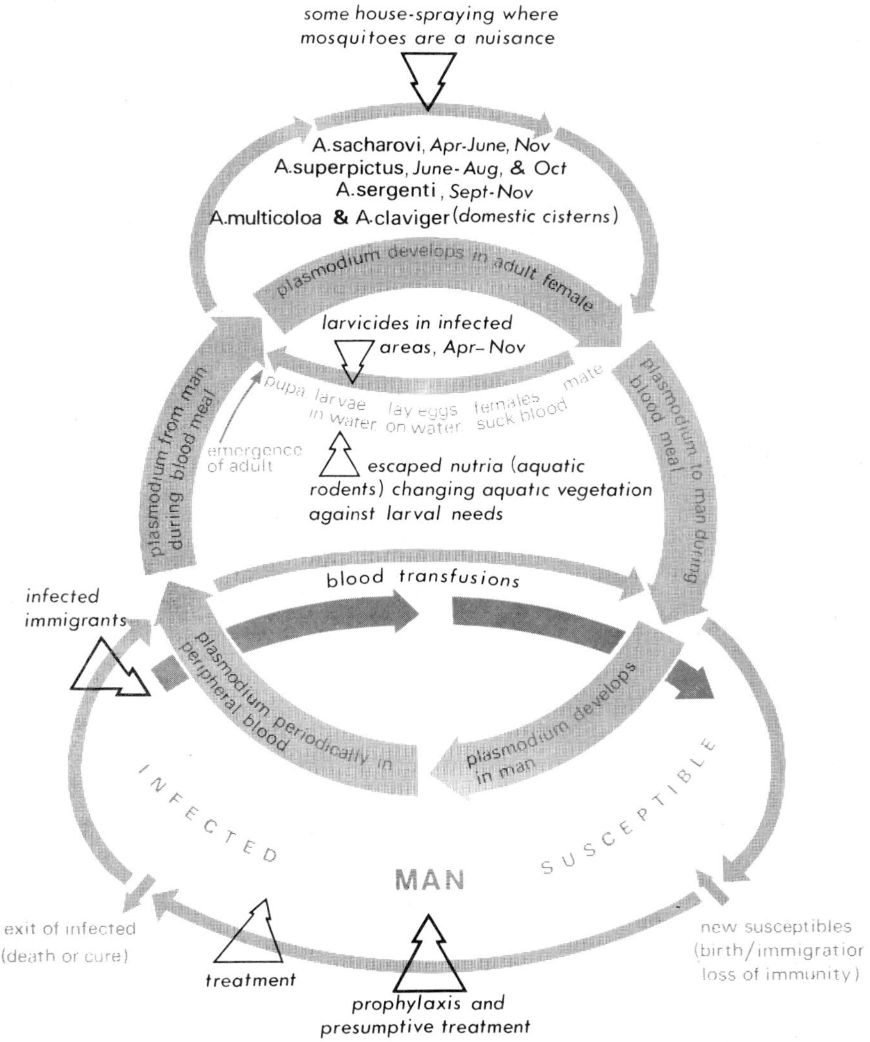

Fig. 3.11 Malaria control campaigns and the malaria cycle: Israel. (Saliternik, 1966, 1954; Ehrlich and Spielberg, 1960; Barkai and Saliternik, 1968).

feature has been the success of escaped nutria (aquatic rodents) in changing the aquatic vegetation in water-bodies and making them less favourable to anopheline larvae.

The second Mediterranean example is another case of multiple

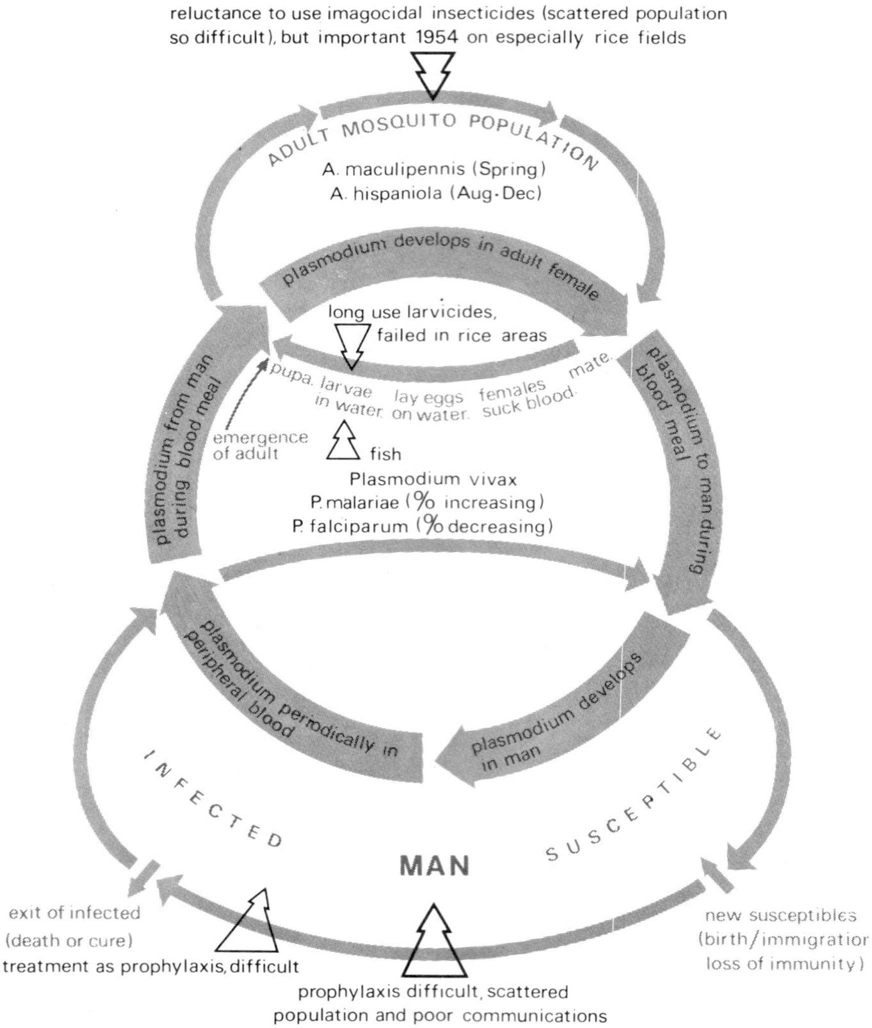

Fig. 3.12 Malaria control campaigns and the malaria cycle: Morocco (Houel and Donadille, 1953; Houel, 1954).

points of attack on the malaria cycle (Fig. 3.12). Morocco is included here, partly because, during the period of strong French influence on health control, there was a particularly strong emphasis on anti-larval measures and an equally marked reluctance to use house spraying.

This was partly due to the scattered nature of the population, poor communications and difficulty in gaining access to all parts of orthodox Muslim households. There is also a legacy of literature which is particularly useful in relation to biological methods of control, particularly by manipulation of the water bodies. The economically important and rapidly extending rice fields were eventually crucial in changing control policy. Biological methods of control, including fish, were only partially successful, and their logical extension in the era of residual insecticides to anti-larval pellets was unsuccessful. Dieldrin granules tended to concentrate their impact at lower levels in the water, killing off culicine larvae which were competitors for resources with *Anopheles maculipennis*, the main vector in rice fields. In this way, *A. maculipennis* multiplied rather than died out. Despite the difficulties imagocidal spraying has been generally successful.

With only two case studies it is difficult to represent the great wealth of material from the long history of malaria control measures undertaken in the Mediterranean world. Spain and Greece have a well-documented literature, as has Italy, not least in the context of the Pontine marshes. To complement the two case studies mention might be made of the attempt to eradicate *Anopheles* completely from Sardinia. Here the main vector *Anopheles labranchiae* was attacked with such success that it might never be able to recolonize its former territory. However, other species such as *A. claviger*, *A. algeriensis*, *A. marteri* and *A. hispaniola* were able to emerge from seclusion where they had lived through the eradication campaign and fill the ecological niches previously occupied by *A. labranchiae*. The parallels with the "wild" strains of *Anopheles gambiae* discussed above (p. 94–5), but occurring in such very different conditions of climate and hydrology, is particularly striking (Loddo *et al.*, 1956).

A comparatively recent case of malaria eradication in a developed western country, viz. the Netherlands, is illustrated in Fig. 3.13. Some parallels to the retreat of malaria from Britain, discussed earlier, or the temperate case in the discussion of the hypothetical malarial continent may be noted. The deltaic parts of the Netherlands constituted a resistant focus of malaria within an area of general retreat of the disease. This was due partly to the hydrological conditions in the delta, and partly to the constant increments of malaria patients associated with the long colonial and trading history

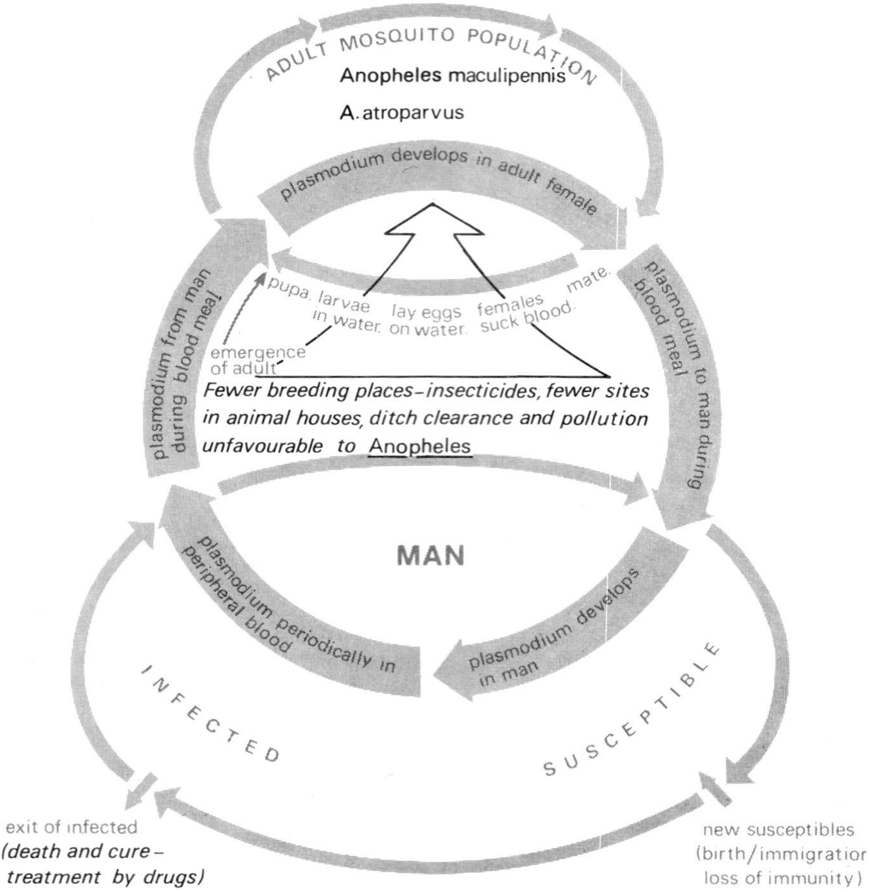

Fig. 3.13 Malaria control campaigns and the malaria cycle: Netherlands (Van Seventer, 1969).

of the Netherlands with malarious tropical areas. The malaria cycle has really been broken in the years succeeding the Second World War. New tools were available for campaigns of treatment and prophylaxis and for anti-larval campaigns, but partly also the retreat of *Anopheles* was due to changes in technology, including agricultural technology. A marked reduction in pig keeping meant a reduced attraction for zoophilic *Anopheles* to the sties which were often sited near dwelling houses. Furthermore, the remaining or new pigsties were sprayed with residual insecticides. Water bodies also underwent changes. Heavy pollution of ditches by anion detergents proved lethal to larvae and mechanical ditch-digging assisted in keeping a free flow of water in ditches. In some other sites a contrary influence was at work with duckweed blanket growth inhibiting the development of larvae.

CONCLUSION

A little less than a century after Laveran's discoveries and almost 80 years after those of Ross and Grassi, the geography of malaria continues to present a fascinating picture, kaleidoscopic and yet with some broad patterns to the observing eye. Along the temperate margins of the world's malarious belt the disease cycle has tended to retreat with improved standards of living and housing. In the mediterranean zone of winter rains and in the tropical summer rainfall zone, it has proved possible to eradicate this global yet paradoxically local disease from wide areas. Some combination of anti-plasmodial treatment or prophylaxis and anti-anopheline larvicidal and imagocidal insecticides have overcome the local ecological web and rhythm of the malaria cycle. Yet resistant foci of malaria remain. In the holoendemic and rainforest climates of the equatorial belt or in extensions of like conditions perennially favourable to anopheline development, malaria eradication has been possible only locally. Here reinvasion from uncontrolled areas is always possible or from reservoirs of the alternate host mosquito in forest refuges away from settlements subject to larvicidal or imagocidal campaigns or else protected by barrier or *cordon sanitaire* projects against the vector species.

In this chapter generalization has been complemented in three ways. First, on the macrogeographic scale by manipulating a model of a hypothetical malarial continent in such a way as to demonstrate the principles of the three-factor but highly multivariate interactions and inter-relationships between man, *Plasmodium* and *Anopheles*; second, by reproducing part of Bruce–Chwatt's world-wide and yet amazingly detailed regional geography of eradication and of anopheline and plasmodial resistance to the new anti-malarial tools; third, by using half-a-dozen case studies thinly strung out between equatorial Africa and temperate western Europe. In some sense, the case studies act as a partial validation of the macro-geographic model of the malarial continent, or of the simple prose generalization. They also throw light and colour on Bruce–Chwatt's inevitably and marvellously condensed regional narrative. Nevertheless, the case studies can be only a very weak and partial validation for the claims advanced in the introduction to this essay for the geographical approach with ecological insights. The ecological web of the malaria cycle has been seen in action, has been seen changing with time and has been seen to have areal or spatial patterns on various scales and this in spite of the local particularities of the cycle and of man-mosquito-*Plasmodium* relationships. These patterns are still imperfectly described but their demonstration is thought to amply justify this contribution.

ACKNOWLEDGEMENTS

Grateful acknowledgement is made to Professor L. J. Bruce–Chwatt of the London School of Hygiene and Tropical Medicine and to the Entomological Society of America for permission to use a long extract from his 1970 paper cited below; appropriate references from his paper are included in alphabetical sequence with the other references to this paper which follow. This extract from Bruce–Chwatt is a much larger proportion of the present paper than would be usual in normal academic convention, but his contribution to knowledge of the geography of malaria since the beginning of the control campaigns seemed to make it necessary, without excluding the possibility of a complementary contribution from a professional geographer like the present writer.

The model of the hypothetical continent is based on an oral paper by the writer to the Commission on Medical Geography at the 1968 New Delhi Congress of the International Geographical Union; but the present treatment owes a great deal to collaboration with Michael Philps, Senior Producer, BBC/Open University, over an experimental "radiovision" programme using this model. The assistance of the BBC graphics designers at Alexandra Palace is also gratefully acknowledged.

The original upon which Fig. 3.2 is based was originally devised by the writer for the Open University Foundation Course in the Social Sciences, D100 Understanding Society, Unit 33, "Demographic Regions of the Indian Subcontinent", and the permission to use this of the Director of

Publishing is acknowledged with thanks. The subsequent treatment of the case studies is based largely on drafts initiated by Alyson Learmonth.

The realization of the maps and diagrams in their present form is due to work by Peter Daniell of the Australian National University and John Hunt of the Open University.

REFERENCES

Andrews, J. M. (1951). Nation-wide malaria eradication projects in the Americas: eradication program in the U.S.A. *J. Nat. Malar. Soc.* **10**, 99–123.

Arthur, J. H. (1965). "Antimalarial Prophylaxis in Primary Schools in E. Nigeria". Wellcome Museum of Medical Science, London.

Barkai, A. and Saliternik, Z. (1968). Anopheline mosquitoes found breeding in Israel in 1963–1965 during the last stages of the malaria eradication project. *Bull. Ent. Res.* **58**, 2, 353–366.

Boyd, M. F. (Ed.) (1949). "Malariology", I and II. W. B. Saunders, Philadelphia and London.

Bruch-Chwatt, L. J. (1954). Problems of malaria control in tropical Africa. *Brit. Med. J.* (Serial No. 4853), 169–174.

Bruce-Chwatt, L. J. (1957). An unusual epidemiology of malaria in S.E. Nigeria. *Trans. Roy. Soc. Trop. Med. Hyg.* **51**, 5, 411–418.

Bruce-Chwatt, L. J. (1959). Malaria research and eradication in the U.S.S.R.: a review of Soviet achievements in the field of malariology. *Bull. W.H.O.* **21**, 6, 737–772.

Bruce-Chwatt, L. J. (1965). Paleogenesis and paleo-epidemiology of primate malaria. *Bull. W.H.O.* **32**, 3, 363–387.

Bruce-Chwatt, L. J. (1970). Global Review of Malaria Control and Eradication by Attack on the Vector. *Misc. Publ. Entomol. Soc. Amer.* **7**, 1, 7–27.

Bruce-Chwatt, L. J. (1970). Malaria zoonosis in relation to malaria eradication. *Trop. Geogr. Med.* **20**, 1, 50–87.

Bruce-Chwatt, L. J., Archibald, H. M. and Haworth, J. (1956–57). Reports of malaria control pilot project in West Sokoto. *In* "Northern Nigeria, Second and Third Annual Reports 1955–56; 1956–57" (mimeo). Yaba, Federal Malaria Service, Lagos.

Coatney, G. R. (1968). Simian malarias in man: facts, implications and predictions. *Amer. J. Trop. Med. Hyg.* **17**, 2, 147–155.

Colbourne, M. J. (1962). A review of malaria eradication campaigns in the western Pacific. *Ann. Trop. Med. Parasitol.* **56**, 1, 33–43.

Coluzzi, A. (1965). Dati recenti sulla malaria in Italia e problemi connessi al mantanimento dei risultati raggiunti. *Riv. Malariol.* **44**, 4–6, 153–178.

Covell, G. (1928). "Malaria in Bombay". Gov. Central Press, Bombay.

Dodge, J. S. (1966). Population movements around local markets in West Sokoto, N. Nigeria. *J. Trop. Med. and Hyg.* **69**, 8, 180–183.

Ehrlich, S. and Spielberg, D. (1960). Alteration of the environment of anopheles larvae by nutria in the Ṇaaman Swamps, Acre District, Israel. *Amer. J. Trop. Med. Hyg.* **9**, 3, 265–268.

Foll. C. V. and Pant, C. P. (1966). The conditions of malaria transmission in Katsina Province, N. Nigeria, and the effects of dichlorvos application. *Bull. W.H.O.* **34**, 3, 395–404.

Foll, C. V., Pant, C. P. and Lietaert, P. E. (1965). A large-scale field trial with dichlorvos as a residual fumigant insecticide in N. Nigeria. *Bull. W.H.O.* **32**, 4, 531–550.

Gad, A. M. (1967). *Anopheles stephensi* Liston in Egypt, U.A.R. *Mosquito News* **27**, 2, 171–174.

Hackett, L. W. (1949). "Malaria in Europe". Oxford Univ. Press, Oxford.

Hamon, J. and Garrett-Jones, C. (1963). La résistance aux insecticides chez des vecteurs majeurs du paludisme et son importance operationelle. *Bull. W.H.O.* **28**, 1, 1–24.

Hamon, J., Mouchet, J., Chavet, G. and Lumaret, R. (1963). Bilan de 14 années de lutte control de paludisme dans les pays francophones d'Afrique tropical et de Madagascar. Considérations sur le persistence de la transmission et perspectives d'avenir. *Bull. Soc. Pathol. Exot.* **56**, 5, 933–971.

Hien Nguyen Thong. (1968). The genus anopheles in the Republic of Vietnam. Bureau of Entomology, National Malaria Program, Ministry of Health, Saigon (mimeo), 205pp.

Hinman, E. H. (1966). "World Eradication of Infectious Diseases." Charles C. Thomas, Springfield.

Houel, G. and Donaldille, F. (1953). Twenty years of antimalaria work in Morocco. *Bull. Inst. Hyg. Maroc.* **13**, 1–2, 3–51.

Houel, G. (1954). Malaria control in rice-growing areas in Morocco. *Bull. Inst. Hyg. Maroc.* **14**, 1, 43–90.

Jadin, J., Fain, A. and Rup, H. (1952). Extensive malaria control with DDT in a rural area at Astrida, Ruanda-Urundi. *Inst. Roy. Colonial Belg. Sect. Sci. Natur. Med. Mem.* **21**, 1, 47pp.

Jerusalem (1953). Ministry of Health Report of the Antimalaria Department for 1950–2 (Saliternik, Z. Director). English Summary (mimeo), 68pp.

Languillon, J., Mouchet, J., Rivola, E. and Rateau, J. (1956). Contribution a l'étude de l'épidémiologie du paludisme dans la region forestière de Cameroun. Paludométrie, espèces plasmodiales, anophelisme, transmission. *Med. Trop. Marseilles* **16**, 3, 347–378.

Learmonth, A. T. A. (1957). Some contrasts in the regional geography of malaria in India and Pakistan. *Trans. Inst. Brit. Geog.* **23**, 37–59.

Learmonth, A. T. A. (1958). Medical geography in Indo-Pakistan: a study of twenty years' data for the former British India, *Indian Geog. J.* **33**, 1–2, 1–59.

Loddo, B., Zambelli, P. and Congiu, A. (1956). Specie anofeliche e reinvasione di teritori disinfestati. *Nuovi Ann d'Igience e Microbiol.* **7**, 2, 117–132, English Summary.

Lupasco, G. and Duport, M. (1968). Modifications de la fauna anophélienne consècutives aux différentes mesures institués. *Arch. Roum. Pathal. Exp. Microbiol.* **27**, 3, 697–706.

Lysenko, A. J. and Beljaev, A. E. (1969). An analysis of the geographical distribution of *Plasmodium ovale*. *Bull. W.H.O.* **40**, 3, 383–394.

Macdonald, G. (1956). Theory of the eradication of malaria. *Bull. W.H.O.* **15**, 3, 369–387.

Macdonald, G. (1957). "The Epidemiology and Control of Malaria". Oxford Univ. Press, London.

Macdonald, G. (1965). Eradication of malaria. *Pub. Hlth Rep. (U.S.A.)* **80**, 10, 870–880.

Maegraith, B. G. (1965). "Exotic Diseases in Practice". Heinemann Medical, London.

Mariani, M. (1956). Sulla sensibilita dell' *A. labranchiae* al DDT dopo sette anni di lotta anthianofelic con insetticidi clorurati in Sicilia. *Riv. Parassitol.* **17**, 3, 171–177.

May, J. M. (1950). Medical geography: its methods and objectives. *Geog. Rev.* **40**, 2, 11–41.

May, J. M. (1951). World atlas of diseases No. 3: malaria. *Geog. Rev.* **41**.

Meyus, H., Lips, M. and Caubergh, H. (1962). The malaria problem at the altitude of Ruanda-Urundi. *Ann. Soc. Belge Med. Trop.* **43**, 5, 77–82.

Pringle, G. (1969). Experimental malaria control and demography in a rural East African community: a retrospect. *Trans. Roy. Soc. Trop. Med. Hyg.* **63**, 417–429.

Prothero, R. M. (1965). *"Migrants and Malaria"*. Longmans, London.

Raffaele, C. and Coluzzi, M. (1957). Richerche sul problema della resistenza degli anofeli agi insetticidi. Nota III. Indogine sulla sensibilità al DDT degli anofeli di varie regioni d'Italia dopo 10 anni di trattamento con insetticidi. *Riv. Malariol.* **86**, 4–6, 177–202.

Russell, P. F., West, L. S., Manwell, R. D. and Macdonald, G. (1963). "Practical Malariology" (2nd edn.). Oxford Univ. Press, London.

Scanlon, J. E. and Sandhinand, U. (1965). The distribution and biology of *Anopheles balabacensis* in Thailand (Diptera: Culicidae). *J. Med. Entomol.* **2**, 61–69.

Sergiev, P. G. (Ed.) (1968). Protozoan diseases. *In* "Manual on Microbiology, Clinical Aspects and Epidemiology of Infectious Diseases", vol. **IX** (4) (in Russian). Medicina, Moscow.

Sergiev, P. G., Rashina, M. G. and Dukhanina, N. N. (1961). Liquidation of malaria in the U.S.S.R. and features of the methods used (in Russian). *Vestnik. Akad. Med. Nauk S.S.R.* **4**, 19–29.

Saliternik, Z. (1954). A comparison between the monthly incidence of primary malaria cases in Israel in the years 1923–1925 and 1950–1952. *Documenta Med. Geograph. Trop.* **6**, 3, 247–251.

Saliternik, Z. (1966). Methods of malaria eradication under the conditions peculiar to Israel. *Israel J. Med. Sci.* **2**, 2, 232–238.

Shortt, H. E., Fairley, N. H., Covell, G., Shute, P. G. and Garnham, P. C. C. (1951). The pre-erythrocytic cycle of *Plasmodium falciparum*. *Trans. Roy. Soc. Trop. Med. Hyg.* **44**, 4, 405–419.

Shute, P. G. (1963). Indigenous malaria in England since the First World War. *Lancet* 14th Sept., 576–578.

Smith, W. D. L. (1956). Malaria and the Thames. *Lancet* 14th April, 433–436.

U.S. Public Health Service (1968). Study of urban malaria in Karachi, West Pakistan (12th Aug.–17th Sept., 1968). Communicable Disease Center, Atlanta.

Van Seventer, H. A. (1969). The disappearance of malaria in the Netherlands (Thesis). University of Amsterdam, Amsterdam.

W.H.O. (1962). Expert Committee on Malaria. *6th Rep. W.H.O. Tech. Rep. Ser.* **132.**

W.H.O. (1965). *W.H.O. Chronicle* **19**, 76.

W.H.O. (1968). Parasitology of malaria: report of a W.H.O. scientific group, Teheran, 16–23, Sept., Geneva. *W.H.O. Tech. Rep. Ser.* **433.**

W.H.O. (1974).ICAS Report on malaria, Geneva.

Zulueta, J. De, Chang, T. L., Cullen, J. R. and Davidson, G. (1968). Recent observations on insecticide resistance in Anopheles stephensi in Iraq. *Mosquito News.* **28**, 4, 499–503.

4. Amoebiasis

R. Elsdon-Dew

There are a number of species of amoebae which may live in the human bowel, some of which are facultative and others obligatory parasites. All of these act as commensal scavengers, feeding on bacteria and food remnants and having a cyst phase which allows transmission to new hosts. However, one of these, *Entamoeba histolytica*, may change its habits and, for some as yet undefined reason, attack the tissues of its host, causing ulceration of the bowel and possibly invading the liver and other organs.

For many years, *Entamoeba histolytica* was considered to be an obligatory tissue-feeder, and thus always pathogenic. Attempts to correlate a patient's presentation with the presence of the parasite led to the amoeba being blamed for a wide gamut of symptomatology, the association in many instances being extremely tenuous. Diagnosis was commonly based on coprological microscopy, often by inadequately trained, uncritical observers.

Even experts were confused. For a long time it was taught that the cysts of *E. histolytica* had a wide size-range, but only some 15–20 years ago it was shown that there were two species of similar morphology and with overlapping sizes. The smaller of these, now known as *Entamoeba hartmanni*, has never been incriminated as a pathogen.

There was yet further confusion. *E. histolytica* can be grown in culture and, when a strain labelled as such was found to grow at room temperature, it was at first regarded as a curiosity and called *E. histolytica* (*Laredo*). However, when it and other strains regarded as "classical" were shown not only to have differing antigenic and enzymatic structure, but to develop contractile vacuoles when grown in hypotonic media, it was appreciated that definitive diagnosis could not be made on microscopical appearance alone. As these Laredo-type amoebae possibly belong to a variety of species, it was wisely decided not to give species rank until the matter had been clarified. Amoebae of this type have been identified in several places. Unfortunately, very few laboratories have appropriate facilities for this highly technical process.

With, on the one hand, the laboratory difficulties and, on the other, the early failure of clinicians to appreciate the difference between lumenal amoebiasis, where *E. histolytica* remains in the gut, i.e. outside of the body, and invasive amoebiasis, where the amoebae are causing disease, the difficulty of forming a global picture can be appreciated.

Quadrinucleate cysts of *E. histolytica*-type have been reported all over the world wherever they have been sought and, though the majority are undoubtedly those of *E. histolytica*, some may have been *E. hartmanni* and some the cysts of facultative parasites of Laredo type. Further, the efficiency and sadly even the *bona fides* of some observers is questionable. No reliance can be placed on most survey records.

The clinical position is no better. The least said about the protean manifestations attributed to the parasite the better, but even reports of amoebic dysentery were completely biased by the unfortunate habit of classing all those cases of dysentery not proved to be bacillary in origin as being due to amoebae, whether or not the protozoan has been found. The same criticism applied to official records.

If, however, one excludes the problematical entity called diffuse amoebic hepatitis, true Amoebic Liver Abscess is a condition unlikely to be mistaken for anything else. It is for this reason that this manifestation has been chosen as the criterion for the prevalence of disease due to amoebae.

If amoebae invade the bowel wall, they may be carried away in the portal blood-stream to be filtered out by the liver. Should they survive, they may set up foci of necrosis of the parenchymal cells of the liver. Pus cells move in to remove the necrotic material left behind by the amoebae and the resultant lesion is commonly termed an Amoebic Liver Abscess, ALA (pedantically a misnomer). Such abscesses are commonly single and usually in the right lobe. Untreated they may reach considerable size with a capacity of a litre or more. They may rupture in any direction—through the skin, into the lung or pleura, into the peritoneum and those in the left lobe may burst into the pericardium. Such a blatant lesion should not be missed.

In such areas where authenticated amoebic dysentery occurs, the ratio of the occurrence of liver abscess to dysentery is of the order of 1:12. Thus if an area reports numerous cases of dystentery and does not report abscesses, the diagnosis of the former is questionable. This underlies the stratagem employed by the author in his assessment of the impact of *E. histolytica* when visiting a number of countries.

A review (Elsdon–Dew, 1968), of the geographical incidence of Amoebic Liver Abscess appeared in *Advances in Parasitology* **6**, and this covered the information available up to 1966. Since that article, there has not only been renewed and more critical interest, but new developments are improving the standard of diagnosis, particularly of Amoebic Liver Abscess.

The advent of scintigraphy (radioactive scanning) has made it possible to locate space-occupying lesions of the liver and this information, taken in conjunction with other features, increases the probability of a correct diagnosis.

Another useful development has been that of serology which requires some explanation. Early attempts at establishing such tests were frustrated by the confusion surrounding the relationship between *E. histolytica* and man. It was only when the distinction between the normal commensal state and the abnormal invasive condition was appreciated that the value of this approach was established. Apparently antibodies arise as a result of invasion, and are not stimulated by amoebae remaining commensal in the gut. However, such antibodies, having appeared, persist for some time after the stimulus of the invading amoebae has been removed. Thus a positive result must be interpreted as indicative of past or present invasion.

A third development has been in therapy. The advent of metronidazole has provided an efficient means of treatment, and a succesful "test of cure" is further evidence of the nature of the infection.

Whereas in the first series the only acceptable criteria of Amoebic

Liver Abscess were post-mortem findings or the aspiration of typical amoebic "pus", the present series includes cases based on the new criteria. In addition, note has been made of other complications, as these seem to occur as isolates.

Country	Source	No. of reports in previous survey	No. of cases	
		AFRICA		
Egypt	Previous Survey, 1968	(7)	34	
	Abd-Rabbo *et al.*, 1973		2	Alexandria
Sudan	Omer, 1972		1	*Situs invertus*
Tunisia	Previous Survey, 1968	(1)	8	in 12 years
	Haddad *et al.*, 1970		4	
Algeria	Previous Survey, 1968	(3)	4	
	Sureau *et al.*, 1968		1	seen in Paris
Morocco	Previous Survey, 1968	(3)	48	(46 prior to 1926)
Senegal	Previous Survey, 1968	(6)	88	
	Sankale *et al.*, 1968		1	Pericarditis
	Payet *et al.*, 1969		11	in five months Scintigraphy
	Carayon *et al.*, 1969		124	in 20 years
Liberia	Miller and Bray, 1966		2	in *Pan satyrus*
	Bada, 1969		1	
Ivory Coast	Pignol *et al.*, 1969		14	Pleuropulmonary. Test of cure
	Charmot, 1969		5	
Upper Volta	Paillet *et al.*, 1972		1	Pericardial tamponnade
Ghana	Danisa *et al.*, 1970		15	
	Haddock and Awadzi, 1970		6	
	Archampong, 1972		4	all ruptures
Sierra Leone	Previous Survey, 1968	(1)	17	Reported by Rowland, 1963 (*vide infra*)
	Rowland, 1967		31	(possibly inclusive)
Nigeria	Previous Survey, 1968	(7)	106	
	Abioye and Edington, 1972		28	in 6179 autopsies
	Matthews *et al.*, 1973		1	seen in Bristol, England
	Nnochiri, 1965		4	
	Odunjo, 1969		43	in 2743 autopsies
	Salako, 1967		78	

Country	Source	No. of reports in previous survey	No. of cases	
Cameroon	Sureau *et al.*, 1968		1	seen in Paris
	Carayon *et al.*, 1969		212	in two years
Zaire	Previous Survey, 1968	(4)	130	
	Sureau *et al.*, 1968		1	seen in Paris
	Wolfensburger, 1968a, b		24	
Ethiopia and Somalia	Previous Survey, 1968	(2)	11	
Uganda	Poltera, 1973		11	cutaneous
Kenya	Previous Survey, 1968	(4)	23	
	Whittaker, 1963		several	Intrathoracic rupture
	Ogada, 1967		1	Rupture into pericadium
Mozambique	Previous Survey 1966	(1)	10	Possible overlap between differing studies
	Ruas and Nunes de Almeida, 1967		50	
	Ruas *et al.*, 1967, 1969		50	
	Jarumilinta *et al.*, 1969		33	
	Ruas *et al.*, 1973		40	
	Viana *et al.*, 1974		20	
	Pedroso de Lima *et al.*, 1967		60	
Rhodesia	Previous Survey 1966	(2)	56	
	Baker and Murray, 1969		1	Oesophageal obstruction
	Axton, 1972		1	Infant
South Africa	*Durban*			
	Previous Survey 1968	(18)	1191	
	Powell *et al.*, 1966		5	
	Powell *et al.*, 1967		50	
	Scragg and Powell, 1968		24	Children
	Powell *et al.*, 1969		50	
	Scragg and Powell, 1970		29	Children
	Powell and Elsdon-Dew, 1971		44	
	Powell and Elsdon-Dew, 1972		70	
	Powell, 1972		285	Metronidazole trials
	Powell *et al.*, 1973a		30	
	Powell *et al.*, 1973b		1	Haemobilia
	Powell *et al.*, 1973c		60	
	Scragg and Powell, 1973		25	Children
	Le Roux, 1969		37	*Empyema thoracis*
	Wainwright, 1972		525	in 20 000 necropsies
	Johannesburg			
	Previous Survey 1968	(2)	12	
	Leigh, 1967		1	*Amoebiasis cutis*

Country	Source	No. of reports in previous survey	No. of cases	
	Norwich and Lieberman, 1969		1	*Amoebiasis cutis*
	Pretoria			
	Bieler *et al.*, 1974		247	Scintigraphy in 8 years
	Cape Town			
	Saunders, 1955		1	*Amoebiasis cutis*
	de Groot, 1963		1	Amoebic Vaginitis
	Watson *et al.*, 1970		8	Children in 10 years
	Cowie *et al.*, 1972		80	1964–69
		ASIA		
Turkey	Massarat *et al.*, 1968		1	seen in Germany
Syria	Previous Survey, 1968	(2)	2	
Israel	Previous Survey, 1968	(7)	109	
	Marberg and Czerniak, 1964		5	
Iran	Mortazavi *et al.*, 1972		4	Scintigrams
Iraq	Previous Survey, 1968	(1)	1	
	Salem *et al.*, 1968		42	Test of cure only
Pakistan	Previous Survey, 1968	(1)		
	Khan, 1969		11	Aspirated
India	Previous Survey, 1968	(22)	(1322)	
	Aikat, 1968		15	A.L.A. in 665 necropsies
	Ansari *et al.*, 1973		1	*Situs invertus*
	Antani and Srinivas, 1970		7	Aspirates in 25 cases
	Banerji *et al.*, 1968		18	All aspirated
	Chari and Gadiyar, 1970		4	Aspirated
	Chhetri *et al.*, 1968		42	All aspirated
	Crawford, 1968		1	Child
			8	in 385 necropsies in 6 years
	Desai *et al.*, 1972		4	with obstructive Jaundice
	Harza *et al.*, 1970		4	with obstructive Jaundice
	Hingorani and Mahapatra, 1964		2	Vaginal Amoebiasis
	Kamat *et al.*, 1968		21	Aspiration test of cure
	Kapoor and Joshi, 1972		98	Necropsy
	Kapoor and Shah, 1972		6	Pericardial
	Kapoor *et al.*, 1972		16	Peritoneal rupture
	Prakash *et al.*, 1969		16	Evaluation of serology
	Sayed and Amin, 1962		1	Balanitis
	Sen, 1949		1	Amoebic Vaginitis
	Singh *et al.*, 1971		1	Left lung
	Subramaniam *et al.*, 1968		10	Aspirated

Country	Source	No. of reports in previous survey	No. of cases	
	Tandon *et al.*, 1966		20	Scintigrams
	Vakil *et al.*, 1970		190	Atypical manifestations
Sri Lanka	Previous Survey, 1968	(4)	257	
	Ramachandran *et al.*, 1971		12	Probably same cases
	Ramachandran *et al.*, 1972		11	
	Ramachandran *et al.*, 1973		11	
Bangladesh	Previous Survey, 1968	(1)	17	
	Islam, 1967		1	"Giant abscess" 6100 ml
	Khan and Muazzam, 1969		4	Aspirated
	Ullah *et al.*, 1970		15	
	Matthews *et al.*, 1973		1	in Britain
Malay States	Previous Survey, 1968	(2)	14	
	Cook, 1970		1	Pericarditis in Britain
Thailand	Previous Survey, 1968	(6)	93	
	Devakul *et al.*, 1967		22	
	Harinasuta *et al.*, 1968, 1969		10	Aspirated
	Savanat and Chaicumpa, 1969		25	Evaluation of serology
	Savanat *et al.*, 1973a		88	Evaluation of skin test
	Savanat *et al.*, 1973b		24	Evaluation of cellular immunity
Indo-China	Previous Survey, 1968	(16)	501	
	Chang *et al.*, 1974		2	seen in U.S.A.
	Griffin, 1973		1	seen in U.S.A.
	Kaminsky *et al.*, 1968		1	seen in U.S.A.
	Sheehy *et al.*, 1968		15	seen in U.S.A.
	Weber, 1971		5	seen in U.S.A.
Indonesia	Previous Survey, 1968	(6)	79	
	McClatchie and Sambli, 1971		3	Amoebic cervicitis
Philippines	Previous Survey, 1968	(7)	180	
Korea	Previous Survey, 1968	(8)	110	
China	Previous Survey, 1968	(5)	354	
Taiwan	Tsai, 1973		2322	ALA in 18 years
	Wang *et al.*, 1973		3	
	NORTH AMERICA			
Canada	Meerovitch and Khan, 1967		3	All at Loon Lake, Saskatchewan
	Miller *et al.*, 1968		1	
	Buchan, 1968		10	

Country	Source	No. of reports in previous survey	No. of cases	
United States (unspecified)	Previous Survey, 1968	(5)	7	Autochonous
New England States	Previous Survey, 1968	(5)	8	Autochonous
Mid Western States	Previous Survey, 1968	(2)	4	Autocthonous
	Marr and Haff, 1971		1	St. Louis
	Schumann *et al.*, 1964		4	Detroit
	Heller *et al.*, 1972		1	Chicago
Western States 105° W.	Nil			
Southern States	Previous Survey 1968	(10)	380	(see text)
	Watson *et al.*, 1972		1	Pericarditis N. Carolina
	Juniper *et al.*, 1971		22	Arkansas
	Juniper, 1971		6	Skin or lung, in above cases
	Le Vine *et al.*, 1968		1	Veterans' Hospital, Houston
Mexico	Previous Survey, 1968	(16)	682	
	Alvarez-Alva *et al.*, 1971		1804	ALA in 278 425 admissions
			114	ALA in 12 171 deaths
	Cuaron *et al.*, 1972		4833	in 8¾ years
	De Leon and Peretes, 1971		1796	1963–70
	González-Montesinos *et al.*, 1972		535	in prophylactic study
	Gutièrrez-Trujillo, 1971		181	in children
	Heller *et al.*, 1972		1	Pericarditis in Chicago
	Hernández *et al.*, 1969		56	
	Jinich and Schnaas, 1971		11	1369 private Mexican patients
			8	8331 estrañeros
	Lombardo and Flores-Barroeta, 1971		93	Autopsies—4 with brain abscess
	Mendoza-Hernández *et al.*, 1969		56	Evaluation of serology
	Munguia *et al.*, 1966		24	Genital cases
	Oritiz-Ortiz and Garmilla, 1973		13	
	Perches and de Leon, 1971		40	Scintilligraphic follow-up
	Villegas-Gonzalez *et al.*, 1971a		11	Brain abscesses in children

Country	Source	No. of reports in previous survey	No. of cases	
	Villegas-Gonzalez *et al.*, 1971b		29	ALA with above
Guatemala	Previous Survey, 1966	(2)	7	
Costa Rica	Previous Survey, 1966	(1)	13	
	Kotcher *et al.*, 1970		8	
	SOUTH AMERICA			
Guiana	Previous Survey, 1968	(2)	7	
Venezuela	Previous Survey, 1968	(2)	4	
Colombia	Previous Survey, 1968	(1)	47	
	Bravo and Botero, 1971		20	(see text)
Peru	Previous Survey, 1968	(1)	1	in 1920
Chile	Previous Survey, 1968	(5)	89	
	Sapunar *et al.*, 1967		1	(see text)
Brazil	Previous Survey, 1968	(4)	6	(see text)
	Huggins, 1971		2	Pernambuco
Argentina	Previous Survey, 1968	(2)	3	
	Meeroff and Meeroff, 1968			(see text)
Uruguay	Previous Survey, 1968	(1)	36	unconfirmed
	EUROPE			
Britain	Previous Survey, 1968	(7)	12	
	Matthews *et al.*, 1973		1	Singapore 23 years ago
	Van Reenen, 1972		2	at Millbank—origin uncertain
France	Previous Survey, 1968	(1)	1	
	Sheehy *et al.*, 1968		1	
Germany	Previous Survey, 1968	(1)	1	
Switzerland	Meyer and Suter-Kopp, 1972		1	Switzerland 16 years
Italy	Previous Survey, 1968	(8)	32	
	Scaffidi and Princi, 1965		6	Pulmonary
	Weaver, 1967		1	seen in London
	AUSTRALIA			
	Sandars, 1966		9	cases in literature
	Morris *et al.*, 1969		1	Autocthonous. Scintigraphy

Country	Source	No. of reports in previous survey	No. of cases	
		OCEANIA		
	Previous Survey, 1968	(1)	3	Hawaii
	ten Seldam, 1970		12	cutaneous cases in Papua
	Norcott, 1973		1	seen in Perth, W. Australia

Table 4.1 Geographical distribution of reported cases of liver necrosis and other complications.

Table 4.1 produces some surprises. Some areas, notorious for Amoebiasis, have provided remarkably little in the way of literature on Amoebic Liver Abscess. However, review of publications is, of course, likely to be biased. In underdeveloped countries, the medical staff may be too busy to report their experiences; where the condition is common, it may not be considered worthy of report, and, in the other direction, where there are enthusiastic observers there may be numerous reports. Nevertheless, positive reports are valid, and these combined with the writer's experience may produce a reasonable picture.

AFRICA

Though Egypt has a bad reputation for Amoebiasis, it is surprising that only two additional cases of Amoebic Liver Abscess have been reported (Abd-Rabbo *et al.*, 1973) since the previous review. Reporting on the four additional cases in Tunisia, Haddad *et al.* (1970) comment on the rarity of the condition. Algeria produced but a single case and that was reported in Paris (Sureau *et al.*, 1968). Almost all the cases from Morocco were reported before 1926 (Elsdon–Dew, 1968). It would seem that the ill-repute of the North-African coast is not deserved. Perhaps this ill-repute was based on troops with previous service in Indo-China. It will have been noted that these countries have a dry climate, but the same applies to the Sudan, where the occurrence of a liver abscess in a patient with reversal of the viscera (Omer, 1972) implies that the condition is common in that country.

From the reports cited in Table 4.1, invasive amoebiasis is common in West Africa. The new reports from the Cameroon, particularly that of Carayon *et al.* (1969) confirm the position reported so long ago by Reichenow (1926). Wolfensburger (1968a, b), working at Kinshasa, confirmed the earlier report by Lambillon and Beheyt (1949) who also reported Amoebic Liver Abscess from Kivu.

The lack of reports from Ethiopia is not in accord with personal conversations with workers in that country. However, during a wartime sojourn of over a year in Addis Ababa, the writer did not see a single case. The reports of complications and of amoebae in unusual sites indicate that East Africa is by no means free of the condition.

The large number of reports from southern Africa are more an indication of the availability of hospitalization and the enthusiasm of the workers than of the prevalence of the disease in that area. It is of interest to note that whilst most early reports came from Durban, there is an increasing number from places with such divergent climates as Cape Town, Lourenço Marques and Johannesburg.

ASIA

Apart from those from Israel, reports from Asia Minor were scanty in both previous and present surveys. A new observation of some weight is that of Salem *et al.* (1968) in Iraq in which the only criterion was "test of cure". Here, however, personal conversations suggest that Amoebic Liver Abscess occurs in both Iraq and Iran. Pakistan shows remarkably few reports in contrast to its neighbours.

India, Sri Lanka and Bangladesh confirm the high prevalence noted in the first review, though only one group reports from Sri Lanka. Reports from Thailand reflect the enthusiasm of the Bangkok medical school.

No doubt, recent military operations have curtailed reports from Indo-China, most being of cases seen in the United States. The report from Sarawak of three undoubted cases of amoebic cervicitis by McClatchie and Sambhi (1971) indicates that, though there are no recent reports of Amoebic Liver Abscess, invasive amoebiasis is a problem in that area.

No references to Amoebic Liver Abscess have been found from the Philippines, Korea and China, though the previous review indicated a high prevalence in these areas—an impression confirmed by the observation of some 130 cases per annum in Taiwan by Tsai (1973).

NORTH AMERICA

Of extreme interest is the isolated focus in north-western Saskatchewan—an area far removed from the tropics. This has been extensively studied by a number of authors (Meerovitch and Khan, 1967; Miller *et al.*, 1968; Buchan, 1968). Epidemiological study has shown a correlation of invasive amoebiasis with density of population in the absence of adequate hygiene—factors noted elsewhere.

The northern United States shows a few cases, probably uncovered by the intensity of medical investigation in that country. The report by Juniper (1971) of cases from Arkansas is well authenticated.

Mexico is recognized as an endemic area and the flush of papers from there is a reflection of the activities of the Centro de Estudios sobre Amibiasis. Worth reading are the Supplements to *Arch. Invest. Med(Mex.)* covering a series of seminarios sponsored by the Centro.

The lack of reports from other Central American States is surprising, though the previous review revealed a similar situation. Schapiro (1956) commented on the rarity of Amoebic Liver Abscess in a zone (Honduras) with a high prevalence of the parasite, and only 50 cases were seen in 25 years at the Gorgas Hospital in Panama.

Reports from the Caribbean are similarly scanty. Cuba featured heavily in early reports of Amoebic Liver Abscess in children.

SOUTH AMERICA

Here the position is strange, the only country reporting large numbers of cases being Colombia (Bravo and Botero, 1971). A recent congress in Medéllin confirmed the situation in Colombia, and will, in due course, swell the literature.

Though there are no reports from Venezuela, it is probable from verbal accounts that invasive amoebiasis is not uncommon.

Though conditions in some parts of Brazil might be considered as likely foci of invasive amoebiasis, reports are scanty and reflect the author's personal observations. In Chile, Sapunar *et al.* (1967) state "*Es un hecho aceptado por todos los médicos clinicos que las frequencia de la amibiasis hepatica es cada menor en Santiago.*" Similarly, from the Argentine, Meeroff and Meeroff (1968) state "Acute hepatic amoebiasis is even more infrequent and has practically disappeared at present. . . . better parasitological diagnosis which has contributed to deflate the 'balloon' of a fictitious clinical problem."

EUROPE

Here most cases discovered are imported. Considered worthy of report (Meyer and Suter–Kopp, 1972) is a case which had not left Switzerland in 16 years. Unreported was an aucthonous case found in Holland by the author.

AUSTRALIA

Subsequent to the review (Sandars, 1966) of nine cases in the literature, only a report (Morris *et al.*, 1969) of a case discovered by scintigraphy has been encountered. Of extreme interest is the report by ten Seldam (1970) of the discovery of 12 well authenticated cases of Cutaneous Amoebiasis in Papua. No reports of other amoebic disease have been encountered.

From this evidence it is apparent that invasive amoebiasis does not have the same wide distribution as does the parasite, confirming the view that some other factor in addition to the parasite is responsible for the disease.

The proven endemic areas are Mexico, Colombia, East, West and southern Africa, India, Sri Lanka, Bangladesh, Thailand, Indo-China, Indonesia, the Philippines, Korea and Taiwan. Isolated foci have been noted in Papua and in northern Saskatchewan. The former may well be a manifestation of a widespread condition (Fig. 4.1).

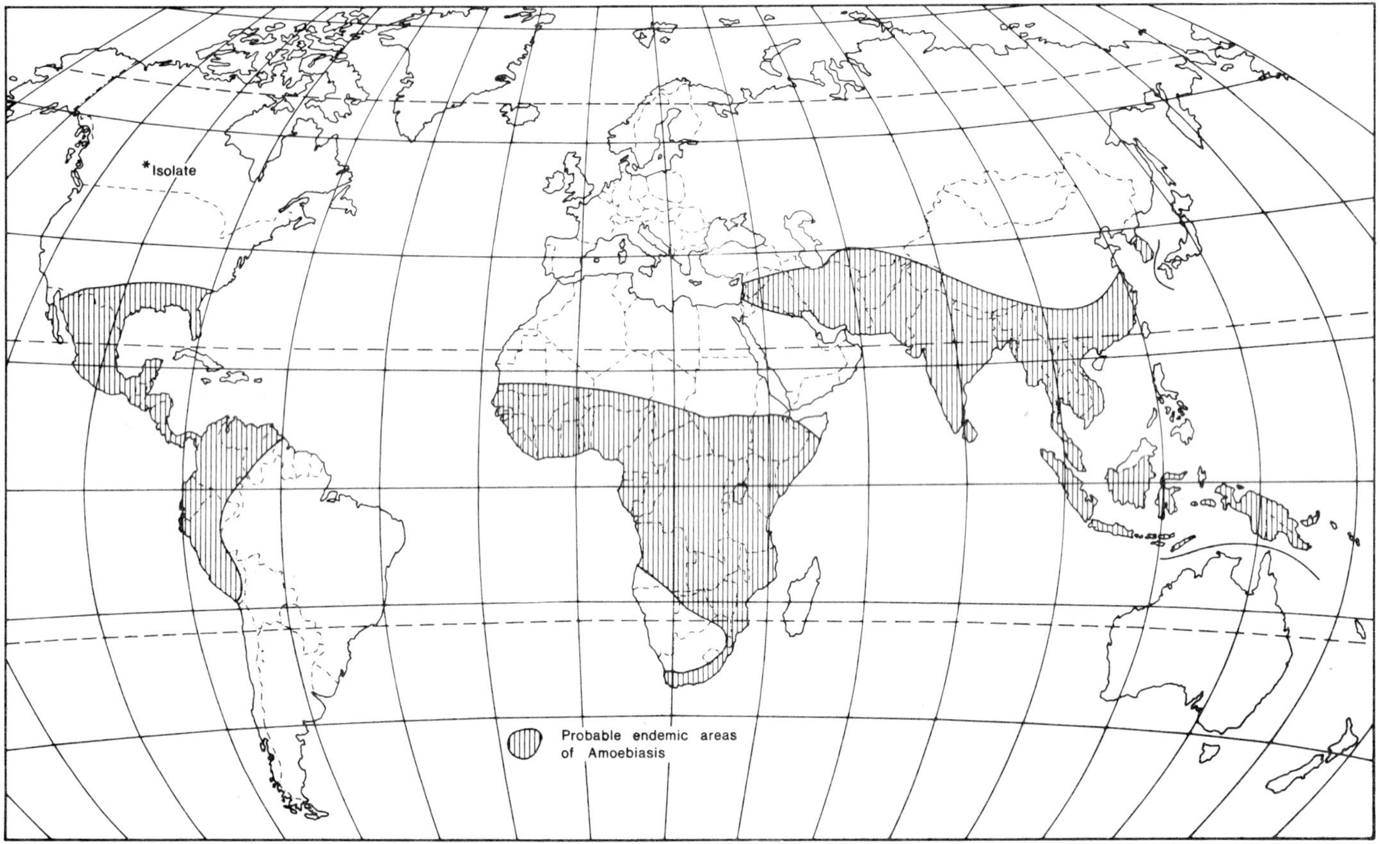

Fig. 4.1 Proven endemic areas of amoebiasis.

The use of reports of Amoebic Liver Abscess is presently the only available criterion of invasive amoebiasis, but this, too, with the advent of metronidazole, will no longer be of much value. Other criteria must be employed. Luckily an appropriate tool has appeared in serology.

Mention has been made that antibodies to amoebae only appear on invasion, and that some of these persist long after the stimulus has disappeared. Thus, the prevalence of these antibodies in a population is an indication of the impact of *E. histolytica* on that population. For example, some 9% of African blood donors in Durban show precipitins whereas less than 1% of their counterparts in Johannesburg show this evidence of invasion by amoebae. The Tswana people (who live in large villages) show a higher prevalence of antibodies to amoebae than do the neighbouring Pedi, who live in isolated kraals. As there are several ways of demonstrating such antibodies, standardization of techniques will be necessary before comparisons can be made.

In conclusion disease due to *E. histolytica* has a much narrower distribution than has the parasite.

REFERENCES

Abd-Rabbo, H., Abaza, H., Hilal, G. and Asser, L. (1973). Further therapeutic studies with low dosage metronidazole. *J. Trop. Med. Hyg.* **76**, 43–44.

Abioye, A. A. and Edington, G. M. (1972). Prevalence of amoebiasis at autopsy in Ibadan. *Trans. Roy. Soc. Trop. Med. Hyg.* **66**, 754–763.

Aikat, B. K. (1966). Amoebic liver abscess—analysis of autopsy and biopsy material. *Indian Practitioner* **21**, 747–748.

Alvarez-Alva, R. and De La Loza Saldivar, A. (1971). Frecuencià del absceso hepático amibiano en hospitales del IMSS de la Republica Mexicana. *Arch. Inv. Méd. (Méx.)* **2** (Suppl. 1), 327–332.

Ansari, Z. A., Skaria, J., Gopal, M. S., Vaish, S. K. and Rai, A. N. (1973). Situs inversus with amoebic liver abscess. *J. Trop. Med. Hyg.* **76**, 169–170.

Antani, J. and Srinivas, H. V. (1970). Clinical evaluation of metronidazole in hepatic amoebiasis. *Amer. J. Trop. Med. Hyg.* **19**, 762–766.

Archampong, E. Q. (1972). Peritonitis from amoebic liver abscess. *Brit. J. Surgery* **59**, 179–181.

Axton, J. H. M. (1972). Amoebic proctocolitis—liver abscess in a neonate. *S. Afr. Med. J.* **46**, 258–259.

Bada, J. L. (1969). Cardiomegaly associated with amoebic liver abscess. *J. Trop. Med. Hyg.* **72**, 247–252.

Baker, N. M. and Murray, J. A. (1969). Oesophageal obstruction due to an amoebic liver abscess. *Cent. Afr. J. Med.* **15**, 129–131.

Banerji, R. N., Basu, A. K. and Ayyar, R. D. (1968). Metronidazole in amoebic liver abscess. *Indian Practitioner* **21**, 737–741.

Bieler, E. U., Meyer, B. J., Jansen, C. R. and Du Toit, D. (1974). The liver in amoebic disease. A report on clinical and scintigraphic observations in 247 patients. *S. Afr. Med. J.* **48**, 308–320.

Bravo, R. C. and Botero, R. D. (1971). Absceso hepatico amibiano. Presentacion de 20 casos tratados con metronidazol. *Antioquia Medica* **21**, 103–108.

Buchan, D. J. (1968). Amoebiasis in Northwest Saskatchewan. Clinical aspects. *Can. Med. Ass. J.* **99**, 683–688.

Carayon, A., Laluque, P., Gruet, M., Fillaudeau, C. and Piquard, B. (1969). Quelques problemès encore posés par l'abcès tropical du foie. *Bull. Soc. Med. Afr. Lge. Fr.* **14**, 209–218.

Chang, S., Hildebrandt, W. and Silvis, S. E. (1974). The accidental discovery that sodium diatrizoate (hypaque) infusion will visualise amoebic abscesses on hepatic tomograms. *Amer. J. Trop. Med. Hyg.* **23**, 31–34.

Chari, M. V. and Gadiyar, B. N. (1970). A new drug (MK 910) in the therapy of intestinal and hepatic amoebiasis. *Amer. J. Trop. Med. Hyg.* **19**, 926–928.

Charmot, G. (1969). Hepatic amoebiasis. *Medicine Today* **3**, 95–98.

Chhetri, M. K., Chakravarty, N. C., Bhattacharyya, B. and Sarkar, S. K. (1968). The treatment of hepatic amoebiasis with metronidazole. *Indian Practitioner* **21**, 742–745.

Cook, A. T. (1970). Hepatic amoebiasis with pericarditis and other complications. *Proc. Roy. Soc. Med.* **63**, 1312–1313.

Cowie, R. L., Hickman, R., Saunders, S. J. and Terblanche, J. (1972). Amoebic liver disease in Cape Town. *S. Afr. Med. J.* **46**, 1917–1920.

Crawford, A. R. (1968). A case of amoebiasis in early infancy. *J. Path. Bact.* **96**, 222–226.

Cuaron, A., Gordon, F. and Landa, L. (1972). La evolución de la cintellographia en el diagnóstico del absceso hépatico amibiano. *Arch. Inv. Méd. (Méx.)* **3** (Suppl. 2), 403–414.

Danisa, K., Ilawole, C. O. O., Saliu-Lawal, M. D., Pearse, S. H. A. and Femi-Pearse, D. (1970). Metronidazole in amoebiasis. *Ghana Med. J.* **9**, 28–30.

De Groot, H. A. Van C. (1963). Amoebic vaginitis. *S. Afr. Med. J.* **37**, 246–247.

De León, A. and Perches, A. (1971). A sociacion de amibiasis invasora del higado con otros padecimentos. *Arch. Inv. Méd. (Méx.)* **2** (Suppl. 1), 387–394.

Desai, H. G., Parikh, V. J. and Antia, F. P. (1972). Obstructive jaundice with amoebic liver abscess. *Indian J. Med. Sci.* **26**, 547–551.

Devakul, K., Areekul, S. and Viravan, C. (1967). Vitamin B_{12} absorption test in amoebic liver abscess. *Ann. Trop. Med. Parasit.* **61**, 29–34.

Elsdon-Dew, R. (1968). The epidemiology of amoebiasis. *In* "Advances in Parasitology" (Ed. B. Dawes), Vol. 6, pp. 1–62. Academic Press, London and New York.

González-Montesinos, F., Lee-Ramos, A. F., Flores-Vazquez, R., Zafra-Ayala, V. and Sainz-Janini, J. M. (1972). Ensayo de profilaxis de la amibiasis invasoria del higado. *Arch. Inv. Méd. (Méx.)* **3** (Suppl. 2), 381–385.

Griffin, F. M. Jr. (1973). Failure of metronidazole to cure hepatic amoebic abscess. *New. Eng. J. Med.* **288**, 1397.

Gutiérrez-Trujillo, G. (1971). Aspectos clinicos de la amibiasis en niños II absceso hepatico. *Arch. Inv. Méd. (Méx.)* **2** (Suppl. 1), 355–360.

Haddad, N., Rebai-Colin, M. T., Potancok, R. and Khemiri, T. (1970). Abcès du foie. Difficultés due diagnostic des formes latentes et des formes compliquées. *Bull. Soc. Path. Exot.* **63**, 126–132.

Haddock, D. R. W. and Awadzi, J. K. (1970). Metronidazole (Flagyl) in invasive amoebiasis. *Ghana Med. J.* **9**, 31–34.

Harinasuta, T., Wiriyawit P., Bunnag, D. and Tejavanija, S. (1968). Clinical trial of Flagyl in amoebic liver abscess. *Indian Practitioner* **21**, 732–736.

Harinasuta, T., Wiriyawit, P., Bunnag, D. and Tejavanija, S. (1969). Clinical trial of metronidazole in amoebic liver abscess. *Medicine Today* **3**, 89–91.

Harza, D. K., Seth, H. C., Elhence, G. P., Hishore, B., Wahal, P. K., Agarwal, S. L. and Asopa, H. S. (1970). Jaundice in amoebic liver abscess. *J. Indian Med. Ass.* **55**, 244–245.

Heller, R. F., Gorbach, S. L., Tatooles, C. J., Loeb, H. S. and Rahimtoola S. H. (1972). Amoebic pericarditis. *J. Amer. Med. Ass.* **220**, 988–990.

Hernández, P. M., Camacho, M. R., Ixcapa, S. T. and Hernandez, D. M. (1969). La reaccion de immuno fluorescencia en el diagnostico de la amibiasis. *Rev. Lat. Amer. Microbiol. Parasitol.* **II**, 97–101.

Hingorani, V. and Mahapatra, L. N. (1964). Amoebiasis of vagina and cervix. *J. Int. Coll. Surg.* **42**, 662–667.

Huggins, D. (1971). Metronidazol (8823 RP) no tratamento do abscesso amebiano do figado. *Hospital (Rio de Janeiro)* **78**, 1255–1266.

Islam, N. (1967). A case of giant liver abscess. *J. Trop. Med. Hyg.* **70**, 68–73.

Jarumilinta, R., Lambert, C. R. and Imhoff, P. R. (1969). Comparative study of the effects of ambilhar and a combination of dehydroemetine and chloroquine in amoebic liver abscess. *Ann. N.Y. Acad. Sci.* **160**, 767–774.

Jinich, H. and Schnaas, F. (1971). Frecuencia del absceso hepático amibiano en clientele particular (communicacion preliminar). *Arch. Inv. Méd. (Méx.)* **2** (Suppl. 1), 333–336.

Juniper, K. Jr. (1971). Amoebiasis in the United States. *Bull. N.Y. Acad. Med.* **47**, 448–461.

Juniper, K. Jr., Worrel, C. L., Minishew, C., Roth, L. S., Cypert, H. and Lloyd, R. E. (1971). Seroepidemiology of amebiasis in Arkansas. *Arch. Inv. Méd. (Méx.)* **2** (Suppl. 1), 445–452.

Kamat, G. R., Johri, B. S., Pathak, V. P. and Tikekar, P. G. (1968). Role of liver function tests and electropheretic patterns of serum proteins in diagnosis and prognosis of amoebic liver abscess. *J. Trop. Med. Hyg.* **71**, 111–117.

Kaminsky, N. I., Singer, F. R. and Cartwright, L. B. (1968). Treatment of amoebic liver abscess with metronidazole (Flagyl). Case report of a Vietnam returnee. *Sthn Med. J.* **61**, 545–546.

Kapoor, O. P. and Joshi, V. R. (1972). Multiple amoebic liver abscesses—a study of 56 cases. *J. Trop. Med. Hyg.* **75**, 4–6.

Kapoor, O. P. and Shah, N. A. (1972). Pericardial amoebiasis following amoebic liver abscess in the left lobe. *J. Trop. Med. Hyg.* **75**, 7–10.

Kapoor, O. P., Nathwani, B. N. and Joshi, V. R. (1972). Amoebic peritonitis—a study of 73 cases. *J. Trop. Med. Hyg.* **75**, 11–15.

Khan, M. A. (1969). Metronidazole in intestinal and hepatic amoebiasis. *Medicine Today* **3**, 64–66.

Khan, A. K. and Muazzam, M. G. (1969). Treatment of amoebic liver disease with metronidazole (preliminary report). *Medicine Today* **3**, 92.

Kotcher, E., Miranda, M. and De Salgado, V. G. (1970). Correlation of clinical parasitological and serological data of individuals infected with Entamoeba histolytica. *Gastroenterology* **58**, 388–391.

Lambillon, J. and Beheyt, P. (1949). L'ambiase hepatique au Congo Belge. *Ann. Soc. Belge Med. Trop.* **29**, 306–327.

Leigh, P. G. A. (1967). An unusual case of acute amoebiasis. *S. Afr. Med. J.* **41**, 543–547.

Le Roux, B. T. (1969). Pleuropulmonary amoebiasis. *Thorax* **24**, 91–101.

Le Vine, M. A., Kahil, M. and Gyorkey, F. (1968). Amoebic abscess on the left lobe of the liver. *Sthn Med. J.* **61**, 415, 419.

Lombardo, L. and Flores-Barroeta, F. (1971). Amibiasis invasora cerebral. *Arch. Inv. Méd (Méx.)* **2** (Suppl. 1), 361–366.

Marberg, K. and Czerniak, P. (1964). Observations of isotope hepatoscanning in diagnosis and treatment of amoebic liver infection. *Ann. Intern. Med.* **60**, 66–78.

Marr, J. J. and Haff, R. C. (1971). Superinfection of an amoebic liver abscess by *Salmonella enteritidis*. *Arch. Intern. Med.* **28**, 291–294.

Massarat, S., Mitzkat, H. J., Streicher, H. J. and Joseph, K. (1968). Amöbenabzseß der leber. *Med. Klin.* **63**, 1217–1221.

Matthews, A. W., Gough, K. R., Davies, E. R., Ross, F. G. M. and Hinchliffe, A. (1973). The use of combined ultrasonic and isotope scanning in the diagnosis of amoebic liver disease. *Gut* **14**, 50–53.

McClatchie, S. and Sambhi, J. S. (1971). Amoebiasis of the cervix. *Ann. Trop. Med. Parasit.* **65**, 207–210.

Meeroff, M. and Meeroff, J. (1968). Caracteristicas clinicas de la amibiasis en el fran Buenos Aires, Argentine. *Bol. Chil. Parasit.* **23**, 131–134.

Meerovitch, E. and Khan, Z. A. (1967). A preliminary report on the serological response of amoebiasis patients from an endemic area in north western Saskatchewan. *Can. J. Publ. Hlth* **58**, 270–274.

Mendoza-Hernández, P., Reyes-Camacho, M., Trejo Ixcapa, S. and Mendez Hernandez, D. (1969). Immuno-fluorescence test in the diagnosis of amoebiasis. *Revta Lat.-Amer. Microbiol. Parasit.* **II**, 97–101.

Meyer, H. A. and Suter-Kopp, V. (1972). Ein fall von nicht-tropischem amobenabszen der leber. Bedeuting der immuno-fluorensenzenuntersuchang fur die diagnostik und der peronalen behendlung met dehydroemetine "Roche". *Schweiz. Med. Wschr.* **102**, 483–487.

Miller, M. J. and Bray, R. S. (1966). Entamoeba histolytica infections in the chimpanzee. *J. Parasit.* **52**, 386–388.

Miller, M. J., Matthews, W. H. and Moore, D. F. (1968). Amoebiasis in northern

Saskatchewan. *Can. Med. Ass. J.* **99**, 696–705.

Morris, J., Cato, J., Walker, A., Na Songkhla, S., Marion, M. and McLaughlin, A. (1969). Liver scanning in the diagnosis and management of hepatic amoebic abscess. *Med. J. Aust.* **ii**, 1301–1303.

Mortazavi, S. H., Nasr, K., Abadi, P., Barekat, R. and Hammick, J. W. (1972). Usefulness of liver scanning—a report of experience in Southern Iran. *J. Trop. Med. Hyg.* **75**, 58–61.

Munguia, H., Franco, E. and Valenzuela, P. (1966). Diagnosis of genital amoebiasis in women by the standard Papanicolaou technique. *Amer. J. Obstet. Gynec.* **94**, 181–188.

Nnorchiri, E. (1965). Observations on childhood amoebiasis in urban family units in Nigeria. *J. Trop. Med. Hyg.* **68**, 231–236.

Norcott, T. C. (1973). Experience with the *Entamoeba histolytica* fluorescent antibody test in Western Australia. *Med. J. Aust.* **ii**, 21–22.

Norwich, I. and Lieberman, B. A. (1969). Amoebiasis of the anterior abdominal wall. *S. Afr. Med. J.* **43**, 1192–1193.

Odunjo, E. O. (1969). Pathological manifestations of amoebiasis in Nigerians. *W. Afr. Med. J.* **18**, 117–120.

Ogada, T. (1967). Rupture of an amoebic liver abscess into the pericardium. *E. Afr. Med. J.* **44**, 228–229.

Omer, A. H. S. (1972). Amoebic liver abscess in situs invertus. *J. Trop. Med. Hyg.* **75**, 42–43.

Ortiz-Ortiz, L., Garmilla, C., Zamacona-Ravelo, G. and Sepulveda, B. (1973). Hipersensibilidad celular en amibiasis II estudio pacientes con absceso hepatico amibiano agudo. *Arch. Inv. Méd. (Méx.)* **4** (Suppl. 1), 191–196.

Paillet, R., Deltiel, C. and Loygue, L. (1972). Tamponnade péricardique par rupture d'abcès amibien du foie. *Bull. Soc. Path. Exot.* **65**, 83–89.

Payet, M., Sankale, M., Bresson, Y., Ancelle, J.-P., Frament, V. and Ballon, G. (1969). Etude scintigraphique de l'amibiase hepatique. *Bull. Soc. Med. Afr. Noire Lgue Fr.* **14**, 194–201.

Pedroso de Lima, J. J., Rego, A. S., Ruas, A., Antunes Dias, F. and Forjas, A. (1967). Colour scanning as an aid in the diagnosis of liver diseases. *Ann. Trop. Med. Parasit.* **61**, 360–364.

Perches, A. and De Leon, A. (1971). El tiempo do resolución centelleográfica del absceso hepático amibiana. *Arch. Inv. Méd. (Méx.)* **2** (Suppl. 1), 401–404.

Pignol, F., Delormas, P. and Coulibaly, N. (1969). Contribution a l'étude de complications pleuro-pulmonaire de l'amibiase: a propos de 14 cas considérés comme amibien, a la suite d'un traitement d'épreuve a la déhydroémétine. *Bull. Soc. Path. Exot.* **62**, 672–689.

Poltera, A. A. (1973). Pseudomalignant cutaneous amoebiasis in Uganda. *Trop. Geogr. Med.* **25**, 139–146.

Powell, S. J. (1972). Latest developments in the treatment of amoebiasis. *In* "Advances in Pharmacology and Chemotherapy" (Ed. S. Garattina *et al.*), Vol. 10, pp. 91–103. Academic Press, New York and London.

Powell, S. J. and Elsdon-Dew, R. (1971). Evaluation of metronidazole and MK 910 in invasive amoebiasis. *Amer. J. Trop. Med. Hyg.* **20**, 839–841.

Powell, S. J. and Elsdon-Dew, R. (1972). Some new metronidazole derivatives. Clinical trials in amoebic liver abscess. Amer. J. Trop. Med. Hyg. **21**, 518–520.

Powell, S. J., McLeod, I., Wilmot, A. J. and Elsdon-Dew, R. (1966). The effect of CIBA 32644-Ba in amoebic dysentery and amoebic liver abscess. *Acta Tropica* (Suppl. 9), 95–101.

Powell, S. J., Wilmot, A. J., McLeod, I. N. and Elsdon-Dew, R. (1967). A comparative trial of dehydroemetine and emetine hydrochloride in identical dosage in amoebic liver abscess. *Ann. Trop. Med. Parasit.* **61**, 26–28.

Powell, S. J., Wilmot, A. J. and Elsdon-Dew, R. (1969). The use of niridazole alone and in combination with other amoebicides in amoebic dysentery and amoebic liver abscess. *Ann. N.Y. Acad. Sci.* **160**, 749–754.

Powell, S. J., Rubidge, C. J. and Elsdon-Dew, R. (1973). Clinical trials of benzoyl metronidazole suspension in amoebic dysentery and amoebic liver abscess. *S. Afr. Med. J.* **47**, 507–508.

Powell, S. J., Sutton, J. B. and Lautre, G. (1973). Haemobilia in amoebic liver abscess. *S. Afr. Med. J.* **47**, 1555–1557.

Powell, S. J., Stewart-Wynne, E. J. and Elsdon-Dew, R. (1973). Metronidazole combined with diloxanide furoate in amoebic liver abscess. *Ann. Trop. Med. Parasit.* **67**, 367–368.

Prakash, O., Tandon, B. N., Bhalla, I., Ray, A. K. and Vinayak, V. K. (1969). Indirect haemagglutination and amoeba immobilization tests and their evaluation in intestinal and extraintestinal amebiasis. *Amer. J. Trop. Med. Hyg.* **18**, 670–675.

Ramachandran, S., Jayawardena, D. L. N. and Perumal, J. R. A. (1971). Radiological changes in hepatic amoebiasis. *Postgrad. Med. J.* **47**, 615–621.

Ramachandran, S., Sivalingham, S. and Perumal, J. R. A. (1972). Hepatic amoebiasis in Ceylon. *J. Trop. Med. Hyg.* **75**, 22–33.

Ramachandran, S., Sivalingham, S. and Perumal, J. R. A. (1973). Concepts in hepatic amoebiasis. *J. Trop. Med. Hyg.* **76**, 39–42.

Reichenow, E. (1926). Zur frage des sitzes von *Entamoeba histolytica* in darm. *Arb. Reichsgesundh Amte* **57**, 136–146.

Rowland, H. A. K. (1967). Amoebiasis in Freetown, Sierra Leone. *Trans. Roy. Soc. Trop. Med. Hyg.* **61**, 706–709.

Ruas, A. and Nunes De Almeida, R. (1967). Serum muco-protein levels in amoebic liver abscess. *Ann. Trop. Med. Parasit.* **61**, 21–25.

Ruas, A., Forjaz, A. and Jarumilinta, R. (1967). Ambilhar in fifty cases of amoebic liver abscess. *Ann. Trop. Med. Parasit.* **61**, 417–421.

Ruas, A., Forjaz, A. and Jarumilinta, R. (1969). Ambilhar in amoebic liver abscess. *Ann. N.Y. Acad. Sci.* **160**, 764–766.

Ruas, A., Ramalho Correia, M. H., Correia Do Valle, J. and Ribeiro, J. A. (1973). RO 7–0207 in amoebic liver abscess comparative study of the effects of RO 7–0207 and metronidazole. *Cent. Afr. J. Med.* **19**, 128–132.

Salako, L. A. (1967). Liver function tests in the diagnosis of hepatic amoebiasis. *J. Trop. Med. Hyg.* **70**, 19–22.

Salem, H. H., Hayatee, Z. G., Awaness, A. M. and Al-Allas, G. (1968). Oral dehydroemetine dehydrochloride in intestinal and hepatic amoebic disease. *Trans. Roy. Soc. Trop. Med. Hyg.* **62**, 406–412.

Sandars, D. F. (1966). Amoebiasis in Australia. *Med. J. Aust.* **ii**, 1073–1078.

Sankale, M., Koate, P., Diop, B., Frament, V., Ancelle, J.-P. and Wade, F. (1968). Péricardite amibienne. *Bull. Soc. Med. Afr. Noire Lgue Fr.* **13**, 982–985.

Sapunar, J., Munoz, M. A. and Castro, J. (1967). Amibiasis hepâtica abierta a los bronquios. *Bol. Chil. Parasit.* **22**, 60–65.

Saunders, S. J. (1955). Amoebic ulceration of the buttock. *S. Afr. Med. J.* **29**, 741–742.

Savanat, T. and Chaicumpa, W. (1969). Immuno-electrophoresis test for amoebiasis. *Bull. W.H.O.* **40**, 343–353.

Savanat, T., Bunnag, D., Chongsuphajaisiddhi, T. and Viriyanond, P. (1973). Skin test for amebiasis. An appraisal. *Amer. J. Trop. Med. Hyg.* **22**, 168–173.

Savanat, T., Viriyanond, P. and Nimitmongkol, N. (1973). Blast transformation of lymphocytes in amoebiasis. *Amer. J. Trop. Med. Hyg.* **22**, 705–710.

Sayed, B. A. and Amin, S. P. (1962). Entamoeba histolytica in urine. *Brit. Med. J.* **i**, 157.

Scaffidi, V. and Princi, P. (1965). Amediasi polmonare. *Giorne. Malattie Infettive Parassit.* **17**, 623–636.

Schapiro, M. M. (1956). Open surgical drainage for hepatic amoebic abscess. *Arch. Surg.* **73**, 780–789.

Schuman, B. M., Block, M. A., Eyler, W. R. and Lucille-De Sault, A. B. (1964). Liver abscess. Rose bengal I^{131} hepatic photoscan in diagnosis and management. *J. Amer. Med. Ass.* **187**, 708–711.

Scragg, J. N. and Powell, S. J. (1968). Emetine hydrochloride and dehydroemetine combined with chloroquine in the treatment of children with amoebic liver abscess. *Arch. Dis. Childh.* **43**, 121–123.

Scragg, J. N. and Powell, S. J. (1970). Metronidazole and niridazole combined with emetine in treatment of children with amoebic liver abscess. *Arch. Dis. Childh.* **45**, 193–195.

Scragg, J. N. and Powell, S. J. (1973). Metronidazole in treatment of children with amoebic liver abscess. *Arch. Dis. Childh.* **48**, 911–912.

Sen, N. C. (1949). Amoebic vaginitis. *Brit. Med. J.* **i**, 808.

Sheehy, T. W., Parmley, L. F., Jr., Johnston, G. S. and Boyce, H. W. (1968). Resolution time of an amoebic liver abscess. *Gastroenterology* **55**, 26–34.

Singh, S. K., Narang, R. K. and Jain, S. K. (1971). Amoebiasis of left lung—a case report. *Indian J. Tuberc.* **18**, 63–64.

Subramaniam, R., Madanagopalan, N., Vijayalakshmi, T. and Shantha, M. (1968). Treatment of metronidazole in extra colonic amoebiasis—a preliminary report. *Indian Practitioner* **21**, 785–791.

Sureau, B., Berrod, J. and Dziubinski, C. (1968). A propos de quatre cas recénts d'amibiase hépatique. Difficultes du diagnostic. *Bull. Soc. Path. Exot.* **61**, 579–585.

Tandon, B. N., Choudury, A. K. R., Tikara, S. K. and Wig, K. L. (1966). A study of hepatic amoebiasis by radioactive rose bengal scanning of the liver. *Amer. J. Trop. Med. Hyg.* **15**, 16–21.

ten Seldam, R. E. J. (1970). Pseudo malignant cutaneous amoebiasis. *Trop. Geog. Med.* **22**, 142–148.

Tsai, Shen Ho (1973). Therapy of amoebic liver abscess in Taiwan. *Amer. J. Trop. Med. Hyg.* **22**, 24–29.

Ullah, W., Chowdury, M. and Sarker, C. R. (1970). Intensive dosage of metronidazole in amoebiasis. *J. Pakistan Med. Ass.* **21**, 120–123.

Vakil, B. J., Mehta, A. J. and Desai, H. N. (1970). A typical manifestation of amoebic abscess of the liver. *J. Trop. Med. Hyg.* **73**, 63–67.

Van Reenen, R. M. (1972). Amoebiasis as a surgical problem. *Trans. Roy. Soc. Trop. Med. Hyg.* **66**, 540.

Viana, R. L., Rego, A. and Antunes Dias, F. A. (1974). Amoebic abscess of the liver. Scanning and selective hepatic arteriography. *S. Afr. Med. J.* **48**, 96–100.

Villegas-González, J., Naranjo-Hernandez, C., Aleman-Velazquez, P. and del Rio-Frias, F. (1971a). Amibiasis invasora certebra en el niño. *Arch. Inv. Méd. (Méx.) 2* (Suppl. 1), 313–320.

Villegas-González, J., Portilla-Aguilar, J. and Angulo-Hernandez, O. (1971b). Localizaciones de la amibiasis invasorica en ninos. *Arch. Inv. Méd. (Méx.)* **2**, (Suppl. 1), 295–306.

Wainwright, J. (1972). Amoebic hepatitis. *S. Afr. Med. J.* **46**, 1176.

Wang, L. T., Jen, G. and Cross, J. H. (1973). Establishment of Entomoeba histolytica from liver abscess in monoxenic cultures with hemaflagellates. *Amer. J. Trop. Med. Hyg.* **22**, 30–32.

Watson, C. E., Leary, P. M. and Hartley, P. S. (1970). Amoebiasis in Cape Town children. *S. Afr. Med. J.* **44**, 419–421.

Watson, R. B., Steel, R. K. and Spiegel, T. M. (1972). Amoebic pericarditis consequent to amoebic abscess of the right lobe of the liver. *Amer. J. Trop. Med. Hyg.* **21**, 889–894.

Weaver, P. S. (1967). Ruptured amoebic liver abscess leading to inferior vena cava obstruction. *Proc. Roy. Soc. Med.* **60**, 136–137.

Weber, D. M. (1971). Amoebic abscess of liver following metronidazole therapy. *J. Amer. Med. Ass.* **216**, 1339–1340.

Whittaker, L. R. (1963). Intrathoracic complications of ruptured amoebic liver abscess. *E. Afr. Med. J.* **40**, 95–104.

Wolfensberger, H. R. (1968a). Amoebiasis: Clinical trials of dehydroemetine late release tables (RO 1.9334/20) compared with parenteral dehydroemetine and niridazole. *Trans. Roy. Soc. Trop. Med. Hyg.* **62**, 831–837.

Wolfensberger, H. R. (1968b). Der amöbenabszeß der leber. *Schweiz. Med. Wschr.* **98**, 965–972.

5. Cholera

H. Jusatz

In the western world, cholera has been known as an acute intestinal infection for about 150 years. The first dissemination of Asian or Indian cholera in a severe epidemic form occurred in almost all the countries of Europe between 1831 and 1835. Since then there have been, from time to time, great cholera movements from India to Europe. Initially these movements took place overland, but later also by way of the shipping lanes, spreading across many countries and occasionally even invading North and South America. But it was not until 1883 that the German bacteriologist Robert Koch, in the course of examining the intestines of a cholera victim, succeeded in discovering the cause of the disease which claimed so many lives during successive cholera epidemics in the course of the 19th century. Koch discovered the micro-organism shaped like part of a screw or a comma, which is now referred to as the *Vibrio cholerae*.

The arrival of a single cholera-infected person in a hitherto cholera-free district is sufficient to cause an epidemic in a country. As cholera has the shortest incubation period of any infectious disease, it attacks man with such speed that the onset of grave symptoms may well occur within only a few hours.

The disease symptoms of cholera may occur on the day of infection by the cholera vibrio or else within the first 5 days of such an infection. These symptoms consist of the abrupt onset of watery bowel movements (the so-called rice-water stools) which recur with ever-increasing frequency and result in an enormous water loss from all tissues and the skin. At the same time there may be vomiting, an acidose will occur together with symptoms of shock and collapse, and body temperature will fall. Without appropriate treatment the disease symptoms continue for 3–7 days. In earlier times, untreated cholera led to death in almost 50% of all cases; nowadays, modern treatment, aimed at making good the loss of fluid, has reduced mortality to about 2%.

Although he elucidated the etiology of cholera, Koch's discovery did not clarify the epidemiology and ecology of the disease. These are characterized by his own words on infectious diseases which, in his view

> are never created by dirt, refuse etc., nor by the sum of factors which have usually been referred to collectively as "poor social conditions" or climatic influences, but surely by the transference of their specific germs, the increase and distribution of which can, however, be favoured by the aforementioned influences.

Here are to be found the great tasks of medical geography; namely to describe and evaluate those factors which *favour* the outbreak of a new cholera epidemic and migration from continent to continent.

Asian or Indian cholera originates in India or, in a wider sense, South Asia. Prior to its migrations, it was completely unknown in Europe and America. In Asia cholera has the character of a nesting disease, i.e. it is endemic in an area in which it has already been known over a very long period and can be considered "at home". Today one speaks of a "natural focus".

Since the beginning of the 19th century, this focus has been located in the delta of the rivers Ganges and Brahmaputra as well as in the delta of the Irrawaddy. With the exception of the present migration, all earlier ones originated from these endemic foci.

To this day it has not been possible to say why the disease, from time to time and at irregular intervals, leaves its home in the Ganges and Brahmaputra valleys and moves from country to country and from one continent to another. These widespread epidemics, which last for several years at a time and cover European, and occasionally African and American countries, are characterized as pandemics. Eight pandemics have so far been recorded, six in the 19th century and two in the present century.

Asian cholera was present in Europe and the U.S.S.R. during the first quarter of the 20th century, but from 1923 to 1943 Europe was free of the disease. The cases of cholera which German and Austrian physicians found among Russian prisoners during the Second World War and among the civilian population of the Ukraine represented an outlier of the then pandemic movement of cholera from India westwards which began in the 1930s. The outbreak in Egypt in 1947 which resulted in 20 000 deaths was a western outlier of this same pandemic of cholera. There were no further advances from India to the west once this pandemic, the seventh, had run its course. Following this pandemic, the disease displayed a regressive tendency in India during the 1950s. This latter pandemic has been vividly presented in cartographic form by Jusatz (1940). The more recent movement of cholera westwards which began in 1961—now regarded as the eighth pandemic (Jusatz, 1973)—is considered later.

Several attempts have been made to explain these quasi-periodic appearances (such as Tchijewski's statements on the influence of sun-spot periods), but it has to be admitted that to date nothing is known either about an inner cause or an external "triggering" to account for such pandemic spreads of cholera.

Allowing for the possibility that cholera in its epidemic form has occurred in India for centuries, as has been supposed by MacNamara (1876) and other researchers, the beginnings of European cholera research relate unquestionably to the fact that cholera did not extend beyond the borders of India and advance to the west via the Khyber Pass until 1816. The movement continued only very slowly *overland* thereafter, not reaching Central-European countries and Britain until 1831.

In retrospect, it is possible to distinguish two further phases in cholera migrations which increased the speed of movement from South Asia to other countries and continents. Since 1865 cholera has moved by *sea* and from that year pilgrims, making their way to and from Mecca in particular, have carried cholera far and wide. A third phase became evident during the course of the present, or eighth, pandemic when *air* transport of infected passengers provided a particularly fast mode of transmission of cholera germs from infected areas to cholera-free areas in the space of hours (Fig. 5.1).

Various cartographic presentations of the routes taken by cholera during the course of pandemics in the 19th and 20th centuries have been attempted, but they have failed to take into account the decisive

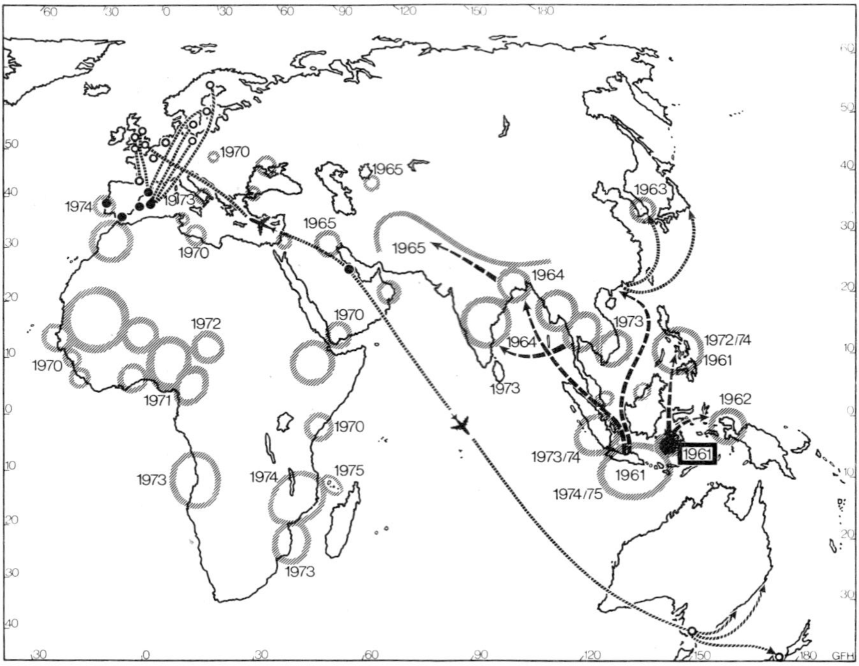

Fig. 5.1 Cholera, 1961–75.

geo-ecological conditions which led to the penetration and establishment of the cholera germ in surroundings alien to it and outside its traditional endemic area in South Asia. Even so, old maps of cholera pandemics in the last century provide many indications of geo-factors in the environment which play a role *favourable* to the advance of cholera into a new territory. In the same way when considering those areas which have remained free from cholera epidemics, it becomes possible to draw conclusions concerning factors which act in a *negative* way. Geo medical analyses of the course of previous cholera pandemics can thus throw light on several favourable, as well as unfavourable, geo factors.

There is little doubt but that *water* is the one geo factor which must be considered as the basis of life, and beyond that as the most frequent transport medium of the cholera vibrios outside the human body. Water is the prerequisite for any diffusion of a cholera infection. Observation of previous epidemics does, however, permit the conclusion that the behaviour of cholera germs varies in its

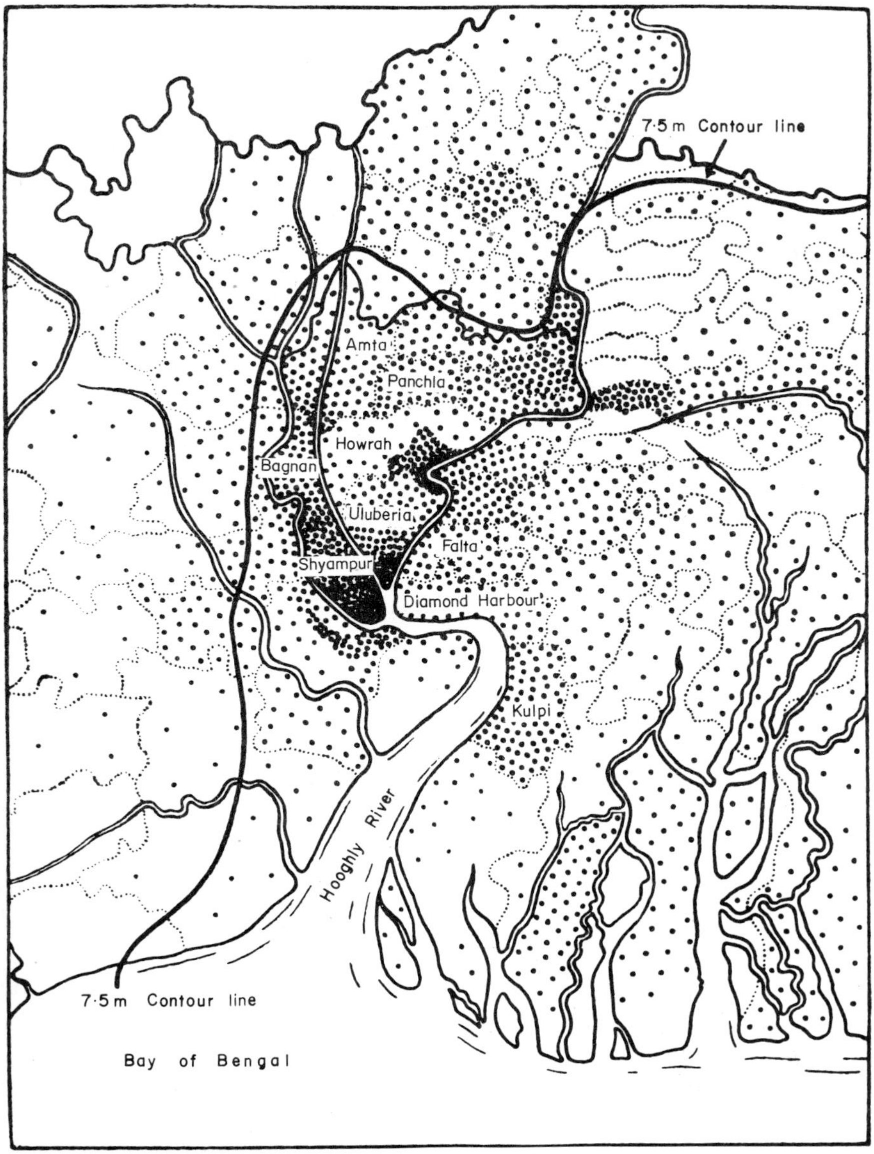

Fig. 5.2 Deltas of the Ganges, Brahmaputra and Irawaddy—examples of areas of "sluggishly-flowing waters" and of cholera endemicity (Krebs, 1936).

relationship to the differing qualities of water as, for example, with drinking water or river water.

In India, for instance, the type of water supply available to the population in the various parts is of great significance in relation to their degree of risk to cholera. It is necessary therefore to analyse the course of epidemics in India by way of correlations between areas of differing water supply (i.e.. wells, tanks or canals) and the number of communities within a district threatened by a cholera epidemic. Ernst Rodenwaldt (1961) considered this to be one of the geomedical causes for the "nesting" of a cholera germ in a region. He wrote: "Endemicity is possible only in areas of stagnating or sluggishly-flowing waters; such areas are plains which are frequently flooded by adjacent rivers and situated at less than 100m above sea-level." The German geographer, Norbert Krebs, described such areas as "the battleground between stagnant rivers and strong tides where salt-water lakes and freshwater swamps mingle." Such a situation occurs in the deltas of the Ganges and Brahmaputra and along the Irrawaddy (Fig. 5.2).

Why is it that the great ports at the mouths of East Asian rivers experience epidemic outbreaks, followed possibly by years or even decades of quiessence, though never by endemic persistence? The explanation is that these ports are not situated in deltas but on estuaries which are subject daily to the brisk movements which accompany the rise and fall of the tide. These rivers enter the sea along drowned valleys between Further India, Java, Sumatra and Borneo. These drowned valleys, once dry land, were flooded when the ice of the last Ice Age melted. The introduction of cholera into these estuarine areas can cause epidemics among the concentrated population, yet no endemicity will occur.

Rodenwaldt (1967), in his geomedical investigations into the course of earlier cholera epidemics, drew attention to another important geo-ecological factor which may explain the differing importance of the waterways (rivers and canals). It relates to the *velocity of the rivers*.

In short, one rule applies. There is a negative correlation between the possibility of persistent cholera and the stream velocity of the waters. The disease gradient is orientated upslope.

In the course of examining the progress of cholera from the mouth to the upper reaches of the Ganges and Jumna, it becomes evident that the density of the epidemic decreases on attaining each successively higher grade of the terrain. Serious outbreaks only occur in places where the water is deliberately made to stagnate, as in Hardwar, in order to allow the crowds of pilgrims to bathe in the holy water.

In its middle course, the so-called "Sack of Assam", the Brahmaputra has but a small gradient for hundreds of kilometres. Braided stretches of river and the formation of stagnant pools result from this. Assam always becomes an area in which cholera breaks out when it arrives there from the coastal delta of the Ganges and Brahmaputra. (Rodenwaldt, 1967).

The gradients of the larger rivers are shown in Fig. 5.3. Most striking is the slowing down of the speed of flow of the Jumna and Ganges between Delhi (280 m above sea-level) and Allahabad (180 m above sea-level). As much as 1000 km from its mouth the Ganges flows at a height of no more than 96 m and, at Bagalpur, it is only 40 m above sea-level.

A third geo-factor, *the quality of water*, also appears to play a role in the endemicity of cholera. This relates more particularly to acidity or alkalinity of the water. From the microbiological viewpoint proof has existed for a long time that cholera vibrios multiply better and remain capable of infecting for a longer time in an alkaline as opposed to an acid milieu. Indian geographers have drawn attention to the high degree of soil and water alkalinity in the Ganges delta. In Bangladesh, it has been established that, in tanks used for the supply of drinking water, algal infestation greatly increases the alkalinity of stagnant water, thereby influencing favourably the living and breeding conditions of cholera vibrios. On the other hand, waters which are known to be especially acid (e.g. the tributaries of the Amazon joining the mainstream from the north) are to be regarded as being negatively correlated.

Hydrological environmental conditions are of great significance in accounting for the movement and distribution of cholera in different geographical areas. Deserts and areas poor in water supply have been largely circumvented by the cholera migrations. Again, settlements in high mountain regions never seem to attract cholera.

The *influence of the seasons* is another factor in any geo-ecological analysis of cholera epidemics. It has long been known that cholera epidemics in Europe collapse at the onset of winter. In the web of ecological conditions cold, snow and frost evidently act as inhibiting factors for the cholera vibrios.

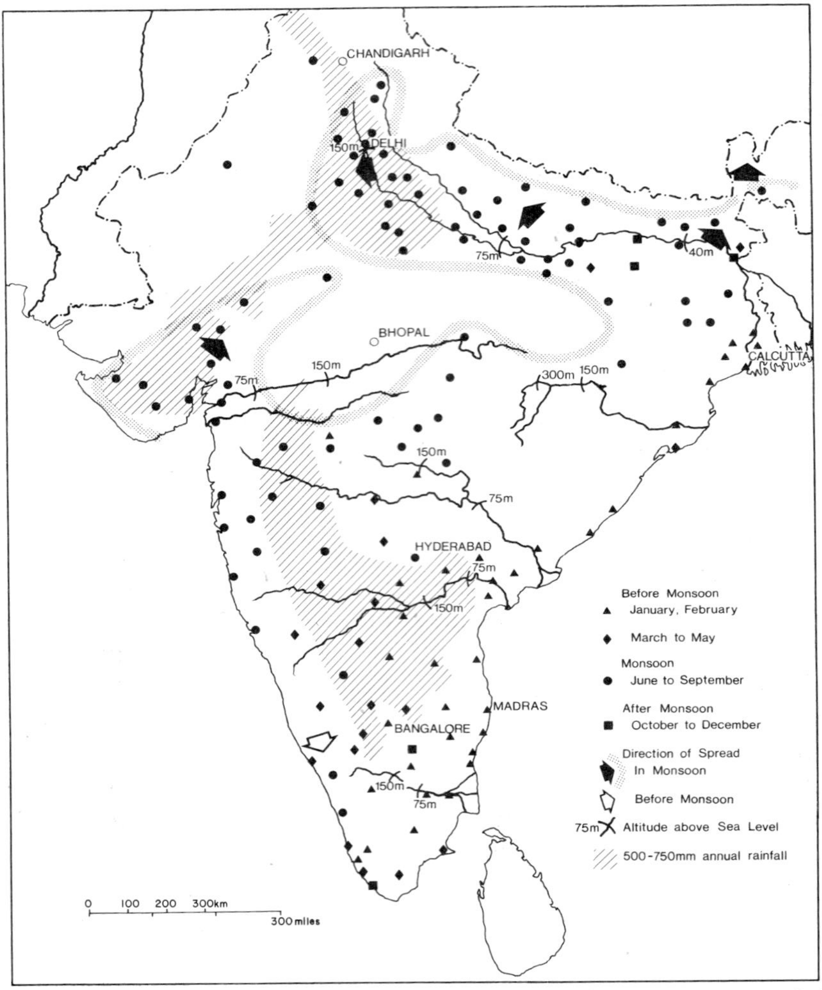

Fig. 5.3 Cholera in India, 1965 giving the months of commencement of the epidemic outbreak (Adapted from Bhatty, 1967).

In India, cholera appears to have a distinctly seasonal character and it is possible to establish a seasonal peak, at least in statistical terms. In the case of the 1962–1966 epidemic, there was a seasonal peak in July coinciding with the peak of monthly precipitation aggregates (Bhatty, 1967) (Fig. 5.4). This peak does not occur every year, nor in every state within India, since the climatic conditions vary appreciably from year to year and throughout the country.

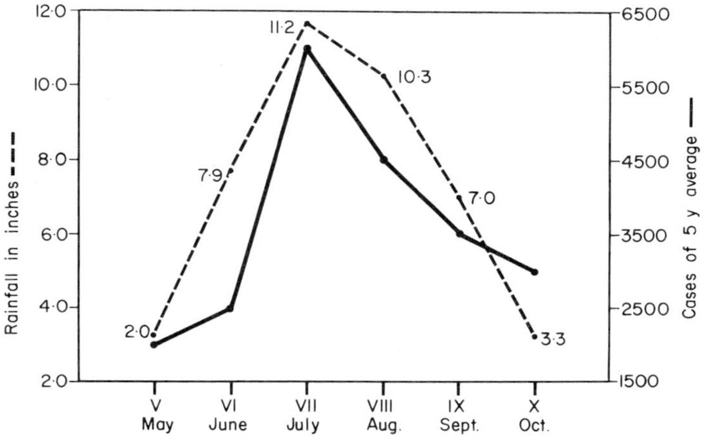

Fig. 5.4 Seasonal factors influencing cholera epidemics in India (Bhatty, 1967).

Even the influence of the monsoon on the distribution of cholera is not the same throughout India since its time of onset and strength varies in the different parts. Whereas in Calcutta the increased incidence of cholera infections takes place in the period *before* the onset of the annual monsoon, the Ganges valley experiences the same phenomenon *during* the monsoon months; epidemics progress more or less from south-east to north-west, as does the monsoon over the same period of time (Fig. 5.3).

Reviewing the course of the great epidemics which have moved across India during the last 150 years and which have developed into eight severe pandemics, one further predisposing factor may be recognized, viz. the *mass movements of people*. Such movements embrace not only military events and movements of refugees but also peaceful mass gatherings and massive religious pilgrimages. In India, this applies particularly to the great annual Hindu and Moslem religious festivals and pilgrimages to ancient holy places. Religious festivals are arranged at intervals of decades and attended by millions of people. Up to the time of the Second World War, these huge festivals often contributed to the epidemic distribution of cholera. Compulsory vaccination of pilgrims and the improvement of the once exceedingly primitive hygienic arrangements for waste disposal have so changed the situation that nowadays there is rarely any further cholera spread following the great festivals or fairs.

The history of cholera as a pandemic infectious disease capable of penetrating all continents has experienced a sudden change during the present century. The explanation of this change might, in retrospect, possibly help explain the mystery of the origins of previous pandemics. The classic Vibrio cholerae has not been involved in the post 1961 migration but rather a biological variant. This is a biotype which can be precisely differentiated microbiologically from the classical Vibrio cholerae. It is known as Vibrio cholerae El Tor and has been recorded in all countries invaded by the eighth pandemic.

The new variant, cholera El Tor, is by no means a new type thrown suddenly into existence by mutation. It was first discovered in 1905 by F. Gotschlich whilst attending pilgrims destined for Mecca at the El Tor quarantine-station on the Sinai Peninsula. The name of the quarantine station was given to this biotype. For decades it was held to be apathogenic since the pilgrims in whom it was found did not fall ill. Even when the Dutch scientist Van Loghem later found this type among the population of a circumscribed area of South Celebes (Sulawesi), albeit with a lower lethality rate than in the case of genuine cholera, this evidence was interpreted as a localized occurrence. Several further epidemics followed on Celebes in which the El Tor vibrio was implicated.

It was not until July 1961 that the El Tor vibrio set out on its great migration, which has now, over the course of some 15 years, extended into Europe and Africa. First disseminated by coastal migration from Sulawesi to the Indonesian islands, it moved thence to the South-Asian mainland. Since then the El Tor vibrio has replaced the classical Vibrio cholerae, the latter having remained in its original endemic home in the delta of the Ganges and Brahmaputra. Fig. 5.5 is a cartographical representation by Bhatty (1967) of the location of the first findings of the El Tor biotype.

Students of medical geography are now presented with the important task of following the course of this, the eighth pandemic of cholera, and producing maps to show its relevant status of spread in the world. This has already been done for the 19th century pandemics by means of cholera maps for individual European countries, and also for the World at large. The maps of the epidemic of 1863–68 which appear in the "World Atlas of Epidemic Diseases" of the Heidelberg Academy of Sciences are an impressive example (Rodenwaldt, 1961).

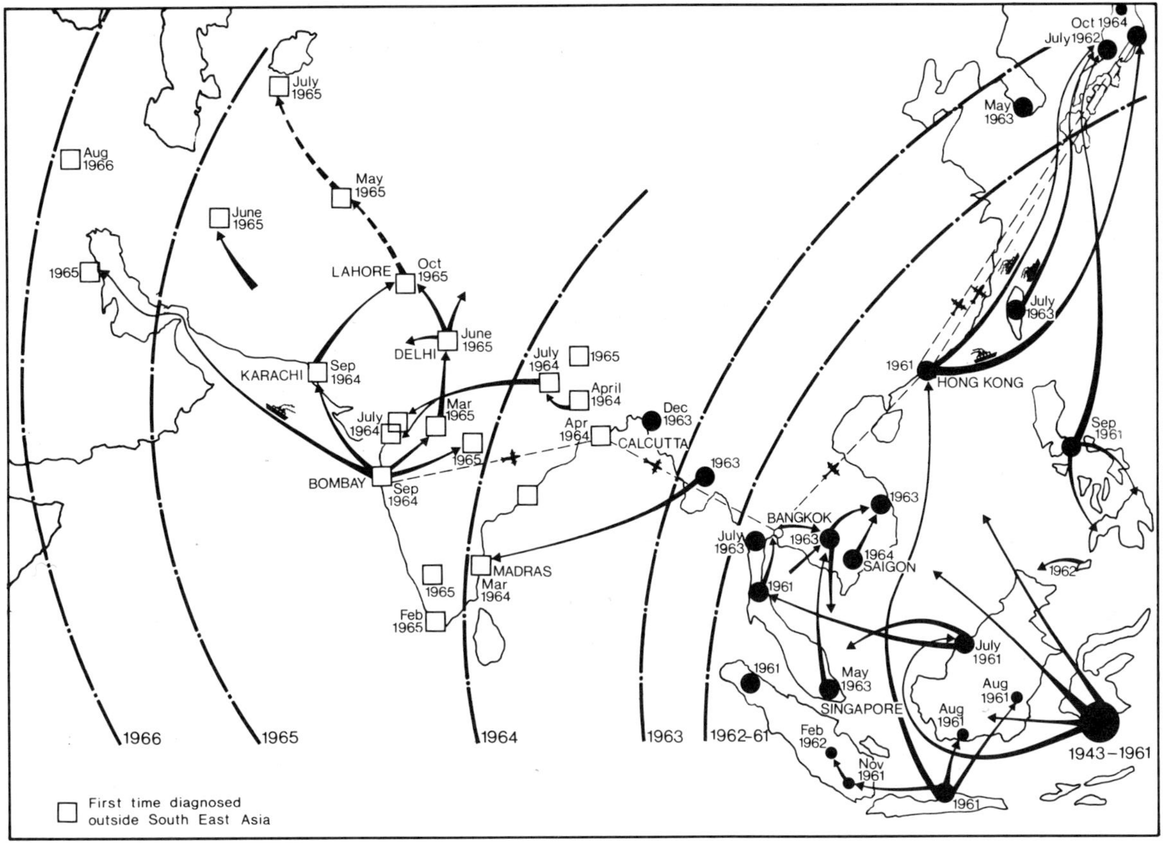

Fig. 5.5 Cholera El Tor pandemic after 1961 (Bhatty, 1967).

Compared with earlier outbreaks certain differences must be noted in the case of the current or eighth pandemic. These differences may influence its future course. Observations to date reveal that the biotype El Tor exerts a much stronger resistance against outside influences than the classical Vibrio cholerae. It remains longer on infected foodstuffs and also in well water and faeces. In addition, because cholerae El Tor excrete over a longer period of time, the excretion of vibrios by infected persons persists over a longer period of time than in the case of classical cholera. For El Tor vibrios the longest recorded period of excretions is that of a woman in the Philippines, involving "Cholera dolores"; she has continued for 8 or more years.

These particular qualities of the cholera vibrio El Tor make it seem probable that cholera may be transported by air to areas which hitherto have been free from the disease but where unhygienic conditions may now allow it to establish itself. Importation by air has to be assumed in the case of the sudden cholera outbreak on the coast of West Africa in 1970. The further dissemination of this West African epidemic was the result of movements of population, particularly by fishermen moving from country to country along the Guinea coast countries to Cameroon. The present pandemic has also extended to Europe: in 1970 there was a locally restricted increase in the number of El Tor cases in eastern Slovakia, a more extensive epidemic in Naples and Bari in southern Italy (1973), and also in Portugal (1974).

Although until now it has not been possible to predict the end of a pandemic, the course followed by all previous pandemics suggests that, after varying periods of epidemic occurrence outside its South Asian foci, no further diffusion of cholera into neighbouring and formerly free countries takes place. It would appear that the virulence of the germs diminishes during the course of a pandemic and the germs themselves seemingly withdraw to their countries of origin. Even in these endemic foci, the annual number of new infections eventually attains a low point and the pandemic ends.

REFERENCES

Barua, Dhiman and Burrows, W. (1974). "Cholera". W. B. Saunders, Philadelphia, London and Toronto.

Bhatty, M. A. (1967). Cholera in South Asia 1961–1966. *In* Series of Theses, South Asia Institute, Heidelberg University, No. 7.

Jusatz, H. J. (1940). Die gegenwaertige Verbreitung der indischen Cholera in der Welt. *Die Medizinische Welt* **14**, 994–996.

Jusatz, H. J. (1968). Die epidemische Verbreitung der Cholera in Suedasien in der Gegenwart. *In* "Yearbook of the South-Asia Institute, Heidelberg University 1967/68", pp. 43–52. Harrassowitz, Wiesbaden.

Jusatz, H. J. (1973). Historical-geographical survey of the 8th pandemic of cholera asiatica. *9th International Congress of Tropical Medicine and Malaria, Athens, Abstracts of Communications* **11**, 19.

Krebs, N. (1936). "Vorderindien und Ceylon". Stuttgart.

MacNamara, C. (1876). "A History of Asiatic Cholera". London.

Pollitzer, R. (1959). "Cholera". W.H.O. Monogr. Ser. No. 43.

Rodenwaldt, E. (1961). The Cholera Epidemic, 1863–1868. *In* "World Atlas of Epidemic Diseases" (Welt-Seuchen-Atlas) (Eds E. Rodenwaldt and H. J. Jusatz), Part I, 13–14. Falk, Hamburg.

Rodenwaldt, E. (1961). Cholera in Asia, 1931–1955. *In* "World Atlas of Epidemic Diseases" (Welt-Seuchen-Atlas) (Eds E. Rodenwaldt and H. J. Jusatz), Part III, 4–6. Falk, Hamburg.

Rodenwaldt, E. (1967). Die Seuchenzüge der Cholera im 19. Jahrhundert. *In* " Der Arzt und der Kranke in der Gesellschaft des 19. Jahrhunderts" (Eds. W. Artelt and W. Ruegg), pp. 201–208. Enke, Stuttgart.

Stock, R. F. (1976). Cholera in Africa. *Int. Afric. Inst., African Environment Special Report* **3**, 1–127. London.

6. Diarrhoeal Diseases

G. Sangster

Although diarrhoea is an important and frequent indicator of disease of the alimentary tract, the cause may lie elsewhere. For example, it can be an expression of disturbed function due to abnormal hormonal influences or a neurological disorder. Thus a wide range of disease is implied by the title of this chapter but the scope will be limited to primary, and mainly infective conditions of the gut. Several well known examples in this category are dealt with elsewhere in this volume—cholera, amoebic dysentery and intestinal schistosomiasis. These by their singular nature and peculiar areal distributions stand out as special problems and, by the same token, lend themselves more easily to detailed study than the several conditions covered in this chapter which are world wide in distribution, extremely common and often trivial. In many countries, they are accepted as inevitable occurrences by the native populations in the way of life and expected by visitors. Nevertheless they remain a significant cause of death, especially in the young and old. It has been estimated that in India about 1½ million infants and young children die yearly as a result of diarrhoeal diseases, excluding cholera.

For several reasons the full extent of the problem is not known with any accuracy. The exact diagnosis may not be available through lack of laboratory facilities. In many countries, if not all, notification is by no means reliable, even when encouraged, with the result that sometimes conclusions from the available data can be only tentative. The International Classification of Diseases is not entirely blameless in this respect. Codification, except when a precise diagnosis can be

	1956	1961	1968		1956	1961	1968
Australia	4.4	4.1	2.7	Israel	18.3	6.5	3.9
Belgium	3.6	3.2	2.5	Italy	16.8	11.6	8.2
Ceylon	41.8	41.5	41.7	Japan	29.0	19.0	5.5
China (Taiwan)	99.2	62.0	17.3	Netherlands	2.5	3.1	3.3
Dominican Rep.	96.3	82.8	87.7	Poland	28.7	13.4	4.1
Egypt (U.A.R.)	685.1	632.8	577.9	Spain	23.4	14.3	9.9
Germany	2.8	3.4	3.5	U.K.	4.6	5.2	4.5
Guatemala	253.7	220.5	234.2	U.S.A.	4.5	4.3	1.5

Table 6.1 Gastritis, duodenitis, enteritis and colitis: death rates per 100 000 population in selected countries, 1956, 1961 and 1968 (W.H.O. data—ICD 7th revision).

given, leaves some freedom of choice and individual and national preferences for certain diagnostic terms may influence classification. Nevertheless, with these reservations, it can be safely said that in the more advanced countries a reasonably clear picture of the basic endemic situation with regard to intestinal infections is available continuously, albeit retrospectively. This is sharpened when special incidents occur. In such situations, attention is drawn to the problem in some of the underdeveloped countries, later rather than sooner. Much effort by national agencies, e.g. laboratory services, is directed towards an improvement in this state of affairs but, while internationally the W.H.O. has achieved success in the control of many important diseases, leading to containment if not eradication, the grumbling problem of intestinal infection remains to be solved in nearly all countries.

Historically diarrhoeal diseases have been a prominent issue in medical and other writings since ancient times when the theories of disease were based on the interaction between "humours" in the individual and common elemental forces in his environment. Endemic and epidemic diseases were appreciated as was the infective nature of some disorders, leading to the practice of quarantine and isolation, both useful measures in certain situations today. The association of putrifaction, human and animal, with the acquisition and spread of infection was considered important, particularly in times of war when such material abounded. Even noxious smells such as arise from drains were regarded as vehicles of infection until less than 100 years ago. Indeed, up to the late 19th century, emanations from the ground (miasmas) were the accepted cause—a view not far removed from the theories of 2000 years earlier when physicians and philosophers were pre-occupied with the elements and physical features (*On Airs, Waters and Places* by Hippocrates). With modification and modernization these are still pertinent to the study of disease. In the case of diarrhoeal diseases, these and other environmental factors play an important role.

CLINICAL AND PATHOLOGICAL FEATURES

To assist the non-medical reader, the following section provides some information on the definition of terms and refers to some clinical and pathological features. In the first instance, diarrhoeal diseases may be considered under two headings—infective and non-infective.

Infective	Non-Infective
Bacteria	
Staphylococcus aureus	Sprue (tropical)
Clostridium welchii	Diverticulosis (-itis)
Escherichia coli	Ulcerative Colitis
Shigellae (*Sh. shigae*, *flexneri*, *sonnei*, etc.)	Crohn's Disease
Salmonellae incl. *S. typhi*, *S. paratyphi* A, B and C	Chemicals
Vibrios	
B. cereus	
Yersinia enterocolitica	
Viruses (Coxsackie, Echovirus, Adenovirus, Rotavirus)	
Protozoa (*Giardia lamblia*, *Balantidium coli*)	

Table 6.2 Diarrhoeal diseases: some causes.

In the first group, which is numerically superior, acute and temporary illness is usual, while in the second, the course may be more prolonged with a tendency to exacerbations or relapses. The term "food-poisoning" is applied loosely to the infective group, especially in the absence of a proven diagnosis such as typhoid fever, bacillary dysentery, etc. Undoubtedly, most of the infective diseases are or can be food borne, but many authorities prefer to reserve the designation "food-poisoning" to those caused by a toxin, bacterial or chemical (Table 6.2).

In both groups diarrhoea of variable degree and character is the principal feature. Vomiting and abdominal pain are frequent accompaniments. When vomiting occurs alone and the patient is fortunate enough to be spared further developments, then a diagnosis of "gastritis" or "duodenitis" is likely to be made—strictly not a diarrhoeal disease. The term "gastroenteritis", which implies involvement of the upper reaches of the gut, is applied when there is diarrhoea and vomiting—or without vomiting, "enteritis". If the lower part of the intestine (colon) is affected, "colitis" (or "enterocolitis") is used. This regional localization may infer an infection of a certain type but unfortunately many organisms do not confine themselves to a particular area in all cases and the position is not clear cut. Although they reside in the intestine (excluding the varieties acting through a preformed toxin), some have a tendency to invade the blood stream (bacteraemia or septicaemia), and thus other organs. This is exemplified by certain members of the salmonella group (*S. typhi*, *S. paratyphi* A, B and C) which regularly enter the blood stream and a characteristic illness follows, typhoid or paratyphoid fever, while the other members normally cause a gastroenteritic illness only. It should be noted that in the early stages of typhoid fever constipation is more likely than diarrhoea. On the other hand, in bacillary dysentery, bacteraemia is rare and the symptoms are produced by the local effect of toxins on the colon. Clostridia (e.g. *Cl. welchii*) act in a similar fashion with additional effects from absorption of toxin but the toxin of one member of this group, *Cl. botulinus*, acts on the nervous system, having little effect on the gut. Thus in botulism, highly lethal but fortunately rare, diarrhoea is only an occasional occurrence.

The most common type of bacterial food-poisoning results from the ingestion of preformed heat stable toxin produced by staphylococci which are common organisms on the skin and in the nose. In this case, bacteriological confirmation may be lacking as the organism may have been destroyed (e.g. by cooking) and cannot be isolated from the sufferer. In a much less common but more serious form of infection with this organism, colonization of the bowel does occur and the organism is recoverable from the faeces. Among the others listed in Table 6.2, none of which constitute serious global problems at present, are the non-cholera, vibrios-organisms almost identical to the prototype, *V. cholerae* (Chapter 5), but producing a milder gastroenteritis as a rule.

In general, the exact diagnosis depends on the laboratory—on the isolation of the organism from faeces and in some instances from blood, which may also furnish confirmatory evidence from specific antibody tests. Thus the availability and quality of such a service must affect the clarity of the global picture as well as the success of control measures. During the past 25 years there has been a steady improvement in this respect and advances in treatment, improved fluid and electrolyte replacement, together with antibiotics, have contributed in no small measure to a general reduction in mortality.

Much less is known of the endemiology of most of the non-infective diarrhoeas which have a varied and indefinite etiology. Indeed, it is only in recent times that interest in this aspect has been aroused, with the exception of tropical sprue.

In this condition, anaemia and other changes due to malabsorption of essential nutrients accompanies diarrhoea. It appears widely in the tropics and occasionally in the subtropics, where it affects newcomers after a variable time, and not infrequently after the person has left the area. The indigenous population may be affected also. Changes in diet play some part in the causation and although no evidence of infection is found, some believe that it is a post-infective state. Seasonal variations occur and it has a possible connection with "Hill Diarrhoea".

On the other hand, ulcerative colitis, which may simulate the dysenteries, is not a disease of tropical climates, as far as is known, but is found mainly in temperate zones, with a high incidence in the U.S.A. and Europe. It may occur at any age but most commonly in young adults. The former sex difference in favour of females is now less marked. Many features suggest that it is an auto-immune process with the colon as the target organ and again a possible association with diet (e.g. milk) has been observed in some patients. In some, cancer of the colon may be a late sequel.

The cause of Crohn's disease (regional ileitis) remains a mystery. Certain similarities to ulcerative colitis exist and the areal distribution is roughly the same.

Diverticulosis and its complications, which affects older adults in advanced countries, is much more common than the aforementioned diseases. In this, the nature of the diet has considerable bearing on the causation—the use of refined foods with low fibre content (roughage), resulting in slow transit times and increased pressure from excessive gas production, contributes to abnormal bowel function. Hence in areas such as Africa, India and most of Asia where coarser foods (which lead to bulkier motions) are used, this condition is rare. According to Painter, the incidence in Scotland is 80 times greater than in Fiji, Singapore and Nigeria. Further evidence confirming an environmental influence is that the rate is much higher in Americans (and Hawaiians) of Japanese stock than in the native Japanese. Also, in Americans of African descent, the incidence now equals that in whites.

Prominent amongst the inorganic chemicals which cause vomiting and diarrhoea are arsenic, antimony, cadmium, copper, zinc and sodium fluoride. While drinking water may contain excessive amounts from natural sources, probably a greater risk of poisoning arises from metal vessels and utensils, made from or containing as impurities these elements which are released by interaction with their contents. Alternatively they may be ingested with food (e.g. animal products and fish) or fruit sprayed for insecticidal purposes. Indeed, the widespread use of pesticides in recent times has complicated the field of toxicology as the effects of the remains of more sophisticated chlorinated hydrocarbons and organophospho-compounds are unfolded, apart from their disturbance of the ecological pattern.

CAUSAL RELATIONSHIPS

Several factors influence the occurrence and behaviour of both groups of disease in a particular case, some more than others. In variable combinations they prepare the way for, assist and perhaps perpetuate the disease process. Also, in the case of infections, the extent of this reaction is dependent on the dose and virulence of the offending organism and the resistance of the host.

As with other infections, the entry of a "new" bowel infection into a community is likely to cause considerable trouble, at least for a time. In other areas where the same organism is endemic, a less serious illness may result, partly through adaptation of the organism and partly from the result of repeated exposure in the individual. However, few intestinal infections give rise to a significant and lasting immunity in which case repeated attacks are common. In some countries with large reservoirs of infection, an almost healthy carrier state develops, thereby perpetuating or increasing the pool.

Age, sex and race

Intestinal infections know no barrier but tend to affect the very young and old most seriously with the result that death rates are highest in these age groups. Direct relationships with race are not very obvious, but one example may be quoted, viz. the strong association of bone involvement (osteitis) by salmonella organisms in sufferers from sickle cell anaemia (due to an abnormal haemoglobin-S) which is distributed genetically throughout Central Africa and parts of the western hemisphere.

Other diseases

The presence of other diseases, although more important to the individual, has some bearing on the behaviour of bowel infections in a community. They may be regarded as factors lowering the resistance of a population and operate adversely in a wide range of infections. Notable examples are avitaminosis and kwashiorkor, both dietary deficiencies seen in their most florid state in the poorer countries.

Almost any abnormality of the gut assists the establishment of infection and may favour its persistence, i.e. a carrier state may ensue. Since the acid barrier of the stomach is an important defence against infection, the absence of effective gastric juice either by non-production (achlorhydria) or by removal of the stomach by operation (gastrectomy) renders the individual more liable to infection with intestinal pathogens.

Socio-cultural

Infants are naturally deficient in respect of the acid barrier of the stomach. They are therefore at greater risk than older children and adults, unless protected by relatively sterile feeds. Ideally such feeds should be of human milk since it provides additional more positive benefits. Indeed, under normal circumstances, the incidence of all bowel infections is extremely low in breast-fed infants. The practice of breast feeding varies widely throughout the world but fortunately infants in the less sophisticated societies tend to receive this protection longer than their counterparts elsewhere. This benefit, however, may be cancelled by other unfavourable factors.

Apart from the adequacy of diet, the preparation, storage and nature of food, governed as they are by local and national habits, may have a considerable influence on the transmission of infection. Such considerations also feature significantly in the aetiology of several of the non-infective conditions. Opportunities for infection occur during the handling and preparation of food in all countries. Where facilities for good hygiene are lacking, these risks are greater. Inadequate preservation leaves a suitable medium for multiplication of organisms and excessive attempts at preservation, often for cosmetic reasons, may lead to chemical food poisoning which may result from contamination during storage, even from the containers themselves. The use of unsuitable utensils and equipment, for example, in amateur wine making, may be dangerous. It is significant that in recent times nearly all incidents of botulism have been traced to defective preservation of foods in the home.

While the ever increasing use of canned products may play a part in the reduction of food poisoning, careful monitoring of possible bacterial or chemical risks is necessary. What happens after tins are opened is obviously of prime importance. Household refrigerators are not plentiful in countries where they are most needed. Even large-scale refrigeration of poultry, for example, is not without hidden perils. After incomplete thawing, organisms may remain viable in internal parts not reached by superficial cooking as by some forms of spit roasting. Many animals harbour organisms pathogenic to man and constitute an important and continuing source of infection (Fig. 6.1). The extent of man's contact with animals varies from place to place—in the home, from a single pet of a town dweller to a greater number in a tent in the desert or under a village hut in Malaysia; at work, in farms, meat shops, abbatoirs, zoos, etc; and in natural surroundings where the range of animals is widest. In advanced countries, several modern practices of commercial benefit have

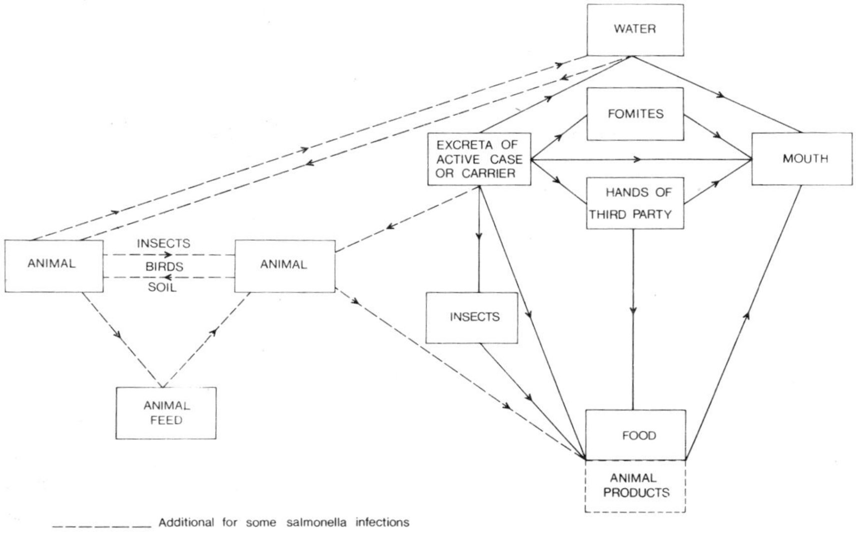

Fig. 6.1 Mode of transmission of intestinal infection.

enlarged and complicated this source, as for example, in methods of rearing livestock and poultry (chicken farming, battery hens) and by the use of fodder unsuspectingly infected and to which antibiotics have been added to stimulate animal growth. By altering the bacterial flora of the intestine, these may create a situation whereby the animal is made susceptible to infection and at the same time encourage the development of resistance in the pathogenic (and other) organisms. When the same antibiotics (usually penicillin, tetracycline and chloramphenicol) are used also to preserve the food, this hazard is increased. With the emergence of strains resistant to one or more of the antibiotics in common use, treatment of the human (or animal) sufferer by these antibiotics is rendered ineffective. For a detailed consideration of the problems raised by this abuse of antibiotics and recommendations for control, the reader is referred to the Swann Report (1969) and the Report of the U.S. Department of Agriculture and the Food and Drug Administration (1969). Undoubtedly the importation of animal foodstuffs from tropical countries has been responsible for the dissemination of certain salmonella organisms in western countries, perhaps more insidiously than the transfer by way of trade in human food from country to country. In most countries, measures to ensure the safety of food at various stages are enforced by law but these can only be as effective as the local standards of food handlers and inspectors permit.

As with other infections, overcrowding is an adverse factor, especially when combined with poor general living conditions. Likewise the movement or migration of large numbers, whether on pilgrimages or as refugees from war, famine, earthquakes and other natural disasters, invariably leads to outbreaks of bowel infections. Special problems arise in war time in barracks and camps and in peace time in large institutions, notably mental hospitals where dysentery may be endemic. Even in general hospitals with overcrowded wards, cross-infection with intestinal pathogens is liable to occur if nursing and other facilities are below standard.

The means used to dispose of excreta vary widely throughout the world, being subject to convenience, density of population, and physical conditions. Promiscuous defaecation is common in many countries, particularly in rural areas. Where community systems are unwarranted for economic and other reasons, privies, bucket systems and septic tanks are used. In this connection, the use of night soil in the cultivation of plants and vegetables which will not be subjected to cooking, e.g. cress, lettuce, etc., opens up another avenue of infection.

In towns and centres of population where more elaborate systems are needed, better control can be exercised and on the whole these are safer, but the most sophisticated depend on the availability of water for operation and final disposal. In many cases the effluent, perhaps untreated, is discharged into a nearby river, thence to the sea from inland areas or directly into the sea from coastal zones. As a result, contamination of shellfish in coastal waters may occur and there is some risk to bathers.

In inland waterways and land-locked seas, chemical and bacterial pollution is intensified, and evidence is accumulating that in time the Mediterranean Sea may reach the same state as exists at present in some inland freshwater areas such as Lake Erie, U.S.A. This is a natural consequence of intensive industrialization which in turn attracts workers and over-stretches existing sanitary facilities to add to chemical hazards. These are by no means confined to fresh water and there is ample evidence that seawater fish may contain toxic substances in excess, the most striking example in recent times being the mercurial poisoning at Minamata, Japan.

Physical environment

The effect of climate is less obvious in the non-infectious diarrhoea, apart from tropical sprue, but has considerable bearing on most of the infective group. Although most of the organisms survive freezing, they may be killed by direct sunlight. Provided that the necessary humidity and nutrients are available, they can survive for long periods in a semi-vegetative state outside the human (or animal) host. Since many remain viable in water for many months, the existence of surface and ground waters which are dependent on rainfall, offers opportunities for such pathogens not only to survive but to be transported from place to place (and person to person). Rain water, properly collected and stored, is of pure quality and safe, especially in rural areas where air impurities are less in evidence.

Geological considerations affect water supplies from other sources. The nature of the terrain determines their collection and distribution. While in most countries large water supplies for urban areas are of reasonable standard, in many regions recourse to such less reliable sources as wells and springs is still necessary. As long as the catchment area of ground waters is free from bacterial or other contamination, such sources are safe if properly managed and used. Soil filtration and other natural processes assist in the provision of wholesome but not necessarily pure water. The mineral content of the water may be affected by the underlying strata as a result of the addition of undesirable elements or an unsuspected geological fault may give rise to contamination from a less clean catchment area. Both of these aspects can be monitored by frequent sampling. In the case of bacterial contamination, use is made of coliform bacterial counts but this unfortunately does not distinguish between *E. coli* from human and animal excreta. Even so by such tests the need for and the required degree of chlorination can be gauged.

Unless obtained near the source water from rivers and streams is in general potentially dangerous. In many countries, these waters contain sewage and yet are used for washing and bathing as well as a supply of drinking water. They can of course be rendered safe by boiling. This method is applicable only to small quantities but it is possible by more elaborate and costly processes to provide a satisfactory supply from impure river water and at the same time conserve the supply by recycling. Lack of water is no less important as an adverse factor by lowering personal and general standards of hygiene.

Less directly, the influence of climate on dietary needs and habits provides varying opportunities for infection in different areas through a variety of agencies—the types and methods of agriculture and animal husbandry, and the presence of vectors, the most important of the latter being the house fly. This common insect, whose reproduction is enhanced manyfold in warmer climates where waste and sewage disposal may be difficult or absent, is not an essential component in the transmission of intestinal infections but there is little doubt that the "filthy feet of faecal-feeding flies" contribute to the generally high incidence in tropical and sub-tropical countries. In these countries, the more equable climate is associated with less marked seasonal variation than in temperate zones. Here, where conditions fluctuate throughout the year and seasonal prevalence is more striking, the peak incidence falls in the warm humid months of summertime—hence the designation "summer diarrhoea" formerly applied to infantile gastroenteritis. This holds globally and leads to striking differences in the timing of the peak incidences between the two hemispheres.

MEDICAL CARE

While effective public health measures related to water supplies, sanitation, housing, etc. are of enormous importance in the control of infective diarrhoeal diseases spread by the faecal-oral route, the extent and quality of other medical services can influence certain aspects, particularly mortality.

For example, immunization against the enteric fevers, which may protect against a small dose of organisms, is at least likely to modify the illness and improve the chances of survival. Before TAB (C) vaccine was first used, and with apparent success, on a large scale in Gallipoli during the 1914–18 war, enteric fever was one of the scourges of armies. In the Second World War beneficial effects were also seen. Since then attempts have continued to improve the efficacy of the vaccine by modification and from controlled field trials, notably in Yugoslavia, the U.S.S.R., Poland and British Guiana, variable degrees of success have been claimed, the average protection rate being 70%. Less use has been made of anti-dysentery vaccines which are, on the whole, less effective than TAB vaccine, although better results have been claimed in recent years.

In some infections, chiefly the enteric fevers, drugs including antibiotics have had a marked influence on the outcome. Fortunately, the most effective antibiotic (chloramphenicol) is comparatively cheap so that poorer countries which need it most are therefore not denied its use. Some disadvantages, however, have occurred and in certain countries, notably South America, resistant *S. typhi* are now appearing. In addition, there is some evidence that antibiotic-treated patients tend to harbour the organism longer and thereby extend the carrier pool. Except in the enteric fevers, there is no strong indication for the use of antibiotics in diarrhoeal diseases.

Since immunization on a scale sufficient to create a high herd immunity has been sporadic and intermittent, it is impossible to evaluate its effect on comparative mortalities, but the effects of chloramphenicol, which began to show about 1950, should have reached a constant level throughout the world, making direct but not retrospective comparisons acceptable.

Clearly all these factors, many of which are interdependent, operate in varying degree from country to country and time to time, but with this group of diseases the most important are good personal hygiene and practices, extended to include food handling, clean food, adequate and pure water supply, and satisfactory means of sewage and garbage disposal. All of these are within the sphere of human control and their universal application could reduce the problem of diarrhoeal diseases to insignificance.

LESS IMPORTANT INFECTIONS

Compared to amoebic dysentery (Chapter 4), the other protozoal infections of the gut are of minor importance. Indeed *Giardia lamblia* is considered by many to be non-pathogenic and merely an opportunistic invader of the upper reaches of the small bowel. In most cases, symptoms are mild and intermittent; prolonged infection may result in a sprue-like syndrome or, in the case of children, failure to thrive. Violent attacks are not common but outbreaks do occur. It is often endemic in children's nurseries and infection is perpetuated through the swallowing of cysts passed in the faeces. The cysts survive in water and may be found in sewage. The distribution is world wide and in some areas, notably eastern Europe, the local strains are more virulent than usual to visitors.

B. cereus, a spore-bearing soil organism, has been incriminated in some outbreaks of food poisoning, particularly in Scandinavia and the Netherlands. Starch, flour and potatoes are common vehicles and elsewhere cooked rice has been involved in outbreaks connected with Chinese restaurants.

Another organism which in recent years has been isolated with increasing frequency from cases of gastroenteritis belongs to the Yersinia species, *Y. enterocolitica*, normally found in animals and soil. It is widely distributed but most human infections have been reported from Scandinavia and South Africa.

As with *V. cholerae*, water plays an important role in the transmission of the vibrio group, at least one of which, *V. parahaemolyticus*, is a common cause of gastroenteritis in the Far East and Pacific area. Being adapted to a marine life, these organisms are to be found in the warm coastal waters of most tropical and sub-tropical countries and even further afield, as for example, off the south-west coast of England. Infection is usually acquired by way of shellfish (crab, shrimps and prawns) and has been introduced from Malaysia and the Far East to distant countries through the importation of frozen sea food. In a similar fashion, air travellers from the same area have been found to be suffering from this infection in widely separated countries but so far the organism has not become established in temperate western countries.

None of the above have created problems of sufficient magnitude to be recognized as major global threats but their significance may be enhanced by the increasing awareness of their presence and the need to search for them in the laboratory.

VIRUSES

To some extent the same applies to viral infections of the bowel. Long suspected as causal agents in the considerable proportion of cases not attributable to bacterial pathogens, viruses have been isolated from a surprisingly low percentage. Those most often found belong to the enterovirus and adenovirus groups, both of which can produce a variety of clinical syndromes. Isolation of these viruses from faeces has been achieved chiefly by tissue culture which is somewhat selective and for technical reasons also restrictive.

In the late 1960s the discovery of the "Norwalk agent" from cases of epidemic winter vomiting intensified the interest in direct examination of faeces by electron microscopy. During the past few years this procedure has revealed the existence of a variety of virus particles, some previously identified by other means. In particular reovirus-like particles, variously described as rotavirus, orbivirus and duovirus from their morphology, have been found in relation to gastroenteritis of infants and young children in all five continents.

Similar, if not identical, viruses have been identified in equivalent illness in young animals (calves, pigs and mice) in many parts of the world. This situation has a parallel in *E. coli* gastroenteritis (see p. 162). More precise classification of these viruses awaits the development of suitable cultural methods which should also provide the tools for confirmatory serological diagnosis.

The clinical illness is indistinguishable from that caused by bacterial infections in nearly all cases. As with bacteria, the usual mode of transmission is ano-oral and waterborne spread becomes a possibility through infected sewage. Food may be infected but no multiplication occurs outside living cells. In certain circumstances, e.g. with adenovirus, infection may be airborne and acquired via the upper respiratory tract. Distribution is world wide.

While it may be shown, in due time, that viruses will account for a further proportion of those cases at present undiagnosed, there is no doubt that bacterial pathogens play a major role in the causation of diarrhoeal diseases.

TOXIN TYPES

Staphylococci

Although first appreciated towards the end of the nineteenth century, scant attention was paid to staphylococci as a cause of gastroenteritis until the 1930s when a high morbidity became apparent. In the post-war period, this type was estimated to be about five times as common as salmonella infections which at that time had assumed considerable importance and were regarded as the main cause of gastroenteritis.

Not all staphylococci produce an enterotoxin and therefore the incidence is dependent on the prevalence of particular strains. From their normal sites of skin and nose, transfer to other persons or inanimate objects is all too easy. Contamination of food may be airborne but more often is effected by hands.

Formerly milk was a frequent vehicle in outbreaks, the infection being introduced at source from the udder or else during delivery to the consumer. With modern mechanical methods of milking obviating contamination from the milker's hands, pasteurization and little human contact up to delivery, it is no longer an important vehicle except in special situations. Some milk products however, such as cheese, are frequently incriminated as are sweets, pastries, meats and, sometimes, canned foods.

The illness produced varies in severity, depending on the dose of toxin absorbed and personal factors. Mortality is low in distinction to that of the rarer enterocolitis which usually follows antibiotic treatment. The distribution is widespread and its apparent preponderance in Europe and North America may be highlighted by the relatively low incidence of other types of food poisoning in these areas.

Clostridia

Up to 1950 nearly all toxin type infections were regarded as staphylococcal in origin. About this time another toxin producing group of organisms was found to be responsible for some outbreaks, the Clostridia, of which *Cl. welchii* is the most common bowel pathogen. Although essentially soil organisms, they may be found in the intestine of healthy men and animals in small numbers and are capable of elaborating toxins with differing actions. In the case of *Cl. welchii*, while preformed toxin may be ingested with the infected food, a continuing source is provided by the organisms when they become established in the gut. Thus the illness is often more severe and prolonged than the staphylococcal variety. Meat and its products are the favourite vehicles in those circumstances which encourage growth, viz. inadequate cooking, slow cooling, delayed consumption or storage at room temperature. The incidence is estimated to be about 10% of the staphylococcal variety but in some countries, notably Norway, it has become the more common type. A particularly virulent form of this infection, Enteritis necroticans, occurs in the highlands of Papua and New Guinea. Here dietary influences are involved; a low protein content leading to enzyme deficiency and an excessive intake of heat-stable enzyme inhibitor contained in sweet potato. This combination leaves one of the important toxin fractions of the organism unmodified.

All members of this toxin-producing group are associated with severe illness, e.g. tetanus and gas gangrene, but *Cl. botulinum* toxin is the most potent. As already stated, bowel symptoms are not a prominent feature of botulism which may be taken as a classical example of food poisoning. Again this organism is an inhabitant of soil, especially uncultivated grassland and, though present in most countries where suitable conditions exist, a dense concentration is seen in certain areas, notably the western states of the U.S.A. and Eastern Europe. Among the wide range of foodstuffs involved in its transmission are home-preserved vegetables and fruits, fish (herring, salmon roe), shellfish (shrimps), meat (especially preserved meat products) and even cheese. Fortunately incidents are infrequent but, even so, a seasonal pattern may be apparent. This is related to the timely use of particular foods, e.g. in winter in the U.S.A. when preserved summer-fruits are ordinarily used.

E. Coli

A large number of strains of this group of organisms which are normal and useful inhabitants of the lower bowel of man (and animals) exists and, in any individual, a continual change-over of strains takes place. Outside the gut they are well known pathogens and over the past 25 years it has been accepted that certain strains are pathogenic in their normal habitat, especially when circumstances favour their upward extension to the small bowel. For several reasons this is more likely to occur in young children, but there is recent evidence that soldiers in the Persian Gulf and Vietnam, young adults, may suffer in this way. Many years ago such infections were found only occasionally in elderly debilitated hospital patients. Indeed, for many years, it has long been suspected that the *E. coli* family and possibly other common bowel organisms such as *Proteus sp* and *Ps. pyocyanea*, are an important cause of travellers' diarrhoea, when none of the well known pathogens, shigella, salmonella, etc. appear to be involved.

Following the demonstration of enterotoxins (thermolabile and thermostable) in some strains of *E. coli*, support for this theory has been strengthened by the recovery of these toxigenic strains from cholera-like illness in the native populations of India and some Far Eastern countries. Identification of these strains is still in the experimental stage and reliance is still placed on antigenic typing, according to the Kauffman–White classification of *E. coli*. Of the several fractions, the "0" antigen with its appropriate number is used as a label, for example 0124, a serotype which has been connected with adult diarrhoea for many years.

Although full awareness and recognition of their role in infantile gastroenteritis did not begin until 1946, suspicion of their pathogenicity in infantile diarrhoea had been raised some 30 years earlier; in fact, an organism associated with "intestinal intoxication" and referred to as "dyspepsie-koli" in Germany in about 1920 proved to be identical with the strain of *B. coli neopolitanum* isolated by Bray in 1942 and with *E. coli 0111* (1946) which may be considered the prototype. Soon other strains, notably 055 and 0119 were identified and isolations were made in widely scattered countries from cases of infantile gastroenteritis which was rampant at that time. Many institutional outbreaks were occurring with case fatality rates of 40–60%, even in advanced countries, a situation comparable to the heyday of summer diarrhoea and a justification for the old term "cholera infantum".

Since 1950 there has been a gradual decline in incidence and a corresponding drop in mortality. Even so, in western countries explosive outbreaks still occur even in well regulated communities, and these are often complicated by institutional involvement (nurseries and hospitals). In such outbreaks a previously unidentified serotype may come to light, e.g. *0142* in 1960, and now nearly 20 enteropathogenic strains are recognized and tested for in most laboratories. Nevertheless several of the earlier discoveries remain endemic in most countries and still produce outbreaks of severe disease.

These hardy organisms, like shigellae, can survive for a considerable time outside the human (or animal) body, in water as well as in a dry state, and are acquired in the same way. Unlike shigellae, however, they are found in animals and indeed certain serotypes are associated with diarrhoeal disease, e.g. "white scours" of calves, a condition analogous to infantile gastroenteritis. Poor hygiene and socio-economic conditions are prominent predisposing factors and the importance of breast feeding in the reduction of this and other bowel infections has been amply demonstrated by many studies which show higher infection rates from the time of weaning onwards. The proportion of the enormous number of infantile diarrhoeas for which these enteropathogenic *E. coli* are responsible cannot be gauged with any accuracy for the reason that few cases are investigated and, with the widening range of tests required, the limited resources of some laboratories do not extend to cover all possibilities.

BACILLARY DYSENTERY (SHIGELLOSIS)

Although Abercrombie gave the first accurate description in 1830, over 30 years passed before it was realized that human excreta were the source of the miasma and it was only in 1898 that the first dysentery bacillus was identified by Shiga in Japan during a severe epidemic (90 000 cases with 20 000 deaths in a 6-month period). Confirmation of the world-wide distribution of dysentery bacilli soon followed and other members of the family, now called shigella, were discovered, notably the bacilli of Flexner, Schmitz, Boyd and Sonne.

Like most bowel organisms, they are capable of surviving in water for long periods and for a time on inanimate objects given favourable conditions. Because it secretes an exo-toxin, *Sh. shigae* is more virulent than the others, giving rise to more severe illness and a higher mortality. To carry identification as far as possible, use is made of the fact that they excrete an antibiotic substance, colicine, with individual characteristics. Colicine-typing is thus another aid to the epidemiologist tracing spread and sources of outbreaks.

Very rarely have dysentery bacilli been recovered from animals other than man in whom it appears to have found conditions most suitable for survival. Insects, however, particularly the house fly, play an important though not essential part in the transmission of the disease from excreta to food, by surface carriage, regurgitation before feeding, or by their own excreta. Increased prevalence is likely in temperate countries during warm moist weather but winter outbreaks can also occur.

In sub-tropical and tropical countries on the other hand where temperature fluctuations are small, epidemics tend to correspond to the fly season and are associated with the rainy season. At such times, there are ample opportunities for contamination of water supplies by overflow from drains and seepage from water-logged soil. At the same time, the enforced alteration of the habits of a village community may lead to a greater concentration of pollution in its midst and to closer contact in dwellings.

In the developed countries overcrowding, with poor or imperfect sanitary conditions, is a common predisposing factor; water-borne spread nowadays is unusual. Thus outbreaks tend to be found in homes for the mentally handicapped, in prisons, schools and other institutions. Outbreaks in schools are associated with the high incidence in young children whose toilet habits may not be foolproof. This is particularly so if proper facilities for hand washing are lacking, a point of particular importance at school meal times. Primary infection of food is rare in the developed countries now though milk-borne outbreaks do occur occasionally. In spite of the benefits of progress in all aspects of public health, dysentery remains endemic where it is least expected. In such circumstances the normal seasonal pattern may be upset resulting in an equally high prevalence in winter as in the summer months. This applies particularly to Sonne dysentery in Europe.

Of the three common varieties, Shiga dysentery has the most limited distribution, with the heaviest concentration in Asia. Westwards it fades out in Eastern Europe, where before 1950 it was endemic in several Baltic states, Eastern Poland, Northern Italy and the Balkans, and eastwards across the Pacific its fringe rests on the western regions of Central and South America. During the past ten years there has been a resurgence of this type in Central America. In El Salvador, for example, it has reappeared after an absence of 40 years. Persistent foci have been noted in neighbouring Guatemala for a long time, and there have been occasional appearances in the southern states of the U.S.A. In spite of importations on a fairly large scale during both World Wars and temporary endemicity in a few areas thereafter, this Shiga type has never become established in Western Europe.

Both Flexner and Sonne organisms are widely distributed and have been isolated in most countries at one time or another. In areas such as India, South America and some Far Eastern States with a high dysentery rate, the Flexner group predominates or at least equals *Sh. shigae* if this variety is present. In many parts of Northern Europe and North America, Sonne infection accounts for most of the cases.

The former high mortality of dysentery (up to 50%) has been curbed considerably over the past 35 years as a result of improved medical care, including drugs and antibiotics. This has been most noticeable in respect of the Shiga variety, from an average of 30% (as exemplified by the disastrous destruction of one-third of the Turkish army after the Gallipoli campaign in 1915) to about 10%. In many areas single figures have been reached since 1950.

While Flexner dysentery has a significant mortality, usually under 5%, that for Sonne is now extremely low. Overall, however, dysenteric infections account for a sizeable proportion of deaths due to diarrhoeal diseases, which latter continue to be high on the list of leading fatal diseases, especially in the youngest age group in some of the less developed countries of the world.

SALMONELLOSIS (OTHER THAN ENTERIC FEVERS)

In contrast to the moderate number of causative organisms in each variety mentioned so far, the salmonella family provide an almost unlimited choice, from over 1500 different organisms, as well as an exercise in topical geography, from Aba to Zurich. Nearly all are labelled with the place name of their original site of isolation. Some bear the name of their animal source, human or otherwise, e.g. *S. thompson*, *S. pullorum*, and a few of the earlier members retain part of the title used prior to reclassification, e.g. *S. enteritidis*, derived from *Bacillus enteritidis* of Gaertner, (1888). At the turn of the century, a second member of the family was associated with an outbreak of food poisoning in the small Belgian town of Aertrycke and called *Bacillus aertrycke*. This organism was found to be identical with that of "mouse typhoid" (Loeffler, 1892), hence its current name, *S. typhimurium*. In fact, it is the most common and widely distributed salmonella in nature, though not the first to be found in animals. This distinction belongs to the bacillus of hog cholera (now *S. choleraesuis*) isolated by Salmon and Smith in 1885.

By virtue of advances in knowledge and improved techniques, an ever-increasing number of strains has come to light and has been shown to cause human disease. Likewise their widespread occurrence in all living species in which they also cause illness has been confirmed. While a few are host-specific, e.g. *S. abortus-ovis* (sheep), *abortus-equi* (horses), *gallinarum* (fowls), most strains have the propensity to interchange their hosts and can occur anywhere. *S. typhimurium*, which may be regarded as nearest to the prototype, remains the most ubiquitous, and *S. dublin* is the most common in cattle.

The ability of these strains to survive in water and soil (for over 280 days) increases their potential and to some extent makes them independent of their animal hosts. Some of the less common types remain restricted to certain areas, though not necessarily confined to a single host. For various reasons, they may be introduced to other parts by human carriers in infected meat, animal products or other foodstuffs. An illustration of this was the rapid increase of exotic types in the United Kingdom during the Second World War. This arose from imported dried egg, mainly from the U.S.A. (Fig. 6.2).

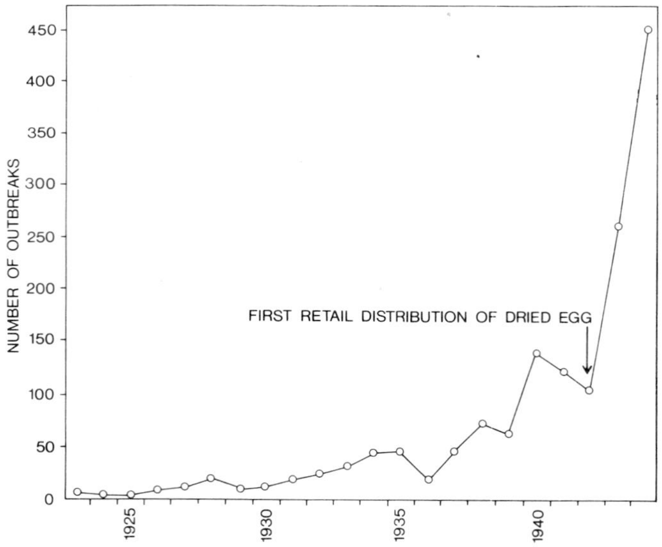

Fig. 6.2 Outbreaks of Salmonella food poisoning in England and Wales, 1923–44 (redrawn from M.R.C. Special Report Series No. 260 by permission of Controller, H.M.S.O., London).

The minor significance of eggs as a vehicle was appreciated earlier in the context of liquid eggs imported from China for use in the bakery and confectionery trades, but it was the sheer volume of the dried product involved which subsequently multiplied the risk and increased the scale. The cause of this striking rise was confirmed later by a similar happening in Western Europe during 1944–45 due to the same medium.

Not only may the infection of eggs be external, leading to contamination on opening, but the organisms may be found inside the shell without any noticeable change in the contents. Poultry birds are well known carriers of salmonella, other than the specifically adapted types, e.g. *S. pullorum*, and duck eggs in particular have often been incriminated. The less commonly eaten gull's egg is also a recognized source. Even turtle eggs are not exempt and through them such birds as the albatross can be infected. For geographical reasons this instance is of minor importance in dissemination, but elsewhere salmonellae have been recovered from many common avian species which may play some part in the cycle. For instance sparrows in the neighbourhood of horse corrals have been found to carry the same strains as the horses.

Transfer of the infection from continent to continent in living animals is limited in extent. It is most noticeable in small animals such as tortoises introduced as pets. In the case of larger animals such as cattle and horses, there is a moderate volume of inter-state traffic. Although salmonellae have been isolated from most mammals, including whales, reptiles, birds and insects, indeed from fleas to elephants, the main problem is centred on those used for food. Reference has been made earlier to the role of animal foodstuffs in the propagation of these and other organisms. Many of the ingredients likely to be infected such as bone, blood, meat and fish meal are of animal origin, and it is significant that the end product often contains a selection of salmonellae. Isolations have also been made from vegetable ingredients such as soya bean and cotton seed meals. In such cases, the likelihood of contamination within factories arises. By the use of phage typing, a particular strain can be traced through animal feed, domestic animal and later to man, thereby confirming this link in the chain of infection.

It follows that ideally the same care should be taken in the preparation of animal foods as to those for human consumption but infection cannot always be avoided when uncooked meat and other ingredients are involved, e.g. horse meat in dog food.

In human infections, foods such as meat and poultry with high protein contents are common sources but cross contamination of other foods is not infrequent. Unpasteurized milk is an occasional vehicle. Perhaps one of the most unusual and unexpected carriers of infection was a carmine dye used during certain bowel investigations in 1967 which involved *S. cubana* and hospital patients in both the United Kingdom and U.S.A. Other medical preparations of animal origin, e.g. pancreatic extract, have been occasionally incriminated.

While most information concerning salmonellosis comes from Europe and the Americas where it is a prominent cause of food poisoning, it is at least an equal and probably greater problem in Africa and Asia. Source names do not give a true and up-to-date indication of the areal distribution. For example, *S. rubislaw* (a district of Aberdeen, Scotland) isolated in 1939 but rarely seen in the United Kingdom since then, accounted for 8% of salmonella isolates in Chad in 1970. Disturbance of the local ecological balance following natural events or human intervention is liable to alter the distribution pattern of the many types to the extent that outbreaks due to exotic types may exceed those caused by established indigenous varieties. Such has been the experience in the United Kingdom in recent years. Whereas in the early 1960s, two-thirds of the outbreaks were due to *S. typhimurium*, by 1972 it was responsible for fewer than half and by 1973 it was in danger of losing its premier position to *S. agona*. *S. agona* was rarely seen before 1970 when it was introduced to the United Kingdom (and also the U.S.A. and the Netherlands) in Peruvian fish meal.

In developed countries, mortality from salmonellosis is generally low—it is about the same level as dysentery, and the majority of fatalities occur in elderly patients suffering from other diseases. It is higher in less developed countries and, where blood stream invasion occurs, the rate is similar to that for the paratyphoid fevers.

ENTERIC FEVERS

Typhoid and the paratyphoid fevers are salmonella infections with special features which distinguish them from the others. Such features include differences in incidence, distribution, host relationships, clinical behaviour and mortality.

The fact that the excreta of sufferers contained the infective agent was first appreciated by Budd in 1856 who, in his full and accurate account of the epidemiology, substituted the "germ" theory for the miasmatic. In 1880 the germ, *Bacillus typhosus*, later *Eberthella typhosa* and now *S. typhi*, was identified by Eberth. The isolation of the paratyphoid organisms came later; A and B at the turn of the century and C in 1919. These latter organisms produce an illness similar in many respects to typhoid but on the whole it is less serious. Sometimes they behave in the manner of the other salmonellae and cause only gastroenteritis.

At the time of their discovery and before, the enteric fevers were extremely common throughout the world. In parallel with dysentery and other infections, they reached epidemic proportions in times of war and natural disaster. In the Spanish-American War, one-fifth of the soldiers in standing camps contracted typhoid and, in the South-African War, casualties from typhoid were greater than from wounds. Gradually, following control measures and improvement in living conditions in most countries, the incidence has declined almost everywhere though at differing rates depending on the speed of progress. This is in contrast to the much greater prevalence of the other salmonellae in similar general circumstances, due mainly to the restricted host range of the typhoid and paratyphoid salmonellas. Typhoid and paratyphoid salmonellas have become adapted to humans. This is particularly so in the case of *S. typhi*, a strain rarely found in animals. *S. paratyphi B*, the most common of the paratyphoid organisms in Europe and America, is the most gregarious. It has been found in cattle, pigs, dogs and fowl. When a case of either disease occurs, it is safe to assume that although the route may be devious it will be traceable ultimately to human source. The picture is thus less complicated than with other salmonellae. Furthermore the enteric fevers are less infectious and there are fewer secondary cases among contacts.

Against this is the tendency for these organisms to persist longer in their special host than the unadapted salmonellae. There is a significant carrier rate, particularly of chronic carriers who may excrete organisms for a period of a year or more. There are in fact several instances of life-long carriage, particularly among females, the most notorious being "typhoid Mary". The sex difference arises because females are the main food handlers and therefore the more likely initiators of outbreaks. Furthermore, the longer life expectancy for women and their higher incidence of gall bladder disease prolongs and encourages biliary carriage. In the majority of infections, the carrier state lasts only a limited time; because excretion may be intermittent the end-point is sometimes indistinct. The importance of carriers in the cycle of infection is particularly evident in areas of low incidence; if unknown and not registered, urgent steps are taken to trace them. In well populated areas where possibly thousands of cases occur annually, there are obvious difficulties in tracing each case. It is only when a special incident occurs that it becomes possible to reach a broad conclusion with respect to source.

Water has always been a dominant vehicle of the typhoid bacillus and it has been involved at some stage or another in many of the large outbreaks. Indeed improvements in water supplies bear a direct relationship to the reduction in incidence in most countries. Nevertheless even when the standard of supply is high at its source, epidemics may still occur through accidental contamination on the way to the consumer either by an unsuspected carrier or leaking pipes. However, it is the irregular and unofficial sources of water that present the main danger.

The following details relating to a minor outbreak illustrate several of the previous points. Over a period of 8 years, eight cases of typhoid fever all due to the same organism, distinguishable by an unusual phage type, occurred in widely separated areas of a Scottish city. The only other common factor was an association with a small river winding its way through the city. One child had fallen into the stream, others, including an adult, had drunk small quantities of its water. By dint of laborious detective work, the origin of the infection was eventually traced to a freshwater drain which entered the stream midway along its 21-mile course. This pipe had been mistakenly connected to the foul water drainage from a group of 12 houses. It transpired that one of the occupants of these houses, an elderly female, was a carrier of the particular organism. The lady had not been abroad nor ill with typhoid fever but had probably acquired the organism from her father 25–60 years previously.

Sometimes water is not immediately or even directly responsible but it can lead to contamination of food. This was the case in the

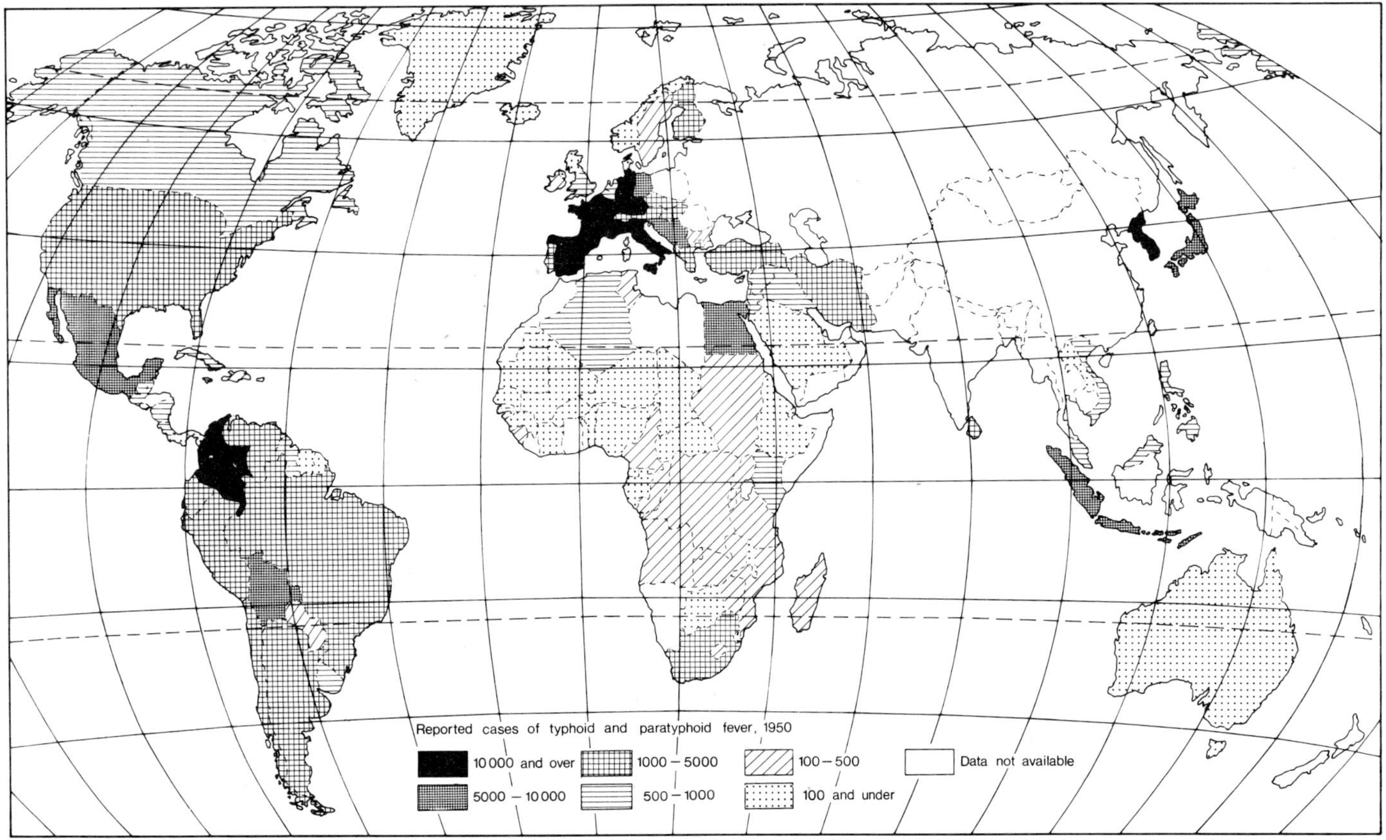

Fig. 6.3 Reported cases of typhoid and paratyphoid fever, 1950.

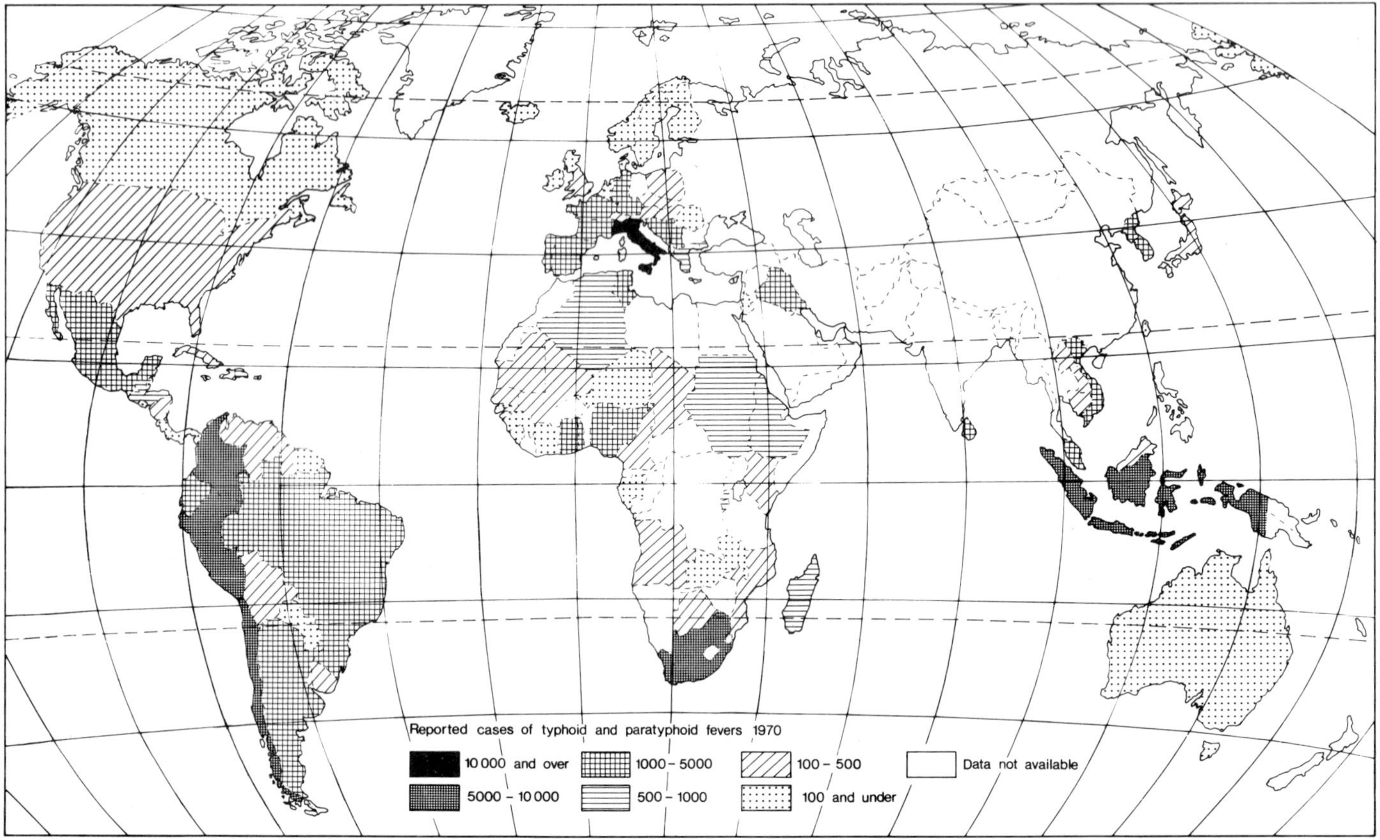

Fig. 6.4 Reported cases of typhoid and paratyphoid fever, 1970.

canning process of corned beef which initiated the large outbreaks in Aberdeen, Scotland in 1964 (over 400 cases) and in several towns in England in 1963. Canned tongue similarly infected was responsible for an outbreak in Pickering, Yorkshire in 1955. As with the other salmonellas, shellfish and uncooked vegetables may be a means of transmission. Unpasteurized milk and products such as ice cream have been involved in many outbreaks. Dried egg is another important source, particularly for the paratyphoid organisms. These organisms have also been disseminated in dessicated coconut from Ceylon and countries further east. Thus bakery products, which may contain egg and confections in which coconut is an ingredient are sometimes implicated in the spread of enteric fevers.

These organisms are still widely distributed but in countries such as those of Northern Europe, they are no longer endemic, except for carriers. Of the small number of cases occurring annually, more than half are the result of infections imported from overseas or even from Southern Europe. Moderate levels of endemicity and extensive tourism associated with the Mediterranean littoral are largely responsible. In Africa, India, the Far East and South America, the incidence of enteric fevers is high. This is largely a reflection of the standard of such factors as water supplies and sanitation. No information is available for a large part of Asia.

In certain areas however, some signs of improvement are apparent, as will be seen from a comparison of Figs 6.3 and 6.4. The latter indicates the current black spots for typhoid but the global picture is far from complete. Indeed this is true of all the conditions covered in this Chapter. Much knowledge and a good understanding of the mechanism of infection are available, but control measures cannot be universally applied. Many of the natural factors which influence the behaviour of these diseases cannot be altered and, of those under human control, progressive improvement can be expected only in a few, and then only as an outcome of socio-economic measures.

FURTHER READING

Christie, A. B. (1974). "Infectious Diseases: Epidemiology and Clinical Practice" (2nd edn). Livingstone, Edinburgh.

Committee on Salmonella National Research Council. (1969). An evaluation of the Salmonella problem. *Nat. Acad. Sci. Washington*, Pub. 1683.

Dewberry, E. G. (1959). "Food Poisoning" (4th edn). Leonard Hill (Books), London.

Hobbs, B. C. (1974). "Food Poisoning and Food Hygiene" (3rd edn). Edward Arnold, London.

Howe, G. M. (1972). "Man, Environment and Disease in Britain". David and Charles, Newton Abbot.

Huckstep, R. L. (1962). "Typhoid Fever and Other Salmonella Infections". Livingstone, Edinburgh.

Lu, F. C. (1973). Wholesomeness of foodstuffs: The role of W.H.O. *W.H.O. Chronicle* **27**, 6.

May, J. M. (1958). The ecology of human disease. "Studies in Medical Geography", Vol. 1. M.D. Publications Inc., New York.

Ordway, N. K. (1960). Diarrhoeal disease and its control. *Bull. W.H.O.* **23**, 1.

Rodenwaldt, E. (Ed.) (1956). "World Atlas of Epidemic Disease" (Welt-Seuchen Atlas), Part I (1952), Part II (1956). Falk, Hamburg.

Seeligher, H. P. (1960). Food borne infection and intoxication in Europe. *Bull. W.H.O.* **22**, 5.

Simmons, J. B., Whayne, T. F., Anderson, A. W. and Horack, H. M. (1954). Global epidemiology. "A Geography of Disease and Sanitation". J. B. Lippincott, London.

Stamp, L. D. (1964). "Some Aspects of Medical Geography". Oxford Univ. Press, London.

Swann Report on the use of antibiotics in animal husbandry and veterinary medicine. (1969). H.M.S.O., London.

Taylor, Joan (1960). Diarrhoeal diseases in England and Wales. *Bull. W.H.O.* **23**, 6.

Van Oye, E. (Ed.) (1964). "The World Problem of Salmonellosis". W. Junk, The Hague.

W.H.O. (1972). "Health Hazards of the Human Environment". W.H.O., Geneva.

7. Tuberculosis and Leprosy

Ian Sutherland

INTRODUCTION

It may at first sight strike a layman as strange that two diseases which are superficially so different as tuberculosis and leprosy should be considered together in the same chapter of this book. Admittedly, both are major infections, widespread throughout the world. Both diseases are of considerable social and economic importance in countries where they are common, because of their particular impact on men and women of working and reproductive ages. Although tuberculosis has a much higher fatality than leprosy (in the absence of effective specific treatment) both diseases often lead to chronic and increasing disablement. Tuberculosis is (or was, until the advent of chemotherapy) much feared as a common and lethal disease; it has been referred to popularly as "the white plague", and as "the captain of the men of death". Leprosy is also feared, partly as a disabling and disfiguring disease but principally because of its Biblical reputation for extreme contagiousness and for the consequent ostracism of those affected. But these similarities are also superficial and are not in themselves sufficient to explain why it is appropriate to deal with both diseases together.

The basic link between them is that they are caused by related bacilli from the genus *Mycobacterium.* Very many species of mycobacteria occur in nature, and many of these appear to be capable of infecting man. However, as will be explained more fully later, infection with mycobacteria (though it may have certain immunological consequences) does not necessarily lead to overt disease, and only two mycobacterial infections are important causes of disease in man. These are infections with the tuberculosis bacillus (*Myco. tuberculosis*) and the leprosy bacillus (*Myco. leprae*). Moreover, there is evidence that the immunological consequences of different mycobacterial infections are themselves interrelated, and this may modify the epidemiology of tuberculosis and of leprosy in areas where these and other mycobacterial infections occur.

This chapter will deal first with tuberculosis and leprosy as separate diseases and then consider the effects of these immunological interrelationships.

TUBERCULOSIS

The infecting organism

Two distinct types of *Myco. tuberculosis* occur, namely the "human" and "bovine" types, so called because they are the principal organisms causing tuberculosis in man and cattle respectively. However, each type is quite capable of infecting and causing disease in the other species, and in certain circumstances infection of man with bovine tubercle bacilli was (and still is) a common occurrence.

Infection of man with human tubercle bacilli is principally by the inhalation of bacilli coughed up by patients with pulmonary tuberculosis. As a result, pulmonary tuberculosis is the commonest form of the disease. However, the bacilli can also travel from the lung and cause disease in other parts of the body, notably in cervical and axillary lymph nodes, in bones and joints and in the genito-urinary system. Disseminated (miliary) tuberculosis and tuberculous meningitis are the two most lethal forms.

Infection of man with bovine tubercle bacilli is principally by the ingestion of raw milk from cows with udder tuberculosis. As a result of this mode of infection, children are particularly at risk and bovine tubercle bacilli usually cause non-pulmonary rather than pulmonary tuberculosis. Indeed, non-pulmonary tuberculosis is sometimes regarded as if it were exclusively bovine in origin and pulmonary disease as exclusively human, but this is an over-simplification. For example, in the Netherlands in 1933–38, when bovine tuberculosis was common in cattle, tubercle bacilli isolated from tuberculous lesions in man were routinely typed. In the small towns and country districts 43% of non-pulmonary and 9% of pulmonary tuberculosis in children (aged under 15 years) was of bovine origin. The corresponding percentages among adults were 22 and 6. In the large towns, the proportions of patients with bovine organisms were smaller, but the same contrasts appeared between non-pulmonary and pulmonary disease, and between children and adults (Ruys, 1946).

Infection and disease

One of the characteristics of tuberculosis which is of particular epidemiological and clinical importance is the existence of a latent stage in which infection has occurred but overt clinical tuberculosis has not developed. In some individuals this latent stage is so short that the infection and the primary lesions it causes appear to progress without interruption into the clinical disease of tuberculosis. However, in the majority of cases, the clinical illness which accompanies infection is so mild that it usually passes quite unnoticed and the primary lesions are self-limiting. This is, nevertheless, a latent stage since tubercle bacilli may remain dormant within the body for many years following the primary infection and may later start to multiply again and cause clinical tuberculosis. Tuberculosis arising in this way is sometimes referred to as *endogenous* (or reactivation) tuberculosis. But in many individuals the latent stage lasts indefinitely and tuberculosis does not develop in later life.

An important further consequence of a primary infection with tubercle bacilli is that the body's immunological status is changed and its resistance to further infection by tubercle bacilli is enhanced. Nevertheless, this enhanced resistance is not a complete immunity. Further infections can occur and the new bacilli may start to multiply and cause clinical tuberculosis. Tuberculosis arising in this way is referred to as *exogenous* (or reinfection) tuberculosis.

Because endogenous and exogenous tuberculosis cannot usually be distinguished from each other nor from progressive primary tuberculosis in their clinical manifestations, the relative frequency of occurrence of tuberculosis arising in these three ways, at different ages and at different times, is not known and has for long been a matter of controversy. It is important nevertheless to appreciate that only a proportion of the cases of tuberculosis which develop are related to *recent* infection or reinfection. The remainder are related to infections acquired some time, perhaps several years, earlier. This is one of the reasons why, despite the highly effective methods which exist at the present time for both the treatment and prevention for this disease, it is not easy to eradicate it completely or rapidly from a community.

Geographical distribution of tuberculosis

Measures of the disease in the community

As with other infections, the occurrence and importance of tuberculosis in the community may be measured in three ways, viz. by prevalance, mortality and incidence. (*Prevalance* is the proportion of the population who are suffering from the disease at a particular time; *mortality* is the number of deaths from the disease in the course of a period of time, usually a year, expressed as a proportion of the population; *incidence* is the number of new cases of the disease starting in the course of a year, as a proportion of the population.) But because tuberculous infection is not necessarily either synonymous or synchronous with disease, there are two further measures of tuberculosis in a community, viz. the prevalence and the incidence of *infection*. (The prevalence of infection is the proportion of the population at a particular time who have already been infected with tubercle bacilli; the incidence of infection is the number of new tuberculous infections occurring in the course of a year, expressed as a proportion of the population.) As will be explained later, the incidence of tuberculous infection is probably the best index of the epidemiological status of a community with regard to tuberculosis.

Prevalence of tuberculosis

Tuberculosis is found in almost every country throughout the world. A few communities, such as those on the Karimui plateau of New Guinea, which were almost completely isolated and unknown until the 1950s, appear to have been free or almost free of the disease until quite recently. Elsewhere the disease is common, though it has been receding for a number of years in most "Western" countries from very high levels during the 19th century and the earlier part of the

20th century. However, there is a basic lack of information on the numbers of sufferers from the disease in many of the countries in which tuberculosis is currently a major health problem; even in those countries in which statistics are compiled, there are wide variations in the definition of what constitutes a "case" of the disease. In consequence, it is not possible to give any reliable indication of the relative prevalence of the disease in different countries.

The W.H.O. (1974) estimates, on the basis of limited prevalence surveys in various countries, that the total number of *infectious* cases of tuberculosis in the world may currently be in the range of 15–20 million. This represents four to six infectious cases per 1000 population.

Mortality from tuberculosis

Statistics of deaths from tuberculosis are more readily collected than statistics on numbers of cases. In the past, tuberculosis mortality provided a good index of the relative importance of the disease in the technically more advanced countries. However, it is in just these countries that the introduction and effective use of specific chemotherapy, from the late 1940s onwards, has had the greatest effect on the mortality from the disease. Before chemotherapy was available, perhaps 50% of all cases of tuberculosis died of the disease; now, the case-fatality in effectively treated cases is well below 1%. In countries with comprehensive treatment services, deaths from the disease represent only a small proportion of the total tuberculosis cases. Mortality statistics thus give a very incomplete picture of the whole tuberculosis problem. Moreover, variations in mortality from country to country may also reflect the efficiency of the treatment services and not solely the size of the tuberculosis problem.

The available data on tuberculosis mortality in 1970 (from various W.H.O. sources) have been summarized in Fig. 7.1. Though there are many countries for which mortality statistics are not available or where the figures are known to be unreliable, the map does illustrate the wide variation in tuberculosis mortality which occurs. Values range from less than 2 per 100 000 in Australia, Iceland and the Netherlands to more than ten times as great in Chile, Hong Kong, Mexico, the Philippines, Poland, Sarawak, Singapore, Taiwan, Thailand, Turkey and South Africa. Despite the lack of reliable quantitative information, mortality from tuberculosis is known to be

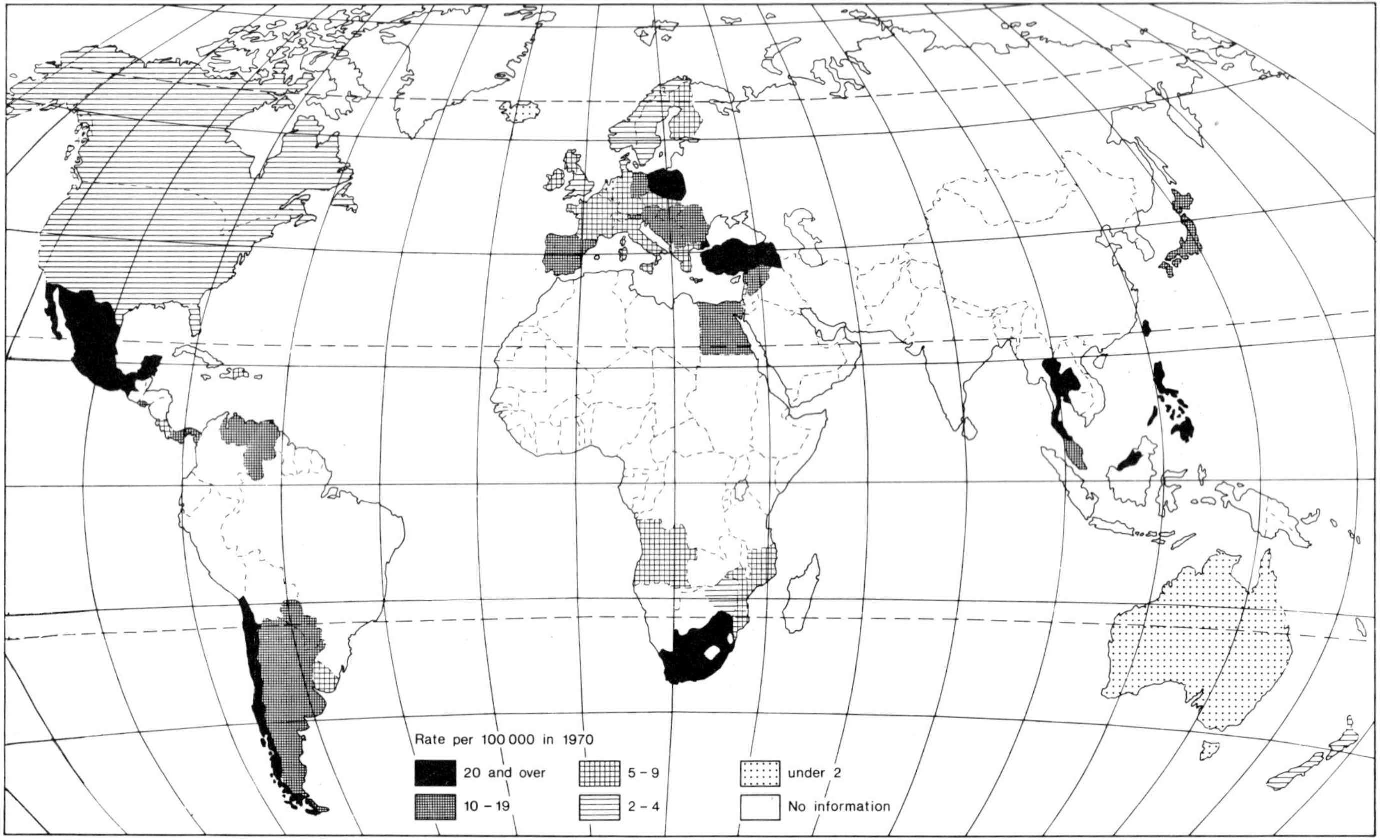

Fig. 7.1 Tuberculosis: mortality from all forms, 1970, per 100 000 population in various countries (based on W.H.O. data).

high in many of the countries which have been left blank on the map (Fig. 7.1).

Incidence of tuberculosis

Because the case-fatality of tuberculosis is so dependent upon the efficiency of the treatment services and the availability of chemotherapeutic drugs, the number of new cases of the disease developing in the course of a year theoretically gives a better indication of the total size of the tuberculosis problem in an area than the number of deaths from the disease. However, the numbers of cases actually reported do not necessarily provide a sound basis for comparisons between areas. Apart from incompleteness of recording, which is to a greater or lesser extent a problem in all areas, standards of diagnosis vary and are dependent on the facilities available. Data for an area where diagnoses are based largely upon clinical criteria may not be comparable with those for an area having extensive facilities for bacteriological or radiographic examinations. Furthermore, special case-finding programmes may temporarily inflate the number of cases detected in a particular period, adding further to the difficulty of making reliable comparisons.

Available data on the annual tuberculosis incidence in the period 1967–70 (from various W.H.O. sources) are summarized in Fig. 7.2. As with mortality from the disease, there is a wide variation in the recorded incidence of tuberculosis, some of the highest figures being found in South-East Asia and some of the lowest in North America, Australia and Scandinavia. It is known that the incidence of the disease is also high in many, perhaps most, of the countries which have been left blank on the map

Prevalence and incidence of tuberculosis infection

The *prevalence* of tuberculous infection can be assessed from the findings of skin tests with an agent prepared from tubercle bacilli and known as tuberculin. Those who have had a primary tuberculous infection, even many years previously, show a characteristic delayed local hypersensitivity reaction about three days after the injection of a small amount of tuberculin into the skin layers. The test has a high "sensitivity", i.e. it identifies a high proportion of individuals who have been infected with tubercle bacilli. However, in some areas, it has a low "specificity", i.e. reactions occur in a proportion of

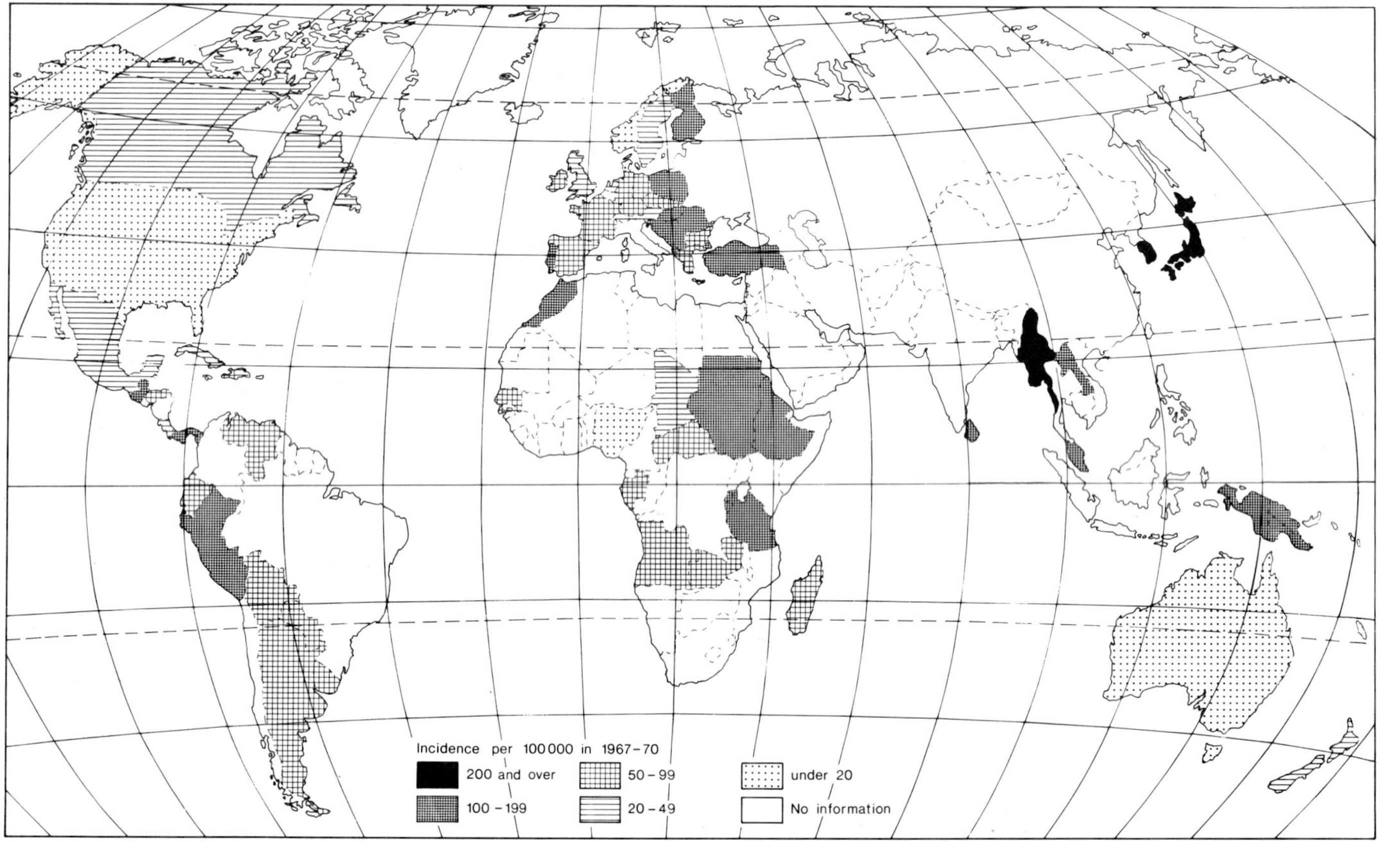

Fig. 7.2 Tuberculosis: incidence. Newly reported cases in one year (between 1967 and 1970) (based on W.H.O. data).

individuals who have *not* been infected with tubercle bacilli (these are usually cross-reactions to infections with other mycobacteria—see below). Nevertheless, with suitable attention to materials and methods, the findings of a tuberculin survey in a representative population group can give a good estimate of the prevalence of tuberculous infection in that population. It should be pointed out, however, that the tuberculin test cannot distinguish between infection with human and infection with bovine tubercle bacilli.

The usefulness of the prevalence of infection as an epidemiological index is limited, partly because it is closely dependent upon the age of the tested subjects (the prevalence is a cumulative measure of past infection and so increases with age) and partly because the tuberculin test cannot distinguish between an infection which took place recently and one which took place many years previously. A figure for the prevalence of infection thus expresses the end-result of the incidence of tuberculous infection over the whole lifetime of the population cohort under study. This incidence may have varied with age, or with calendar time, or both.

For epidemiological purposes, the *incidence* of tuberculous infection is probably the most meaningful index of the impact of tuberculosis on a community. It is a direct measure of the capacity of existing cases of tuberculosis to maintain the disease in the community by causing new tuberculous infections. Incidence of infection is thus more immediately relevant to the current and future epidemiological situation than the incidence of new cases of the disease, which will reflect infections some years previously as well as recent infections.

The incidence of tuberculous infection can be measured directly, by repeating tuberculin tests in the same individuals. Alternatively, it can be measured indirectly from figures for the prevalence of infection. However, a change, or trend, in the incidence of infection can only be assessed satisfactorily if more than one representative tuberculin survey has been made in the area at different times.

Secular trends in tuberculosis

In most of the countries in which reliable tuberculosis statistics have been available for a number of years, there is evidence, both from mortality and incidence rates, of a decrease in tuberculosis. This decrease is often substantial. It is, however, uncertain whether this applies in developing countries, with their increasing populations, small budgets and few facilities for disease control. Although some information has been obtained on the extent of the tuberculosis problem in many such countries, principally from recent surveys of the prevalence of tuberculous disease and tuberculous infection, there is very little knowledge as to whether tuberculosis in those countries is an increasing, static or decreasing problem.

Trends in the incidence of infection

The incidence of infection provides a particularly useful measure of the trend of tuberculosis in an area. Figure 7.3 shows the available information on both the incidence (or risk) of tuberculous infection and its trend with time in a number of areas between 1915 and 1970 (data from Sutherland, 1976). Three groups of areas may be distinguished. First, there are areas showing a high risk and a moderate downward trend in the incidence of infection during the years preceding the Second World War, namely France, the Netherlands, Prague and Vienna. Second, there are areas with a low risk and a substantial downward trend in the incidence of infection

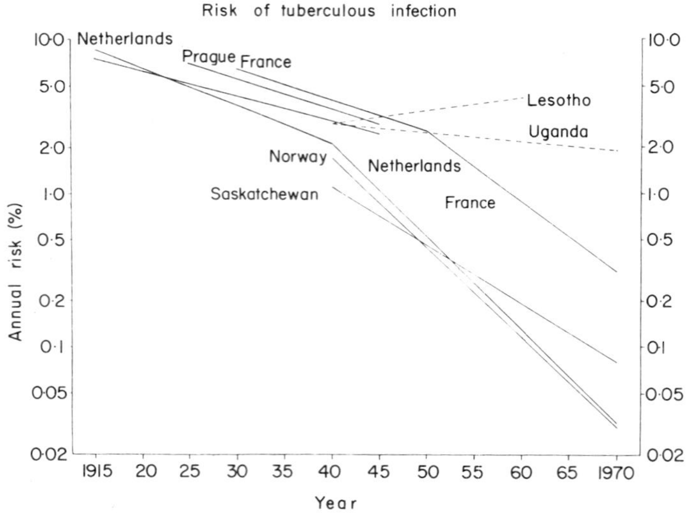

Fig. 7.3 Secular trends in the incidence of tuberculous infection. Annual percentages infected with tubercle bacilli in different areas, 1915–70 (Sutherland, 1976).

during the years following the Second World War, namely France, the Netherlands, Norway and Saskatchewan. Third, there are areas with a moderate incidence of infection, showing no important trend in the incidence with time, namely Lesotho and Uganda.

A clear contrast emerges, therefore, between the European and North American experience on the one hand, where the incidence of tuberculous infection has been decreasing for many years, particularly so since 1950, and on the other the African experience, where the incidence of infection has remained virtually unchanged since 1950 (in the absence of intensive control measures against the disease). It is probable that the high risks of infection in the European experience before the Second World War, exceeding those in the African experience today, were due partly to the substantial additional risk of bovine tuberculosis infection in all those areas at that time. There is now little risk of bovine tuberculous infection in most of Europe and North America, and little risk in the two African countries.

Changes in the age and sex pattern of the disease

In parallel with the decrease in the incidence of infection in Europe and North America, there has been a notable change in the age and sex pattern of the mortality and incidence of tuberculosis. The mortality from tuberculosis in these areas used to be high at ages 0–4 years, fell to a minimum at ages 5–9 years and rose to a peak in the age group 15–24 years, especially among females. Above this age, the rates decreased steeply again in both sexes and, above the age of 45 years, mortality was substantially greater in males than in females. This pattern applied to the incidence as well as to the mortality of the disease and persisted in England and Wales until the beginning of the Second World War. Since then, the peak at young adult ages has virtually disappeared. From being a disease primarily affecting young adults, tuberculosis has become largely a disease of old men. The explanation is mainly a consequence of the decrease in the incidence of tuberculosis infection. At younger ages, most of the cases stem from recent infections. These are now very much less frequent than previously in these areas. In the older age groups, however, a substantial proportion of the cases represent endogenous reactivation of infections acquired many years previously; the incidence of tuberculous infection. At younger ages, most of the proportion of the population who have had a previous infection is also high, in consequence of the high incidence of infection they experienced in their early years. Eventually the proportions at advanced ages who have had a previous infection will decrease substantially, and the incidence of tuberculosis at these ages may then also be expected to decrease substantially. The higher incidence of tuberculosis among older men than among older women indicates that previously infected men have a higher risk than women of developing endogenous disease.

Factors influencing the geographical variations and secular trends of tuberculosis

Organism

(a) *The human and bovine types of the tubercle bacillus* In areas where tuberculosis in cattle is common and where the opportunity exists for the infection of humans through the consumption of raw milk, then the total incidence of infection, by bovine and by human tubercle bacilli, is likely to be higher than in an area where milk is pasteurized or cattle tuberculosis is uncommon or has been eradicated.

(b) *Variations in virulence of the human tubercle bacillus* In some parts of the world, principally in South-East Asia, strains of human tubercle bacilli are found which are of reduced virulence in guinea pigs compared with the strains found in Europe (Mitchison, 1970). It is not known, however, whether these strains are of reduced virulence in man.

Host

(a) *Genetic susceptibility* The mortality of tuberculosis in England and Wales (as in other European countries) has been decreasing for more than a century. A much-discussed explanation for the decline is that genetically more susceptible individuals in the population have been gradually eliminated, leaving behind a more resistant population. It is generally accepted that this cannot be the sole explanation of the decline, but (if there *are* variations in genetic susceptibility to infection and disease in tuberculosis, which is not established) this factor could have contributed to the decrease.

(b) *Acquired immunity* As explained earlier, a primary infection with virulent tubercle bacilli, if it does not lead to progressive tuberculosis, confers an enhanced resistance or partial immunity to further infection with virulent tubercle bacilli.

An enhanced resistance to infection with virulent tubercle bacilli, falling short of a total immunity, may also be conferred on an uninfected individual, either artificially by vaccination or naturally by infection with another mycobacterium. The effects of such acquired immunity on the incidence of tuberculous infection and disease will be discussed more fully on pp. 190 *et seq.*

(c) *Nutritional status* Those with a poor nutritional status have an enhanced susceptibility to tuberculous infection and disease. Differences in the nutritional status of populations living in different areas will consequently contribute to geographical variations in the disease.

(d) *Intercurrent infections* Miller (1973) discusses geographical variations in the clinical manifestations of tuberculosis and suggests that the differences between the clinical types of tuberculosis seen in tropical regions and in present-day Britain are due principally to differences in nutrition and in the frequency and severity of intercurrent infection.

Environment

(a) *Social and economic factors* Because tuberculosis is a disease principally spread by droplet infection the whole complex of social and economic factors which influence the proximity of diseased and uninfected subjects are relevant to the *size* of the tuberculosis problem. Of these factors physical crowding is clearly predominant. More importantly, such socio-economic factors are particularly relevant to the *trend* of the disease. In an environmental situation in which 100 infectious cases of tuberculosis cannot infect sufficient numbers of individuals to generate ultimately as many as 100 new infectious cases of tuberculosis, the disease must decline and will do so progressively even if there is no further improvement in the environmental situation (Frost, 1937). Conversely, if the situation favours the generation of more than 100 new infectious cases, tuberculosis will increase.

(b) *Treatment* The extent to which cases of the disease are detected, early and treated promptly and effectively by chemotherapy, is of primary importance to the trend of the disease. A reduction in the period of time for which cases of the disease are infectious will reduce the risk of infection for the uninfected and so reduce the ability of tuberculosis to maintain itself in the population.

LEPROSY

The infecting organism and the disease

Leprosy is caused by the leprosy bacillus, *Mycobacterium leprae*. In contrast to the relative ease with which the tubercle bacillus can be grown in the laboratory and will multiply in a range of experimental animals, the leprosy bacillus has not been grown as yet outside living tissue; only recently has it been found to multiply in the footpads of mice (and then only to a limited extent), and in a species of armadillo. These experimental limitations have hampered considerably the study of the disease and, in consequence, many aspects of leprosy are much less well understood than they are in tuberculosis.

The sites principally affected by the leprosy bacillus are the skin and the peripheral nerves. Progression of the lesions leads to anaesthesia in affected areas and to deformities, particularly of the hands and feet. There are two main types of the disease, tuberculoid and lepromatous. They are distinguished, largely on clinical grounds, from the appearance and distribution of the lesions. Disease which is intermediate between these two types (borderline leprosy) is also found, but this tends to be unstable in its characteristics and to change into one of the two main "polar" types. Tuberculoid leprosy tends to be self-limiting (and may disappear without treatment, especially in children), and few bacilli are found in the skin lesions, though in other patients with this type of leprosy the disease may gradually progress and cause deformities. The impression is, however, of a chronic disease fairly well controlled by the immunity of the host. In contrast, lepromatous leprosy is usually progressive, disfiguring and disabling with many bacilli found in the skin lesions, and extensive involvement of the nerves. The impression is that of a progressive disease in a host with few immunological defences. Although it is consequently suspected that genetic factors may influence the type of leprosy which an infected individual will develop, this has not been firmly established.

Because of the extensive involvement of the skin in leprosy, it has been assumed, until recently, that the disease was spread by direct contact from person to person and that the principal route of infection was the skin. The disease has also been widely regarded (in modern times) as much less infectious than tuberculosis. However, there is evidence now (Rees and Meade, 1974) that the numbers of tubercle bacilli in the sputum of infectious tuberculosis patients are similar to the numbers of leprosy bacilli in the nasal secretions of lepromatous leprosy patients and that the attack rates of the two diseases in family contacts in similar circumstances are also similar. This suggests that the method of spread and the portal of entry for the leprosy bacillus may be the same as for the human tubercle bacillus, viz. airborne infection via the upper respiratory tract.

Infection and disease

Because the responsible organisms are both mycobacteria, it has been tacitly assumed that the same pattern of infection and disease occurs with leprosy as with tuberculosis. In other words, it is believed that a primary infection with leprosy bacilli does not usually result in overt clinical leprosy but rather confers some protection against the subsequent development of the disease and that there is often a long, latent period between infection and overt disease. This is little more than an argument by analogy and direct evidence of its validity is lacking. (In addition to the difference in the clinical and pathological manifestations, the analogy between the two diseases breaks down also in the response of the bacilli to chemotherapeutic drugs, e.g. DDS is of little value in tuberculosis and isoniazid of no value in leprosy, yet each is a powerful drug in the treatment of the other disease.)

Geographical distribution of leprosy

Prevalence of leprosy

Leprosy is now largely confined to tropical and sub-tropical areas of the world; in most temperate zones the only patients are those who have contracted the disease elsewhere. The W.H.O. has estimated, from a large number of surveys of variable reliability, that the total number of cases in the world is currently at least 10 million (Bechelli and Dominguez, 1966, 1972), of which perhaps a quarter are cases of lepromatous leprosy.

The estimated prevalence of leprosy in different parts of the world is shown in Fig. 7.4. (from Bechelli and Dominguez, 1966). (It should be noted that areas left blank on this map represent areas with the lowest prevalence of the disease, not, as in Figs 7.1 and 7.2, areas for which no estimate can be made or for which no data are available.) The proportion of cases which are of the lepromatous type varies widely. It is of the order of 10% in tropical Africa, 30% in Asia and 60% in the Americas. The reasons for these variations are as yet unknown.

Mortality and incidence of leprosy

Although leprosy is such a widespread and disabling chronic disease, the mortality specifically attributable to it is not high. Because the disease is most common in the developing countries, little reliable information is available, either on the mortality or the incidence of the disease in different areas, and no figures can usefully be given to supplement the general impression provided by Fig. 7.4.

Secular trends in leprosy

Bechelli and Dominguez (1972) estimated that the world total of cases of the disease in 1970 was not greatly different from the total in 1965. However, in view of the limitations of anti-leprosy drugs and the characteristics of the disease, they considered that leprosy might take decades to control with present methods and that consequently 5 years was too short a period in which to detect a trend in the disease.

This is a global assessment of the position, and there are indications that the disease may be decreasing in some areas. There is, however, a dearth of reliable evidence on this matter.

INTERACTIONS BETWEEN MYCOBACTERIAL INFECTIONS

Vaccination against tuberculosis

The fact that a primary infection with virulent tubercle bacilli confers an increased resistance to subsequent infection provides the rationale for vaccination against tuberculosis. BCG vaccine consists of artificially attenuated, bovine-type tubercle bacilli which are no longer capable of causing tuberculosis in man. The result of

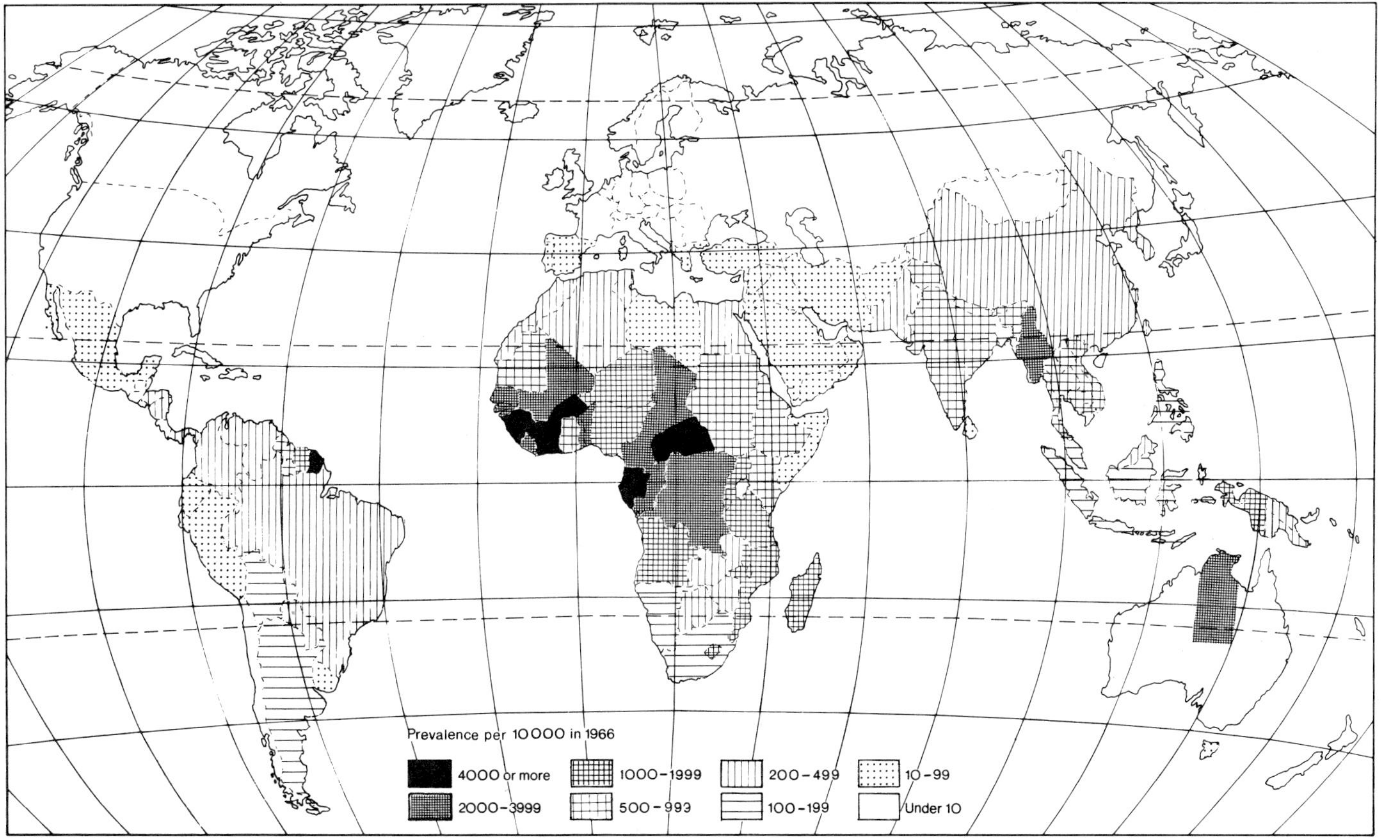

Fig. 7.4 Prevalence of leprosy: numbers of sufferers from the disease per 100 000 population in different countries (based on Bechelli and Dominguez, 1966).

vaccinating an uninfected subject is thus an innocuous primary infection which confers an increased resistance to subsequent infection with virulent tubercle bacilli. The extent of the increased resistance varies with the particular strain of BCG, but it can be substantial, preventing up to about 80% of the cases of tuberculosis which would otherwise have occurred.

Similarly, vole bacillus vaccine consists of a species of naturally-occurring mycobacterium (*Myco. microti*) which does not cause disease in man but confers on the vaccinated subject an increased resistance to subsequent infection with virulent tubercle bacilli. The extent of the resistance is similar to that provided by a potent BCG strain. This phenomenon of "cross-resistance", conferred by infection with one mycobacterium to subsequent infection by another, is of considerable relevance to the geographical pathology of both tuberculosis and leprosy.

Vaccination against leprosy

The prospect that a primary infection with BCG might also provide cross-resistance to subsequent infection with *leprosy* bacilli has led to studies of BCG vaccine against leprosy, but with puzzling results. A strain of BCG which has a high protective efficacy against tuberculosis in Britain has also been found to have a protective efficacy against non-lepromatous leprosy in Uganda. This same strain, for reasons which are not understood, shows very little protective efficacy against leprosy in Burma. Another strain of BCG gives moderate protection against leprosy in New Guinea.

Naturally-acquired resistance against tuberculosis

Infection with leprosy bacilli

It is not known whether a primary infection with the leprosy bacillus confers any protection against subsequent infection with the tubercle bacillus.

Infection with other mycobacteria

As already stated, there are many species of mycobacteria, other than the tubercle bacillus and the leprosy bacillus, which are capable of infecting man naturally. Several of these mycobacterial infections occasionally result in overt disease. The two most important in this respect are *Myco. ulcerans*, which causes skin ulcers, known in Uganda as "Buruli ulcer", and *Myco. intracellulare*, which causes a disease resembling pulmonary tuberculosis, known as "Battey disease". The numbers of cases of these diseases are trivial compared with those of tuberculosis and leprosy. Most of these infections, however, reveal their occurrence (but not their identity) only indirectly; if those infected are skin-tested with tuberculin (prepared from human tubercle bacilli) many of them show weak "cross reactions" to this antigen. There is virtually no information on the nature or geographical distribution of different species of these "atypical" mycobacteria.

Indirect evidence suggests that some of these natural mycobacterial infections confer a degree of protection against tuberculosis, in particular those occurring in south-eastern U.S.A. (where disease due to *Myco. intracellulare* occurs) and those occurring in Britain. This protection does not seem to be as great as that conferred by BCG.

Naturally-acquired resistance against leprosy

There is evidence that in Uganda a primary infection with tubercle bacilli confers protection against non-lepromatous leprosy. Its extent is similar to the protection conferred by BCG vaccine against leprosy in the same area. On the other hand, other mycobacterial infections occurring in Uganda do *not* appear to confer any protection against leprosy.

Vaccination superimposed on naturally-acquired resistance

There is some experimental evidence that if more than one mycobacterial infection is given to the same animal, their protective effects are not additive. In particular, BCG vaccination, superimposed on a mycobacterial infection which confers a lesser degree of protection than BCG, confers enough additional protection to bring the level up to that conferred by BCG alone, but no higher. The presence in an area of a mycobacterial infection with some protective efficacy against tuberculosis or leprosy may therefore not only affect the natural epidemiology of the disease in the area, but may also affect the extent to which the epidemiological pattern can be further modified artificially by vaccination.

CONTROL OF TUBERCULOSIS AND LEPROSY

Epidemiologically, tuberculosis and leprosy are both slow-moving diseases. It is a characteristic of most other infectious diseases that the prevalence of the disease in an area may change rapidly from one level to another. It is thus relatively easy to distinguish between periods when the disease is endemic and periods when it is epidemic in the same area. With tuberculosis and leprosy, however, the main contrasts in prevalence are geographical, it being relatively easy to distinguish between areas where the disease has a high level of endemicity and areas where it has a low level of endemicity. A change from one prevalence level to another in the same area is less easily detected because it is necessarily a slow process, measured in years rather than in months or weeks. However, a trend, once established, tends to persist. It is for this reason that assessments of the tendency of these diseases to increase, remain static or decrease in an area are at least as important in the understanding of the epidemiological situation in the area as are assessments of the endemic level.

From the foregoing sections, it is clear that the endemic level of either disease in an area is the result of the action and interaction of many factors. These include the virulence of the infecting bacilli, the opportunities for airborne infection or contagious spread, the occurrence of tuberculosis in cattle and the opportunities for infection by this organism, the general environmental (and perhaps the genetic) resistance of the individual to infection and disease, including his nutritional level and status in regard to intercurrent disease, the possibility that an acquired cross-resistance to the specific infection has been conferred naturally by a primary infection with another mycobacterium, or artificially by vaccination, and the rapidity and effectiveness of treatment of infectious cases. In some areas, the totality of these factors will favour a high level of endemicity, in others a low level.

Whether the level is changing or static in an area depends

ultimately on the balance between the factors favouring the further transmission of the disease to uninfected subjects, and those which discourage it. Frost (1937) pointed out the key role of the isolation of the infectious case of tuberculosis as a means of preventing the spread of this infection.

> However, for the eventual eradication of tuberculosis, it is not necessary that transmission be *immediately* and *completely* prevented. It is necessary only that the rate of transmission be held permanently below the level at which a given number of infection spreading (i.e. open) cases succeed in establishing an equivalent number to carry on the succession. If, in successive periods of time, the number of infectious hosts is continuously reduced, the end-result of this diminishing ratio, if continued long enough, must be extermination of the tubercle bacillus.
>
> Bearing in mind this principle, it is a fair inference that in this country (U.S.A.) as a whole we have already reached the stage at which the biological balance is against the survival of the tubercle bacillus, for year by year the mortality from tuberculosis is decreasing . . . This means that under present conditions of human resistance and environment the tubercle bacillus is losing ground, and that the eventual eradication of tuberculosis requires only that the present balance against it be maintained.

It is clear that as far as tuberculosis is concerned, the situation in many other countries is basically similar to that outlined above for the U.S.A. in 1937, and has been so for many years. Estimates of the secular trend in the risk of tuberculous infection, though at present available for only a handful of countries (Fig. 7.3), confirm this. They also suggest that the eradication of bovine tuberculosis as a source of infection, coupled with the introduction of effective chemotherapy for the disease since the Second World War have, in developed countries, tipped the balance even further against the survival of the tubercle bacillus. In these countries, there is no special need to intensify existing tuberculosis control measures, though they should be made more economical and efficient; the disease is losing ground rapidly and there seems little likelihood of any reversal of that trend.

Figure 7.3 also provides a reminder that these trends are not by any means universal. There are probably many other developing countries in which the tuberculosis situation, as in Uganda and Lesotho, shows little or no sign of improvement or where it may be deteriorating. The figures suggest that in developing countries since the Second World War, the reduction in general mortality levels (which in turn has stimulated the increases in population), together with limited budgets for tuberculosis control measures, are factors which are tending to tip the balance towards the survival of the tubercle bacillus. In such countries, the urgent need is to develop more intensive tuberculosis control programmes in order to counteract this tendency.

Less information is available for leprosy than for tuberculosis but the same considerations apply. In most of those mainly tropical and developing countries in which leprosy has a high prevalence, it is probably wise to conclude that, as with tuberculosis, there have not been major improvements during the past 20 or 30 years. In all these countries, there is a need to monitor the endemic levels, both of tuberculosis and leprosy, in parallel with the introduction and implementation of effective control policies.

REFERENCES

Bechelli, L. M. and Dominguez, V. M. (1966). The leprosy problem in the world. *Bull. W.H.O.* **34**, 811–826.

Bechelli, L. M. and Dominguez, V. M. (1972). Further information on the leprosy problem in the world. *Bull. W.H.O.* **46**, 523–536.

Frost, W. H. (1937). How much control of tuberculosis? *Amer. J. Publ. Hlth* **27**, 759–766.

Miller, F. J. W. (1973). Regional differences in tuberculosis in children, with special reference to India and W. Africa. *Tropical Doctor* **3**, 66–71.

Mitchison, D. A. (1970). Regional variation in the guinea-pig virulence and other characteristics of tubercle bacilli. *Pneumonologie* **142**, 131–137.

Rees, R. J. W. and Meade, T. W. (1974). Comparison of the modes of spread and the incidence of tuberculosis and leprosy. *Lancet* **i**, 47–49.

Ruys, A. C. (1946). The influence of war conditions on bovine tuberculosis in man in Amsterdam. *Mon. Bull. Minist. Hlth* **5**, 67–71.

Sutherland, I. (1976). Recent studies in the epidemiology of tuberculosis, based on the risk of being infected with tubercle bacilli. *Adv. Tuberc. Res.* **19**, 1–63.

W.H.O. (1974). W.H.O. Expert Committee on tuberculosis, ninth report. *W.H.O. Tech. Rep. Ser.* **552**.

8. Diphtheria

J. A. Forbes

Age cannot wither her, nor custom stale Her infinite variety;
(Anthony and Cleopatra II, V 28).

An ubiquitous disease of antiquity, diphtheria is one of the historic scourges controlled, albeit tenuously, in some countries but still prevalent amongst the major populations of the world.

Few diseases attracted more attention both lay and scientific prior to the extensive use of vaccine in developed countries; lay attention induced by fear, scientific by the variety of diphtheritic phenomena as well as the mortality rates.

The derivation of the name of the causal organism, *Corynebacterium diphtheriae*, so elegantly described by Christie (1974), which preserves the three ancient Greek words denoting "a club-shaped rod or bacterium that produces a membrane in the throat", is at once explanatory and interesting.

The geography of diphtheria is that of scholarly descriptions and successful investigations of the disease which in modern times have been centred largely in the countries influenced by Koch and Pasteur, although ancient observations of the disease were made in Rome and Spain (Parish, 1968).

That the name is derived from the Greek, by way of the French, diphtérite and later, diphtérie, does not imply that the pestilence was worse in France or Greece any more than the connotation of the Spanish, French and Italian disease occurring in the wake of Columbus was true of these countries.

French writers dominated the early relatively modern literature on diphtheria, from Guilome de Bailou who described an epidemic in Paris in 1576 to Bretonneau who recognized its infectivity and coined the name in 1826. In America too, Samuel Bard published a classical description in 1771.

Klebs, Eberth and Loeffler added another European facet to the geography of the disease with their contributions to its initial bacteriology, and in 1888 Roux and Yersin, at the Pasteur Institute in Paris, showed that the organism produced an exotoxin which is responsible for the disease itself.

In Germany, Von Behring developed an antitoxin which was used initially to treat the disease in Berlin in 1891, and by 1895 horse serum antitoxin was being used in England and the U.S.A. as well as in France and Germany with dramatic results. Dr. Bela Schick of Vienna and later of New York who, in 1913, contributed the skin test for susceptibility to diphtheria, provided an important epidemiological tool for studying the disease.

Active immunization progressed in the 1920s when, in 1923 again as a part of the Pasteur heritage, Ramon showed that formalin-treated toxin was an antigenically-effective immunizing agent. The introduction of toxin-antitoxin and toxoid immunization, by no means an uneventful task, added geographic facets to the history of diphtheria immunization in the 1920s with tragedies involving a mortality in countries as diverse as in the U.S.A. and Austria through faulty manufacture and in Australia through staphylococcal contamination of an open ampule.

In 1931 refinements in the preparation of Diphtheria toxoid in England by Glenny, Pope, Waddington and Wallace, who found that the antigenicity of toxoid was enhanced by alum precipitation, allayed fears about the safety of the vaccine and led to its more extensive use. Extensive control of diphtheria, coinciding as it did with the introduction of antibiotics, led some to the fallacious use of antibiotics to treat the disease which, being caused by the exotoxin, requires a specific antitoxin for its amelioration. Erythromycin, however, is the effective drug of choice for clearing the carrier state (Haight and Finland, 1952; Forbes, 1954).

Recent observations (Sgouris *et al.*, 1969) suggest that preparation of human diphtheria immune globulin may be possible to replace the horse serum preparation, at least for use in relatively small doses as a prophylactic, if the volumes required for appropriate dosage preclude its use in the treatment of the disease. The toxigenic effects of diphtheria β-phage on non-toxigenic *Corynebacterium diphtheriae in vitro* has aroused discussion for more than a quarter of a century. Although hypotheses incriminating phage in the conversion of non-toxigenic to toxigenic strains *in vivo* as a fundamental epidemiological factor were commonly discussed, it is only in recent years that this hypothesis, still lacking final proof, has achieved scientific respectability. Apart from the successful antibiotic treatment of carriers, the principles of treatment and control have advanced little since the 1930s.

It is ironical that the efficient control of diphtheria should breed and illustrate novel problems for the well-immunized community with the development of professional disinterest in the diagnosis and management of the disease associated with lay complacence in the absence of a continuing epidemic threat. The consequent penalty of recurrent outbreaks in pockets of unimmunized children has been experienced in most "immunized" countries in which uninitiated professional reaction often leads to over investigation and under immunization. These emphasize the need for specialized Communicable Disease Hospital Centres to maintain skills in the management of inevitable recurrences of formerly common epidemic problems, as well as their other important functions.

Wherein lies the fascination of diphtheria? Is it for some the concept of a disease caused by an exotoxin which has an affinity for the myocardium and the nervous system, produced by organisms proliferating at a focus of infection in the throat? Is it the somewhat astonishing appreciation that antibiotics are of no value in the treatment of the disease itself, which requires the administration of specific diphtheria anti-toxin, anti-exotoxin which also curiously has a potent anti-bacterial effect in degrading the focus of infection? Is it the pattern of the disease after bacterial activity has subsided, in the development of later lethal lesions in myocarditis and the clockwork progression of paralyses for as long as 8 weeks? Is it the hypothetical implications of immunizing with a modified exotoxin to promote a herd immunity, which initially aroused emotive argument and gloomy predictions of excess carrier rates which have been dispelled by its effectiveness in practice?

For others the concept of phage-induced toxigenicity *in vivo* provokes interesting epidemiological speculation. Sir McFarlane Burnett (1973) is one of these and in the context of an Influenza Symposium, made the following comments.

Finally, a word about diphtheria, which I shall call the most extraordinary of all virus diseases. For those who remember what they were taught about the diphtheria bacillus and its toxin, I hasten to add that a virus disease due to phage β of the diphtheria bacilli is responsible for the production of diphtheria toxin. Some of the details are still not clear, but it appears highly probable that the structure of the toxin is genetically determined by the virus nucleic acid and that toxin may be liberated only by that fraction of bacilli in which the normally temperate phage is stimulated to proliferate and lyse the bacillus.

Recent studies by Pappenheimer and Gill (1973) clarify, for those versed in biosynthesis, the role of the *tox* gene of β-phage and the molecular mechanisms involved in the pathogenesis of diphtheria.

Since the *tox* gene of β-phage does not influence β-phage replication, a reduction in carriers of toxigenic diphtheria in an immunized population will be a function of the numbers game. Cases of diphtheria liberate many more β-phage infected toxigenic organisms than do carriers, a proportion of whom will be spreading non-toxigenic organisms which incidentally will not be immunizing or reinforcing the immunity of their recipients. In an immunized community, the net result will presumably be a reduction of the proportion of toxigenic carriers until the coincidental appearance β-phage in a pocket of unimmunized children.

Additionally, since the toxicity of *Corynebacterium diphtheriae* cultures may decline on keeping and since toxin is not produced in the presence of β-phage until the inorganic iron content of the culture medium is largely depleted, slavish reliance on the routine tests for the toxicity of isolates for public health purposes may be delusive.

The role of bacteriophages in the pathogenesis of diseases due to other toxin-producing bacteria, including cholera, tetanus, botulism, streptococcal and staphylococcal diseases, is coming under scrutiny. It seems by no means unlikely that extension of the work done on, and the thought stimulated by diphtheria may revive the interest shown in bacteriophages in the 1920s and yield new concepts of the pathogenesis, virulence and epidemiology of other bacteria.

REFERENCES

Burnet, F. M. (1973). Influenza—this disease. *Med. J. Aust.* (Spec. Suppl.) **1**, 3–6.

Christie, A. B. (1974). "Infectious Diseases Epidemiology and Clinical Practice". Churchill Livingstone, Edinburgh, London and New York.

Forbes, J. A. (1954). Treatment of persistent diphtheritic infection with erythromycin. *Med. J. Aust.* **11**, 501.

Haight, T. H. and Finland, M. (1952). Laboratory and clinical studies on erythromycin. *New Engl. J. Med.* **247**, 227.

Pappenheimer, A. M. Jr. and Gill, D. M. (1973). Diphtheria. *Science* **182**, 353–358.

Parish, H. J. (1968). "Victory with Vaccines". E. and S. Livingstone, Edinburgh.

Sgouris, J. T., Bolk, V. K., Angela, F., Portwood, L. and Gottshall, R. Y. (1969). Studies on diphtheria immunoglobulin prepared from outdated human blood. *Vox Sang.* **16**, 491–495.

9. Venereal Diseases

R. R. Willcox

INTRODUCTION

Influence of population concentration

Today venereal diseases are the most common infective diseases affecting man, except for the common cold. They affect all sectors of society. As with other communicable diseases, their distribution depends on the inter-relationship of geographical, historical, climatic, cultural and economic circumstances combined with social advancement and behavioural patterns.

The social conditions pertaining in the larger towns and cities ensure not only an increased number of cases but a higher incidence of disease. For example, in data from selected cities in the U.S.A. only 33.6–34.0% of the total population contributed 70.5–73.2% of the reported venereal disease (Fig. 9.1).

Influence of population mobility

The venereal diseases have traditionally affected the seaman and soldier through the mediary of prostitutes. Highest rates of infection are still found around military encampments, particularly in times of war. Until relatively recently, extremely high rates were found among the military personnel in Korea, Thailand and Vietnam (Fig. 9.2). The sailor has repeatedly been shown to be appreciably more prone to infection than the same age-groups of the home population.

However, the principal traveller is no longer the seaman but the

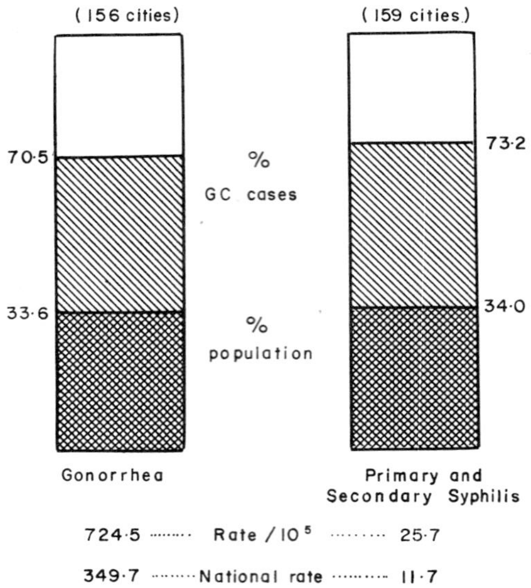

Fig. 9.1 Concentration of venereal disease in urban areas in the U.S.A. (data from *Amer. Soc. Hlth. Ass.*, 1973)

tourist. Although many of these consort with each other while abroad there is nevertheless a considerable inter-country exchange of disease.

In 1971, it was estimated that there were some 171 million tourists in the world, 126 million being in Europe. There are also more than

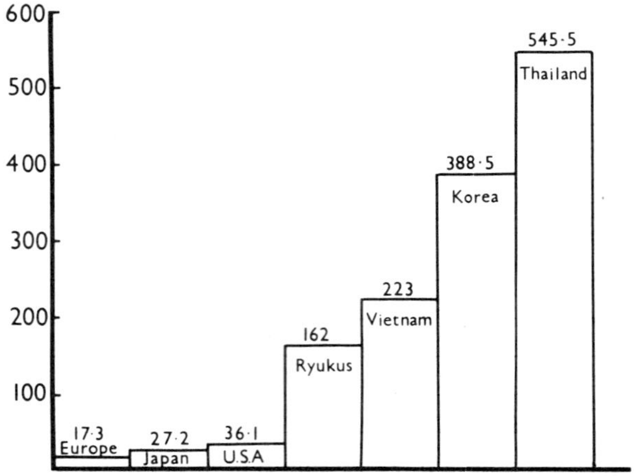

Fig. 9.2 Incidence per 1000 per annual mean strength of venereal disease in U.S. Army (1970 data from Greenberg, 1972).

10 million immigrant workers in Europe, half of whom return to their own countries each year.

Universally, much higher rates of infection are encountered amongst immigrant groups than in the home population of, for example, England and Wales (Fig. 9.3).

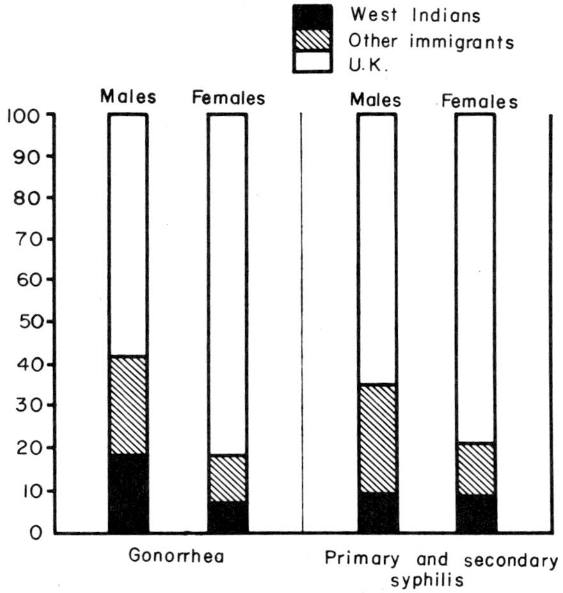

Fig. 9.3 Percentage distribution of venereal disease amongst immigrants and others in the United Kingdom (1968).

Influence of social change

So-called "civilization", resulting in homogenization of society and breaks in traditional home, religious and cultural ties, is occurring in all continents. Less profound effects from such changes have been claimed for some well-disciplined communist countries such as China though precise data are difficult to obtain.

Social changes are reflected more particularly in the reduced role of the prostitute in some Western countries such as the U.S.A., Canada and the United Kingdom. Prostitution in these countries is responsible now for only 10–20% of infections in males; it nevertheless still plays a significant role amongst seafarers and foreign visitors. Elsewhere prostitutes remain the major source of infection. In the West Pacific region, the Far East (e.g. Thailand, Hong Kong and Japan), most countries of South America and Africa, together with certain others in Europe (including Portugal, Italy and to a lesser extent France) prostitutes are responsible for up to 80–90% of the infections.

Difficulties in assessment

It is not possible to contrast the data of one country with those of another. While most countries provide some information concerning the cases of syphilis and gonorrhoea treated in their governmental institutions, the vast and unknown majority are treated and unrecorded elsewhere, e.g. in private practice, by pharmacists and quacks, or even by self-treatment.

Standards of diagnosis also affect the statistics. In some developing countries, inexperienced para-medical personnel label all cases of genital sore as "syphilis" and of genital discharge as "gonorrhoea"; the true picture may be very different. In developed countries with good reporting requirements such as pertain in, say, Sweden, there is compulsory reporting of positive findings from laboratories. Such reporting inevitably boosts numbers in such countries relative to those which lack such elaborate arrangements.

Venereal disease statistics can only claim to reflect comparative, sometimes misleading, trends within the same country since often, when rates are calculated, even on realistic data, they may be presented differently, e.g. per 100 000 total population or of a particular age-group.

THE TREPONEMATOSES

The treponematoses are contact diseases evoking indistinguishable antibodies caused by morphologically-similar organisms which comprise venereal and endemic syphilis (*Treponema pallidum*), yaws (*Treponema pertenue*) and pinta (*Treponema carateum*). Only venereal syphilis is transmitted sexually. Also *Treponema cuniculi* is responsible for a naturally-occurring venereal treponematosis (cuniculosis, pallidoidosis) in rabbits and another treponeme (*Treponema Fribourg Blanc*) has been found in the *cynocephalus* monkey in some yaws areas which may represent an animal reservoir of the condition.

It is postulated that the pathogenic treponemes arose originally from free-living organisms in water or mud (of which *Treponema zuelzerae*, which shares some antigenicity with *Treponema pallidum*, still remains an example) and these became adapted to man in the manner of the saprophytic spirochaetes which may be found in dirty mouths and wounds, in the bowel and elsewhere. Some believe the human diseases to be caused by the same organism, producing varying clinical patterns in different environments; others that the organisms concerned are closely allied, the spread and extent of each being determined by environmental circumstances.

Venereal syphilis is ubiquitous, yaws is found in the low-latitude areas between the tropics of Cancer and Capricorn, endemic syphilis in the adjacent semi-arid regions and pinta in Central America and the northern part of South America (Fig. 9.4). Venereal syphilis recognizes no class barriers but the others are diseases of the under-privileged.

PINTA (CARATE; MAL DEL PINTO; "BLUE STAIN" DISEASE)

Geographical distribution

This disease is found today amongst the primitive under-privileged Indians in remote jungle areas of Central America and the northern part of the South American continent. It is most prevalent in Mexico, Venezuela, Columbia, Peru and Ecuador. It has also been reported in Argentina, Chile, Cuba, the Dominican Republic and Haiti. The disease is not known for certainty outside the Americas.

Evolution of pinta

Pinta, which is spread by skin to skin contact, has been regarded as the first of the endemic treponematoses. It is virtually confined to the skin, producing an initial and subsequently satellite or more remote lesion (pintides) of various colours ranging from pink, brown, blue and black, finally becoming achromatic. It is believed that the disease originally arose in the Afro-Asian land mass and was carried by man

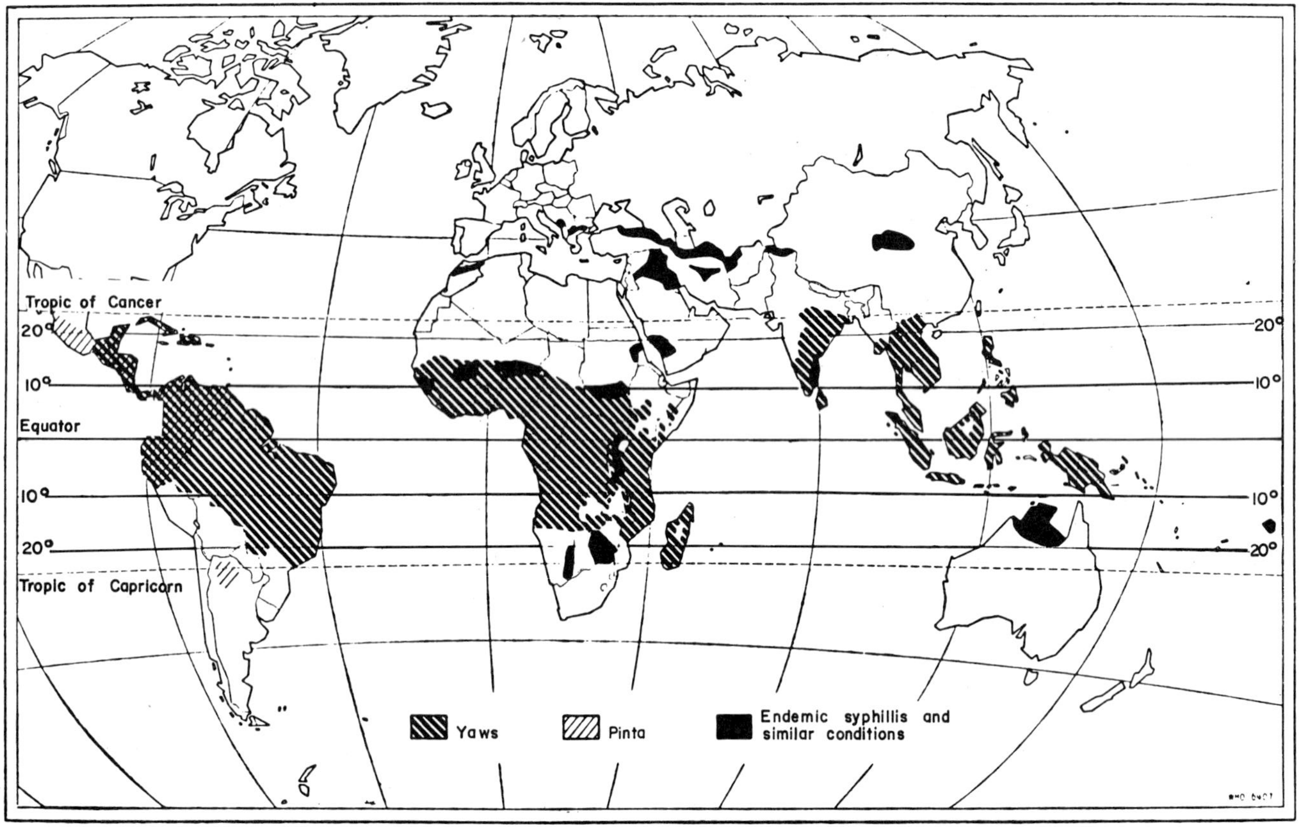

Fig. 9.4 Treponematoses (courtesy of W.H.O.).

to the Americas in his earliest migrations over the then ice-free land bridge across the Bering Straits. Its present localization has been attributed to this region being largely excluded from the mainstream of migration and evolutionary change in the manner of the unusual finches and other birds found by Darwin on the Galapagos Islands.

With such developments as the opening up of jungle territories by air and by road, changing social customs such as the wearing of more clothes by primitive Indians and the beneficial effects of penicillin, the future trend is towards the disappearance of pinta and its replacement by venereal syphilis against which it confers immunity.

YAWS (FRAMBOESIA, PIAN)

Evolution

It is thought that pinta evolved into yaws when the humid warm climate developed in Afro-Asia around 10 000 B.C. Others have suggested the reverse process. The new environment ensured the selection of mutant organisms producing the characteristic exuberant skin lesions which remain infective for long periods of time. Trauma occasioned by the absence of clothes and sweaty skins ensured its rapid spread in primitive tropical communities and it quickly became mainly a disease of childhood.

Clinical aspects

Yaws, unlike pinta, has serious complications remote from the skin including osteo-periostitis and hyperkeratosis of the feet ("crab yaws") in the early infection and gummatous ulcerative lesions of skin and bone in the late disease, including destruction of the nose and palate (gangosa). By its effects on economic potential, it breeds poverty which in turn breeds more disease.

Geographical distribution

Twenty years ago it was estimated that there were approximately 50 million cases of yaws existing between the tropics of Cancer and

Capricorn. The disease was found in the northern South America (Brazil, Venezuela, Colombia, Ecuador and British and French Guiana), in the Caribbean area (including the Dominican Republic, Jamaica and Tobago and Haiti). In Haiti, 50% of the population was affected—the world's highest prevalence.

Half of the world total of cases was believed to exist within the tropical belt of Africa, while in South-East Asia, it was prevalent throughout Indonesia, Malaya, Thailand and those countries which are now called Laos, Cambodia and Vietnam. Scattered pockets also existed in Southern India, Burma and Sri Lanka (Ceylon). It was also found in Northern Queensland, Australia, and many islands of the Western Pacific (including the Phillipines, New Guinea and the Gilbert, Ellis and Solomon Islands), sometimes with high incidence.

Decline in prevalence of yaws

Yaws has declined in prevalence following economic and social advancement. The process has been markedly accelerated by W.H.O.-assisted mass campaigns in the West Pacific Region (e.g. in the former Netherlands New Guinea, New Hebrides, Philippines, Western Samoa, Solomon Islands and Tonga), South East Asia (e.g. in Cambodia, Indonesia, Laos, Malaya and Thailand), Africa (e.g. in Nigeria, Sierra Leone, Togo and Upper Volta) and in the Americas (e.g. in Ecuador, Haiti and Paraguay). In these campaigns—in addition to those against endemic syphilis—more than 368 million examinations have been made of 154½ million persons and in excess of 47 millions have been treated with penicillin as clinical cases, latent cases or contacts.

Prevalences found at the time of the initial mass campaigns (1952–1956) included 4.1% in Togo, 3.0% in Western Samoa, 1.9% in Eastern Nigeria, 0.13% in Southern Thailand and 0.10% in the Philippines. By 1961–1966, these percentages had been reduced to 0.11, zero, 0.07, 0.06 and 0.04 respectively. In other countries (e.g. Papua and New Guinea and Venezuela), new clinical cases became rare although in some areas they are again increasing. However FTA and TPI-test reactors are still found in some children, probably indicating that low level transmission persists.

SYPHILIS

Evolution

Possibly around 8000 B.C., a further evolution occurred in the more arid regions which bordered on the yaws areas. The drier climate, though still warm, was frequently cold at night and necessitated the wearing of clothes. With the protection thus offered and the lesser prevalence of exuberant lesions on the now dry skins, the organisms could only survive by producing infective lesions of mucous membranes. These, as a result of direct contact by kissing or indirectly by the use of fingers or communal drinking vessels, still resulted in childhood spread. Infected children retained the latent childhood disease through to maturity and were thus not susceptible to venereal syphilis.

Geographical distribution

Endemic syphilis under the name *bejel* or *balash* has been studied in recent times in a number of Middle-Eastern countries, usually in desert or near desert regions. In Africa, it is found in the north in countries bordering the Sahara desert and in the south in those countries around the Kalahari desert (under the name *njovera* in Rhodesia and *dichuchwa* in adjacent Botswana). The disease is also encountered in the Transvaal in the South-African Karoo.

Foci of endemic syphilis were present in Europe in Bosnia (Yugoslavia) even after the Second World War. Between the two World Wars, the disease extended over wide areas of southern U.S.S.R. (e.g. the Ukraine and Uzbekistan) and in the then Palestine. The many historical examples in Europe include the *button scurvy* of Ireland, the *sibbens* of Scotland, the *radesyge* of Norway, the *Dithmarsh Evil* of Schleswig-Holstein, and the *spirocolon* of Greece. Doubtless the disease was widespread in Europe in pre-Columbian times.

Emergence of venereal syphilis

A most effective W.H.O.-assisted mass campaign based on penicillin has been conducted against the endemic syphilis of Bosnia. Initially in 1948–1951, there were 2.3% of infectious cases in the localized populations affected but the disease has now been eradicated. Other W.H.O. campaigns against endemic syphilis have taken place in Botswana (then Bechuanaland) and Iraq. Following such campaigns, new populations emerge which are susceptible to venereal syphilis.

Without such campaigns venereal syphilis emerges from endemic syphilis only when primitive customs and unhygienic habits are discarded, enabling some young persons to become susceptible by escaping the childhood infection. During the period of transmission, while some unhygienic habits persist, both non-venereal and venereal infections are found together with older persons now being affected by the former as the prevalence of the childhood infection wanes.

Should there be any deterioration in social conditions accompanied by overcrowding, venereal syphilis may well "spill over" once more to the children. Isolated small, usually family, examples have been periodically described in a number of countries including Austria, Hungary, India, Scotland, South Africa and the U.S.A.

VENEREAL SYPHILIS

The distribution of venereal syphilis is world wide except for those areas where the endemic treponematoses are found. Following peak levels during or immediately following the Second World War, many of the areas of venereal syphilis experienced a marked decline in incidence—over 95% in some countries. In recent years, however, there has been a slight to moderate regression.

Geographical distribution

Africa

Syphilis remains common throughout Africa. In a few countries, it is still emerging from endemic syphilis. It is particularly prevalent in Ethiopia (Abyssinia) where in some areas 40% sero-positivity has been found. In Fez (Morocco), early syphilis increased threefold between the years 1960 and 1968. In Uganda, 7–16% of sero-positive reactors have been found amongst blood donors.

In some countries syphilis incidence has been overstated since chancroid, herpes and other genital sores may be diagnosed as "syphilis" on clinical grounds and serological results confused by past yaws. In some countries, e.g. Chad, Mali and Senegal, the numbers had decreased in 1972–1973 compared with 1965.

The Americas

In 1962, when the syphilis rate in North America was calculated as 63.9 per 100 000 of the population, that of Central America was assessed at 77.3 and that of South America (excluding Brazil) as 47.8.

In Canada in 1970, 892 cases of infectious syphilis were notified. This was slightly less than in the previous year.

In the U.S.A., where four-fifths of cases are unreported, the rate per 100 000 for reported infectious primary and secondary syphilis was 21.6 in 1950. This fell to a low point of 3.8 in 1957. Subsequently, there was a rise to 12.3 in 1965, falling to 9.3 in 1969, but increasing again to 12.1 (11 080 reported cases) in 1973. Rates in that year were highest in South Carolina (29.6), Georgia (26.4 per 100 000), Florida (26.4) and New York (19.9); they were lowest in Montana (0.7), South Dakota (0.7), North Dakota (1.0) and Wyoming (1.1) (Fig. 9.5).

In Trinidad and Tobago in 1972, there were 141 reported cases of primary and secondary syphilis compared with 8071 of gonorrhoea. In Guadeloupe, 10% of sero-reactors were found in expectant mothers and 3.9–9.4% amongst assorted patients in Guyana.

Asia and the Western Pacific region

In Thailand in 1970, the rate for infectious syphilis was 12.99 per 100 000 in the population over 15 years of age (2528 cases). High rates of infection have been reported from parts of India, particularly around Bombay. In Sri Lanka, where it was estimated that three times as much venereal disease was treated outside clinics and not reported, the recorded rate was 6.6 per 100 000 in 1970/71 compared with 8.8 per 100 000 in 1965/66.

In the Western Pacific region, the W.H.O. reported in 1968 that following the post-war decline there had been recent increases in parts of Australia, New Zealand, Fiji, Japan, Malaysia and Vietnam. Increased sero-positivity rates had also been encountered in Korea and Taiwan. Decreases were reported in Hong Kong (after an earlier

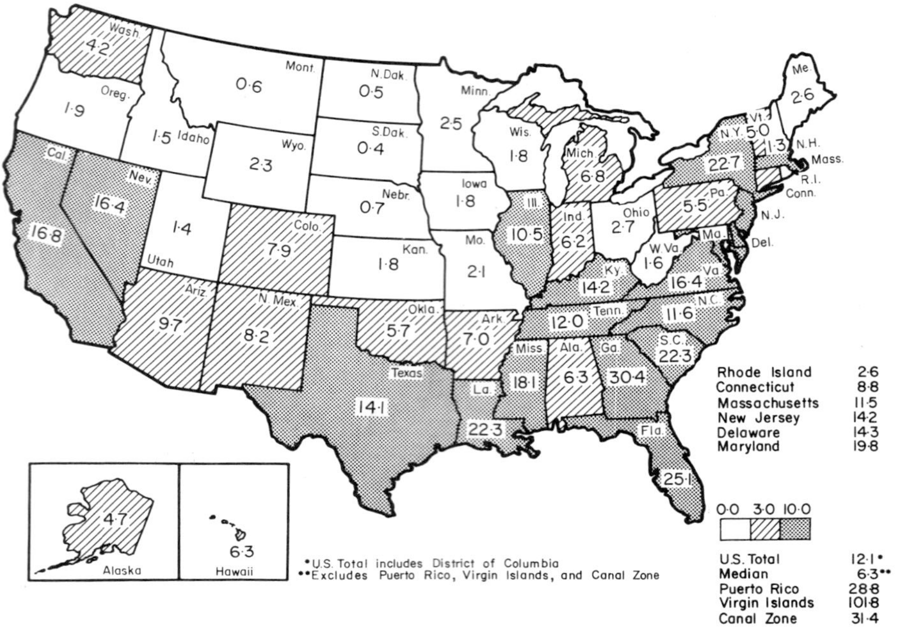

Fig. 9.5 Primary and secondary syphilis case rates per 100 000 in the U.S.A. in the fiscal year, 1973. (Reproduced with permission of Technical Information Services, Bureau of State Services, Center for Disease Control, Department of Health, Education and Welfare, U.S.A.)

rise), the Philippines, Singapore (to a slight extent) and smaller areas such as French Polynesia, New Caledonia, Papua and New Guinea, the Trust Territory of the Pacific Islands and Western Samoa.

Some sero-positivity rates on routine tests on expectant mothers in this region are shown in Table 9.1.

The percentages of sero-reactors found in students in the same years included 3.5 for Korea, 2.6 for Singapore, and 0.2 for Japan (in which country 1.1% of positives were found in premarital tests). Amongst soldiers the figure in Taiwan was 5.4, Korea 2.8 and New Caledonia 0.6 while no less a proportion than 21.2% was obtained amongst blood donors in Korea. This latter figure must to some extent reflect the methods of testing in use.

In the Western Pacific region also, there are a number of examples (which include Tahiti and Papua and New Guinea) of syphilis appearing where it was previously seldom seen following the near disappearance of early yaws. Indeed, in Papua and New Guinea, there is a considerable recently-occurring outbreak of syphilis along the new road traversing the Highlands from the port of Lae in the east to Mount Hagen in the centre. Prostitutes and lorry drivers contribute to the latitudinal spread which occurs in proportion to the sexual permissiveness of the local population being especially marked amongst the promiscuous Chimbu.

Europe

In 1950–1954, W.H.O. data from 20 countries showed highest case rates for Spain, 18.8 per 100 000, followed by Austria, 17.0 per 100 000, and Yugoslavia, 16.6 per 100 000; lowest rates were recorded for Belgium and Hungary, 1.5 per 100 000 respectively. By 1955–1959, data per 100 000 from 23 countries placed Poland at the top (16.1) followed by Spain (5.8); lowest rates were reported from Finland (0.6), Scotland (0.6) and Hungary (0.3).

There has been a rise in incidence in many countries following the low points reached in 1955–1959 (Fig. 9.6) and the situation in 1974 resembles that of 1950–1954. The problem is still a considerable one particularly in Poland and in Romania.

	Year	Test	Tested	Percentage positive
Korea	1966	VDRL	330	6.9
Taipei City	1967	VDRL and Kahn	1 555	6.6
Vietnam	1967	VDRL	11 060	6.4
Taiwan	1967	VDRL	17 610	3.0
New Caledonia	1967	Kline, Kolmer	988	1.5
Japan	1967	Ogota WR	609 607	1.1
Hong Kong	1967	VDRL and RPCFT	55 012	0.3
Singapore	1967	Unspecified	12 983	0.3
Philippines	1966	Unspecified	3 586	0.08
Sri Lanka	1970	VDRL	29 120	2.0
Thailand	1969	VDRL	38 973	10.3
Trinidad and Tobago	1972	VDRL	15 859	3.1

Table 9.1 Routine serum tests on expectant mothers in selected areas.

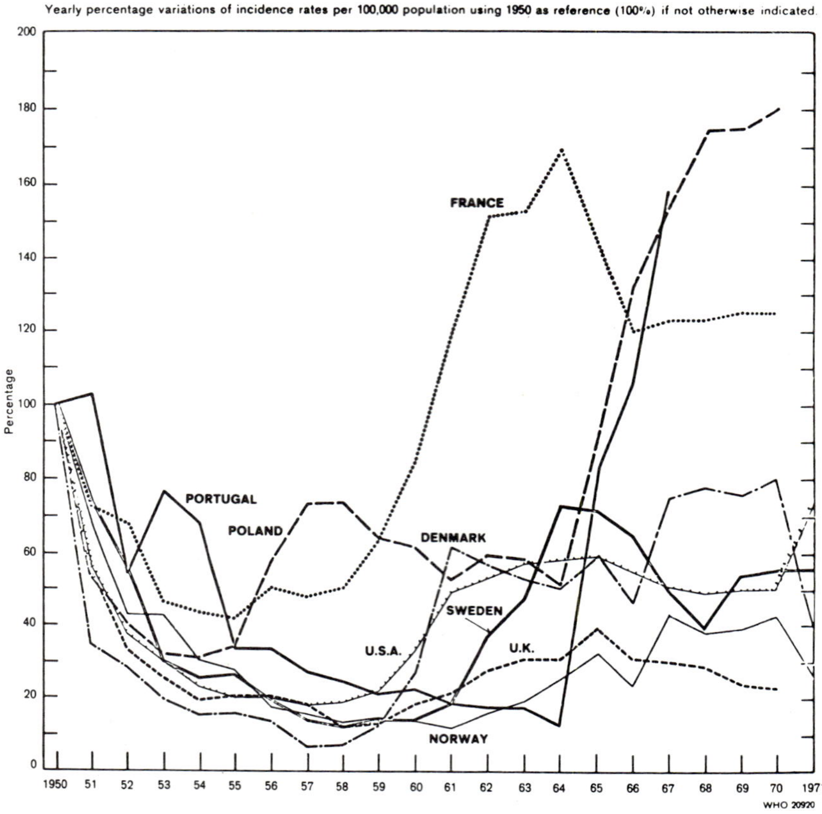

Fig. 9.6 Reported primary and secondary syphilis 1950–71 (W.H.O. data).

In the United Kingdom, there were 17 675 cases of acquired syphilis under one year in 1946, which fell to 704 in 1958 but rose again to over 2000 in 1965. Until recently, the disease has been contained below this figure: but the rate of 4.59 per 100 000 in 1973 was substantially greater than the 3.64 for 1967. In 1973, positive serological tests amongst primiparae ante-natal patients in different parts of the country varied from 0.036% to 0.124%.

In France the rebound was higher. The 15 000 reported cases in 1946 fell to 1837 in 1959 but increased to 4039 in 1967. In East Germany in 1972, the infectious syphilis rate was 3.2 per 100 000 being highest (13.3) in Berlin and lowest (0.7) in Neubrandenberg. In

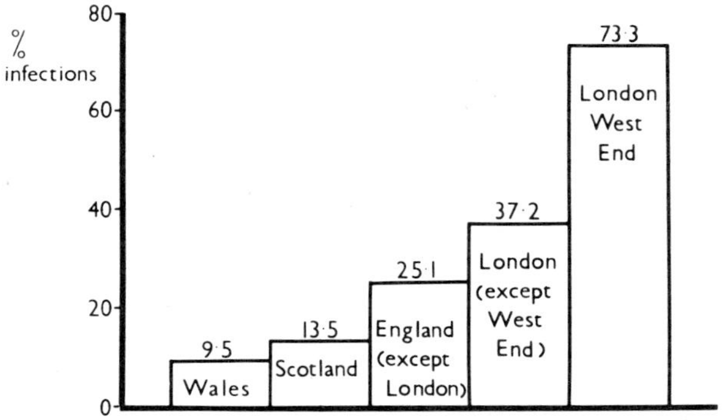

Fig. 9.7 Primary and secondary syphilis: incidence of homosexuality in the United Kingdom in males.

Poland, there were 2681 cases of early syphilis in 1955, 7435 in 1965 rising to no less than 16 383 in 1971 with a subsequent fall to 6654 in 1974.

Influence of homosexuality

In Great Britain in 1971, for example, no less than 42.4% of the infections with primary and secondary syphilis were homosexually acquired. This percentage was lowest in Wales (9.5%) and Scotland (13.5%); highest was in London (62.1%) with an even greater concentration (73.3%) in five clinics in the West End of the capital (Fig. 9.7). Indeed in London, with only 13.7% of the United

Region	No. in thousands	Percentage	Percentage of total primary and secondary syphilis	Percentage of homosexual infections
London	7379	13.7	50.5	74.0
Remainder of England	38 491	71.5	39.3	23.2
Scotland	5228	9.7	4.5	1.0
Wales	2723	5.1	5.6	1.8
Total	53 821	100.0	100.0	100.0

Table 9.2 Percentage of total primary and secondary syphilis in males and of total homosexual infections according to population in the United Kingdom (data from *Br. Coop. Clin. Group*, 1973).

Kingdom's population, were found no less than one-half of the reported male cases of primary and secondary syphilis and nearly three-quarters of the national total of infections known to have been contracted homosexually (Table 9.2).

Decline in the complications of syphilis

In addition to bone changes and gummata as found in yaws, syphilis has the serious late complications of cardiovascular and neurosyphilis and it may also be congenitally transmitted. Since the introduction of penicillin, the numbers of cases with late complications, and deaths from the disease, have markedly declined (Fig. 9.8).

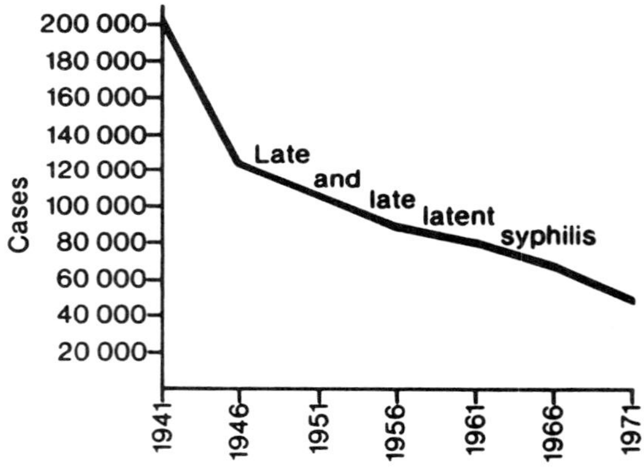

Fig. 9.8 Decline in late syphilis in the U.S.A.

Although congenital syphilis has been reduced to an almost insignificant problem in developed countries (e.g. in U.S.S.R. and the United Kingdom only 16 cases under 1 year were reported in 1971), in some other areas (e.g. Ethiopia, Uganda and Mexico) it remains a problem.

GONORRHOEA

Gonorrhoea is a discharge-producing inflamation caused by the gonococcus. Untreated, numerous complications arise, such as urethral stricture and epididymitis in the male, salpingitis with sterility in the female and arthritis, rheumatism and iritis in both sexes. It may also cause ophthalmia neonaturum which has been responsible for much of the world's blindness.

The complications of gonorrhoea are now uncommon in developed countries where antibiotics are generally available. In developing areas, however, where patients either do not seek treatment or enlist the help of practitioners of "native medicine", or else receive inadequate treatment by pharmacists, they remain a significant health problem.

Geographical distribution

Gonorrhoea is ubiquitous. As with syphilis, peak rates were recorded in many countries during or just after the Second World War. These had fallen by 50–70% by 1956–1959 but since then there has been an alarming world-wide sustained upsurge and, in some areas the peak wartime figures have already been surpassed.

Africa

Gonorrhoea is rife throughout Africa, affecting all social groups. One quarter of the students in some universities in Uganda and Nigeria (as in Sweden in Europe) have been reported to be affected with urethritis annually.

Americas

In 1962, the gonorrhoea rate for North America was assessed at 139.8 per 100 000, for Central America at 111.1 and for South America (excluding Brazil and Argentina) at 150.7.

In Canada, the numbers of cases doubled between 1960 and 1970. In the U.S., there were 303 922 cases in 1950 (204.0 per 100 000) which fell to 216 476 cases in 1957 (129.8 per 100 000). By 1973, however, there had been an increase to 809 681 reported cases (392.2 per 100 000), although the actual number, including those treated by private practitioners, was believed to be nearer 2½ million. Highest rates per 100 000 were obtained in South Carolina (896.6), Alaska (886.9), Georgia (764.2), Florida (683.9), and Tennessee (673.3); lowest rates were in Vermont (88.1), New Hampshire (93.9), North Dakota (110.2) and Iowa (120.9) (Fig. 9.9). The 1974 figures were even greater (874 161 cases).

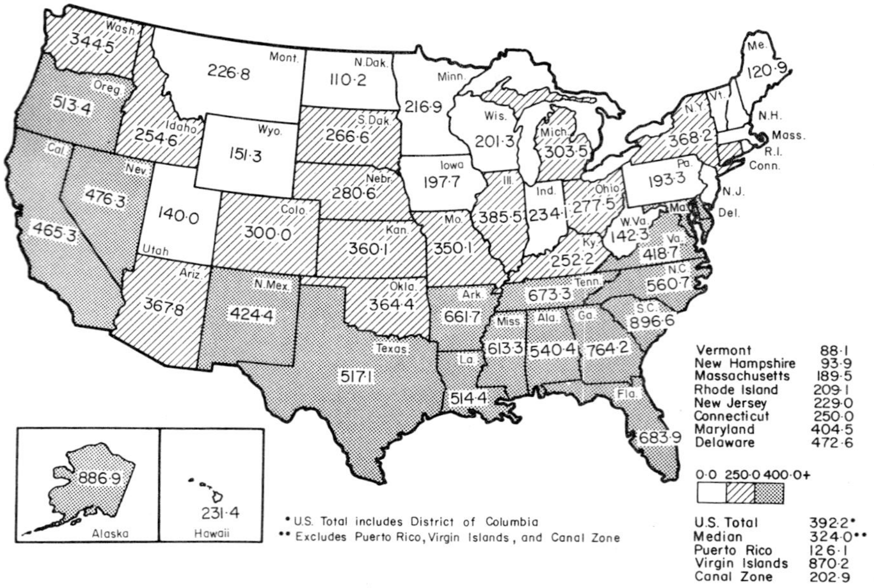

Fig. 9.9 Gonorrhoea case rates per 100 000 in the U.S.A. in 1973 fiscal year. (Reproduced with permission by Technical Information Services, Bureau of State Services, Center for Disease Control, Department of Health, Education and Welfare, U.S.A.)

Asia and Western Pacific region

In the Western Pacific region of W.H.O., the percentage increases in the prevalence of gonorrhoea between 1960–1967 with the reported 1967 figures in brackets were Western Samoa 597.1 (244), Philippines 268.7 (4397), Fiji 152.6 (962), New Zealand 142.4 (2305)—where incidentally the number of cases had nearly tripled between 1955 and 1956—Vietnam 108.3 (2066), Australia (6 states only) 55.9 (7712), Trust Territory of the Pacific Islands 42.7 (488), Hong Kong 12.9 (7344) and Singapore 3.5 (2617)—where, in 1971, the total proven gonorrhoea rate was estimated at 373 and the total urethritis rate at 877 per 100 000; falls were recorded in Japan and New Caledonia. The fact that more cases should be reported from New Zealand than Vietnam, in which country in 1960 the U.S. medical authorities estimated that 40 000 cases of gonorrhoea were occurring in the civilian population *each week*, further emphasizes the virtual uselessness of venereal disease statistics for comparative purposes.

In Sri Lanka, the gonorrhoea rates per 100 000 were 31.0 in 1970/71 compared with 23.3 in 1965/66. In Thailand in 1970, which contained military forces from without the country, the gonorrhoea rate had soared to 515.73, per 100 000 population over the age of 15 (100 396 cases), from 5.79 (1101 cases) in 1953 (Fig. 9.10).

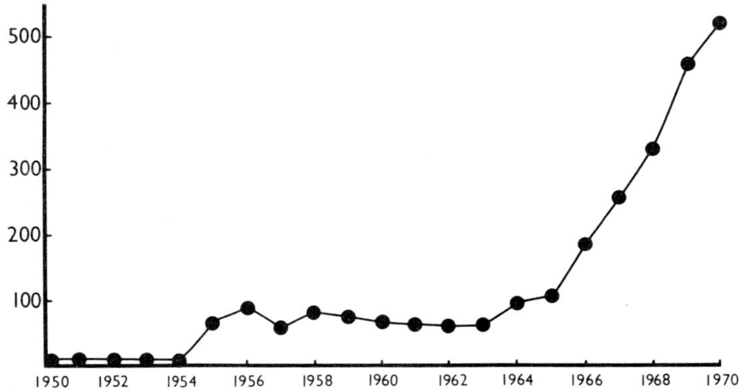

Fig. 9.10 Increase in gonorrhoea in Thailand. Case rates are per 100 000 population over 15 years of age (57% of total).

Europe

By 1960–1965, an increasing prevalence of gonorrhoea over a 5-year

A World Geography of Human Diseases

Erratum

On page 219, line 18, Poland should read Finland.

in 1946 fell to 17 536 by 1954. Since that time there has been a practically unbroken increase. In England alone, there were 58 645

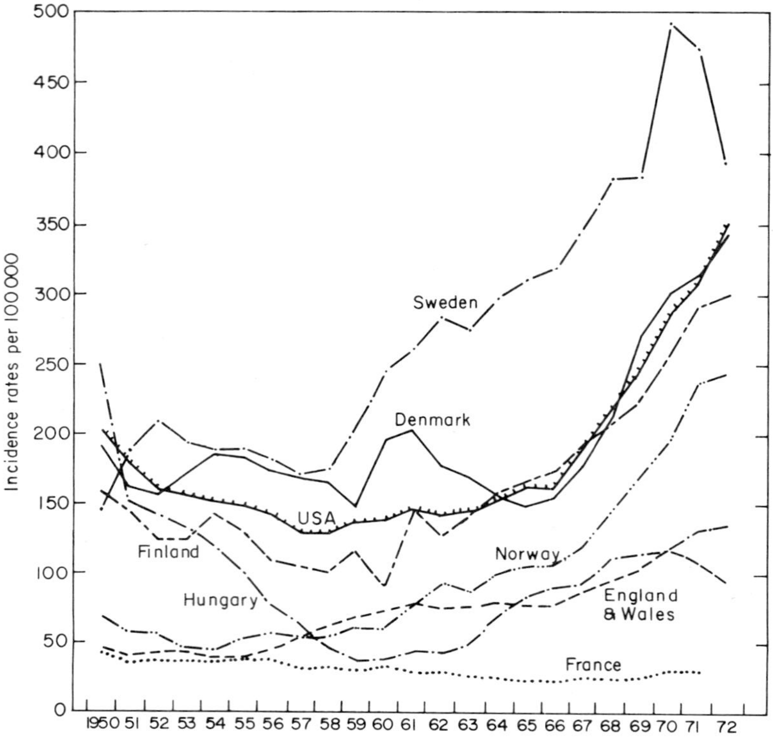

Fig. 9.11 Gonorrhoea incidence trends in Europe (W.H.O. data).

cases in 1973, a rate per 100 000 of 126.10 compared with 81.17 in 1966.

Epidemiological factors

Factors leading to the failure to control gonorrhoea lie in the frequent asymptomatic infection in the woman and in the passive homosexual male, together with those stemming from its short incubation period and consequent rapid spread. Changing modes, earlier sexual awakening, modern contraceptive devices and more varied sexual habits also contribute. Oral sex is now commonplace and mouth infections with gonorrhoea—reported in up to 6–10% of patients with genital gonorrhoea in Denmark and elsewhere—are being increasingly recognized. In a recent series of tests at St. Mary's Hospital, London, oral sex had been practised in the previous three months by 41.0% of 105 female gonorrhoea contacts and rectal sex by 18.1%.

Male homosexuals were recently responsible for 4.0% of the infections in males in Wales, 4.1% in Scotland and 10.5% in England as a whole. They were responsible for 19.9% in London and as much as 27.6% in the clinics of the West End of the city (Fig. 9.12).

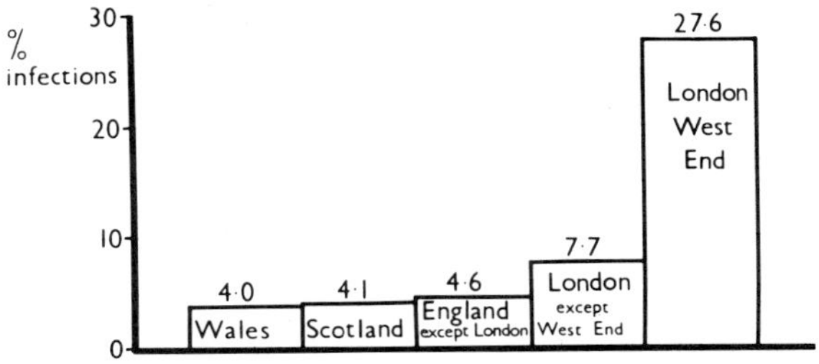

Fig. 9.12 Gonorrhoea incidence of homosexuality in males in the United Kingdom.

Another important factor in the increasing failure rates is the development of resistance of the gonococcus to penicillin. The degree of resistance varies geographically, being worse in the Far East and Africa than in the United Kingdom and Northern Europe (Fig. 9.13). The importance of this factor is related to frequent sexual interchange amongst promiscuous groups in some areas, to the degree of self treatment or treatment by pharmacists with inadequate doses of antibiotics and to the extent of the basic free clinic facilities available to the population to "mop up" and dispose of failing cases.

Recently some totally resistant strains have been encountered.

NON-GONOCOCCAL URETHRITIS

Non-gonococcal ("non-specific") urethritis is a condition usually recognized in males only in which the gonococcus cannot be found in the urethral discharge. About 1% of presumably inherently susceptible patients develop the serious systemic rheumatic and other complications of Reiter's syndrome.

A proportion of cases may be associated with intra-urethral sores and tumours (including urethral stricture), with diseases of the

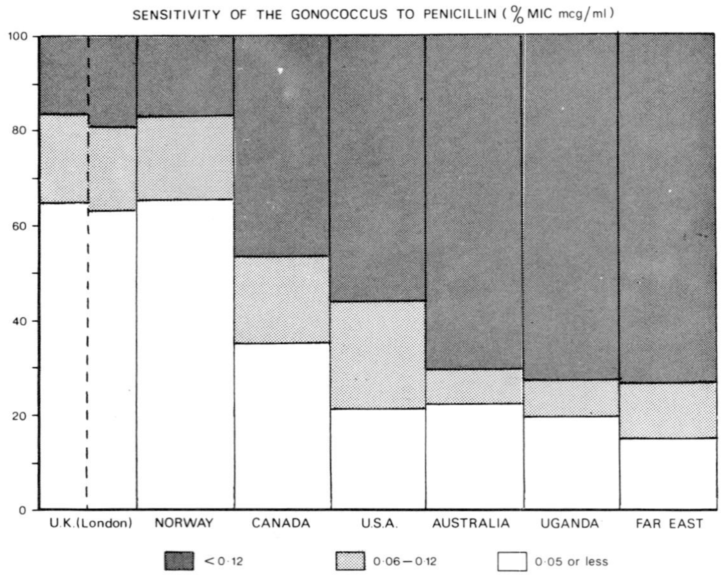

Fig. 9.13 Resistance of the gonococcus to penicillin.

urinary tract (e.g. cystitis from all causes, including bilharziasis), with such known agents as *Trichomonas vaginalis*, *Candida albicans* and *Herpes simplex* virus. However, none of the causes apparently operates in 70–90% of patients. Mycoplasma may be isolated but, albeit sexually-transmitted, they have uncertain significance.

For many years, inclusions resembling those of the genus now called *Chlamydia* have been found in the urethral epithelial cells of affected patients. Using modern techniques of tissue culture, such can be isolated in approximately 40% of the cases. The agent resembles that of trachoma and of inclusion conjunctivitis and is sometimes termed "TRIC agent". The disease may occur on its own or follow treated gonorrhoea, in which case it is presumably due to double infection.

Geographical distribution

The condition is world-wide but there are varying degrees of recognition according to diagnostic standards. Not being statistically reportable in most countries, there are few reliable figures of incidence. In the United Kingdom, where there is a close network of clinics and the disease has been reportable since 1951, the numbers of cases rose steadily from 10 794 in that year to 46 912 in 1970. The rise has been even more marked following changes in reporting classification criteria (Fig. 9.14).

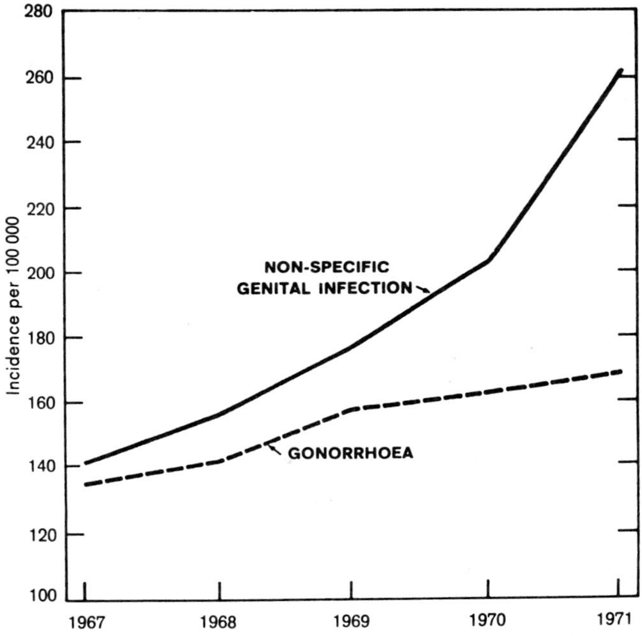

Fig. 9.14 Rising prevalence of non-gonococcal urethritis in England and Wales.

As mild or asymptomatic cases may occur in males and, because of the so-far practical impossibility to demonstrate its presence in females in routine practice, there is an almost complete absence of control measures against it. With the present extent of modern travel it must surely be assumed that the genital transmission of chlamydia occurs on a global basis from Alaska to Auckland, and from Vladivostok to Valparaiso.

Non-gonococcal urethritis was first generally accepted as an entity in the United Kingdom during the Second World War. At this time, thousands of troops were admitted to hospital for early morning smears and the gonococcus was found wanting. At the end of the

Second World War, it was reported that gonorrhoea was becoming penicillin-resistant in the Far East. The U.S. Surgeon General sent a team to Hawaii, the Philippines, Korea and Japan which reported that gonococci were recovered from only 9% of so-called penicillin failures. Spot examinations of 2000 men in these areas showed that whereas 1.22% had gonorrhoea 12.4% had non-gonococcal urethritis. Furthermore, in a routine check of enlisted men who had never left the U.S.A., this condition was found to be five times more common than gonorrhoea. However, the disease is not reported statistically from clinics and no collated civilian data are available.

Elsewhere reports from individual physicians and clinics emphasize its prevalence throughout Central, East, West and North Africa, countries surrounding the Mediterranean, Europe, the Caribbean and Central and South America, as already noted in the United Kingdom.

W.H.O. reports indicate that the disease is more prevalent than gonorrhoea in Sydney, New South Wales, Korea (four times more so), Japan and New Caledonia, and probably so in Laos, but less so in Hong Kong, Singapore, Sri Lanka (rate 3.9 per 100 000 in 1970/71), Taiwan and the Philippines where the two diseases alternate for supremacy.

Epidemiology

The TRIC agent has been found in material from cases of non-gonococcal urethritis in males and in their female consorts (in whom the condition "inclusion cervicitis" has been recognized by colposcopy) and in some cases of opthalmia neonatorum. It is also responsible for inclusion conjunctivitis in the adult. The fact that the organism is very similar or else the same as that of trachoma has led to the postulate that trachoma—which causes greater havoc in the eye amongst poor people in unhygienic surroundings—is itself often genitally spread.

Non-gonococcal urethritis is a disease of the permissive society. It affects all social groups and is frequently contracted from friends (who pronounce themselves horrified that they should be thought to harbour a venereal-transmitted agent). The role of chlamydia in the common condition of non-specific proctitis in male passive homosexuals has yet to be elucidated.

CHANCROID

Chancroid (soft chancre, soft sore, ulcus molle, chancre mou) is an auto-inoculable, sexually-transmitted disease caused by a bacillus the *Haemophilus ducreyi*. It is characterized by necrotizing ulceration and inflammatory enlargement with suppuration of the regional lymph nodes. Once a very prevalent disease with world-wide distribution, it remains common now only in certain tropical and subtropical countries; elsewhere it has become or is becoming rare.

Geographical distribution

Africa

The true incidence of chancroid is unknown in those areas where diagnostic facilities are limited, where (without dark-field or serum tests) cases of genital sore tend to be diagnosed clinically as "syphilis" and where serological findings are confused by previous yaws. The author in 1956, reviewing the then available evidence from African countries, noted that the number of cases of gonorrhoea compared with those of chancroid was less than 10 to one in certain medical faculties of present-day Botswana, Ghana, Nigeria and the then French Dahomey and French Somaliland. The chancroid condition comprised no less than 18 and 26% respectively of all the venereal infections encountered in venereal-disease clinics in Accra (Ghana) and Salisbury (Rhodesia).

The disease has always been endemic in North Africa, and especially so in Morocco. Many cases were encountered amongst troops stationed there during the Second World War. Chancroid is prevalent in Ethiopia.

The Americas

Though, at present, found more commonly in South and Central America, chancroid was once endemic in the south-eastern states of the U.S.A. Recent data from the U.S.A. (Table 9.3) show the marked rise associated with the Second World War, the subsequent decline and recent slight resurgence.

Asia

According to the W.H.O., chancroid was prevalent in 1959 in

Year	Cases	Case rate per 100 000
1941	3384	2.5
1947	9039	6.4
1956	2322	1.4
1961	1595	0.9
1966	950	0.5
1968	827	0.4
1971	1507	0.7
1974	1064	0.5

Table 9.3 Chancroid cases reported by State Health Departments in the U.S.A. (U.S.P.H.S., 1975).

Cambodia, Hong Kong, Laos, Singapore, Taiwan and Vietnam. In a number of these countries, it was more prevalent than syphilis. It was reported as rare in Australia, New Zealand, French Polynesia and the Philippines. Declining prevalence rates were also reported from Hong Kong, Korea, Philippines, Singapore, Taiwan and Japan. In Japan, rates per 100 000 had fallen from 52.3 in 1947 to only 3.4 in 1956. By 1969, cases were still being encountered in Fiji, Hong Kong, New Caledonia, Vietnam and Singapore. In Singapore there were 478 cases in 1967, 36 of them seamen.

The disease was encountered amongst U.S. servicemen in Japan, Okinawa and Korea. It is endemic in Vietnam and in some military units it was second only to gonorrhoea in venereal disease incidence; the same has been noted for clinical patients in New Delhi, India. In Sri Lanka, in 1970/71 the rate was 5.2 per 100 000 compared with 6.6 for primary and secondary syphilis.

Europe

Chancroid is becoming uncommon in Europe now, but at one time it was endemic in the Mediterranean region, especially in Italy (where large numbers of troops were infected during the Second World War). In 1912, in the British Army at home, the case rate for chancroid per 1000 was 8.3 compared with 18.7 for primary and secondary syphilis and 29.5 for gonorrhoea; in the British Navy, the respective rates per 1000 in that same year were 19.4, 28.9 and 57.6. In England and Wales in 1974, only 45 cases were reported (40 in males) compared with 295 (285 in males) in 1955 and 1075 (1048 in males) in 1925.

Similar low numbers have been recorded in recent years from other European countries. In France, on the other hand, there has been a recent slight rise; only 38 cases were reported in 1968 and 69 in 1969 but 93 cases (83 in males) were encountered in 1970.

Epidemiology

Chancroid has been regarded as a disease of the un-enlightened and common poor. It is a condition of the unclean and unwashed and affects only the most indiscriminate of promiscuous men and women. It is commonly caught from prostitutes and found most frequently in seaports. In the East, the prostitute remains the principal source of infection. The prevalence of the disease commenced to decline in many areas a half century or more before the introduction of the sulphonamides, the first effective drugs, due probably to improved water supplies, improved hygiene and possibly better nutrition.

As with other sexually-transmitted diseases, chancroid is a disease of young adults. The excess numbers of reported male cases compared with female cases may be due to the fact that the female can remain an infective carrier after the lesions have healed.

GRANULOMA INGUINALE

Granuloma inguinale (Donovanosis, ulcerating granuloma of the pudenda, granuloma venereum, sclerosing granuloma, granuloma pudendi tropicum) is a usually rare, slowly progressive, auto-inoculable, mildly contagious disease, characterized by velvety, beefy granulations usually affecting the genitalia and surrounding skin. Metastatic spread to the bones occasionally occurs. It is caused by *D. granulomatis (Calymmatobacterium granulomatis)*, an encapsulated organism, at one time believed to be a protozoon, but now shown to have properties in common with Gram-negative bacteria.

Geographical distribution

Africa

It has been reported as endemic in West and Central Africa but is not encountered in large numbers. The author found 17 cases in 1948 during a survey over a period of 6 months in the, then, Southern Rhodesia. It has been stated to be rare in Ethiopia where other venereal diseases are common.

Americas

The disease has been endemic in the past in some countries of North, South and Central America and the West Indies (including Jamaica); epidemics have been reported from South America. In the U.S.A., it has always been more prevalent in the south (including Florida) than in the north, but there has been a 95% reduction in the total of reported cases since 1947 (Table 9.4). No cases were reported in Trinidad and Tobago in 1972, and it is very rare in Mexico.

Year	No. of cases	Rate per 100 000
1941	639	0.4
1947	2403	1.7
1951	1637	1.1
1961	296	0.2
1966	164	0.1
1971	103	0.1
1974	51*	0

* There were 24 728 cases of primary and secondary syphilis in this year.

Table 9.4 Granuloma inguinale in the U.S.A. (U.S.P.H.S., 1975).

Asia

Although the disease has been stated to exist in Southern China, Indonesia, Northern Australia and Southern India, it appears to be particularly prevalent in Madras State in South-East India and in New Guinea, although it is possible that a local interest taken in the condition by interested physicians has tended to attract and emphasize its presence. Certainly, in Madras State, individual physicians have recorded over 100 cases encountered in a single year but others have also found smaller numbers in the Punjab and in the Himachal Pradesh in north west of India. Even in southern India, the hospital incidence has been described as "negligible" compared with that of syphilis and gonorrhoea. Granuloma inguinale is still seen occasionally in Northern Australia and is very rare in Singapore and Sri Lanka.

Epidemics have been reported in Papua and New Guinea and also in the western part of New Guinea (formerly Dutch New Guinea, later West Irian, now part of Indonesia). The condition was first recognized in the early 1900s when it was usually mistaken for chancroid. In 1925, no less than 25% of a population examined were found to be infected; in 1946, some 422 cases were encountered in 8761 persons examined compared with 362 cases of gonorrhoea.

In Papua and New Guinea in the year ending March 1971, 813 cases of granuloma inguinale were reported from limited reporting facilities compared with 3285 of gonorrhoea, 1946 of syphilis, 20 of lymphogranuloma venereum and four of soft chancre. No less than 746 of these cases (compared with 851 of gonorrhoea, 45 of syphilis and none of the other conditions cited) were encountered in the Central district including Port Moresby where Donovan bodies may be found in approximately 12.5% of cervical cytology specimens. The disease is apparently less prevalent in other parts of the Territory. In the Central Highlands and Chimbu Districts, only 22 cases of granuloma inguinale were seen although 60% of the national total of reported cases of syphilis were found in these areas where, as already noted (p. 213), an outbreak of venereal syphilis is occurring along the new highway. When a diagnosis of genital sores is made only on clinical grounds, the early lesions of syphilis and of granuloma inguinale may be very confusing.

Europe

In recent years only individual cases have been reported from Holland, East Germany, the United Kingdom and elsewhere, and mostly in immigrants. Thirteen (8 in males) were seen in the venereal-disease clinics of England and Wales in 1974 compared with 16 (13 males) in 1962.

Epidemiology

Though possible, no proof of racial susceptibility has been forthcoming to date. There is also some dispute as to how disease is spread. Its common association with other venereal disorders, although favouring direct sex transmission, may only reflect a common economic stratum. Another view is that *D. granulomatis* is a bowel inhabitant which normally causes no local lesions but grows on skin injured by trauma or bacterial inflammation and that skin lesions result from auto-inoculation with faecal material.

There is certainly a strong link with the practice of anal coitus. 80% or more of some reported series have been in male homosexuals. In the epidemic amongst the Marandmois tribe in Dutch New Guinea, in the 1920s the disease was associated with the widespread indulgence in sexual orgies, including pederasty.

Metastatic spread to the bones (including the vertebrae) has been reported from the U.S.A. and Jamaica. Although the associations of granuloma inguinale with malignancy has not been accepted in all areas, that the condition is pre-malignant is a belief held by the majority of those who have studied the disease in Jamaica. In addition, serological reactions to *D. granulomatis* antigens have been found in a significant proportion of patients with penile cancer in those areas where granuloma inguinale is endemic.

LYMPHOGRANULOMA VENEREUM

Lymphogranuloma venereum (lymphogranuloma inguinale, lymphopathia venereum, Nicolas-Favre disease) is a venereal disease of the lymph channels characterized by a small fleeting primary lesion, followed by the development of a usually suppurative adenitis. In the male, the lymph glands most commonly affected are those of the inguinal region (*climatic bubo; poradenitis*) and if the glandular destruction is severe this may be followed by elephantiasis of the penis and scrotum. In the female, the intra-pelvic and para-rectal glands are frequently involved with peri-proctitis and proctitis. Inflammatory stricture of the rectum may result or involvement of the connective tissue may lead to polypoid growths and vulvar elephantiasis (*esthiomène*).

The causative agent belongs to the genus *Chlamydia* (Bedsonia), members of which are responsible for a wide range of infections in the animal kingdom. In man, these infections include lymphogranuloma venereum, trachoma and non-gonococcal urethritis caused by Group A organisms which have glycogen-containing inclusions and psittacosis of Group B which do not. These organisms are no longer classified as "viruses" since they are not ultra-microscopic, reproduce by binary fission and are affected by sulphonamides and some antibiotics.

Geographical distribution

Lymphogranuloma venereum seems to be a dying disease; it tends to be found in sailors and port prostitutes. National statistics, especially in developing countries, are more usually related to available diagnostic facilities than to true prevalence. Figures for 1952 from a W.H.O. survey are shown in Table 9.5; procurable data have been more scanty since that date.

	Territory	Cases
Africa	French West Africa	2042
	Cameroons (Fr.)	861
	Madagascar	679
	French Equatorial Africa	597
	Belgian Congo	304
	Tanganyika	53
	Togoland	7
America	U.S.A.	1200
Asia	French settlements in	
	India	394
	Japan	208
Europe	United Kingdom	69
Oceania	New Caledonia	26

Table 9.5 Lymphogranuloma venereum: cases reported in 1952 (W.H.O., 1954).

Africa

The disease is encountered throughout most of the continent and is endemic along the West African coast (including Ghana and Nigeria), Central Africa (including Rhodesia) and in Madagascar. It is said to be rare in Ethiopia.

The Americas

It is prevalent in the ports of South America, especially Brazil and also in the West Indies. Sixteen cases were reported from Trinidad and Tobago in 1972. The numbers of reported cases seen in the U.S.A. (military cases excluded) are shown in Table 9.6.

Fiscal years	Cases	Rates per 100 000
1941	1381	1.0
1944	2858	2.2
1946	2603	1.9
1951	1332	0.9
1956	602	0.4
1958	436	0.3
1961	842	0.5
1966	625	0.3
1968	349	0.2
1971	615	0.3
1974	374	0.2

Table 9.6 Lymphogranuloma venereum prevalence and incidence in the U.S.A. (known military cases excluded). (U.S.P.H.S., 1975.)

A marked increase in the number of cases was noted during the Second World War. This increase reached a peak of 2858 cases in 1944. There followed a fall to 436 cases in 1958 with subsequent fluctuation. In 1971, the incidence per 100 000 was similar to that of 1957–1959. The most recent rise has been attributed to the return of troops from South–East Asia.

Asia

Lymphogranuloma venereum exists in most countries of Asia, e.g. Cambodia, Fiji, Hong Kong, India, Korea, Laos, New Caledonia, Pakistan, Singapore, Thailand and Vietnam, but has become rare in Sri Lanka, Japan, Papua and New Guinea and the Northern Territories of Australia.

Europe

A few cases are encountered in North-European countries (e.g. the United Kingdom, France and Finland), usually amongst sailors or men is shown in his first General Order of the Peninsular War, which included the instruction that there were to be six women to every 100 men (drawn by lot before embarkation amid screams and swooning), the men to have one pound of biscuits and one pound of meat every day, with wine added if the meat was salt; the women to be on half rations and no wine, however salt the meat.

A more recent biography that I have enjoyed is Michael Holroyd's *Augustus John*—a fascinating and sympathetic portrait of an impossible man, forgiven much because he was an artist (in the same way that Elizabeth Longford forgave *Byron* many of his excesses because he was a poet), but not forgiven by Holroyd for not fulfilling his potential to become a great artist. Caught in a vicious circle, he was unable to paint really well when he was sexually frustrated (which he didn't allow very often), but lacked the drive to do so when he was satisfied. Books about the Bloomsbury group and about their friends (such as Augustus John, Lady Ottoline Morrell, and Bertrand Russell) usually interest me, perhaps because they are within living memory.

After all these I came back to the last and most gripping volume of *The Raj Quartet*, in which Paul Scott gathers together all the strands of this long and satisfying saga about India; I hope that others will enjoy it as much as I have, because one of the pleasures of reading is to share books by exchanging ideas about them with friends. One of the difficulties of writing about reading is that, as I read more and more, my choice constantly changes and in a few months' time it may well be quite different; and the never-ending flow of books, old and new, ensures that the luxury of a good read will be with us for as long as our eyes hold out.

Chang and his colleagues look at prognostic indices for patients in circulatory shock, and Jennett and Teasdale look at the prognosis of neurosurgical patients. To define the role of intensive therapy, and to measure its successes and its failures, we need such evaluations.

A controlled trial of intensive care is almost impossible and, with increased technology, it is here to stay. This book will help all who run these units and, equally, those who only use their facilities occasionally. The only criticism I have is of the continuing use of abbreviations. The editor refers to his own outstanding institute as the WIG—I hope it covers him with confusion.

JOHN NORMAN

Universal disorders

A World Geography of Human Diseases. Ed G Melvyn Howe. (Pp 621; £24.) Academic Press. 1977.

Doctors have been fascinated by the geography of human disease since Hippocrates wrote in *On Airs, Waters and Places*:

> "Whoever wishes to investigate medicine properly should proceed thus . . . When he comes into a strange city, he ought to consider its situation, how it lies to the wind and the sun, and consider the waters the people use . . . For if he knows these things well he cannot miss knowing the diseases peculiar to the place".

Some of the reasons for the interest are clear: firstly, the fascination of far-off places and the pattern of life of other endemic foci. Such techniques are very dependent on geographic skills and now, after 11 years, success in this worldwide campaign can be announced.

Tuberculosis provides an interesting contrast to smallpox: a slowly-developing infectious disease that has been one of the major scourges of mankind and still remains an important source of morbidity, incapacity, and death. The true incidence of such diseases cannot be determined accurately and the best measure available to estimate their importance is mortality, but this is a defective measure because death may occur after many years of active disease and hence the control of such diseases is difficult to establish and precarious to maintain. The prevalence of tuberculosis depends on the virulence of the infecting organism, the social and economic opportunities for airborne or contagious spread, contact with animals and milk products, the nutritional standards of the total population, primary and acquired resistance, effective treatment of proved cases, and immunisation of those at risk of contact. So complex a system can never be disentangled entirely and the changing levels in different areas prove to be an important indicator of what factors are most effective in influencing change of prevalence.

The world pattern of chronic diseases is more difficult to determine than that of infectious diseases. The analysis of cancer depends on worldwide cancer register reports, which enable valid estimates to be made of the incidence of these diseases; but for cardiovascular disease inevitably most of the work relates to mortality reports. The geographic complexities of the relation between death from heart diseases and hardness of water, temperature, rainfall, and latitude might have been usefully examined in much more depth in a book dealing specifically with the geography of disease, as this association is based primarily on geographic evidence.

The GLI, along with several other similar hospitals in London, was founded at a time when midwifery was beginning to take on respectability. It is not clear what inspired John Leake, already the designer of a pair of obstetric forceps, to put forward his plans in 1765, but the hospital opened two years later with 20 beds. From the first, one of its functions was regarded as teaching and Leake wrote a number of textbooks. Under his liberal guidance some 300 women were soon being delivered each year, of whom 10% were single, and even larger numbers on the "district." In spite of recurrent financial difficulties progress was steady and by the end of the century those two great libertarians, Fox and Wilberforce, were vice-presidents of the hospital. Because of pressure on space a new and larger hospital had to be built in the 1820s, and all went well until disaster struck in 1877. The hospital had to be closed because of an outbreak of puerperal fever, dissension broke out between the older more conservative obstetricians and their younger progressive colleagues, and committees of inquiry were set up. All was not lost, however, because the year after that Joseph Lister was appointed to the consulting staff and served the hospital for 34 years, the last 15 as its president. Within 10 years maternal mortality had fallen to a third of its former rate. Years of consolidation followed, with further enlargement of the hospital, the development of a modern training school for midwives, and increasing numbers of deliveries on the "district."

The Great War had little impact, but in 1939 patients had to be evacuated to Hertfordshire and only antenatal work and domiciliary deliveries continued in London. After the war, rebuilding of bomb-damaged buildings was hardly completed before the National Health Service was born, and the fate of the GLI was settled. Even before the bicentenary celebrations in 1965, which ironically seem to have passed without record, there

H CAMPBELL

Midwifery with a human face

Doctor John Leake's Hospital: A History of the General Lying-in Hospital, York Road, Lambeth, 1765-1971. Philip Rhodes. (Pp 400; £12.) Davis-Poynter. 1977.

Hospital histories are as exciting as detective stories, especially if you know the institution. As a student and young doctor I used to walk past the grand portico of the General Lying-In Hospital (GLI) on my way to and from Waterloo Station. I went inside the building only once or twice on visits, but something of the atmosphere remains still. So I picked up Professor Rhodes's attractively produced history with keen anticipation and discovered a minutely detailed account of the rise and fall of an obstetric centre of excellence during the last 200 years. Almost all the minutes of board meetings have survived, so it has been possible to document the numbers of mothers delivered, maternal and child mortality, appointments of medical and nursing staff, names of illustrious governors and patrons, and, above all perhaps, the dedication and financial expertise that kept the charity going for so long. Professor Rhodes provides background information on the state of the country and of medicine and midwifery at different periods, and is continually forced to point out the contemporary ring to many of the frustrations and problems that the board faced. The striking contrast between technical progress and the dead hand of bureaucracy is well illustrated: a doctor of 1774 would be quite unable to understand the present-day practice of obstetrics, but would have no difficulty in recognising the false assumptions behind the phenomenon of "reorganisation." place for a small, isolated, specialist hospital, destroy the GLI in 1971. Was this, one wonders, another example of the demise of midwifery with a human face. If so, Professor Rhodes's book is not only a memorial to a noble and humane institution but becomes in a sense an artefact like those early obstetric forceps now confined to museums.

ALEX PATON

More specific than general

Immunology in Medicine: A Comprehensive Guide to Clinical Immunology. Ed E J Holborow and W G Reeves. (Pp 1185; £25.) Academic Press and Grune and Stratton. 1977.

A book entitled *Immunology in Medicine* is timely: for too long the explosive growth of immunology fell outside the sphere of medical practice itself. In the 'sixties a very good understanding of the fundamental immunological processes was achieved, but, although some attempts were then made to determine the clinical relevance of exotic studies in the mouse, only in the last two or three years have immunological aspects of clinical disease become more useful to the clinician.

The strong tendency for theoreticians to decide that any aberration of normal processes constitutes a disease, and then to make armchair decisions about such a disease, is not confined to immunology. The next unfortunate step has been to look for clinical pictures that superficially resemble the aberrant state, and then to decide that these must be the causal factors in the disease. In immunological diseases, or those that masquerade as them, commonly assumptions are made that disease is caused by abnormalities of the immune system rather than by its

Recent Advances in Intensive Therapy. No 1. Ed I McA Ledingham (Pp 257; £10.) Churchill Livingstone. 1977.

Most hospital physicians and surgeons will have a few patients who need very high levels of medical and nursing skills, and time, if they are to survive. Traditionally, such patients would be looked after near the sister's desk on the Nightingale ward. Increasingly during the last 20 years, in the hope of better results, they have been grouped together in areas which allow a concentration of the necessary skills. This is an appropriate time to review the progress of such intensive therapy units and Dr Ledingham has gathered together an interesting collection of essays.

Some describe specific problems such as upper gastrointestinal haemorrhage, pancreatitis, or poisoning with paraquat, paracetamol, or salicylates; but each such essay explores the problems deeply and will make the reader assess his own standards of knowledge and practice. A second theme in these essays is a look at some regimens used in intensive therapy. Mueller, for example, describes the place of intra-aortic balloon pumping in cardiogenic shock. The problems of transporting critically ill patients are also appraised, with the Glasgow approach—taking care to the patient rather than the other way round—having much to commend it.

A third theme is, perhaps, the most valuable: intensive therapy is extremely expensive and, as might be expected, in some units the mortality and morbidity are high. Should all critically ill patients be looked after in such high care areas? Many units will not usually accept patients with terminal cancer, but is that correct? Should we be able to assess better how the high grade care and technology of intensive care is going to improve survival rates and the quality of life? These essays examine such questions. Civetta looks at the overall selection of patients for intensive care in an attempt to help select those who will be helped;

The difficulties faced by geographic pathologists or by geographers interested in pathology are formidable. A major problem is that of diagnosis of disease in different societies, in different cultures, and with different languages. Although the profession of medicine is relatively homogenous in its methods of diagnosis and in its classification of diseases, inevitably there are wide variations in the standards of diagnosis among different countries. Medical services, the number of doctors available, and, above all, the statistical support systems for recording the frequency of disease will also vary. A more subtle difficulty is the awareness of disease in different cultures, and what deviations from normality are considered appropriate to the medical profession.

The World Health Organisation has greatly encouraged work on the geography of disease by its own detailed studies on smallpox, cholera, malaria, and on cancers and cardiovascular diseases. The interplay between the skills of geographers, social scientists, epidemiologists, pathologists, physicians, and surgeons, has helped to develop many interesting studies.

Professor G Melvyn Howe, the editor, has gathered together 24 contributors—almost all of them of British origin—who have each examined the geographic pattern of the worldwide dispersion of a specific disease, or group of diseases. Such a symposium necessarily means that the standard will vary widely but it does mean that a recognised authority is able to deal with a topic with which he is fully conversant.

The chapter on smallpox eradication, although brief, is an excellent illustration of the contribution of geography to the control of a disease. In 1967, WHO decided on a policy of genocide against variola major which was then endemic in Africa, Asia, and South America. At first the aim was mass vaccination of total populations, but, although the campaigns met with great success, by 1973 it was clear that these alone would not eradicate the disease, and the emphasis moved to identifying local areas of infection and placing a cordon sanitaire around recent immigrants. The disease is seemingly more prevalent in South-European countries such as Portugal, Spain and Italy.

In the venereal disease clinics in England and Wales, the numbers of cases between 1952–1954 was 63–76 annually. The number of cases rose to between 96 and 102 annually during the years 1960–1963. Since then they have fallen by more than half to 36 in 1969, to 47 in 1971 and 46 in 1974. Of 982 cases reported in the 15-year period 1960–1974, 884 were males and 98 females, the majority of the male patients contracting their disease overseas.

Routine skin and complement-fixation tests on venereal-disease patients in London have shown 2–11% of reactors. These cases may only indicate past infection; some confusing low grade sero-positivity may be present in patients with non-gonococcal urethritis.

Epidemiology

A high incidence of past or present infection has been found in prostitutes. In published series from Brazil and Portugal, as many as 60% of certain groups (though more particularly among older women) have been shown to be reactive to skin and complement-fixation tests. The association of proctitis with lymphogranuloma venereum has been noted for many years and an appreciable incidence of positive tests has been reported from the U.S.A. in the male homosexual, more especially those with abscesses and fistulae.

Disabling chronic lesions in the male may ensue, including urethral stricture, but particularly in the female where, apart from rectal stricture and fistulae (which may sometimes be associated with intestinal obstruction), polypoid growths and vulvar swelling, there may be destructive ulceration with tissue loss and consequent urinary and faecal incontinence. Moreover, the incidence of subsequent malignancy is high enough to warrant a high index of suspicion towards such a development.

REFERENCES

General

Amer. Soc. Hlth Ass. (1973). "Today's VD Problem—1973". New York.

Greenberg, J. H. (1972). Venereal diseases in the armed forces. *Med. Clinics N. Amer.* **56**, 1087–1100.

Guthe, T. and Willcox, R. R. (1971). The international incidence of venereal diseases. *Roy. Soc. Hlth J.* **97**, 123–133.
W.H.O. (1972). The inter-county spread of venereal disease: report of a working group. W.H.O. Regional Office for Europe, Copenhagen.
Willcox, R. R. (1970). Immigration and venereal diseases. *Brit. J. Vener. Dis.* **46**, 412–422.

Treponematoses

Grin, E. I. and Guthe, T. (1973). Evaluation of a previous mass campaign against endemic syphilis in Bosnia and Herzegovina. *Brit. J. Vener. Dis.* **49**, 1–19.
Guthe, T. and Idsoe, O. (1968). Rise and fall of the treponematoses. II endemic treponematoses of childhood. *Brit. J. Vener. Dis.* **44**, 35–48.
Guthe, T. and Willcox, R. R. (1954). Treponematoses a world problem. *Chron. W.H.O.* **8**, 37–114, (special number).
Hackett, C. J. (1963). On the origin of the Human Treponematoses. *Bull. W.H.O.* **29**, 7.
Hudson, E. H. (1958). "Non-venereal syphilis". E. and S. Livingstone, Edinburgh.
Medina, R. (1967). Pinta. *Derm. Ibero Lat. Amer.* (*Engl. Ed.*) **1**, 121.
Rhodes, F. A. and Anderson, S. E. J. (1970). An outbreak of treponematosis in the Eastern Highlands of New Guinea. *Papua New Guinea Med. J.* **13**, 49.
Willcox, R. R. (1972). The treponemal evolution. *Trans. St. John's Derm. Soc.* **58**, 21–37.

Venereal syphilis and gonorrhoea (see also General References)

British Co-operative Clinical Group (1973). Homosexuality and venereal disease in the United Kingdom. *Brit. J. Vener. Dis.* **49**, 329–334.
Bro-Jørgensen, A. and Jensen, T. (1971). Gonococcal tonsillar infection. *Brit. Med. J.* **4**, 660.
Department of Health and Social Security (1972). Report of the Chief Medical Officer, 1972. H.M.S.O., London.
Pan American Health Assoc. (1965). International Travelling Seminar on Venereal Diseases to the U.S.A., Report, Washington D.C.
Willcox, R. R. (1972). A world wide view of venereal disease. *Brit. J. Vener. Dis.* **48**, 163–176.
W.H.O. (1968). Report of Second Regional Seminar on Venereal Disease Control. W.H.O. Regional Office for the Western Pacific, Manila, Philippines.
W.H.O. (1975). *W.H.O. Stat. Rep.* **28**, 118–125, Geneva.

Other sexually-transmitted diseases

Chlamydial Infection. *Brit. J. Vener. Dis.* Dec. 1972, 48, (papers by Darougar *et al.*, 416; Dunlop *et al.*, 421, 425; Oriel *et al.*, 429; Richmond *et al.*, 437; Vaughan-Jackson *et al.*, 445; Dwyer *et al.*, 452).
Favre M. and Hellerstrom, S. (1954). The epidemiology, aetiology and prophylaxis of lymphogranuloma inguinale. *Acta Dermato-Venereol.* 34, (Suppl.) 30.

Goldberg, J. (1964). Studies in granuloma inguinale: VI, some epidemiological considerations of the disease. *Brit. J. Vener. Dis.* **40**, 140–145.

Greaves, A. B. (1963). The frequency of lymphogranuloma venereum in persons with perirectal abscesses, fistulae in ano, or both, with particular reference to the relationship between peri-rectal abscesses of lymphogranuloma origin in the male and inversion. *Bull. W.H.O.* **29**, 797–801.

Harkness, A. H. (1950). "Non Gonococcal Urethritis". Livingstone, Edinburgh.

Maddocks, I. (1967). Donovanosis in Papua. *Papua New Guinea Med. J.* **10**, 49–54.

Rajam, R. V. and Rangiah, P. N. (1954). "Donovanosis, Granuloma Inguinale, Granuloma Venereum". W.H.O. Monogr. Ser. No. 24, Geneva.

Sigel, M. (1962). "Lymphogranuloma Venereum. Epidemiological, Surgical and Therapeutic Aspects Based on a Study in the Caribbean". Univ. of Miami Press, Florida.

United States Public Health Service (1975). VD Fact Sheet—1974, U.S. Dept. Health, Education and Welfare, Public Health Service, Atlanta.

Willcox, R. R. (1956). Importance of chancroid in Africa. *J. Roy. Army Med. Cps* **102**, 15–27.

Willcox, R. R. (1974). Chancroid, granuloma inguinale and lymphogranuloma venereum. *In* "Recent Advances in Sexually Transmitted Diseases" (Ed. R. Morton and J. R. W. Harris). Churchill-Livingstone, London.

W.H.O. (1954). *Epidem. Vital Stat. Rep.* **11**, 417.

W.H.O. (1959). Report on the First W.H.O. Venereal Disease Control Seminar of the Western Pacific Region, Manila, Philippines.

10. Measles

A. P. Ball

When the summer is hot and dry . . . and the rains come on very late, then the measles quickly seize those who are disposed to them; but all these things admit of great differences by reason of the diversity of countries . . . so that they happen in other seasons besides these (Rhazes, Arabian physician *c.* A.D. 850).

Measles is prevalent worldwide as an endemic children's disease. In the densely populated areas of the western world, it is subject to epidemic fluctuations and seasonal variations in incidence which are most marked in the temperate zones. In the Old World, the disease has been documented since earliest times notably by the physician Rhazes who drew an incomplete distinction between measles and smallpox. Confusion in diagnosis continued for a further eight centuries, until in England in the 17th century Thomas Sydenham finally delineated the two diseases. Measles had been classified separately from smallpox for the previous 50–100 years but the criteria were such as to invalidate earlier data.

The disease has remained unchanged in its major features but variation in severity has occurred down the centuries. Following exploration of the earth from the 13th century onwards, severe outbreaks have occurred in previously unexposed populations. These epidemics in "virgin soil" areas continue to the present day but such areas are now few and the disease has assumed global proportions.

Variation in the severity of the disease in exposed areas of the world has now occupied a fairly clear socio-geographical distribution and is determined to an extent by geographical factors. This pattern is being altered both passively and actively by man himself and, the influence of man on his environment through social change and medical care, including vaccination, has become a major factor. The virus, the contemporary disease, its distribution and geographical variations will be discussed, followed by an assessment of factors associated with, or determining, these variations.

THE VIRUS AND THE DISEASE

The virus

The causative agent of measles is a roughly spherical viral particle. The individual virus particle contains a nuclear core of RNA (Ribose nucleic acid) which is surrounded by a coat of protein and an outer layer of protein and fat. It is a member of the myxovirus group which produce in man a variety of illnesses including influenza and mumps. However the measles virus most resembles myxoviruses which produce animal diseases, notably canine distemper and rinderpest. These viruses produce diseases in animals having similarities to measles in man. The virus is easily grown in the laboratory and in the clinical disease patients develop a rapid rise in antibodies to measles virus which are again easily demonstrable in the laboratory by techniques using serial blood samples. These methods aid the diagnosis in atypical cases and are useful in assessing the susceptibility or previous exposure of individuals or populations. They are, however, usually unnecessary since the developed disease is so easily diagnosed clinically.

The virus is adversely affected by heat and ultraviolet radiation in terms of its viability but no agency, natural or artificial, has succeeded in changing the structure of the virus such that the disease produced differs from the original. Vaccine strains of the virus which have been attenuated—decreased in virulence in the laboratory—produce a much less severe response; this is a variation in intensity only and not in basic type. Infection with the wild virus or the living attenuated vaccine strain produces identical high level immunity and an attack confers complete immunity to further infections which lasts many years. Virus variation therefore does not occur and in consequence no "new" virus epidemics appear. This contrasts with the influenza viruses whose mutations are responsible for periodic pandemics. Measles epidemics are occasioned by other factors.

The disease

Measles is the most unpleasant of the childhood diseases and is no less so in adults. The mode of spread is by droplet emission from the upper respiratory tract of an infectious case to the nose of a susceptible contact. There is some evidence to suggest the conjunctiva as an alternative portal of entry but, as tears are drained from the conjunctiva of the eye into the nose through the duct system, it seems most likely that the nose is the initial site of the infection.

After contact, the disease incubates for a period of about two weeks and then manifests itself as an upper respiratory catarrhal disorder. This is known as the prodromal phase and is characterized by congestion of the lining tissues of the upper respiratory tract, hypersection of mucus and conjunctivitis. This leads to the picture of the child with reddened streaming eyes, nasal discharge, cough, laryngitis and an engorged reddened mucosal lining of the mouth. On this mucous lining there occur small pinpoint clusters of white spots known as Koplik's spots. These are diagnostic of measles but, unlike the catarrhal symptoms, they disappear when the external rash or exanthem appears.

The prodromal phase, associated with continuous fever, continues for 2–3 days before the external rash appears, often associated with a further rise in temperature. The rash is a blotchy, red to purple, raised eruption appearing initially behind the ears and thereafter spreading rapidly on to the face and thence longitudinally down the body and limbs. The rash reaches its peak about 4–6 days after the onset of the condition and the affected child presents a picture of abject misery.

All manifestations then begin to regress and in the uncomplicated cases the temperature begins to fall. The rash fades in the order it appeared, commencing with the face, but leaves behind a faint brown stain in the distribution of the lesions. This is often associated with a fine desquamation of superficial dead skin. This phenomenon is much less severe than the profuse desquamation seen in Nigerian children (p. 245). It is not associated with the complications seen in the latter cases and occurs at a later stage in the illness.

The uncomplicated case in the developed countries takes about 10 days to run its course, but complications can and do occur. These are almost all the effect of secondary bacterial infection by the upper respiratory tract flora of the patient, *Staphylococcus aureus* and *Streptococcus pneumoniae*, and comprise bacterial conjunctival infection, middle ear infections and pneumonia. All are amenable to antibiotic therapy and seldom affect the ultimate good prognosis. Rare complications of non-bacterial origin include encephalitis of various forms and a potential link between measles in childhood and later development of the crippling disease multiple sclerosis.

EPIDEMIOLOGY

No evidence of a carrier state exists in measles and the disease spreads from infectious cases to susceptible contacts directly. Thus a continuous chain of susceptibles is required to maintain the presence of the infection. In densely populated areas, this undercurrent of continuous endemic infection is interrupted at intervals by periodic epidemic fluctuations. In practice, this periodicity of epidemics tends towards a 2–3 year cycle with a peak seasonal incidence in the winter of "measles years" superimposed. This periodicity is related to the percentage of immunity of the "at risk" community as a whole, a factor referred to as "Herd Immunity". Brincker (1938) has shown that, in the case of measles, if herd immunity remains at 80% or greater, the disease continues on a low level endemic basis, but when the level falls to 60% or less, epidemic fluctuations in incidence may be expected to occur.

In a continuously exposed community, the "at risk" group of susceptibles can only be those previously unexposed. This group, the herd non-immunes, consists of a fixed number of susceptibles who, for some reason, escaped previous infection together with an expanding population of children born since the previous epidemic. Thus, as time passes, this group of susceptibles, made up largely of young children, increasingly dilutes the previously immune population until herd immunity drops below 80% and approaches 60%. An epidemic then occurs leaving a higher proportion of immune individuals in its wake and the cycle begins again. This explains not only the periodicity of the disease, but also the predominance of young children affected in an epidemic. The above pattern, however, is typical of Western developed society only and patterns elsewhere differ markedly.

GEOGRAPHICAL DISTRIBUTION

Developed countries

The preceding description of the disease and its epidemiology represent the current status of the measles virus and its effect on the population of the developed countries. It has become a mild disease with mortality rates of less than 0.01% and although, even to the present, children from lower social class backgrounds continue to have a slightly higher incidence of complications, the overall complication rate is minimal. The present position is a recent phenomenon since measles in 18th and 19th century Britain and other developed countries resembled closely the severe disease which is seen in the isolated areas and underdeveloped countries of the world in recent years.

Measles is known to have fluctuated in severity over the centuries. In the London epidemic of 1674, it caused more deaths than smallpox but thereafter decreased in virulence only to reappear as a more serious infection in the 19th century. This is in part a tribute to Jennerian vaccination which, by eradicating smallpox, allowed the weak children previously taken by that disease to live long enough to contract measles and maybe die of it. However, the measles epidemics of 19th century Glasgow and London were no respectors of persons, weak, strong or otherwise and took a particularly severe form not unlike that recently described as occurring in Nigeria in the early 1960s.

It is tempting to draw a relationship between the recurrence of measles in Britain in its severe form and the advent of the Industrial Revolution. The shift of population from the isolated rural areas into the developing industrial conurbations with their overcrowded and poor living conditions may well have created an epidemic situation associated with factors determining the severity of measles to be discussed later.

Global spread

At present measles is a world-wide endemic disease except in areas of extreme isolation. Isolated areas are now few and yet the area of the known world has expanded maximally only within the last few hundred years. The question arises as to whether measles has always been a world-wide disease or, as is thought, has spread gradually to its present global distribution. The presence of measles in the Old World has been established at least as far back as the 9th century A.D. when it was described by Rhazes. Research being undertaken into the antibodies possessed by Egyptian mummies will almost certainly establish its presence in that country many centuries B.C.

Measles has no natural reservoir, relying instead on a continuous supply of susceptible hosts to remain endemic in a community. After the Tahitian epidemic of 1951, the disease vanished within months not to reappear until the next imported epidemic in 1960. The island population of 35 000 was apparently insufficient to maintain endemicity. Outbreaks in the Faroes, 65 years apart, showed a similar phenomenon and recent studies have suggested that a population in excess of 100 000 in close geographical proximity is required to maintain endemicity if outside contact is not a factor. It seems unlikely that the indigenous populations of the New World in the time of the Age of Discovery would have been of a size to maintain the disease within the population. Evidence from the Spanish colonization of Mexico and the Central Americas, related to the high attack rate and severity of the disease suffered by the local populations when exposed to the disease through the incoming conquistadors, suggests that these people had not suffered from the disease before and were thus a truly "virgin" population.

Wherever frontiers have been pushed outward and new lands discovered there have been typical "virgin soil" outbreaks in the local populations after their first meeting with civilization. Darwin, in 1836 during the voyage of the *Beagle*, comments on the gradual extinction of the Australian aborigines by measles which had been brought to that country by European colonists. Such epidemics have occurred world wide; in Amazonia in 1749, Hudson Bay in 1846, Tasmania in 1852, Fiji in 1875, but such areas have always been recognized as not having suffered previous exposure after the event. Recently, Peart (1954) described an outbreak among Canadian

Eskimos in Ungava Bay, Northern Quebec Province where there had been no previous measles. Gajdusek (1963), when studying this problem in Micronesia (Mariana, Caroline, Marshall and Gilbert island groups) found a tribe who were proved by serological analysis to have had no previous exposure to measles but then suffered a typical "virgin soil" epidemic of the disease after extraneous infection.

It would seem, from the factors described, that measles spread from the Mediterranean cradle of civilization as a result of colonization of the New World and contact with previously unexposed tribes. The infection then either died out as the colonizers moved on or else became established in populations increasingly absorbed into the colonist communities.

Previously unexposed communities

Previously unexposed areas are constantly diminishing as communications improve but, when the measles virus makes contact with these areas of isolation, a typical pattern ensues irrespective of geographical location. In such "virgin" communities, the attack rate is 100%, all susceptibles contracting the disease. The only exceptions are survivors of a previous epidemic at some stage in the past. This 100% attack rate contrasts with the 85% attack rate amongst susceptibles in endemic areas. The lower rate for the latter is due to the prevalence of sub-clinical infection leading to a proportion of the supposed susceptibles being in fact immune.

The isolated "virgin" community represents a total epidemic situation. In the Faroes, the epidemic of 1846 attacked 6000 of the 8000 population and, almost without exception, the 2000 who escaped infection were immunes surviving the epidemic of 65 years earlier. In the Fijian outbreak of 1875, an almost 100% attack rate resulted in a 25% mortality and even in 1951 the South Greenland epidemic, once again having an attack rate of almost 100%, had a complication rate of 45%, fortunately with a much lower mortality.

Virgin populations may be geographically isolated; they can also be created, often by wars. In the American Civil War, 70 000 troops died of measles to which they had not previously been exposed and to which they were exposed *en masse* in camps and prisons. In the Boer War, women and children refugees from the veld were placed in large camps near to cities and the resulting outbreaks assumed virgin soil features of high attack rate and extreme severity. Later in the 20th century, troops of the Highland Division stationed at Bedford, made up largely of men from the remote West Highlands of Scotland suffered an epidemic with the usual 100% attack rate. Prior warning had been given and in one unit, 104 cases were assessed as susceptible: of these 102 contracted the disease and later questioning of relatives revealed that the two who did not contract the disease had probably been previously exposed.

The pattern of high attack rate and extreme severity is confirmed in the present day by Gajdusek's study of the patterns of measles amongst many isolated tribes in Micronesia. An important factor in these outbreaks is the extremely high complication rate. This is paralleled by the mortality rate which until recently often attained 20%. Virgin populations evidently suffer a severe form of measles which is characterized by severe laryngitis, broncho-pneumonia and enteritis. This severity appears to have no racial associations as similar patterns are seen in ethnically diverse areas of isolation. However, isolation itself may be a factor in the severity of the disease, though the level of socio-economic development rather than the geographical location may be the critical parameter. Vaccination studies in the 1960s have shown an exaggerated response in previously unexposed populations and it has been suggested that some unknown genetic factor may be absent in unexposed populations leading to a peculiarly severe reaction to the wild virus. Virgin populations constitute a group at high risk of developing severe measles and this has been recognized in W.H.O. vaccination programmes.

Developing countries

Severe measles has long been associated with the tropics but it is now known to be present in most areas of the Third World. The severe form of the disease, as well as being observed in "virgin" outbreaks, is seen typically in Africa, India, South America and South-East Asia. The bulk of Asia produces little in the way of reliable statistics but mortality rates ranging from 14–22% in West Africa, 5% in the rest of Africa and thirty times that of Europe in South America in the early 1960s indicate the severity of the disease in these areas. Such figures closely resemble those reported in the study of the City of Glasgow during the years 1807–1812 when measles accounted for 10% of all deaths in the city, and later at the turn of the century when the measles mortality rate was still 5%. These figures are taken from an age when the Scots population were living at a subsistence level not unlike that of the developing nations today.

Few areas in the early 1960s, however, could compare with mortality rates in Western Nigeria (Morley *et al.*, 1963). The 25% mortality in measles was associated with the major complications of pneumonia, obstructive laryngitis and dysenteric diarrhoea. The disease itself is associated with an enhanced rash which is a confluent deep dusky-red eruption. It does not resemble the "black measles", a haemmorrhagic variant, but may well resemble the severe cases described by Rhazes in the 9th century A.D. Rhazes wrote that "the measles which are of a deep red and violet colour are of a bad and fatal kind" and his view is confirmed by Morley (1969) who found that the mortality in Western Nigeria was related to the severity of the rash and subsequent desquamation. This severe desquamation occurring early in the illness, and described in Britain in the last century, is associated with a similar series of changes in the larynx, bronchi and intestine which lead to the fatal complications described above. Thus the severity of the desquamation is a good guide to prognosis, and to the severity of the problem in affected countries of the developing world.

PREDISPOSING FACTORS

Measles exhibits three main patterns in the world today.
1. Endemic disease in the developed countries associated with low complications and mortality rates subject to epidemic fluctuations.
2. Epidemic disease in isolated virgin populations with an attack rate of 100% and high complication and mortality rates.
3. Severe endemic disease in developing countries with manifestations resembling the condition in Britain prior to the 20th century.
These variations are now considered in terms of various parameters.

Climate

In the temperate zones, measles has a higher incidence in the colder months, reaching a peak in January and February which is most marked in an epidemic year. This phasic annual incidence is less marked in the tropics and tends to occur in different seasons. In India, for instance, the peak incidence of measles occurs between March and June (hot season) and the abrupt decline in incidence in July correlates well with the onset of the monsoon. These findings suggest that colder months may enhance activity of the disease and that rainy seasons or high humidity may have an adverse effect on the virus or its transmission. Although in the laboratory the virus is preserved by cold and killed by heat, it is doubtful whether these factors can be related to climate, as the temperature extremes in the laboratory are not greater than those of geographical variation. It is more likely that it is not the virus, but the host response to virus or other factors determined by climate that affect the outcome. Careful study must therefore be directed towards the effect of climate on the human host, both in individual response and in herd response.

There is no evidence to suggest that any parameter of climate other than extreme cold exposure, which reduces the blood white-cell count and hence lowers resistance to infection, influences individual response to an infective challenge by measles virus. Climate does, however, have a pronounced effect on the behaviour of human populations, being a major determinant of their life style. Movement of peoples is often dictated by climate and this has been studied in Nigeria by Morley (1969). In this area, a peak incidence of severe measles is seen in the middle of the dry season, declining, as in India, with the onset of the rainy season. In the dry season, the people leave their isolated farms and congregate in the villages for festivals during which time the susceptible children are living in close proximity allowing spread from endemic cases to epidemic proportions. The coming of the rainy season necessitates return to the farms and the situation returns to the normal endemic undercurrent of cases. Climate is operating through the shift of population as a determinant of the incidence of measles infection.

Similar climatic pressures on the population may be operative in the temperate zones which have their peak incidence in mid-winter. The tendency of the population to crowd together in the wetter, colder months may encourage spread to the susceptible population. Most childhood infections spread in schools. In Britain, the re-opening of schools in January after the Christmas holidays followed by a latency period of some 2–3 weeks during which time the susceptibles are contracting and incubating the disease, may account for the highest incidence in late January and early February. This does not explain why this happens only in the term following Christmas, but the predominance of indoor teaching may be a factor determined by climate.

The ideal study of the effect of climate would obviously be best conducted in a country with a gradient of climatic conditions, ranging from tropical to temperate zones. Chile fulfills these criteria and climatic factors have been studied by Ristori and his colleagues. The country, a narrow strip nearly 3000 miles long, was subdivided into a northern zone, between latitudes 18°S and 32°S; a central zone, between latitudes 32°S and 38°S.; and a southern zone, between latitudes 38°S and 54°S. The northern zone where the climate is arid and warm showed an overall mortality from measles of 13.1 per 100 000, the central zone with a cold, dry winter and warm, dry summer a mortality of 22.9 per 100 000 and the southern zone with a heavy rainfall, prolonged winter and extremes of temperature a massive mortality of 46.7 per 100 000.

On the basis of these figures, it would seem that humid, low temperature climates predispose to severe measles. The authors of this study point out, however, that, proceeding in a southerly direction in Chile, living conditions worsen in terms of standard of agriculture, housing, sanitation, nutrition and medical care. The suggestion that measles severity may be influenced by extreme cold directly conflicts with the incidence of severe measles in Nigeria and India coming in the dry hot season. The remarkable similarity of "virgin soil" outbreaks in many climatically unrelated areas tend to negate the possibility of climate acting as a direct factor on measles incidence and severity.

The evidence suggests that climate exerts an indirect effect through its relationship with socio-economic development and with population movement.

Race

A superficial view of morbidity and mortality patterns would suggest that the black races suffer an ethnic predisposition to severe measles but a consideration of the global picture and history of the disease shows that this is far from the case. It has been shown that outbreaks in virgin communities have the same severity regardless of the race involved, and have occurred with equal ferocity and frequency amongst Caucasians, Micronesians, Eskimos, Black Africans and many others. Further, in areas where white and black populations live side by side, such as in the U.S.A. and in British immigrant areas, the severity of measles is similar providing that both groups are living in identical socio-economic circumstances.

The present day disease in the developed countries of Anglo-Saxon and Caucasian population types has been stated to be a modern phenomenon. The fact that descriptions of 19th century British measles so closely resemble the severe measles seen in the Third World today emphasizes that it is the level of economic development and not skin pigment which influences disease patterns, and the differential mortality in different social classes within a racial group further exemplifies this.

Beliefs and customs of peoples may influence the course of events and this may account for the apparent severity of measles in some areas. The belief that measles is due to sorcery or a malignant goddess is still widely held both in Africa and Asia. Neither is the Western World free of such myths, since for many years the belief was held in Europe that childhood measles was the effect of the mother's failure to menstruate during pregnancy and that the rash was due to the appearance of the retained "bad blood".

Current attitudes in Nigerian tribes can adversely affect prognosis, measles being accepted as a natural consequence of childhood and therefore not a matter for medical attention. It is also thought that feeding should be kept to a minimum during the attack. This may precipitate marasmus or kwashiorkor.

Cultural habits of races may also influence the course of disease. The long house villages of Brunei and population aggregations of nomadic tribes tend to encourage outbreaks by virtue of human proximity and the association between plague, pestilence and pilgrimages is well known. Food sharing customs and common utensils have been implicated in Eskimo outbreaks.

Race therefore confers no predisposition or immunity to the ravages of the measles virus but the custom and culture of an individual race or races may be a factor in the epidemiology of the disease. That race is unimportant is confirmed by the similar response of a variety of peoples to measles vaccination.

Socio-economic environment

The severe form of measles in the developing nations and its relationship and similarities to the severe measles of the Western World one hundred years ago has been discussed. The differing severity of measles in these areas appears to be directly related to the socio-economic implications of under-development, just as the lessening severity of the Western World appears related to advancing development.

Studies in Britain still show that low social class is linked to higher morbidity and mortality in measles, but this has been recognized for a long time. Glasgow at the turn of the century had a mortality of 9% for children coming from families living in one room (the "single-end" of the tenements), whereas children from homes of four rooms had a mortality of only 2%. Current studies in Lagos have provided comparable results.

This factor of available living space is of course but one aspect of the problem, the increased mortality reflecting the low standard of living. Resources are limited and, in many developing countries, the critical factor is food. Climate, type of agriculture, traditional food preferences and religious taboos contribute to this problem, but all too often the situation is not one of choice but of absolute lack.

Most countries affected by severe measles have either a cereal-orientated agricultural economy, or to a lesser extent collecting economies such as hunting and fishing. Few have organized livestock farming. Agriculture is limited by the use of primitive implements and is hampered by climatic upheavals with the result that famine is not uncommon. War and insurrection exacerbate the situation, and central government together with voluntary organizations may, by attempting to westernize methods, reduce output of basic foodstuffs further. Those factors result in a large percentage of the population living below subsistence level, and in primitive housing with poor sanitation, which together with lack of adequate medical resources, must influence the course of many diseases, including measles.

Basic lack of foodstuffs leads to the condition of protein-calorie malnutrition in childhood, which in its most severe manifestations leads to the syndrome of kwashiorkor. This condition is characterized by a failure of growth, swelling of the trunk and lower limbs, muscle wasting, skin changes, anaemia and associated vitamin deficiency states. Milder forms of protein calorie malnutrition result in impairment of resistance and response to infection. Numerous reports stress the relationship of this condition to severe measles with a high complication rate and resultant mortality. One of the most striking features of the disease and its relation to measles in Western Nigeria in the early 1960s was the considerable weight loss provoked by an attack of measles in the malnourished child, in some children sufficient to precipitate kwashiorkor. Thus protein-calorie malnutrition predisposes to severe measles and is itself precipitated into a severe form by the attack of measles to which it has predisposed the child. The local custom of restricting food intake to a minimum of carbohydrate in children with measles may also have influenced this outcome. It is of interest that a similar abrupt weight loss occurred in malnourished children in Great Britain prior to the 20th century and carried a poor prognosis.

Severe measles in the tropics is almost exclusively found in areas where the population exist at subsistence level or below. The more "well-off" children in these areas do not suffer the same severity of an attack of measles. Severe measles correlates with a low order of socio-economic development, a primitive agriculture and childhood malnutrition. Wherever these factors co-exist, severe measles will occur in the population.

Human influences

Evidence has been presented which reveals measles to be a worldwide cause of morbidity and mortality. Both areas of isolation and the developing countries constitute groups at risk from severe measles and although enhanced socio-economic status is the ideal goal, prevention by vaccination has proved a simpler solution. In 1963, the W.H.O. set up a scientific group on measles which recommended that W.H.O. should coordinate a series of field trials of living attenuated measles vaccines in countries with different climates. Vaccines for measles have been pioneered by Enders and others and in preliminary trials have been shown to be effective and safe.

Calculations suggested that in an endemic area a vaccination rate of 40–50% of children born every year would be necessary to prevent epidemic fluctuation and that, to eradicate the disease and prevent reintroduction, a vaccination rate of 80–90% would be required.

Vaccination programmes were organized world-wide with emphasis on under-developed "at risk" areas. Reactions and effect were remarkably similar in all population groups studied with similar vaccines. Some vaccines were discontinued after they had been shown to produce high temperatures and rashes, a form of modified measles, but the remaining vaccines which produced a mild febrile reaction only were shown to produce a 95% or better response in terms of production of immunity.

Over 3 million doses of vaccine have now been dispensed in Nigeria alone and the effectiveness of the W.H.O. programme is endorsed by the precipitate reduction in morbidity and mortality and the resulting closure of "measles" wards in West-African hospitals. Measles is no longer a problem. Similar experience was found in the U.S.A. where after the introduction of vaccination, measles became a relative rarity. It has re-emerged recently due to a lower vaccination rate but still represents only a fraction of the previous problem.

The similarity of reactions to, and development of high level, long-lasting immunity with, similar vaccines in differing countries and geographical areas such as Canada, Czechoslovakia and Nigeria adds weight to the assertion that race is of little relevance in the pathogenesis of severe measles. However, a study of vaccination in American Indians has shown an apparent racial difference. In this study, previously unexposed Indian populations showed a higher mean temperature response to vaccination than control groups. No evidence of other factors determining this abnormal temperature response could be found and an apparent racial idiosyncrasy appeared to be present. However this was an isolated population with respect to measles and their exaggerated response compares with the severe reaction to wild virus in other virgin populations which has been described. The authors of this study suggest that exposed populations have evolved an unknown genetic factor which modifies the course of the disease, which such isolated populations have had no chance to evolve. This is a highly arguable hypothesis and the question of this apparent idiosyncrasy remains unsettled.

Measles vaccination after some 10 years of clinical usage in various forms now appears to be safe, reliable and, in comparison with the cost of dealing with outbreaks such as have occurred in the past, is inexpensive. The morbidity from measles world wide has been drastically reduced in all areas in which vaccination has been made available and in many areas has been reduced from an endemic to a sporadic problem.

MEASLES AND NEUROLOGICAL DISEASES

Increasing evidence links measles in childhood to the subsequent development of subacute sclerosing panenchephalitis (SSPE) and multiple sclerosis (MS) in some patients. The hypothesis relates to an age-dependent host response to childhood challenge by the measles virus. This virus is almost certainly responsible for SSPE, the risk being increased amongst those who develop measles in infancy. The virus enters the brain during the childhood illness, producing no symptoms and remains latent for a period of up to 5 years. For reasons unknown, the virus then reactivates and this is followed by convulsions, spastic paralysis and death within a matter of months. Racial factors appear to operate in the development of SSPE which is more common in the black races, Arabs and Sephardic Jews. The poor of any race also appear to have a higher risk.

These racial factors contrast sharply with those found in MS which is commoner in the affluent white races and rare in Arabs and Sephardic Jews. MS has an interesting worldwide geographical distribution, the disease exhibiting an increasing incidence with increasing latitude. The high risk zones, where attack rates of over 50 per 100 000 of the population are found, all exist outside latitudes 40°N and 40°S, compared to an equatorial incidence of 5 per 100 000 of the population. Geographical areas may thus be high or low risk. It has been suggested that measles in childhood, not in infancy as with SSPE but at a later pre-adolescent stage, may influence the risk of subsequent development of MS. Alter (1976) has recently reviewed this hypothesis, and has quoted immigrant studies showing that, although adult immigrants retain the risk of development of MS associated with their country of origin, younger immigrants who move before or at adolescence acquire the risk associated with their country of adoption. This supports the concept of an adolescent or pre-adolescent factor influencing the development of MS. In the tropics where the risk of MS is low, measles is acquired early in life whereas in temperate areas measles tends to attack older children when it is associated with a higher risk of MS. The mechanism of this increased risk in older children is at present unknown but is presumed to be an age-dependent factor in the host response to the measles virus. The peculiar geography of MS is explicable when these factors are considered.

Further evidence linking measles to MS has come from antibody studies which have shown that patients with MS have higher levels of measles antibody than other people. Miller (1973) has found an association between measles antibody, present in the cerebro-spinal fluid, and MS, which does not occur in other subjects. It is suggested that, as with SSPE, virus invasion of the brain during childhood measles and subsequent episodes of reactivation after many years is causally related to MS. The period of latency between brain infection and reactivation appears to be at least 20 years.

To provide substantiation of the relationship between measles and MS, it would seem reasonable to look at a measles epidemic occurring 20 years ago, in a previously unexposed population, and to assess the incidence of MS then and now. South Greenland, a potentially high risk area, has a much lower than predicted incidence of MS and it is tempting to suggest that this is related to lack of previous exposure to measles virus before the epidemic of 1951. This being so and 20 years having elapsed since that epidemic, the first case of a rising incidence of MS should soon begin to occur. This would provide fairly strong evidence of a causal relationship.

If such a relationship is proven then MS, currently the commonest crippling neurological disease, may be preventable by measles vaccination; indeed the mass vaccination programmes both in developed and developing countries undertaken from the 1960s onwards might be expected to produce a decline in the incidence of MS over the coming two decades. Future study must be directed to this possibility for therein lies hope for the eradication of MS.

REFERENCES

Adels, B. R. and Gajdusek, D. C. (1963). Survey of measles patterns in New Guinea, Micronesia and Australia, with a report of new virgin soil epidemics and the demonstrations of susceptible primitive populations by serology. *Amer. J. Hyg.* **77**, 317.

Alter, M. (1976). Is multiple sclerosis an age-dependent host response to measles. *Lancet* **1**, 456.

Amer. J. Dis. Children (1962). World wide importance of measles (Symposium). **103**, 219–281.

Black, F. L., Hierholtzer, W., Woodall, J. P., Pinhiero, F. (1971). Intensified reactions to measles vaccine in unexposed populations of American Indians. *J. Infec. Dis.* **124**, 306.

Brincker, J. A. H. (1938). A historical, epidemiological and aetiological study of measles. *Proc. Roy. Soc. Med.* **31**, 807.

Christie, A. B. (1969). "Infectious Diseases: Epidemiology and Clinical Practice". E. and S. Livingstone, Edinburgh.

Cockburn, W. C. (1969). World problems in viral vaccines. *Brit. Med. Bull.* **25**, 121.

Gordon-Smith, C. E. (1972). Changing patterns of disease in the tropics. *Brit. Med. Bull.* **28**, 3.

Lancet (1974). Measles and multiple sclerosis. **1**, 247.

Lancet (1971). Measles in vaccinated communities. **2**, 910.

Miller, J. H. D. (1973). In symposium: viral diseases. *Proc. Roy. Coll. Phys. Edinburgh.*

Morley, D. C. (1969). Severe measles in the tropics. *Brit. Med. J.* **1**, 297, 363.

Morley, D. C., Woodland, M. and Martin, W. J. (1963). Measles in Nigerian children. A study of the disease in West Africa and its manifestations in England and other countries during different epochs. *J. Hyg. Camb.* **61**, 113.

Peart, A. F. W. and Nagler, F. P. (1954). Measles in the Canadian Arctic. *Can. J. Publ. Hlth* **45**, 146.

Rhazes, (A.D. 1850). A treatise on the smallpox and measles. *Proc. Sydentian Soc. Lond.* (1848), (Translation).

Spillane, J. D. (1972). The geography of neurology. *Brit. Med. J.* **2**, 506.

W.H.O. Technical Report (1963). W.H.O. Scientific Group of Measles. Measles Vaccines Series No. 263.

11. Smallpox

A. B. Christie

Few diseases have been more dreaded throughout the world than smallpox. It has engendered fear and distraction among the masses, alike in developed and informed communities as in isolated, bewildered tribes meeting the disease for the first time. By contrast, in countries where for centuries the disease has been endemic, it is sometimes accepted as an inescapable fact of life, or of death. It has indeed slain its millions throughout the ages. Yet smallpox is possibly not a highly infectious disease. When a patient suffers from smallpox, even if he dies from it, he probably does not infect more than two or three people and these are usually members of his own family or household or people he has been in very close contact with. There is thus a paradox somewhere in the behaviour of smallpox, this great disease which can at one time smoulder as a family or village infection yet at another blaze forth as a widespread epidemic. To resolve the paradox, the smallpox virus must be studied, how it affects its victim and how it behaves both inside and outside his body: in other words, the aetiology, ecology and epidemiology of the disease must be studied.

AETIOLOGY

The pox viruses

The virus of smallpox, or variola, belongs to the pox groups of viruses. The group includes the viruses of variola major and variola minor (p. 267), the viruses of vaccinia, cowpox and monkeypox, as well as the somewhat mysterious white pox viruses (p. 269). Seen under the electron microscope, these viruses are all brick-shaped and they cannot be distinguished one from another morphologically or by serological tests. On culture on the chorio-allantois of developing chick embryos, some of them can be distinguished by the different ceiling temperature at which they grow and by the type of pock they produce on the chorio-allantois, whether haemorrhagic or not: but intradermal inoculation into rabbit skin may be required to distinguish the smallpox from monkeypox virus, and the white poxes may still be difficult or impossible to differentiate. These points are of importance when considering the problems of world eradication of smallpox (p. 266).

Entry of the virus

Smallpox virus enters the body via the mucous membranes of the upper respiratory tract. It may also enter through the conjunctiva, for virus can certainly pass out of the body through the conjunctiva (p. 260), and it is therefore probable that it also passes in the opposite direction. Once inside the body it finds its way to the reticulo-endothelial cells in many organs and there it multiplies for 12 days without inconveniencing its host in any way. This is the incubation period. At the end of 12 days, the virus re-enters the bloodstream and its presence there causes in most patients a severe prodromal or pre-eruptive illness. It seems to leave the bloodstream quickly because, except in fulminating cases, it cannot be grown from the blood of a patient after the second day of the illness. It invades many organs of the body and can cause severe, even fatal, damage therein. Indeed, in severe, fulminating, haemorrhagic smallpox, the virus often kills the patient before it has itself a chance to escape from the body, and such patients are usually not infectious. In most cases, however, the virus finds its way to the mucous membranes of the respiratory tract and to the cells of the skin. In both these sites, its presence causes inflammatory reactions. Deep in the skin there is first of all a dilatation of the blood capillaries. Soon the overlying epithelial cells begin to swell and stretch their walls. The walls rupture and several adjacent cells run together, forming first the maculo-papules and later the vesicles and pustules that are characteristic of the disease. The roof of these skin lesions is formed by the horny layer of the skin epithelium, and as long as this layer remains intact, as it often does, virus cannot escape to the outside. If the roof bursts or is broken the contents escape and these are full of smallpox virus. All the pustules eventually dry up and are finally shed as scabs, leaving behind a pock mark on the skin. These scabs still contain virus, and this virus, along with any that may have escaped from broken blisters or pustules contaminates the environment of the patient.

Escape of the virus

The mucous membranes of the upper respiratory tract are far more delicate than the skin. They are not covered by any horny layer. The inflammatory reaction caused by the virus is the same as in the skin but, as the cells swell, they quickly burst through and discharge their contents on the surface of the upper respiratory tract. Such ruptured lesions can often be seen on the soft palate and uvula and there are probably many unseen in the upper trachea and larynx. This means that virus is now present in the secretions of the throat and mouth and it can very readily escape from the patient's body. Virus reaches the cells of the skin and the respiratory tract simultaneously so that the inflammatory reactions occur at the two sites at the same time. This means that the rash is appearing on the skin at the same time as the cells are swelling in the respiratory mucous membranes. Virus escapes from the latter and renders the patient infectious, but the early rash is already present on his skin. In other words, the patient is not infectious before the rash appears on his skin. Perhaps, because the cells can swell a little more quickly in the delicate mucous membranes than in the tough skin, virus might escape just before the first spots appear on the skin, but this is unlikely to be more than, at the most, 12 hours earlier. This is an important point for two reasons. First, if the disease is suspected in the patient before he gets his rash then steps can at once be taken to protect those around him; those steps will be successful. Second, patients who do not develop the skin rash are not infectious.

Infectious or non-infectious

These latter patients are of two very different types. The first type is the patient almost, but not completely, immune because of previous vaccination. His immunity is not high enough to suppress multiplication of the virus in his body: the virus spills over into the bloodstream. The patient suffers from the symptoms of the pre-eruptive fever but his immune mechanisms take over in time to neutralize the virus before it can reach the mucous membranes or the skin and the illness aborts before any rash appears. The patient has suffered from smallpox without the rash, *variola sine eruptione*. He is not infectious because the virus cannot get out of his body. The second type of patient is the one who has no immunity to smallpox. In his body, the virus multiplies exceedingly and, when the virus spills over into the bloodstream, the viraemia is so intense that it overwhelms and kills the patient before the virus has time to penetrate the skin or mucous membranes. There may be, and usually is, a rash on the skin, but it is a fiery reddening of all the skin, often with blotches of blood in it: it is sometimes called *purpura variolosa*, but it is a prodromal rash, not the true focal rash of smallpox. This is haemorrhagic or hypertoxic smallpox. The patient dies but he is not infectious for the virus dies with him, trapped inside his body.

The missed case

A slight difference in the immune status can greatly affect infectivity. A patient may have an immunity just a little lower than the patient with *variola sine eruptione*. In such a patient, a small amount of virus gets through to the mucous membranes and the skin: it may be enough to cause only one or two spots on the skin. The writer has seen a patient with only one spot. The patient suffers from modified smallpox, i.e. smallpox modified by vaccination. He may be no more ill than the patient with *variola sine eruptione* but he has virus on his mucous membranes and he can be infectious. He is infectious only to very close, intimate contacts, because he excretes only very small amounts of virus; but he is a dangerous person because, having very little outward evidence of the disease, very few and often very atypical spots, his illness is quite likely not to be diagnosed for what it is until one of his intimate contacts goes down with smallpox a fortnight later; and this contact may go down with severe or even fatal smallpox. Time and again in the history of smallpox outbreaks, a modified case is missed in this way.

A second difference in immune status is when a patient has immunity just a little higher than the patient who dies of hypertoxic smallpox as already described. The patient with the slightly higher immunity survives the intense viraemia. The virus bursts through to his skin and mucous membranes. The patient develops the true rash of smallpox and virus abounds on his mucous membranes. He is highly infectious. He may die within a day or two before the rash has time to mature and be recognized, or he may survive for a week or more, or even recover: in such a case, the rash, though profuse, may be flatter and more velvety than in a typical case of smallpox and its nature may not be recognized by an inexperienced doctor.

Clinical types

Five different clinical varieties of smallpox have to be considered and it is not possible to understand the sometimes baffling spread of smallpox, unless all five are taken into consideration. There are *variola sine eruptione* and *purpura variolosa*, the one a trifling condition, the other fatal, but both non-infectious: there is modified smallpox, the patient with only a few spots, very slightly infectious but very liable to be missed, and so a danger to close contacts: there is the patient with haemorrhagic smallpox who survives the initial viraemia, is highly infectious, but can be missed: and the ordinary typical case of smallpox, infectious but easy to recognize and unlikely to be overlooked.

ECOLOGY

Outside the body

Virus escapes from the body of the smallpox patient mainly from his mouth and throat. Droplets from the patient's mucous membranes land on the mucous membranes of someone near him and this person then gets smallpox. There is no doubt that this is the main way in which smallpox spreads. When skin spots break down or scabs are shed virus again escapes and contaminates the environment, on bed clothes, in floor dust, etc.; these are a less important but not neglible source of infection. Virus is also excreted in the patient's urine and obviously urine could contaminate bed clothes or the hands of a careless nurse, but there is no evidence that this is an important method of spread. Virus can escape from the conjunctiva, especially if the patient has conjunctivitis. The main importance of this route is that sometimes a contact with a high degree of immunity has conjunctivitis as his only symptom of smallpox and, like the patient with only one or two spots, he can be the missing link in an otherwise unexplained spread of the disease (Downie *et al.*, 1969; Kempe *et al.*, 1969; Sarkar *et al.*, 1973).

Effect of weather and climate

How does the virus fare outside the body? Most of the drops from the patient's mouth fall within a few feet. If it has not reached the mucous membranes of another person the virus falls on the bed-clothes or into the dust around the bed and soon becomes dried. How long can it survive and how dangerous is the dried virus? At room temperature and relative humidities such as are found in Britain, say 20°C and 58–75% relative humidity, the virus has survived for 12–18 months in bales of cotton or in crusts. In Madras, in bedding or clothes kept bundled in a cool dark room or box, it has survived for 60–70 days. In bales of cotton kept at 30°C, the virus has survived for 6 weeks when the relative humidity was 84%, for 2 months at a relative humidity of 73% and for 3 months at relative humidity of 58%. Sunlight kills it quickly. In bedding exposed to indirect sunlight, virus survives for a few days but for only a few hours in direct sunlight. All these findings are relevant to the spread of smallpox. Infected laundry can obviously be dangerous to those who handle it, and a laundry worker has in many outbreaks gone down with smallpox. A patient's bedroom can be contaminated with virus and remain so for several days; the occasional nurse or cleaner may have been infected in this way. But none of these ways are of major epidemic importance; they account only for the odd case now and then. (Christie, 1974; W.H.O., 1972a.)

Airborne spread

Can fine droplets from a patient's mouth or can virus in dust be wafted through the air and infect a contact at some distance from the source of infection? This is one of the great unresolved controversies of medicine. There is no doubt that smallpox virus can get out from smallpox hospitals but there is a great unwillingness to allow that it can do so on its own. Yet there are cases where it has been very difficult to explain the spread of the virus in any other way. A boy aged 2 years lived 400 yards away from the writer's smallpox hospital in which there was a patient with severe smallpox: the child had been confined to his house for 2 weeks suffering from mumps. The day he was infected was the first day he had been out of doors; he had been taken in a wheelchair to a barber's shop even farther away from the hospital. There was absolutely nothing to connect him with the smallpox hospital except the prevailing wind, and this blew from the hospital towards his home. Yet every other conceivable agent, not excluding cats and starlings, was blamed for the transfer of virus. Could it not have been air-borne? (Christie, 1974).

Inside a hospital in Meschede in Germany, the virus spread from one patient in a single room and infected 16 other patients throughout the three-storey hospital block and also a visitor who stood in the entrance hall for only 15 minutes. Smoke tests showed that air currents passing through the building corresponded well with the direction taken by the virus (Wehrle *et al.*, 1970), yet there were some who still contended that air spread was inconceivable and that doctors or nurses must have carried the virus from the one patient to the others. The truth is that smallpox normally spreads by face to face contact of one patient with another but there are occasions, admittedly rare, when the virus may be wafted in a current of air, smuggled around in a bundle of clothes or inhaled in the dust of a patient's bedroom.

Spread in a community

It has already been stated that smallpox is not a highly infectious disease (p. 255). It spreads within the house or the hut. In an African village, cholera can sweep through the compounds within hours or days since it is transmitted in drinking water. Measles can spread through all the younger children in the village within a few weeks for measles is infectious in the prodromal period, before the patient is too ill to run around. But smallpox smoulders inside the mud-hut, passing slowly from one unvaccinated member of the family to another, and then perhaps on to some other person in a neighbouring hut. If the village is remote, the virus may never get outside it, and, indeed, in the early days of the smallpox eradication scheme (p. 266), pockets of infection persisted in remote African villages because villagers were unwilling to travel to a vaccination assembly point and field vaccinators were reluctant at first to penetrate too far into the bush (Imperato *et al.*, 1973). When there is some communication between villages or when villagers journey now and again with their produce to neighbouring market townships, then smallpox virus can get around. A villager with one or two spots takes the virus with him to the market and can pass it on to a stranger and that stranger can take it back with him and sicken in some distant village or town (Al-Tikriti and Jurji, 1973). Smallpox is then on the move.

EPIDEMIOLOGY

Behaviour in different communities

The arrival of smallpox in the new village or town is likely to remain a mystery, for how can a chance contact be traced in the swarm of life in a tropical market? Moreover, the new arrival may get smallpox in a mild, unrecognized form and so, too, may the one or two people he first infects. It is often not until the third or fourth generation of cases that the first florid, unmistakeable case of smallpox is seen. By that time, infection may have spread widely among the population. An outbreak of smallpox, widespread and apparently unexplained, has broken out. Just how such an outbreak will develop depends on the type of population affected, on its previous experience of smallpox, history of vaccination, degree of overcrowding, type of housing or lack of it, movement of population, standard of medical organization and perhaps even on the beliefs and traditions of the people. Most likely there will be no devastating epidemic. Mild cases will occur side by side with severe cases while other people will escape altogether because of a previous attack or of vaccination. Mortality is likely to be around 25% so that 75% of those affected will survive and be immune. The virus will have increasing difficulty in finding new victims and will tend to attack the youngest children being born into or added to the community and who have no experience of the disease. The outbreak will tend to smoulder and crackle rather than blaze forth. If the population is large enough and the birth rate high enough, the infection may establish itself in the population, never quite dying out, but every now and again becoming more lively and active. In other words, smallpox becomes endemic in the population and part of its normal pattern of disease. The survival of smallpox as a disease of man has depended on this ability to establish itself in endemic areas.

Smallpox in a previously unexposed population

In a completely "virgin" population with no previous experience of the disease and poor or non-existent medical facilities, the disease has sometimes descended as an overwhelming scourge and virtually eliminated it. This probably occurred when the disease was first introduced into the Americas in the early 15th century when whole tribes were wiped out by smallpox (Dixon, 1962). For the virus of smallpox such devastation is self-defeating, because smallpox virus infects only man and if an agent of infection destroys all its hosts, it too dies out in the process. Smallpox has survived as a world disease by sparing most of its victims and continuing to spread from one to another in established endemic areas. From these areas, it can spread only with the help of man, its sole host.

Effect of travel

The case of a villager leaving his tropical compound and carrying smallpox virus into a neighbouring market town has been considered. The virus can accompany man on much longer distances and the history of the epidemiology of smallpox is full of accounts of the spread of the disease over vast areas of the world. Before the era of rapid travel, this spread was often across land masses, being carried by armies, bands of pilgrims or migrating populations. The disease was probably present in China 1000 years B.C., it may have accompanied Alexander's army into Persia and India and it may have spread from Abyssinia (Ethiopia) to Mecca in an invading army in the sixth century A.D. (Dixon, 1962).

Travel by sea in the early days was a slow process and passengers and crew members had time to sicken and die or recover on the voyage between one continent and another. However, the virus of smallpox can persist in clothes and bedding (p. 260). One large outbreak in South Africa in the 18th century began among those who washed clothing from an infected ship from India although there were no longer any infectious patients on board. In modern times, smallpox has often crossed the sea in ships from the Far East, Africa, South America and elsewhere in Europe. Sea travel is faster now and often a seamen or a passenger still has clearly visible signs of the disease on arrival in Europe. In such instances measures can be taken from the outset to contain the disease. By air travel, however, a passenger can have crossed the world within 24 hours of being infected: he is perfectly well on arrival and will not become ill with the pre-eruptive fever until he has been another 11 days in his new environment. The chances of his passing on the infection before the nature of his illness is diagnosed are thus much greater, especially so in a country where smallpox has become a rare, imported disease. Once the first cases of smallpox are diagnosed, strict measures can be taken to limit the spread. In a modern developed country with an efficient medical service, such measures prove successful and importation does not result in uncontrollable epidemics. This is because smallpox spreads in a developed country in exactly the same way as in a primitive village. The virus passes from the respiratory mucous membranes of the infectious patient to the mucous membranes of his close contacts, there is an incubation period of 12 days, and if these contacts can be traced, vaccinated, and kept under surveillance, the medical team will eventually catch up with the slow-spreading virus which must then die out in its new environment.

Smallpox in a developed country

There is no doubt that it is this intense surveillance that contains smallpox virus and prevents its spread in a modern, developed community. The essence of the method is to throw a ring of vaccinated contacts around each possible infected person. If the ring is complete the virus cannot break through it, for it cannot establish itself and multiply in a fully vaccinated immune person. There may have to be several rings after one importation of the disease; some rings may have to be much wider than others, depending on how much start the virus has had in different areas. But if the mode of surveillance is dogged and thorough, there is never any need for mass vaccination. Indeed, in a modern developed community mass vaccination is usually the result of propaganda by ill-informed mass media. It leads to the vaccination of thousands of people who have not been exposed to the virus. Many of these will suffer inconvenience or worse as a result of vaccination. The control of the outbreak will still depend on the vaccination and surveillance of only those few who *have* been exposed to the virus.

The effect of weather and climate on smallpox is not very great. Smallpox is not, like malaria or yellow fever, confined to areas of the world where climate and other environmental factors favour the survival of some mosquito or other intermediate host of the infecting agent. Smallpox can spread in any part of the world where people are gathered together close enough for the virus to pass from one to the other. The disease has, in the past, been endemic in developed countries which are now free of it. In Britain in the last two centuries it was, indeed, rarely absent. It was the cause of much illness and many deaths and there were times of great incidence when few families, at least in the big towns escaped. In the first 30 years of the present century, there were still thousands of cases, albeit latterly the disease was mainly variola minor, a much milder variety of smallpox. It is not easy to explain fully why the disease has died out in developed countries. It is probably due, in the main, to improved hygiene and other conditions of life: as these became better for the people, life became worse for the virus. The disease began to show the signs of obsolescence. As Creighton said

> It first left the richer classes, then it left the villages, then it left the provincial towns to centre itself in the capital: at the same time it was leaving the age of infancy and childhood. Of course it did none of these things absolutely: but the movement in any one of these directions has been obvious as in any other (Creighton, 1891–4).

Diseases do appear to decline and fall without the intervention of specific scientific measures. Scarlet fever has become a trivial disease in Britain in the last 30 years for no obvious reason at all, and measles is now a much milder disease than it was in Britain 40 years ago, though it is still deadly in some underdeveloped countries. The same thing has probably happened with smallpox in the Western World.

Effect of vaccination

Has vaccination had anything to do with the great decline? Vaccination certainly protects a person against smallpox: the duration of protection varies with the individual, from a few years to very much more. A patient rarely dies of the disease within 10 years of successful vaccination. It would therefore be foolish to claim that vaccination has had no effect in the decline of the disease in the population. Had every individual in the population been vaccinated, and possibly revaccinated, this would probably have led to the eradication of the disease in that population; but nothing like this level of vaccination has ever been achieved in Britain, in spite of legal compulsory measures. Only a minority of the population has been vaccinated. Long before the repeal of compulsory infant vaccination in Britain in 1948, less than 40% of the infant population was vaccinated. Even this proportion might have had the effect of shifting the incidence of the disease from infancy and childhood, one of Creighton's criteria of obsolescence, but it is most unlikely that it would have brought about the disappearance of the disease. Vaccination may, then, have been one modifying factor but it can scarcely have been a major one. That this is true may be seen from the behaviour of the disease in less favoured countries where, in spite of a considerable amount of vaccination, the disease has remained endemic. Between 1962 and 1966, five hundred million vaccinations were carried out in India yet the disease continued to spread: 5–10% of a population always escaped, mainly children under 15 years, and these unvaccinated persons gave the virus its chance to survive.

ERADICATION

The eradication programme

Because of the success of control measures in developed countries in preventing the spread of smallpox and of bringing imported outbreaks to an end, the W.H.O. decided, in 1967, to introduce an intensive world-wide programme aimed at the eradication of the disease. At that time, smallpox was endemic in 30 countries. Most African countries south of the Sahara were included; Afghanistan,

India, Indonesia, Nepal and Pakistan; and Brazil in South America. At first, the aim was mass vaccination and mobile teams vaccinated masses of people. The campaign met with success, but not complete success. By 1973, there were only five endemic areas left, Ethiopia and the Sudan, India, Pakistan and Nepal, but in these areas the disease was still spreading. It became clear that mass vaccination alone would not eradicate the disease in those areas (Henderson, 1972, 1973; W.H.O., 1972a, b). The emphasis passed to the accurate reporting of cases and to the meticulous surveillance of patients and the vaccination of contacts. Just as a vaccination ring is placed round one imported case in Europe so a ring had to be placed round an endemic focus in a village or compound in Ethiopia, Nepal or in any of the other endemic areas. The surveillance teams had to be highly mobile, ready to move in and vaccinate contacts if they were to keep ahead of the virus. The virus could be contained even in a remote village if unvaccinated contacts could be prevented from moving out. By the autumn of 1975, smallpox was eradicated from every area in the world except Ethiopia where the campaign still goes on (1976) (Fig. 11.1).

A reservoir in nature

The war in the Indian continent in 1972 disrupted the already primitive living conditions in Bangladesh and smallpox virus spread rapidly in the disorganized population. This certainly slowed down the eradication campaign but the work of eradication went on, and there is little doubt that success will be achieved. Two factors favoured success; the first was that, from the vaccination point of view, smallpox is a single antigenic virus: the second was that smallpox has only one host, man, and there is almost certainly no reservoir of smallpox virus infection in nature.

Variola major and variola minor viruses are both smallpox viruses: vaccinia virus is closely related. All three have slightly different growth and other laboratory characteristics, but they share common antigens and vaccination protects against all three. Camelpox is a related virus but can be distinguished from smallpox virus by differing growth patterns on a range of cell tissue cultures (Baxby, 1974). Monkeypox virus cannot be distinguished from smallpox virus when grown on chick embryo but, when injected intradermally

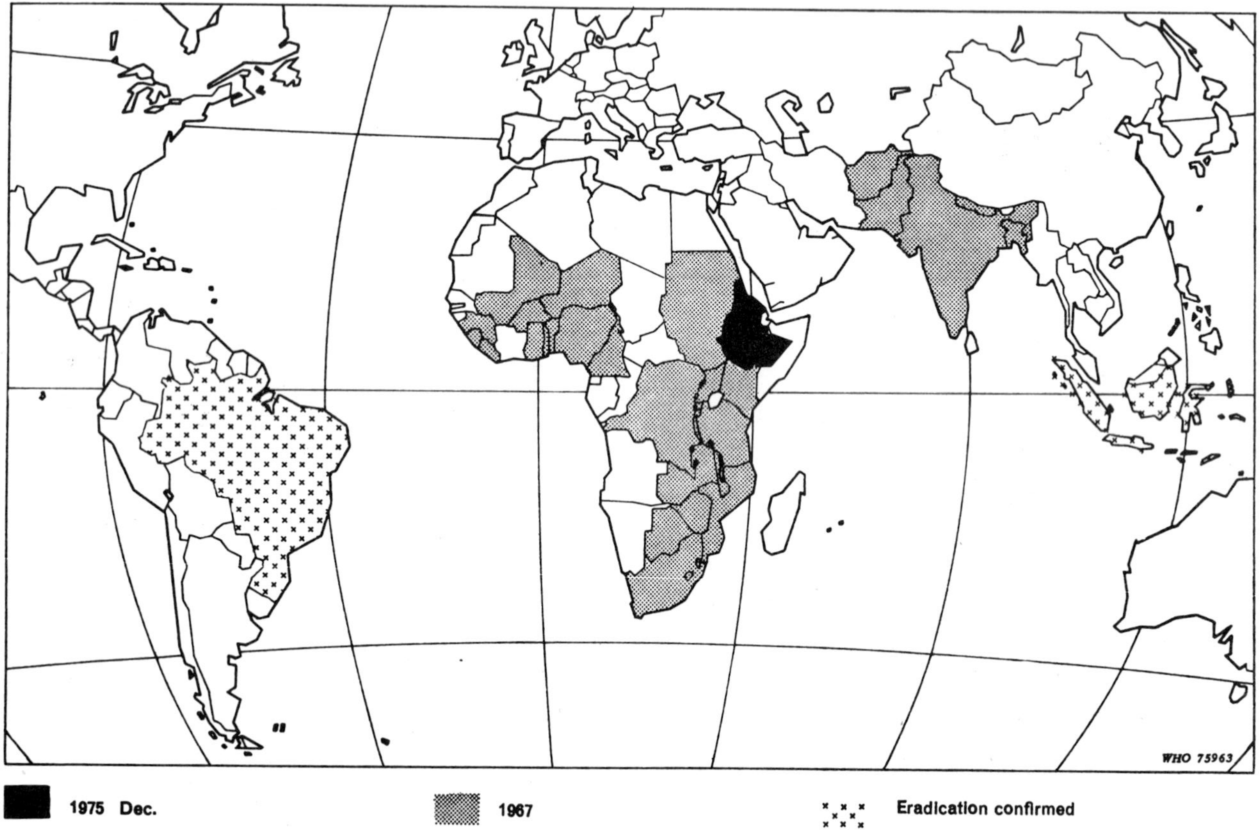

Fig. 11.1 World status of smallpox, December 1975 (W.H.O. data).

into rabbits, the two viruses behave differently (Marrenikova *et al.*, 1972; Cho and Wenner, 1973). Monkeypox virus can be spread to man, but not readily. The virus was first isolated in 1959, and since then 10 outbreaks have been reported in captive monkey colonies: in no instance did the disease spread to man. However, there have been at least 14 cases of monkeypox diagnosed in man in Africa but, in only one case, was there evidence of spread from one person to another: all the others had had very close contact with live monkeys or their carcases. The disease in man cannot be distinguished *clinically* from human smallpox but it can be distinguished *virologically* (Foster *et al.*, 1972; Lourie *et al.*, 1972). The discovery of these cases, so like smallpox, in an area from which it was believed the disease had been eradicated came first as a shock, but its true nature is now known. It may remain a diagnostic problem, though a rare one, for monkeypox seems to be a rare infection in monkeys in the wild. Other strains of poxviruses known as white poxviruses have been isolated from monkey kidney. These are almost impossible to distinguish from smallpox virus, but they seem not to have caused any disease either in monkeys or in man (Gispen and Brand-Saathog, 1972). Neither monkeypox virus nor white poxvirus represents a reservoir of smallpox virus in nature; all evidence seems to show that no such reservoir exists. Smallpox is a disease of man, and of man only. Throughout history, it has plagued its only host. Its end is in sight.

REFERENCES

Al-Tikriti, S. K. and Jurji, F. J. (1973). Smallpox eradication in Iraq—1972. *Bull. Endem. Dis.* **14**, 7.

Baxby, D. (1974). Differentiation of smallpox and camelpox viruses in cultures of human and monkey cells. *J. Hyg.* (*Camb.*) **72**, 251.

Cho, C. T. and Wenner, H. A. (1973). Monkeypox virus. *Bact. Revs.* **37**, 1.

Christie, A. B. (1974). "Infectious Diseases: Epidemiology and Clinical Practice" (2nd edn). Churchill Livingstone, Edinburgh.

Creighton, C. (1891–4). "A History of Epidemics in Britain", Vol. II, p. 617; quoted by Greenwood, M. (1930) in *J. Roy. Stat. Soc.* **93**, 233.

Dixon, C. W. (1962). "Smallpox". Churchill, London.

Downie, A. W., Fedson, D. S., St. Vincent, L., Rao, A. R. and Kempe, C. H. (1969). Haemorrhagic smallpox. *J. Hyg.* (*Camb.*) **67**, 619.

Foster, S. O., Brink, E. W., Hutchins, D. L., Pifer, J. M., Lourie, B., Moser, C. R., Cummings, E. C., Kuteyi, O. E. K., Eke, R. E. A., Titus, J. B., Smith, E. A.,

Hicks, J. W. and Foege, W. H. (1972). Human monkeypox. *Bull. W.H.O.* **46**, 569.
Gispen, R. and Brand-Saathof, B. (1972). "White" poxvirus strains from monkeys. *Bull. W.H.O.* **46**, 585.
Henderson, D. A. (1972). Epidemiology in the global eradication of smallpox. *Int. J. Epidem.* **1**, 25.
Henderson, D. A. (1973). Eradication of smallpox: the critical year ahead. *Proc. Roy. Soc. Med.* **66**, 493.
Imperato, P. J., Sow, O. and Benitieni—Fofana (1973). The persistence of smallpox in remote unvaccinated villages during eradication programme activities. *Acta Tropica* **30**, 261.
Kempe, C. H., Dekking, F., St. Vincent, L., Rao, A. R. and Downie, A. W. (1969). Conjunctivitis and subclinical infection in smallpox. *J. Hyg.* (*Camb.*) **67**, 631.
Lourie, B., Bingham, P. G., Evans, H. H., Foster, S. O., Nakano, J. H. and Herrmann, K. I. (1972). Human infection with monkeypox virus: laboratory investigation of six cases in West Africa. *Bull. W.H.O.* **46**, 633.
Marrenikova, S. S., Seluhina, E. M., Mal'ceva, N. N., Cimiskjan, K. L. and Macevic, G. R. (1972). *Bull. W.H.O.* **46**, 599.
Sarkar, J. K., Mitra, A. C., Mukherjee, M. K., De, S. K. and Guha Mazumdar, D. (1973). Virus excretion in smallpox. *Bull. W.H.O.* **48**, 517.
Wehrle, P. F., Posch, J., Richter, K. H. and Henderson, D. A. (1970). An air-borne outbreak of smallpox in a German hospital and its significance with respect to other recent outbreaks in Europe. *Bull. W.H.O.* **43**, 609.
W.H.O. (1972a). W.H.O. Expert Committee on Smallpox Eradication, second report. *W.H.O. Techn. Rep. Ser.* **493**.
W.H.O. (1972b). The smallpox problem. *W.H.O. Chronicle* **26**, 393.

12. Yellow Fever, Dengue and Dengue Haemorrhagic Fever

A. W. A. Brown

These mosquito-borne diseases, due to the yellow fever and dengue arboviruses of the Group-B type, are confined to tropical and semitropical regions inhabited by vectors belonging to the subgenus *Stegomyia* of the genus *Aedes*. At the present time, yellow fever causes recurrent epidemics in Africa and more sporadic infections in South America. It originates in monkeys, the principal reservoir hosts. The disease is still absent from Asia. Dengue, independent of the wild monkey host, is now endemic among human populations in the Caribbean area while the more serious disease, known as dengue haemorrhagic fever (DHF), now causes epidemics in the cities and towns of South-East Asia. The present situation is different from that of a century ago, when severe epidemics of yellow fever recurred throughout the Caribbean area but were not reported from the interior of tropical Africa, and when dengue was epidemic in the southern U.S.A. and being reported from eastern Asia for the first time. Clearly, the medical geography of these diseases cannot be considered in isolation from their history. Their geographical limits are determined by the climatic conditions that allow the survival and multiplication of their *Stegomyia* mosquito vectors. Since all the evidence indicates that the principal vector, *Aedes aegypti*, originated in tropical Africa, the geography of these arbovirus diseases (Fig. 12.1) is best understood by accepting that this vector spread from an African origin, and that human life-styles determine the extent of its infesting the human environment.

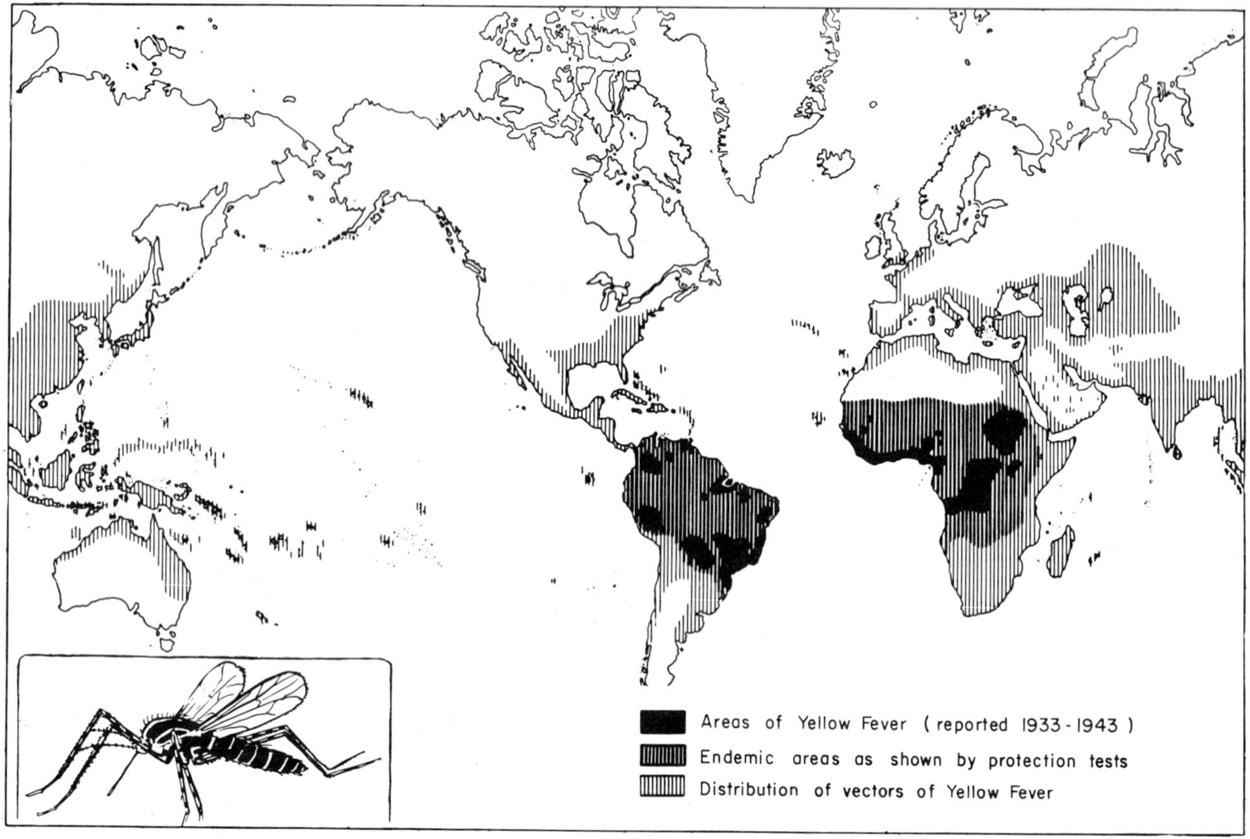

Fig. 12.1 Yellow fever and *Aedes aegypti*, 1945 (Ash and Spitz, 1946).

MOSQUITO VECTORS

Aedes aegypti

In its wild state in tropical Africa, *Aedes aegypti* is a forest mosquito. The larvae breed in tree holes and the adults often feed on monkeys. More than any other species of *Stegomyia*, it proved capable of colonizing human settlements, the larvae breeding in jars of stored drinking water and the adults feeding on man. In towns and cities, *Aedes aegypti* did not breed in the polluted waters of drains and cesspools but rather in barrels, cisterns, flower vases, ant traps, a great variety of discarded containers and more recently in old motor-vehicle tyres. Colonies would develop and persist in the water casks of sailing vessels so that, during the three centuries of the notorious Middle Passage of the slave trade, this African species would be repeatedly introduced into the Caribbean islands and adjoining mainland, the ports and hinterland of eastern Brazil, and later the Amazon river system. In South America, where there are no native species of *Stegomyia* mosquitoes, the arrival of *A. aegypti* in certain inland localities is so recent that it can be dated, e.g. Bucaramanga, Colombia in 1909, and Santa Cruz de la Sierra, Bolivia in 1919.

In its spread into Asia from the East-African ports, *A. aegypti* came into competition with an Asiatic species of *Stegomyia*, namely *A. albopictus*. While both species transmitted dengue in Asia, neither of them acquired the yellow-fever infection. By 1903, *A. aegypti* had established itself in Singapore and at Port Swettenham but nowhere else on the Malayan peninsula; by 1955, it still was not to be found in many of the inland villages. It reached Hong Kong some time after 1902 and Haiphong in 1915. In the last half-century, *A. aegypti* has been observed to have progressively replaced *A. albopictus* in Calcutta, Kuala Lumpur, Semarang and the cities of Thailand, and developed far greater infestations. Further east, the colonization by this vector of certain Pacific islands is quite recent:— Nanumea and Funafuti (Ellice Islands) and Treasury Island (Solomons) during the Second World War and Niue in 1972.

Whereas the adults of *A. aegypti* in the forests, villages and towns of Africa are jet black with white stripes (described as the subspecies *formosus*), sporadic populations in the African ports and coastal sail-boats are orange in colour. This light form, observed also in ports on the Red Sea, in South Arabia, the Seychelles and Mauritius, was described as form *queenslandensis* from a population at Burpengary near Brisbane. Both forms coexist on the Makonde plateau of south-eastern Tanzania and in certain villages north of Mombasa, *formosus* in the bamboo stumps and treeholes, and *queenslandensis* in the large water jars in the huts where they had bred continuously for decades if not centuries. On the Makonde plateau, where in 1956 an epidemic due to the type-A chikungunya virus had been transmitted by *A. aegypti*, the domestic light forms have been found to be more anthropophilic and less zoophilic than the feral dark forms. Populations of the *queenslandensis* form have occasionally been found in isolated inland locations in Sudan, Algeria and interior West Africa. The populations now inhabiting Asia and the Americas are of an intermediate mahogany colour, conforming with the description of the type form* (typicus) of *Aedes aegypti*.

By the 1930s *A. aegypti* had extended its range to southern Japan, Australia and most of the larger islands of the Pacific (Fig. 12.2). It was present along the coasts of the Mediterranean and even along those of the Black Sea. It reached the Caspian Sea at Baku and, on the Atlantic coast, it extended as far as the Bay of Biscay. In North America, populations were established as far north as Cairo, Illinois and Norfolk, Virginia, with transitory infestations reaching the latitudes of St. Louis and Boston. On the Pacific coast, it was present in San Diego, San Francisco and even coastal British Columbia. The entire Caribbean area was heavily infested. A survey revealed that *A. aegypti* could be found in more than 50% of the houses in most of the towns and cities of northern Colombia. In South America, this vector had penetrated to the headwaters of the Amazon and Parana river systems and throughout eastern Brazil south to Montivideo and Buenos Aires, with an outlying population in Bahia Blanca; on the west coast it extended south to Antofagasta, with outlying populations in Coquimbo and Valparaiso.

The zone of the earth permanently colonizable by *A. aegypti* lies between the 10°C isotherm for July in the southern hemisphere and the 10°C isotherm for January (or somewhat north of it) in the

* Specimens from Kuala Lumpur were designated as neotypes of *A. aegypti* in 1962 (P. F. Mattingly, *Bull. Zool. Nomencl.* **19**, 208–219), the original description of "*Culex aegypti* Linnaeus", as published by Hasselquist in 1762 from Egyptian material being clearly applicable to *Aedes caspius*.

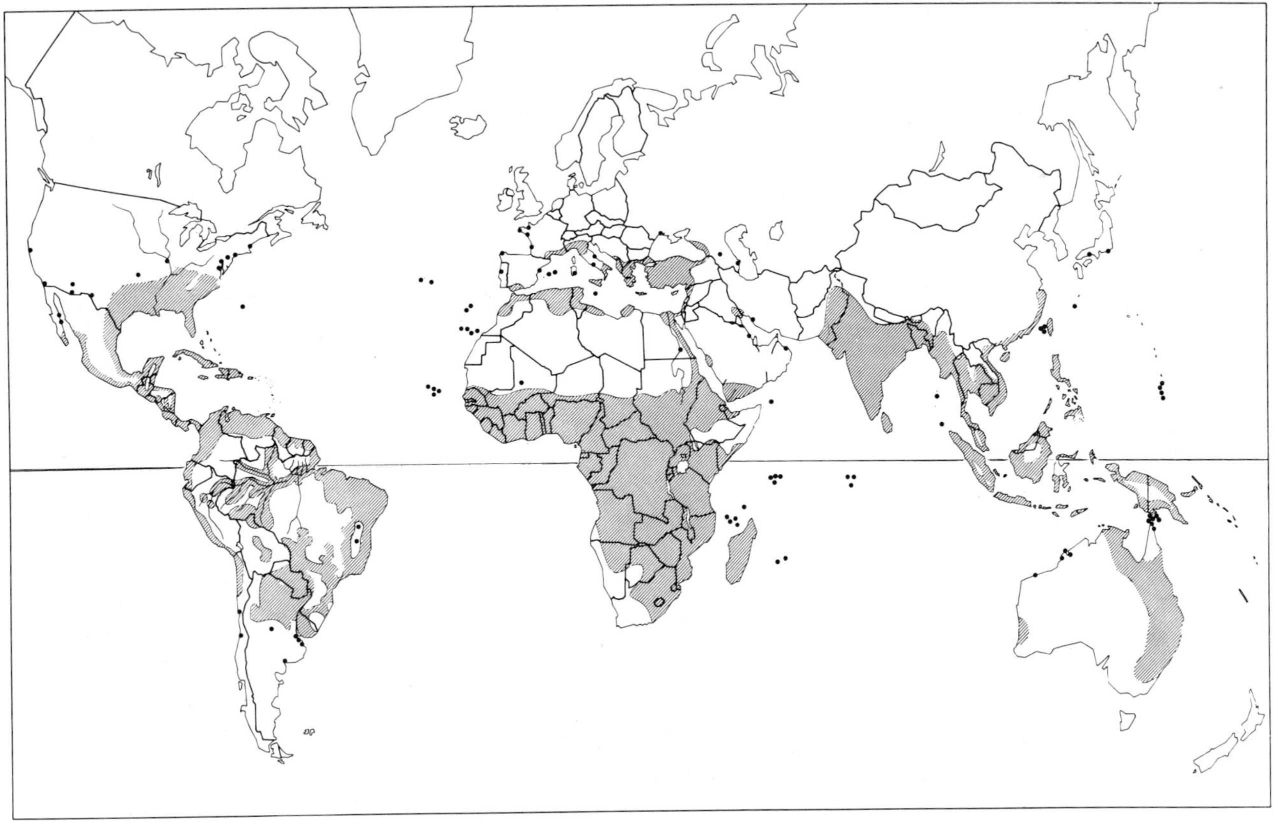

Fig. 12.2 *Aedes aegypti* at the maximum extent of its world distribution (*c*. 1930).

northern hemisphere. At 10°C, the adults enter a dormant state while at 4°C a 1 hour exposure is fatal. The eggs, resistant to desiccation maintained for over a year, can also survive freezing temperatures for at least 9 days when in the dry state. The larvae, although they can survive a few hours of freezing, die after a couple of days at temperatures below 5°C. Populations in Oklahoma and southern New South Wales can overwinter successfully in the dry egg stage; in Texas and Alabama larvae as well as eggs have been found to survive in such protected situations as cisterns and fire barrels. For *A. aegypti* to breed continuously, a temperature of at least 18°C is necessary.

The middle of the 20th century has seen a marked regression in the distribution of this vector, particularly during the decade 1946–55 when the insecticide DDT had not yet engendered resistance (Fig. 12.3). In South America, *A. aegypti* was eradicated from Bolivia by 1948; it was no longer found in Brazil by 1950 and eradication was formally declared in 1953. Eradication was confirmed in Chile, Peru, Ecuador, Paraguay and Uruguay by 1955 and in Argentina by 1959. In Central America, eradication was clearly achieved in Panama, Costa Rica and Nicaragua by 1955 and in El Salvador, Guatemala and Honduras by 1957. An eradication programme was started in the U.S.A. in 1964, but was discontinued in 1968; during this period some progress was made towards eradication in Mexico.

In the Mediterranean area, *A. aegypti* has almost completely disappeared, the only recent records here being Algiers and Gabes, Tunisia in 1960 and Desenzano in Northern Italy in 1972. Searches for this species in Greece and Israel have proved negative. It has not been found in Egypt since 1946, and has been eliminated from the Red Sea ports of Massawa, Assab and Djibouti. It is now absent from Hong Kong, the Ryukyu Islands and Japan, and eradication has been achieved in the Mascarene Islands and on Oahu among the Hawaiian Islands. *A. aegypti* has also been eradicated from the Azores, the Canary Islands, Sao Vicente in the Cape Verde Islands and Bermuda.

The entire Caribbean area (with the exception of Bonaire, Aruba, Saba, St. Eustatius and the Cayman Islands) remains infested. The southern limits of this American infestation are in the Guianas and in Colombia where, since 1969, the entire Magdalena valley has been reinfested; in the U.S.A. the distribution is bounded by latitude 36°N in Tennessee and North Carolina and by longitude 100°W in Texas. From 1965 to 1971, local infestations appeared successively in Mexico,

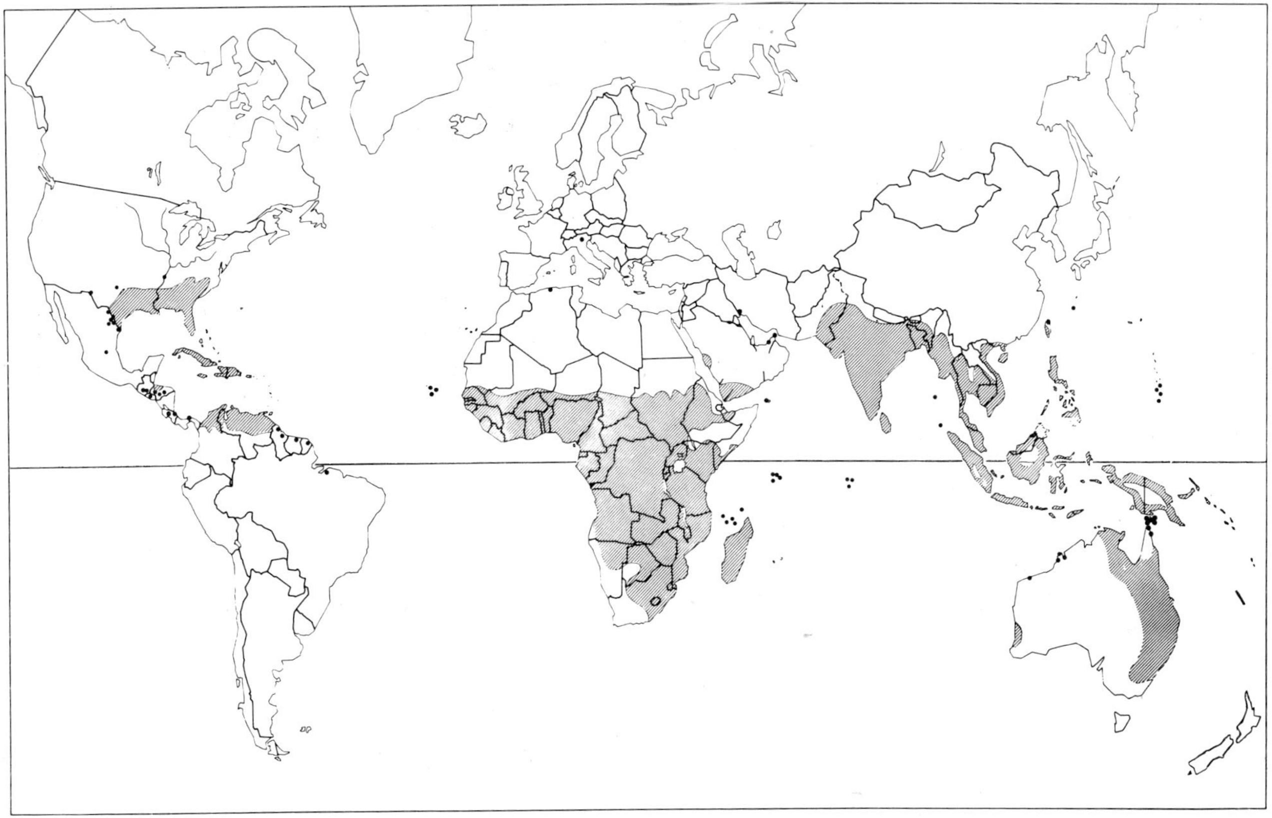

Fig. 12.3 Present day distribution of *Aedes aegupti* (*c.* 1970).

El Salvador, Guatemala, Para state of Brazil, Honduras and Panama; they also appeared in Buenos Aires and the Escuintla area of Costa Rica, but were quickly eliminated. The traffic in used tyres from the U.S.A. was frequently suspected as the source of these reinfestations.

The density of infestation by *Aedes aegypti* in villages, towns and cities is measured by empirical indices.

1. House index: percentage of houses positive for the species.
2. Container index: percentage of water-holding containers that are positive for larvae of the species.
3. Breteau index: number of positive containers per 100 houses.

In order that the results may be expressed in map form, densities are then expressed on a scale of 1–9. Those density figures are derived from one or more of the above indices according to a conversion table based on figures obtained in places where three indices were simultaneously determined (Table 12.1). Some indication of the epidemiological significance of density level has been obtained in two instances: for yellow-fever transmission in the 1965 epidemic at Diourbel, Senegal, which occurred in places with container indices above 30 and Breteau indices above 50 (density figure 5) and not in those with Breteau indices below 5 (density figure 1); and for DHF transmission in Singapore where it was found to be most prevalent in those quarters where the house index exceeded 15 (density figure 4).

Approximately 10 000 records of the presence or absence of *A. aegypti*, or of its density, have been processed by the W.H.O. for display in computer print-out maps on a scale of 1–8 million. The map for the Guinea-coast countries (Fig. 12.4) shows the vector to be

Density figure	House index	Container index	Breteau index
1	1–3	1–2	1–4
2	4–7	3–5	5–9
3	8–17	6–9	10–19
4	18–28	10–14	20–34
5	29–37	15–20	35–49
6	38–49	21–27	50–74
7	50–59	28–31	75–99
8	60–76	32–40	100–199
9	77 <	41 <	200 <

Table 12.1 Density figures corresponding to the larval indices found.

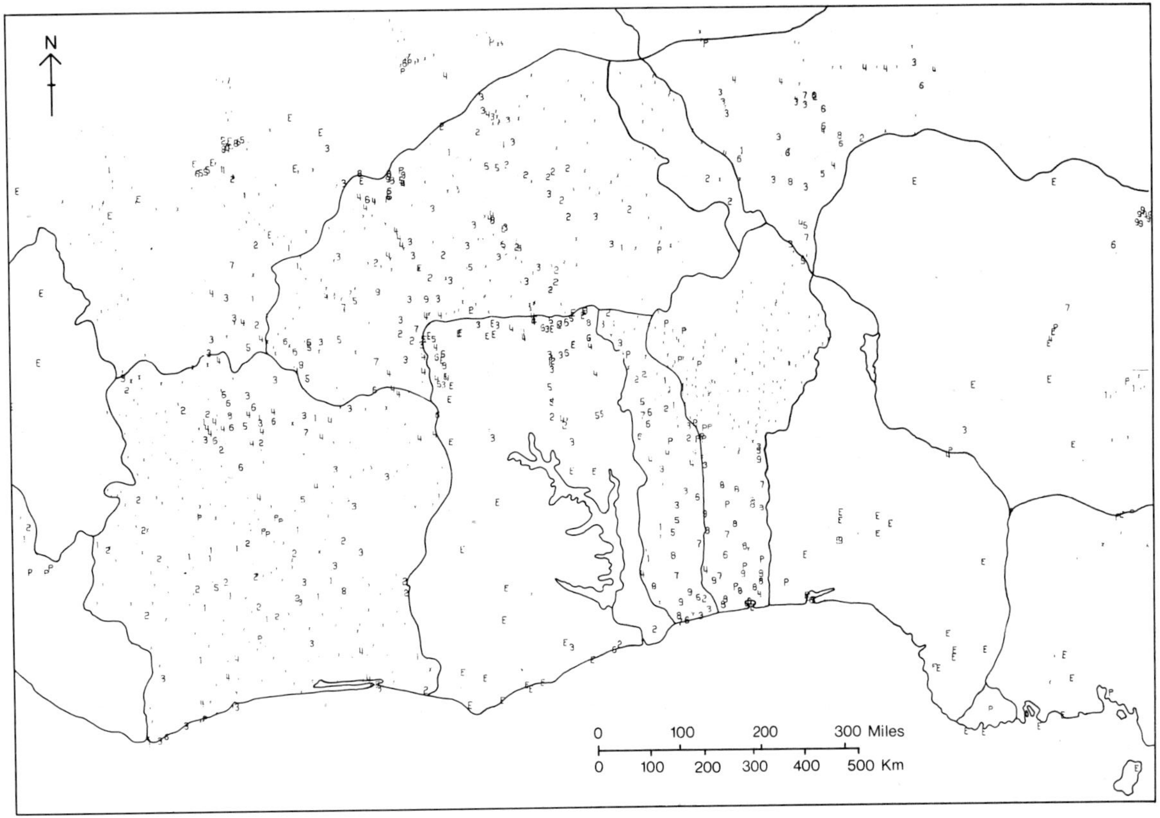

Fig. 12.4 Densities of *Aedes aegypti* in the cities, towns and villages of West Africa (computer print-out map, explained in text).

present in densities of value 5 or greater in south-eastern Mali, western Upper Volta, south-western Niger, northern Nigeria, northern Ghana and southern Togo and Dahomey. In these areas, the domestic water-supplies are stored in large jars and breeding continues unabated throughout the dry season. The same situation applies in western Senegal and northern Cameroon, while in northern Ivory Coast the vector breeds in pots of plant infusions made for medicinal purposes; in central Upper Volta the breeding is mainly in discarded jars and is confined to the wet season. Indices are also high in coastal Gabon. Further south, in Luanda in Angola, site of a yellow-fever epidemic in 1971, the average container index was 52 (density figure 9). In East Africa, consistently high indices have been found only in villages north of Mombasa and at Mtwara and Newala in south-eastern Tanzania. In Madagascar, where small emptiable pots are used for water storage, *A. aegypti* is not abundant.

In Asia, extremely high indices are present in the cities and villages of the Mekong delta and around the Gulf of Thailand (Fig. 12.5) where the house indices usually exceed 80 and the Breteau indices exceed 200 (density figure 9). The larvae breed in the large ceramic jars of drinking water placed inside or just outside the house and in the little water-filled tins used as ant traps under the legs of tables and cupboards. In the Philippines, Breteau indices of 50–100 are found in the coastal cities, being as high as 500 at Davao, Mindanao. Although *A. aegypti* is becoming scarce in Taiwan and Australia, Breteau indices of 25–50 still occur on the Torres Strait Islands. Indices exceeding 50 have been found in Fiji and Western Samoa. Density levels are now increasing in Tahiti, New Caledonia and the New Hebrides.

A. aegypti is sporadic in northern Borneo but it is abundant in Java, the house index exceeding 80 at Semarang. In the Malay peninsula, house indices have increased somewhat over the levels of 20–65 found in towns in 1955. In Cambodia and up-country Thailand, the Breteau indices usually exceed 100 in the towns and 20 in the villages. Whereas indices are high in southern Burma (average container index 35 at Rangoon), in Bangladesh the house indices seldom exceed 20. *A. aegypti* is omnipresent in eastern India, sporadic in western India, and uncommon in southern India and Sri Lanka.

In the Caribbean area, the density levels are considerably abated by chemical-control operations, formerly with DDT, now with

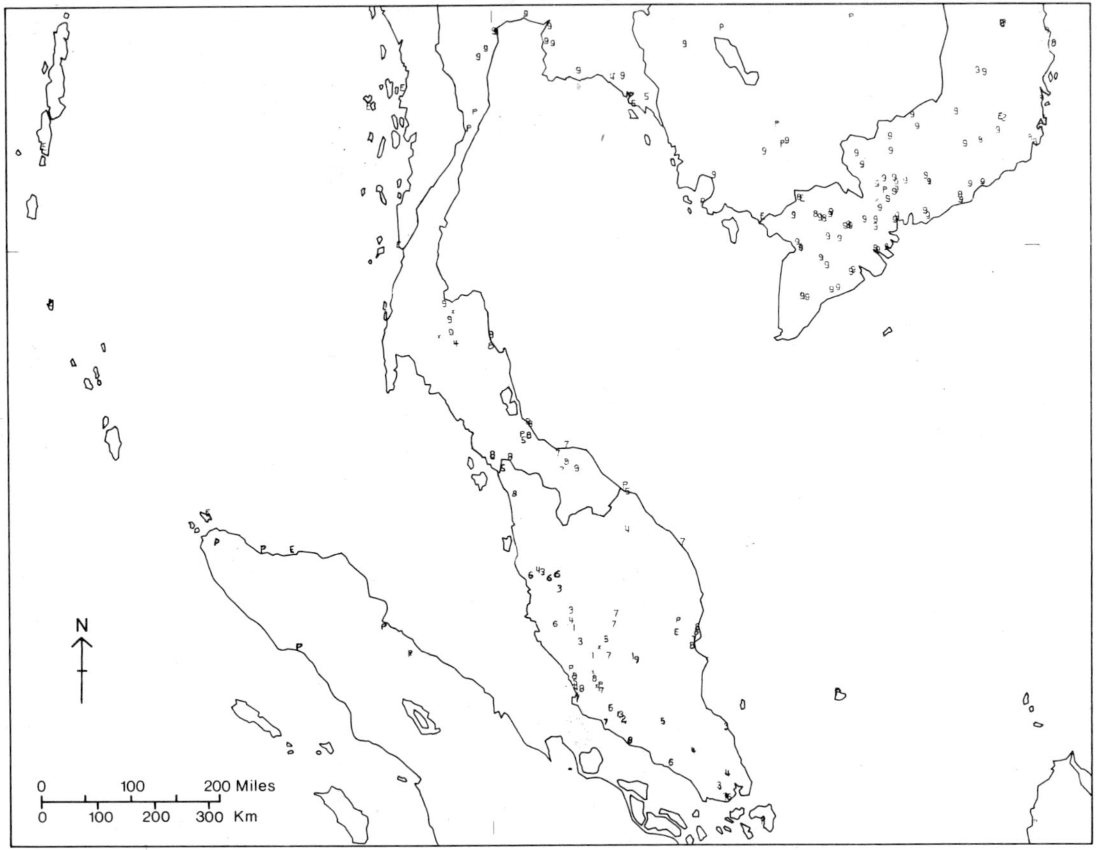

Fig. 12.5 Densities of *Aedes aegypti* in the cities, towns and villages of South-East Asia (computer print-out map, explained in text).

fenthion and temephas (Abate). In the communities of western Venezuela, house indices were thereby reduced from an average of 12.4 in 1967 to 1.0 in 1971. In 1970, the house indices in southern Jamaica ranged from 21 to 47; in 1972 the indices were 2 in Grenada, 5 on Montserrat, 12 on St. Vincent, 4 in Georgetown and 3 in Cayenne. Some domestic jars are found to be infested but the main breeding is in discarded containers, old motor vehicle tyres and in boats. In the U.S.A. the highest infestations have been found in Alabama. Here 23 of the 64 communities examined in 1964 had house indices exceeding 10. More sporadic infestations were found in Florida, Georgia and South Carolina, usually in the poor part of town, in old car tyres and discarded containers.

OTHER STEGOMYIA VECTORS

Two species breeding in tree-holes are the principal vectors of yellow fever among monkeys in Africa, and from monkeys to man; the yellow-fever virus has frequently been isolated from field-collected pools of these species (Fig. 12.6). *Aedes africanus* is characteristic of the rain-forest. Its distribution is limited to areas where the annual rainfall exceeds 1000 mm (40 inches). Its northern limit is about latitude 13°N, extending from Senegal to western Ethiopia. In East Africa its biting is limited to monkeys in the forest canopy but, in West Africa, it bites man at ground level in the bush country. *A. luteocephalus* extends from the forest into the savanna and even to the Sahel where the annual rainfall is less than 375 mm (15 inches). Thus its northern limit is about latitude 17°N across Africa from southern Mauritania to Eritrea. It enters villages to bite man in the savanna zone; it occasionally breeds in artificial containers. A third tree-hole breeder, *A. metallicus*, has been proved by experiment to be capable of transmitting yellow-fever virus among monkeys. Its distribution in the south and east of the continent betrays its oriental affinities.

Aedes simpsoni is the most common and widely-distributed *Stegomyia* in Africa. It ranges from Dakar and Eritrea south to the border of Cape Province. Although occasionally found in tree holes, the larvae characteristically breed abundantly in the leaf axils of plants such as bananas, pineapples, false bananas (*Musa ensetta*) and

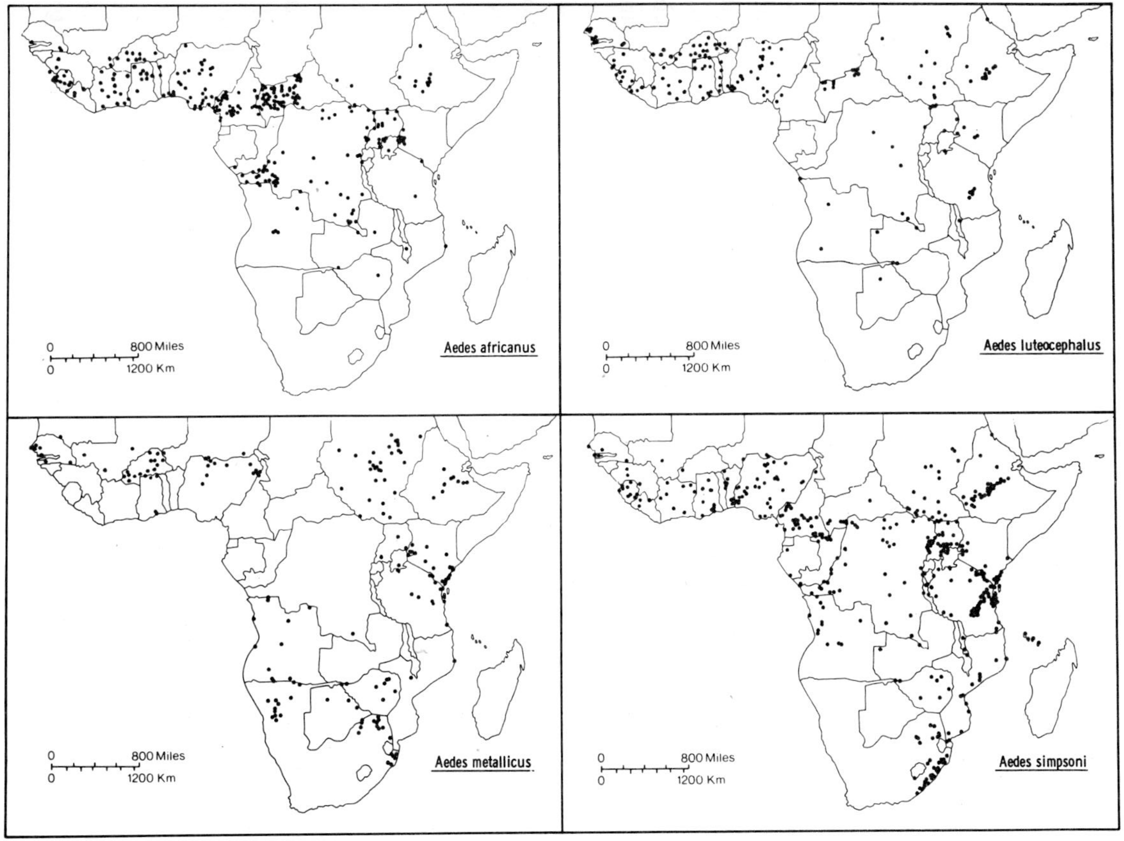

Fig. 12.6 Distribution records of African vector species of *Aedes* (*Stegomyia*).

cocoa-yams (*Colocasia* spp), and thus are characteristic of crop cultivations in forested areas. Limited to regions where the rainfall exceeds 500 mm (20 ins), *A. simpsoni* has not been found in southern Angola nor South-West Africa but it does extend to the Comores Islands, stopping short of Madagascar. In West Africa, it seldom bites man but in Ethiopia it is anthropophilic and proved to be an important yellow-fever vector in the Omo valley, where collected pools of *A. simpsoni* were frequently found positive for yellow-fever virus.

The species *Aedes vittatus*, breeding characteristically in rock holes bordering riverbeds in Africa, has been proved experimentally to be capable of transmitting yellow-fever virus. It was suspected as having been an important vector during the 1940 epidemic in the Nuba Mountains of Sudan. It is also common in the drier parts of India, often breeding in domestic pottery, where it could well be a vector of dengue viruses. It has an extraordinarily wide distribution, in Asia extending east to Indo-China and Hainan Island and in Africa north through Tibesti in the Sahara and into Europe as far as Spain and southern France (Fig. 12.7).

The Asiatic species *Aedes albopictus* breeds commonly in tree holes, bamboo stumps, leaf axils and rock pools. It is also peridomestic, breeding in artificial containers in the immediate vicinity of houses. It has frequently been found positive for one or other of the dengue viruses. Its distribution extends from Pakistan to Korea and Japan, and from Madagascar and the Indian Ocean islands to Timor and Celebes, i.e. just east of Wallace's Line which separates the Oriental from the Australian zoogeographical region. Eastward in the Pacific, the species has been introduced into the Bonin and Mariana Islands, Guam (where it has replaced the indigenous *A. guamensis*), Taiaro Island in the Tuamotu archipelago and Oahu Island, Hawaii. Here it remains as a dengue vector while *A. aegypti* has been eradicated. It is capable of transmitting yellow-fever virus among monkeys in the laboratory.

The sylvan species *Aedes scutellaris* extends from the Philippines and Indonesia eastward to Papua and New Guinea. It was proved to be a dengue vector in the 1944 New Guinea epidemic. The closely-related *A. polynesiensis* extends from Fiji east to French Polynesia. Laboratory experiment has shown it to be an effective vector of dengue virus. The member species of this *scutellaris* complex are

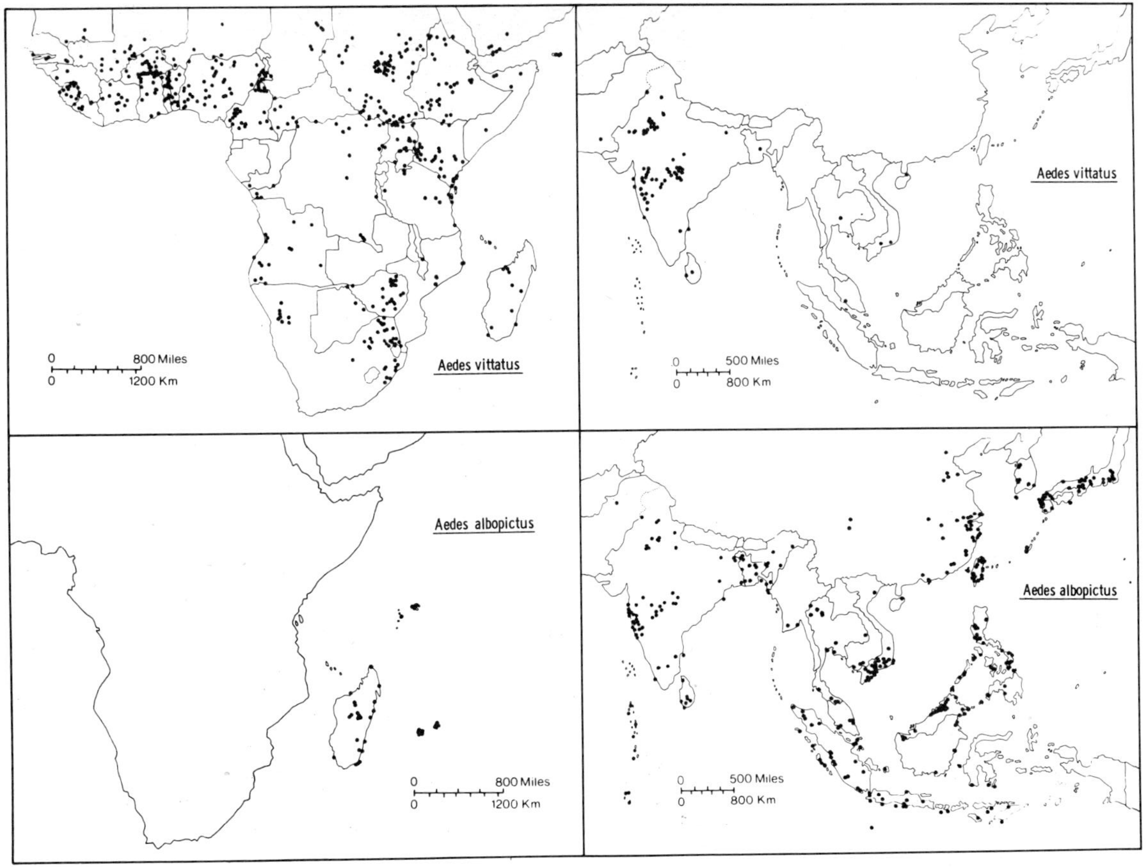

Fig. 12.7 *Aedes vittatus* in Africa and Asia and of *A. albopictus* in Asia and Madagascar.

essentially tree-hole breeders which infest a wide variety of sites, such as plant axils, crab holes, coconut shells, canoes, artificial containers and even puddles and wells.

OTHER CULICINE VECTORS

Three species of *Aedes* outside the *Stegomyia* subgenus are implicated in the transmission of yellow fever. *A. (Aedimorphus) dentatus* was found positive for yellow-fever virus in the Ethiopian epidemic and was the most common man-biting mosquito at Marsabit in northern Kenya. *A. (Aedimorphus) stokesi*, a tree hole mosquito which has been proved capable of transmitting yellow fever, is a frequent man-biter in Ethiopia, but has pronounced zoophilic habits in West Africa. *A. (Diceromyia) taylori*, also found to be a vector by experiment, is an anthropophilic tree-hole breeder with a distribution similar to that of *A. metallicus*. Virtually indistinguishable from its very close relative *A. furcifer*, it was prominent during the Nuba Mountains epidemic.

The species *Eretmapodites chrysogaster* extending from Senegal east to Ethiopia and south to Natal, breeds after the rains in small collections of water in fallen leaves, snail shells, etc. The adults are sylvan and diurnal, occasionally biting man; they have been demonstrated to be capable of transmitting yellow-fever virus. Several other closely-related *Eretmapodites* species occur in West and Central Africa.

Mansonia africana is the most common man-biting species in the rain-forest areas of Africa. It has proved capable of transmitting yellow-fever virus in experiments. The larvae breed in aquatic weeds, inserting their siphons into the vascular tissue. In deep forest, where there may be no *Stegomyias* present, this *Mansonia* may keep the yellow-fever virus circulating among monkeys.

MAMMALIAN RESERVOIRS

African species

Among the Old-World monkeys, species in the family Cercopithecidae comprise the main reservoirs of yellow fever in

Africa. The most important genus is *Cercopithecus* which includes the guenons. *C. aethiops*, the green or vervet monkey, is an arboreal species common in gallery forest in the Guinea savanna zone extending from Senegal to western Ethiopia. This species is also present in East Africa from Kenya south to Cape Province, which in the latter distribution is shared by the diademed guenon, *C. mitis*. In the rain forest of the Congo basin and coastal West Africa, the most important species are *C. mona, diana* and *nictitans*. Both the vector *Aedes africanus* and the reservoir *C. aethiops* are most active in the tree-tops at dawn. Serological tests have shown 29–35% of this species of monkey to have been yellow-fever positive in Uganda, 33% in Nigeria and 71% in southern Sudan. It was the main mammalian reservoir seeding the recent epidemics of yellow fever in Ethiopia and Senegal.

Among cercopithecids, the patas monkey *Erythrocebus patas* is an important terrestrial species, widely distributed in dry savanna areas from Senegal to Sudan. Implicated in the 1965 Senegal epidemic, it was heavily involved in the 1969 yellow-fever epidemic on the Benue plateau of Nigeria. Two species of mangabeys, the grey-cheeked (*Cercocebus albigena*) and the sooty mangabey (*C. torquatus*), are important yellow-fever reservoirs; the former species is arboreal and extends from Uganda to Cameroon, the latter is terrestrial and extends from Cameroon to Liberia.

The baboons are cercopithecids that, from their habit of leaving the forest to raid plantations, offer a route for carrying the yellow-fever virus. *Papio anubis*, the most common baboon between Nigeria and East Africa, proved 30–40% positive in Uganda and 80% positive in Sudan. *P. papio*, a common West African species, was 16% positive in Guinea, 87% positive in Gambia and was involved in the Senegal epidemic. In contrast to baboons, chimpanzees are not sufficiently numerous to be significant reservoirs of yellow fever.

In the family Colobidae, the northern guereza *Colobus abyssinicus* is an important reservoir, being the only monkey from which yellow-fever virus has been isolated in the field. It extends from western Nigeria to Ethiopia and Uganda, where it has shown a high incidence of yellow-fever antibodies. The southern guereza *C. polykomos*, which extends from Senegal to the Congo basin and Tanzania, is also an important reservoir.

Among the Lemurioidea, the bush-baby *Galago senegalensis* is widely distributed in wooded areas throughout tropical Africa except the rain forest, and has shown an average of about 10% yellow-fever positivity in Nigeria, Rhodesia and the Kenya coast; the antibody incidence was slightly higher in *G. crassicaudatus*, found only south of the Equator, in data from Rhodesia, Kenya and Zanzibar. A third species, *G. demidovi*, is refractory to yellow fever, while the potto *Periodicticus potto* is too rare to be important epidemiologically.

Other possible reservoirs of yellow fever in Africa include bats and rodents, antibodies having been found in *Epomorphorus* during the Ethiopia epidemic and in *Arvicanthis* during the Senegal epidemic.

Asiatic species

Among the Old-World monkeys, the macaques are reservoirs of the dengue viruses in Asia and potential reservoirs for yellow-fever virus. The rhesus monkey *Macaca mulatta*, the ideal subject for laboratory research in yellow fever, is distributed from the Indus valley to the China coast and is also abundant in the Ganges valley. In southern India and Sri Lanka, it is replaced by *M. sinica*, while other species of *Macaca* are found in South-East Asia and the Philippines. The Barbary ape of North Africa, *M. sylvanus*, is also susceptible to yellow-fever virus.

American species

Among the New-World monkeys, the family Cebidae comprises the main reservoirs of jungle yellow fever, the most important being species of *Alouatta*, *Ateles* and *Cebus*. The howler monkeys, *Alouatta*, are most susceptible to yellow fever and the epizootic preceding the 1954 Trinidad epidemic was detected by deaths of the red howler, *A. seniculus*, in the forest. The rufous-handed howler, *A. belzebul*, is an important reservoir in South America north of the Amazon, while the black howler, *A. caraya*, is distributed throughout eastern Brazil south to Uruguay; the brown howler, *A. fusca*, is found in Bolivia, Paraguay and Corrientes (Argentina), and *A. palliata* of Central America extends north to Yucatan.

By contrast, the capuchin monkeys in the genus *Cebus* are important reservoirs that do not die from yellow fever. The brown capuchin, *C. apella*, extends south from Trinidad to the extreme south of Brazil. Among the many species of *Cebus* are those which extend north to British Honduras. Among the spider monkeys, *Ateles*, all of which are susceptible to jungle yellow fever, the most important reservoir species are *A. chamek* in southern Peru and Bolivia, *belzebuth* in north-eastern Peru and southern Colombia and *hybridus* in northern Colombia. A succession of *Ateles* species extends through Panama into Central America, the northern limit being that of *A. vellerosus* at Tamazunchale, 160 km south-west of Tampico, Mexico.

Other Cebid reservoirs of yellow fever include the squirrel monkey, *Saimiri boliviensis*, of the upper Panama basin, the night monkey, *Aotes trivirgatus*, of the Amazon basin and the masked titi, *Callicebus personatus*, of eastern Brazil. In the family Callitrichidae, the marmosets of the genus *Callithrix* are important as reservoirs in eastern Brazil. These little monkeys are killed by the infection. The most important species of this coastal area is the common marmoset, *C. jacchus*, in the north and the black-pencilled marmoset, *C. penicellata*, in the south.

There are no monkeys present in the Greater Antilles nor in most of the Lesser Antilles. Among other possible reservoirs elsewhere, the opossum *Didelphis marsupialis* gave evidence of yellow fever in the endemic focus at Muzo in eastern Colombia where no monkeys exist.

YELLOW FEVER*

This lethal disease is characterized by a high fever of about 3 days duration accompanied by intense headache and muscle pains, which recurs some days later with a drop in pulse and jaundice in mild cases, and in severe cases with liver necrosis, visceral haemorrhage, toxic nephrosis and a "black vomit" of blood and bile. It is frequently fatal among adults but it is mild in children. Apparently, it is less severe in Africans than in other races. The viremic period, during which the patient can infect the vector *Stegomyia* mosquitoes, is during the 3 days of fever, following an incubation period of 3–6 days after the initial infective bite: the extrinsic incubation period in the

* We are grateful to Dr. Paul Bres, Virus Diseases Unit, W.H.O., Geneva for his critical reading of the following sections.

mosquito is usually 10–12 days, but it can be as short as 4 days under especially favourable conditions.

Yellow fever first came into prominence in the Caribbean area and the Gulf of Mexico, where an epidemic broke out in Guadeloupe in 1648 and spread to Campeche and inland to Merida in Yucatan (Fig. 12.8). The infection was considered to have arrived from St. Kitts and from Barbados. This would be the first port of call of slave traders on the Middle Passage from Africa, the introduction of sugar cane in 1641 requiring the importation of field hands*. Subsequently, epidemics occurred in Cuba (1649), St. Lucia (1665), New York (1668), Boston (1691) and Charleston (1699). The severe Caribbean outbreak of 1699 brought yellow fever to Vera Cruz in Mexico and to Cadiz in Spain in 1700. Another Cadiz epidemic in 1730 followed the return of a Spanish fleet from Cartagena in Colombia where, in 1741, a British expedition lost 8431 out of 12 000 soldiers from the disease. Yellow fever reached Guayaquil, Ecuador in 1740, Surinam in 1760 and New Orleans in 1791; in 1761, it became endemic in Havana. Along the coast of West Africa the first recorded epidemic occurred among British troops at St. Louis, Senegal in 1778. Within the following century 10 epidemics were recorded from Senegambia (St. Louis, Bathurst and the island of Goree, off Dakar) and 12 from Sierra Leone (especially the Bulam area); four epidemics occurred at Luanda, Angola, three on the Gold Coast and one on the Benin coast, five on the Canary Islands, three on the Cape Verde Islands, and two on each of the islands of Ascension and Fernando Po. Epidemics would also occur among Europeans on ships anchored off the West-African coast.

The arrival in 1793 of "Bulam fever" at Grenada ushered in the great pandemic of 1793–1804. It commenced in the lesser Antilles and Venezuela, later striking the Atlantic ports of the U.S.A. from Charleston to Boston and finally bringing yellow fever to the Spanish coast from Cadiz to Barcelona, and also to Majorca and Morocco. The pandemic coincided with the first phase of the Napoleonic wars and, in the period 1795–98, French forces in Santo Domingo, Guadeloupe and Martinique lost 30 000 men to the disease. The Americans observed that their epidemics always began and often

* The "yellow scourge", described by Oviedo and by Las Casas as fatal to Spanish conquistadors along the Caribbean coast of South America in the 16th century, may have been indigenous jungle yellow fever.

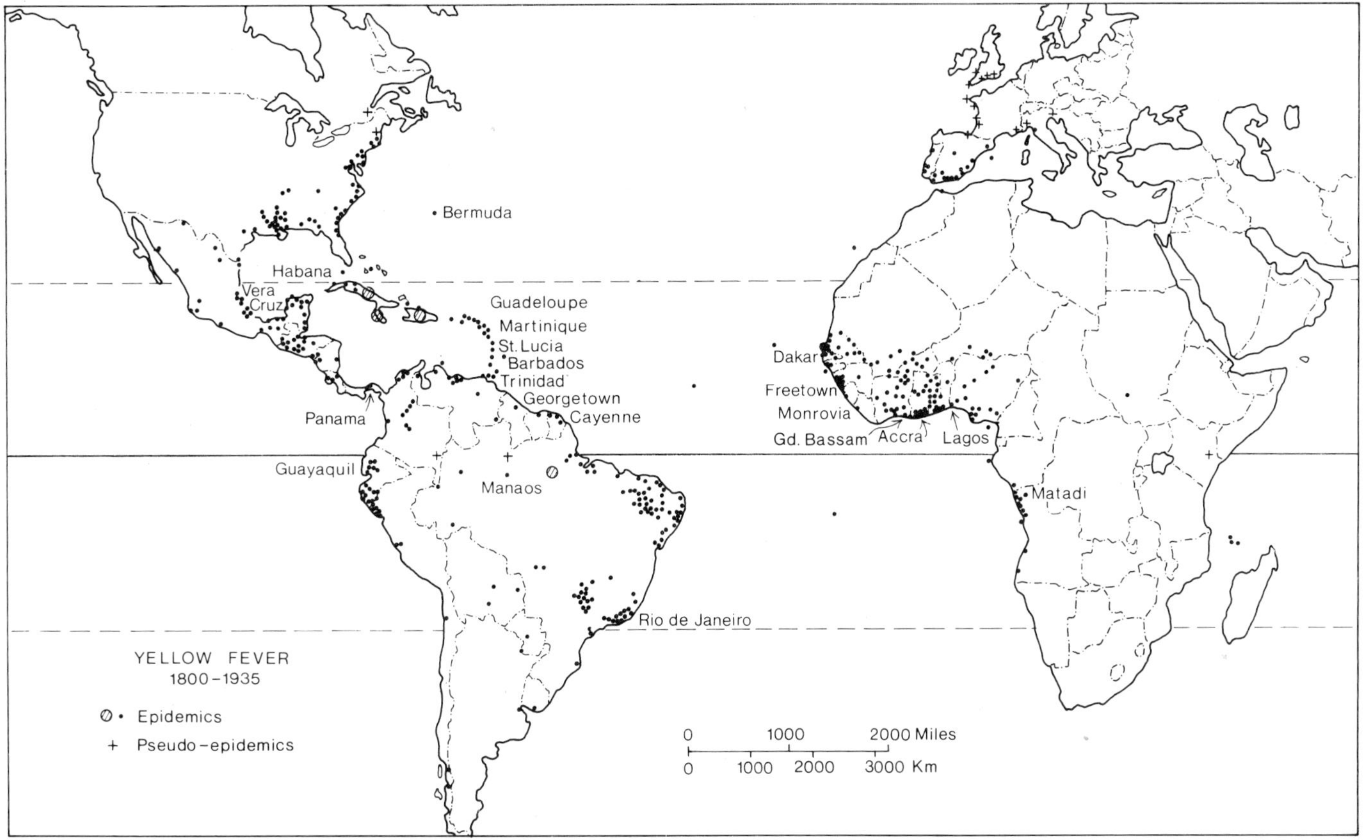

Fig. 12.8 Locations of yellow-fever epidemics, 1800–1935 (Strode, 1951).

remained confined to the low-lying streets crowding the quays; their records allow the conclusion that the vector mosquito had survived one winter (1797–98) in New York, three winters (1796–9) in Philadelphia and was perennial in Norfolk and Charleston. Once fire-barrels had been replaced by piped water in Philadelphia and Baltimore in 1821, the transmission of yellow fever there ceased.

Writing in 1833, Hirsch described seven pandemics of yellow fever in the 19th century.

1. 1818–20 Antilles, Venezuela, Guyana, Louisiana to Massachusetts, Cadiz to Valencia.
2. 1837–40 Antilles, Guyana, Texas to South Carolina (including Florida).
3. 1852–53 Antilles, Mexico, Texas to Pennsylvania, north to Arkansas and Tennessee (Memphis), Bermuda.
4. 1855–56 Antilles, French Guiana, Texas to New Hampshire, Bermuda.
5. 1866–69 Antilles, French Guiana, Nicaragua, El Salvadore, Texas to Florida.
6. 1873 Southern U.S.A. northwards to Memphis, Tennessee.
7. 1875–78 Antilles, Mexico, southern U.S.A. northwards to Memphis.

During the second pandemic, British garrisons in the Lesser Antilles and Guyana suffered the loss of 15–69% of their strength to yellow-fever fatalities. The third pandemic was particularly severe in the Antilles, and the fourth was important in Texas. The seventh pandemic, which was severe on the east coast of Mexico, caused 13 000 deaths in the U.S.A. in 1878. Sailing ships leaving the Caribbean and infested with *Aedes aegypti* could become travelling epidemics not only of yellow fever but also of dengue, as recorded for H.M.S. *Scout* out of Tobago in 1866. Such vessels arriving in northern harbours became the source of temporary transmission of yellow fever in Portsmouth, New Hampshire (1798), Portland, Maine (1801), Halifax, Nova Scotia (1842, 1861), Quebec City (1864), St. Nazaire, France (1861) and Swansea, Wales (1865).

Yellow fever first appeared in Brazil in 1849 when a ship from Havana brought it to Bahia (now Salvador). It also appeared in Rio de Janeiro (1849), Belem, Paraiba, Recife and Alagoas (1850), Ceara and San Luis de Maranhao (1851), southwards to Santos and Santa

Catarina state (1850), and westwards up the Amazon to its junction with the River Negro (1855). Subsequently, five epidemics occurred along the coast of Brazil between 1859 and 1876 and further south in Montevideo (1857), Buenos Aires (1868), Asunción (1869) and Corrientes province (1870).

By the end of the 19th century, yellow fever was endemic in the Lesser Antilles, Yucatan and the South-American shore of the Caribbean. The great ports of Havana, Vera Cruz, Panama, Guayaquil, Bahia and Rio de Janeiro were permanent endemic centres where virtually all surviving citizens were immune and all newcomers were in danger of contracting the disease. Outside the tropics, seasonal epidemics were liable to occur in New Orleans, Buenos Aires and Montevideo. With the finding of the U.S. Yellow Fever Commission in 1900 that *Aedes aegypti* was the vector, the fearsome history of this disease during the previous 250 years could be understood in terms of the spread of this mosquito in stored water. The elimination of Havana as an endemic centre, following the mosquito-control operations directed by General Gorgas in 1901, showed the way to the termination of this epoch of urban and shipboard yellow fever in the Americas.

Thus, when the pandemic of 1905 commenced, it was immediately arrested in Havana. Its appearance in New Orleans and other southern U.S. ports, where it caused some 1000 deaths, was followed by anti-*aegypti* operations that made it the last yellow fever outbreak in the U.S.A. (Fig. 12.9). The endemic centre at Rio de Janeiro—where, on average, 500 persons died each year from the disease—was similarly eliminated. Yellow fever elimination by means of mosquito control was achieved in Panama-Colon (1906), Vera Cruz (1907), Cuba (1909), Guayaquil (1919), Peru, Guatemala, Nicaragua, Honduras (1921), Yucatan (1922) and El Salvador (1924). Control activities in the Brazilian ports of Bahia, Belem, Recife and Manaos were similarly successful; the local up-country outbreaks of 1926 were controlled by 1927. An epidemic in Sergipe and Pernambuco states and in Rio itself in 1928 stimulated a campaign aimed at complete eradication of the vector. As a result, transmission of the disease had virtually ceased in the ports and the countryside of Brazil by 1934 and with it the elimination of urban yellow fever from the Americas.

However, in 1932, studies in the Canaan valley of Espiritu Santo state, Brazil, where yellow fever was present in the absence of *A.*

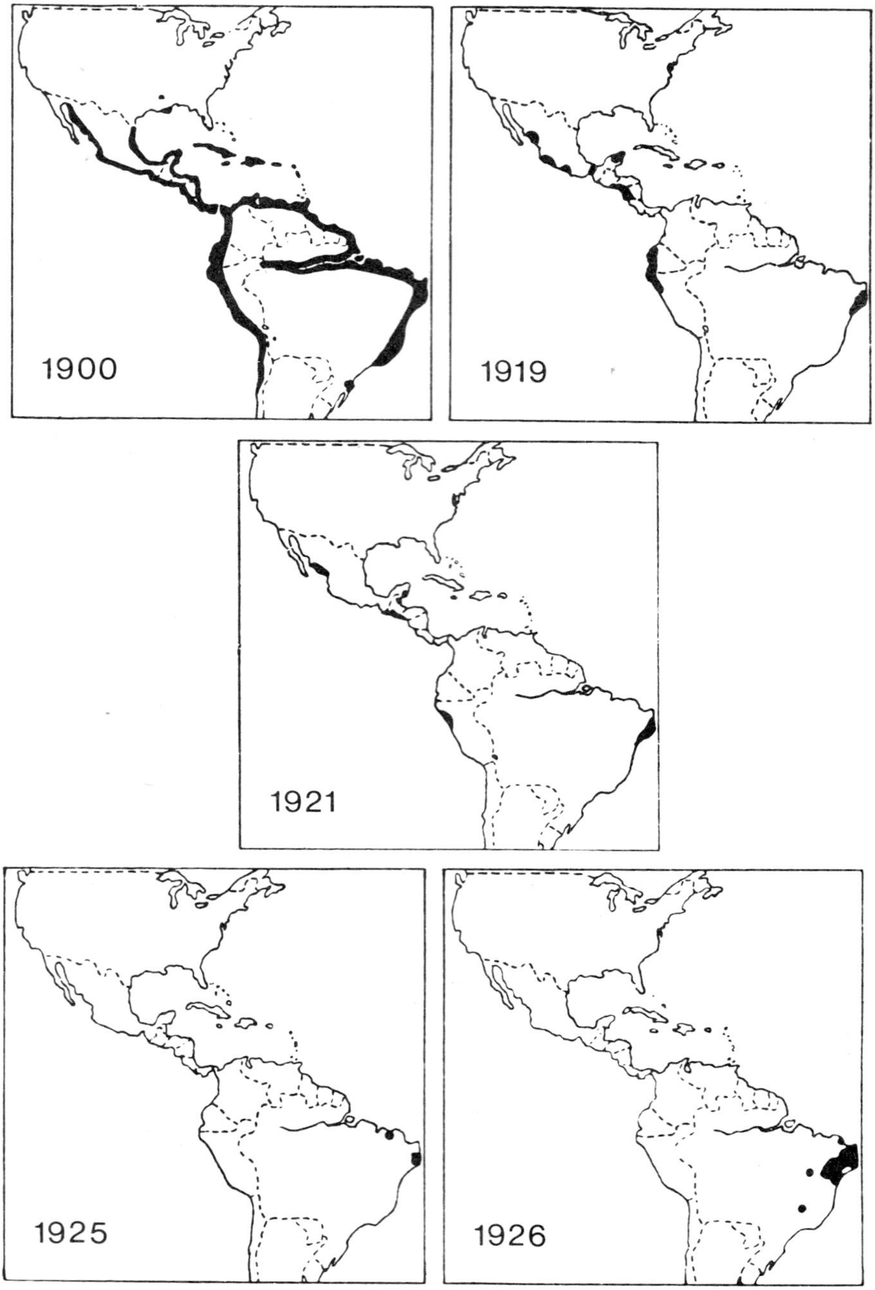

Fig. 12.9 Decline of yellow fever in the Americas, according to Annual Reports of the Rockefeller Foundation, 1900–26 (Biraud, 1935, see Strode, 1951).

aegypti revealed that monkeys were harbouring the virus, which could be transmitted by wild Culicine mosquitoes such as those in the genus *Haemagogus*. From this source, woodcutters could be infected and thus engender outbreaks in country towns where *aegypti* still survived. A wave of this jungle yellow fever among *Cebus* monkeys, which it does not kill, could be detected moving southward (at 200 km/month in active seasons) from Mato Grosso, Goias and Minas Geraes states (1934) into Sao Paulo and Parana states (1936) and Paraguay and the hinterland of Rio de Janeiro state (1938), accounting for 937 human deaths in the period 1934–42. Two subsequent waves passed south from Mato Grosso down to the Parana river system in 1943–44 and 1950–53 respectively. Another wave moved through southern Bolivia in 1950, causing at least 230 deaths, repeating patterns observed there in 1912 and 1931. Evidently, jungle yellow fever had been the origin of *aegypti*-transmitted outbreaks at Labrea, Xapuri and Sierra Madureira in the remote parts of Brazil lying north of Bolivia, and those at Bucaramanga and Socorro, Colombia.

In 1948, an epizootic wave fatal to *Ateles* and *Alouatta* monkeys commenced in eastern Panama and crossed the canal into western Panama (1951), Costa Rica (1951–52), Nicaragua (1953–54), Honduras (1954), Guatemala and British Honduras (1955), to reach the Mexican border (Yucatan) in 1956; of the 98 human deaths recorded, the majority were in Costa Rica. A previous wave had evidently passed through Central America in 1912. An outbreak of jungle yellow fever occurred in 1954 in Trinidad and neighbouring Venezuela, decimating the howler monkeys and causing several thousand human infections; but neither in Caracas nor in Port of Spain, where *A. aegypti* still persisted, did urban yellow fever break out.

Mato Grosso, standing at the divide between the Amazon and Parana river systems, is the focus of jungle yellow fever that threatens southern Brazil (Fig. 12.10). The yellow-fever virus isolated there, apparently indigenous, differs from the yellow-fever virus of West Africa by lacking one of the full complement of antigens. The Amazon and Orinoco basins probably constitute endemic reservoirs of jungle yellow fever among monkeys; the eastern Panama jungle, the Magdalena valley of Colombia and the Ucayalli valley of Peru constitute foci, with smaller foci among the marmosets of the Ilheus

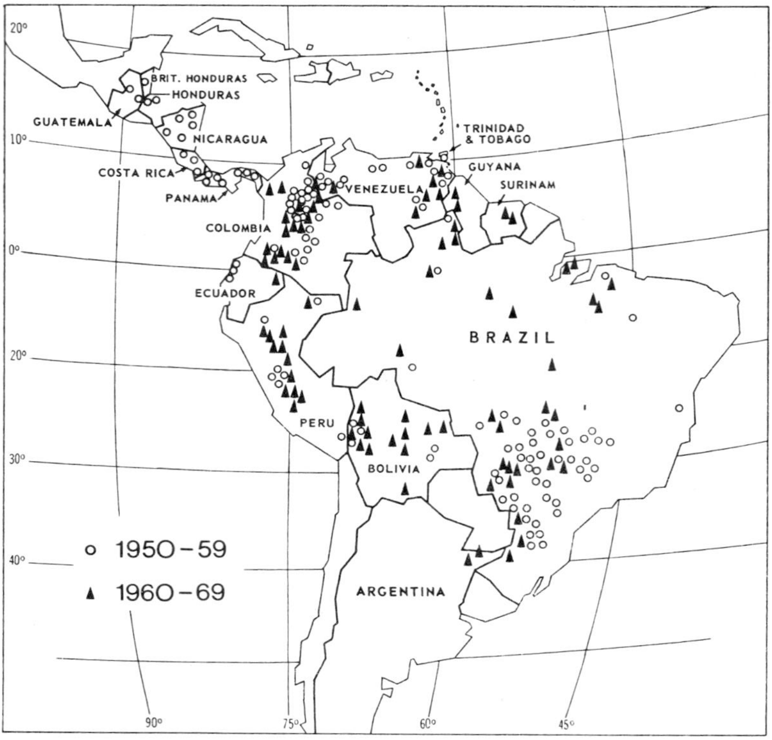

Fig. 12.10 Notified cases of yellow fever in the Americas, 1950–69 (W.H.O., 1971).

area of eastern Brazil and with the opossums of Muzo, Colombia. Jungle yellow fever continues to cause about 100 human cases per annum in South America (Table 12.2). It is no direct threat to the Antilles, where monkeys are absent, but the persistence of *A. aegypti* in Colombia, Venezuela and Trinidad and its reintroduction into Para state, Brazil, poses the hazard that epidemics of urban yellow fever might again develop in this region.

In Africa, the epidemic of 1926–28, which struck the west-coast towns from Dakar to Luanda (especially Accra and Lagos), stimulated a systematic collection of morbidity figures. The data for 1931–35 showed 314 cases (198 fatal), 154 of which were Europeans. They were confined to West Africa from Nigeria to Senegal and inland to Haute Volta and southern Niger, except for two cases in Moyen Congo and one in Sudan. Urban outbreaks followed in Bathurst (1935), Dakar and Accra (1937) and rural Ghana (1933,

	1951–55	1956–60	1961–65	1966–70	1971–75
Colombia	77	109	61	33	53
Ecuador	42	0	0	0	0
Peru	31	16	181	121	26
Venezuela	47	18	23	5	29
Brazil	319	43	30	32	94
Bolivia	26	59	114	105	45
Argentina	0	0	2	52	0
Total	542	245	411	348	247

Table 12.2 Number of deaths due to jungle yellow fever in South America notified during 5 year periods between 1951 and 1970.

1937). Serological surveys of yellow-fever antibody incidence by mouse-protection test made between 1932 and 1948 (Fig. 12.11) revealed that immunity rates were high in West Africa, very low in Ethiopia, and zero in Somalia, Madagascar and South Africa.

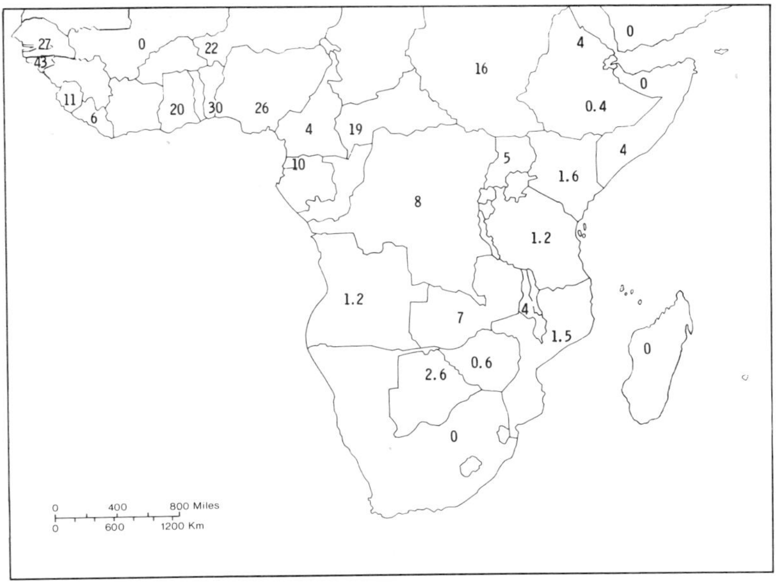

Fig. 12.11 Surveys of yellow-fever immunity in sample populations of African countries: % positive by mouse-protection test (Smith, 1951).

In 1940, the arid Nuba Mountains area of south-western Sudan was struck by an epidemic involving more than 15 000 cases. Nigeria experienced epidemics in the Ogbomosho (west-central, 1946), Jos Plateau (north-central, 1951) and Ngwo (east-central, 1951–2) areas, each involving thousands of cases; smaller outbreaks were recorded in Nigeria in 1953, 1955 and 1957. Cases of yellow fever were reported from Sierra Leone and Ghana in each year during the period 1953–55, and a large epidemic in Ghana, occurring in 1955 at Kintampo, midway between the coastal and northern endemic centres, was succeeded by smaller outbreaks in 1956, 1959 and 1963. There were at least 60 cases in north-eastern Zaire (Fig. 12.12) in 1958, 23 of which were fatal.

In the Blue Nile province of Sudan, 88 deaths from yellow fever were reported from the Kurmuk area in 1959, and 98 deaths immediately across the border in Ethiopia. In 1960–62, the most disastrous epidemic of modern times struck south-western Ethiopia, where among its 1 million inhabitants there were 3000 deaths notified and there had probably been 30 000 deaths among 100 000 cases of yellow fever. In the Didessa valley, the virus was transmitted from

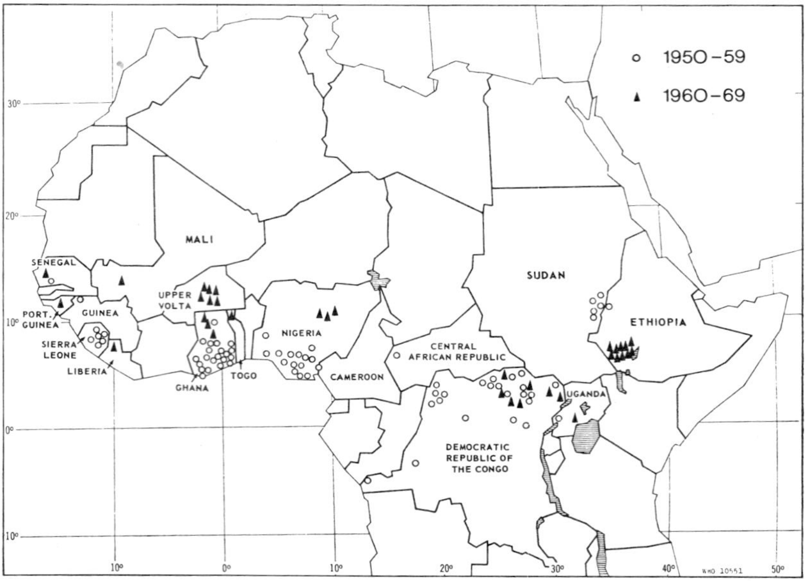

Fig. 12.12 Notified cases of yellow fever in Africa, 1950–69 (W.H.O., 1971).

monkeys by *A. africanus*, and in the Omo valley by *A. simpsoni* breeding in the false-banana plantations, *A. aegypti* being absent. In 1966, a new Ethiopian outbreak further east near Lake Abaya in the Rift Valley, where *aegypti* was abundant, caused some 350 deaths.

Subsequent to a programme of mass vaccination from 1940 to 1960, yellow fever had been almost completely silent in francophone West Africa, except for a small outbreak in Senegal in 1953. In 1965, an urban-type epidemic broke out in the vicinity of Diourbel, Senegal, in which 216 deaths were reported; the estimated 20 000 cases (2000 fatal) were nearly all among children born since 1960. This epidemic probably originated from jungle sources in Guinea-Bissao, where six fatal cases had occurred in the previous year. In 1967, two cases of jungle yellow fever were diagnosed in up-country Liberia.

In 1969, yellow fever became epidemic in the interior of West Africa. The northern focus in Ghana became active, with 61 cases (21 fatal) followed by 12 cases (seven fatal) the next year. In the Ouagadougou area of Upper Volta, where monkeys were massively infected, 136 human deaths were recorded among an estimated 3000 cases; *A. africanus*, *luteocephalus* and *taylori* introduced the infection into the villages, where *aegypti* took over as the vector. On the Bandiagara escarpment of southern Mali, there were 21 cases (12 deaths) of sylvan origin; several cases were notified from upcountry Togo. The most severe 1969 outbreak was on the Benue plateau of north-central Nigeria, centred on Jos, with 208 cases (60 fatal) recorded, which may have involved 50 000 cases and 1000 deaths. *A. luteocephalus*, *africanus* and possibly *vittatus* were more important than *aegypti* as vectors. In 1970, there was an epidemic in the southern Benue and Okwogo areas with probably more than 1000 cases; deaths from yellow fever were also reported from Cameroon and Equatorial Guinea. In 1971, an outbreak occurred at Luanda, Angola, with 65 cases (42 fatal) recorded, and two deaths were reported from Gemena in north-western Zaire. At least 10 deaths were reported from an outbreak in the South-Eastern state, Nigeria, in 1974.

In East Africa south of Ethiopia, yellow fever has been extremely rare. In Uganda, only two fatal cases are known, at Toro (1952) and Kampala (1964): despite an enzootic maintained among monkeys by *A. africanus* in the Bwamba forest of western Uganda, only one human case (1941) is known there and it was not fatal. In Kenya, only two cases have been detected in the last 15 years, at Kitale and in the Langata forest near Nairobi. A serological survey in 1968 found about 15% of the population to be positive for antibodies at Marsabit and Lokitaung in northern Kenya but negative further south at Garissa. At Gede on the Indian Ocean coast, a few of the monkeys and 20% of the bush-babies (*Galago* spp.) proved to be positive for antibodies.

Yellow fever has never occurred in Asia. It is remarkable that during the Indian Ocean pandemic of dengue in 1870–73, at the height of the Zanzibar slave trade, yellow fever was not introduced into India. At present, *aegypti* populations are high in villages near Mombasa and in south-western Tanzania, and *simpsoni* is abundant on the slopes of Kiliminjaro and on the Tanzanian coast, but there is no evidence of the presence of yellow fever in western Tanzania, Comores, Madagascar, Zanzibar or Seychelles. On the other side of the Arabian sea, *A. aegypti*, *vittatus* and *albopictus* are present in western India but not abundant; monkeys (*Macacus rhesus*) extend as far north and west as the Indus valley. From the Persian Gulf to the South Arabian coast to Somalia, monkeys are absent and *aegypti* is present but only sporadically. Strains of *aegypti* from India, Malaya and Java have proved fully capable of transmitting the virus. Of the 876 human sera examined by the mouse-protection test in the 1932–48 survey, only two were positive and they were from Indians that had never left the country. Although it is likely that cross-immunity from the other group-B viruses, especially dengue, WN and Zika could afford protection against the eastward spread of yellow-fever virus, it seems most reasonable to believe that as Soper pointed out many years ago, "yellow fever does not exist in Asia simply because it has not been introduced there".

In the present-day era of air travel, passengers infected in Africa or South America could easily reach any part of tropical Asia or Oceania undetected during the incubation period of 3–6 days before symptoms of the disease would become recognizable. Therefore, all countries in which *A. aegypti* or other *Stegomyia* vectors could exist require that a traveller from an infected area produce a valid certificate of vaccination; those countries lying wholly or partially within the proven yellow-fever endemic zones are considered to be infected areas (Figs 12.13 and 12.14). At the same time, efforts are

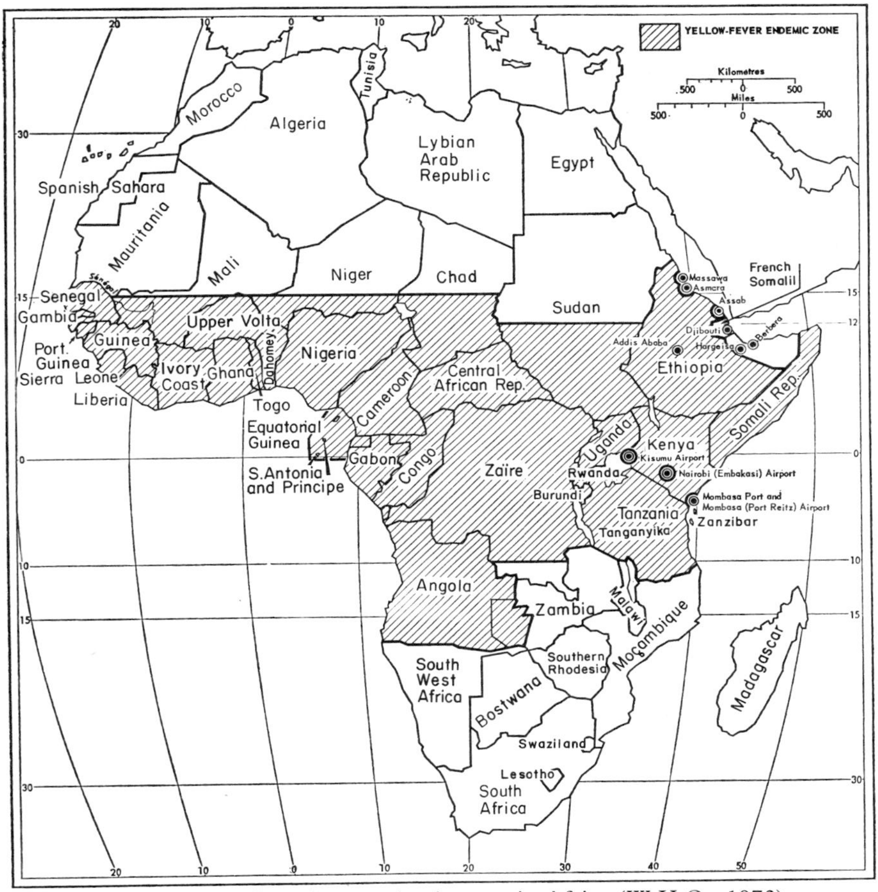

Fig. 12.13 Yellow-fever endemic zone in Africa (W.H.O., 1973).

made to keep international airports free of *A. aegypti*, and sea-ports controlled at least to the point where the house index of this species is less than 1. Travel from international airports such as Lagos and Dar es Salaam, which are extremely difficult to keep free from *aegypti* at all times of the year, could pose a hazard to India were it not for the fact that the Indian airports are continuously kept *aegypti*-free. Since it was found that nearly 10% of the *aegypti* mosquitoes experimentally embarked on aircraft survived to reach a destination one day later, the International Health Regulations require aircraft leaving an *aegypti*-infested area for an *aegypti*-free area to be disinsected by aerosols before take-off or by insecticidal vapour during

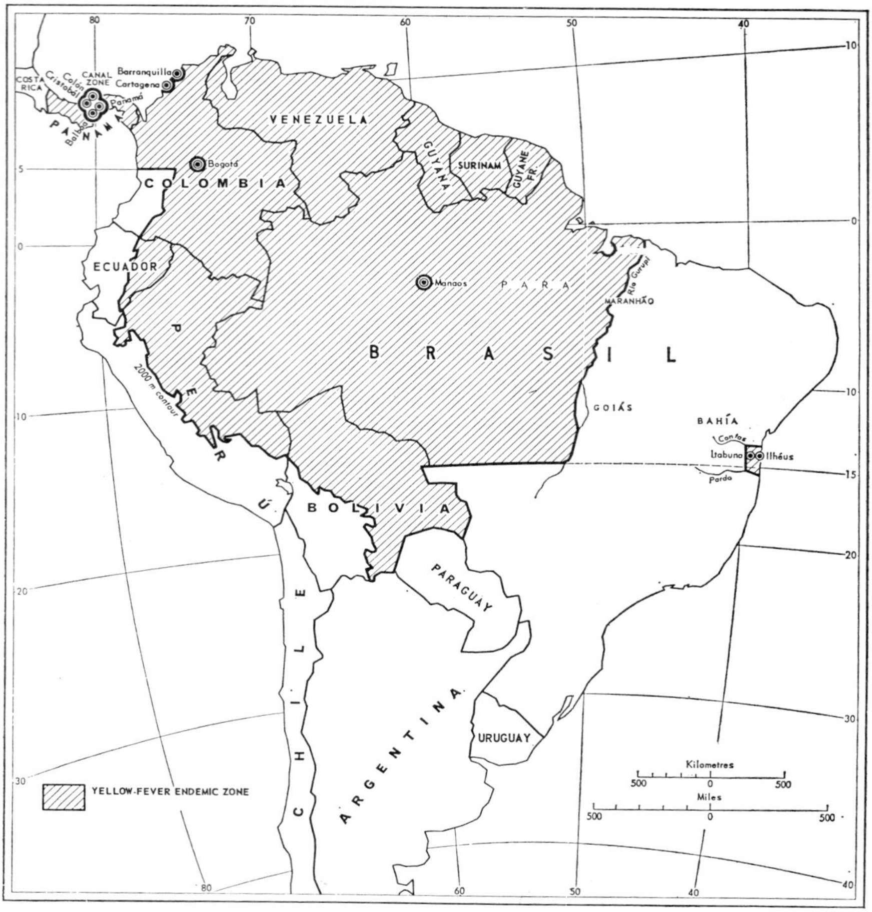

Fig. 12.14 Yellow-fever endemic zone in Central and South America (W.H.O., 1973a).

flight; aircraft leaving a yellow-fever infected area are to be similarly disinsected no matter what the destination. National health authorities may also take action to ensure that *Aedes aegypti* is not introduced in ships arriving at their ports.

DENGUE*

This non-fatal disease, due to one or other serotype of the dengue

* We are grateful to Dr. (Col.) Philip K. Russell, Director, Communicable Disease Division, Walter Reed Army Institute of Research, Washington D.C. for a critical reading of the following sections.

virus, is characterized by a high fever of about 4–7 days' duration, with severe pains in the joints, which may often recur a few days later. The viremic period is the 3 days starting 12 hours before the onset of fever; the extrinsic incubation period in the *Aedes aegypti* vector is 8–11 days, which can remain infective for 6 months. Transmission of dengue can derive from just one or two infective bites but it ceases at temperatures below 20°C.

As early as 1635, a non-fatal fever called *coup de barre* (an expression denoting lumbar pain) was known to attack new European arrivals to the Caribbean islands of Guadeloupe and Martinique. It was the opinion of Carlos Finlay that dengue was present in the Caribbean in the 17th century, by which time the slave trade had already transported more than a million Africans to the Antilles and neighbouring South America. Subsequently, epidemics of dengue, which characteristically affect large numbers of people, could be readily recognized and identified in varous parts of the world (Fig. 12.15).

The records collected by Hirsch and others allow the following eight pandemics, of 3–7 years' duration, to be discerned in the period between 1779 and 1916.

1779–1784 First year (a) Cairo and Alexandria*, (b) Djakarta; second year (c) Madras south to Pondicherry, (d) Philadelphia; final year (e) Cadiz and Seville.

1824–1828 First year (a) Suez, (b) Pondicherry north to Calcutta; second year (c) Chittagong, Rangoon and Ganges valley up to Benares; third year (d) Virgin Islands, Curacao, Jamaica and Savannah; final year (e) Lesser Antilles, northern Colombia, Cuba and Vera Cruz, (f) New Orleans, Pensacola, Charleston and Bermuda. This pandemic had been preceded by an outbreak in Lima, Peru in 1818 attacking an estimated 50 000 persons.

1845–1851 First year (a) St. Louis and Goree on Senegal coast, (b) Cairo, (c) Rio de Janeiro; third year (d) Calcutta and Kanpur, (e) Hawaii; fifth year (f) New Orleans; sixth year (g) U.S. coast from Brownsville to Charleston and inland to Augusta, Georgia and Woodville, Mississippi; final year (g) Reunion and Mauritius, (h) Tahiti. Dengue returned to Lima in 1851 and Cadiz in 1867, and subsequently appeared in Benghazi (1853), the Canary Islands (1865) and Port Said (1868).

* That this Egyptian epidemic was due to dengue is doubted by Theiler and Downs (1973).

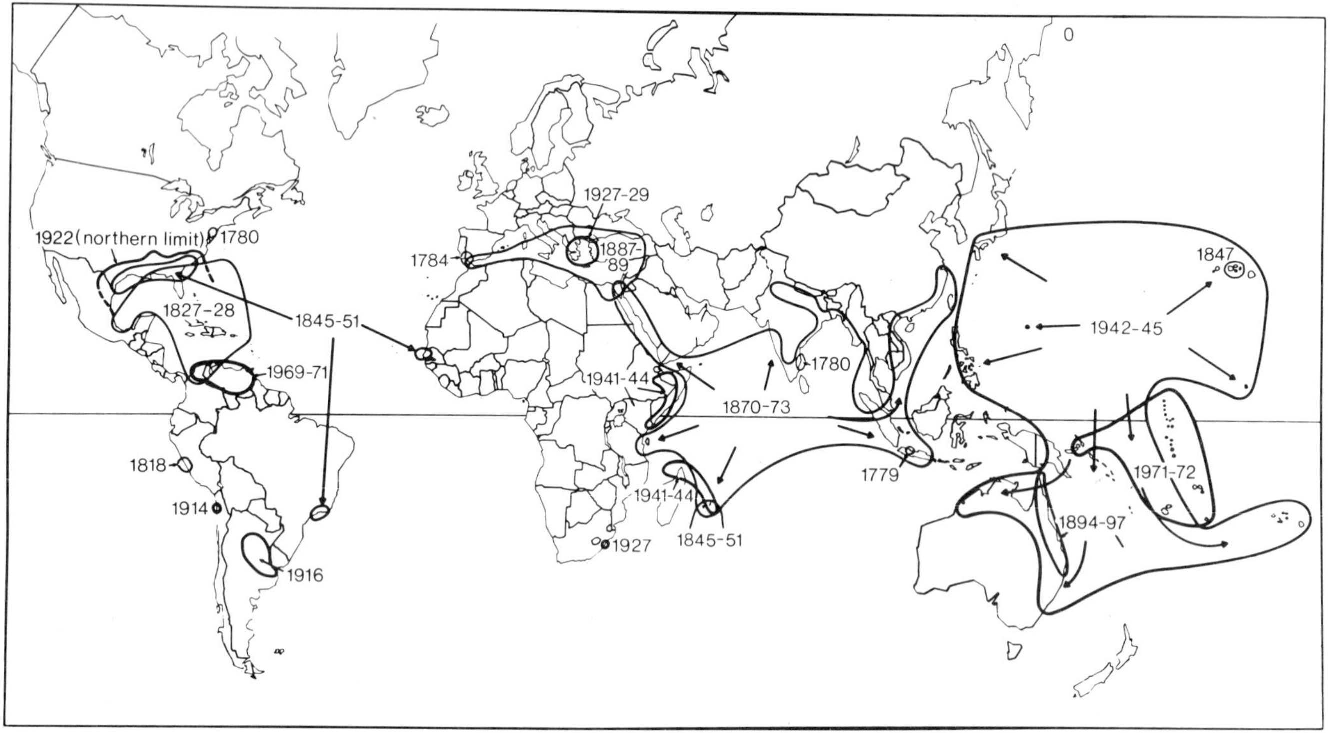

Fig. 12.15 Epidemics and pandemics of dengue, 1780–1972.

*1870–1873** First year (a) Zanzibar and Dar es Salaam; second year (b) Port Said, Jiddah, Mecca and Aden, (c) Bombay and Poona, (d) Calcutta; third year (e) Ganges valley as far as Ludhiana, (f) Kerala coast from Calicut to Quilon, (g) Madras, Dacca, Rangoon and Singapore; final year (h) Java, (i) Indo-China, (j) Amoy, Taiwan and Shanghai, (k) Reunion and Mauritius, (l) Louisiana, Alabama and north to Vicksburg, Mississippi. This great pandemic was followed by a period of silence until 1880, when dengue appeared in Crete, Beirut, Cairo and the Red Sea ports.
1887–1889 First year (a) Gibraltar; second year (b) Cyprus; final year (c) Greek islands, southern Turkey, Syria, Palestine and Nile delta, (d) Istanbul on the Bosporus and Varna and Trabzon on the Black Sea.
1894–1897 First year (a) Thursday Island in Torres Strait; second year (b) Townsville and Charters Towers, Queensland, (c) Indo-China and Hong Kong; final year (d) entire Queensland coast from Cooktown to Brisbane.
1901–1907 First year (a) Hong Kong, Canton, Bangkok, Singapore, Rangoon and Calcutta; second year (b) Ganges and Irrawaddy valleys; fourth year (c) Shanghai, (d) Brisbane and Thursday Island, (e) Florida, Texas and Panama; fifth to final year (f) Caribbean and Gulf pandemic from Mississippi to Colombia and Cuba.
1912–1916 First year (a) Panama; second year (b) Meerut in northern India; third year (c) Iquique, Chile; final year (d) northern Argentina, (e) Queensland and northern New South Wales.

From consideration of the first dates of recorded epidemics (Table 12.3), it may be concluded that, at the beginning of the 19th century, dengue had established itself in the Caribbean, probably as a result of the African slave trade, and was present in India and Java. The dengue outbreaks of 1779 in Philadelphia and of 1828 in several U.S. ports were due to infections brought by sailing ships. The pandemic of 1828 carried dengue into the interior of India, and that of 1850 carried it into the interior of the U.S.A. and later to Tahiti and the Mascarene Islands. The 1870–73 pandemic, starting in East Africa, carried the disease from Indonesia to Indo-China and China; it is

* The epidemics in Zanzibar in 1870 and 1823, and in India in 1824, 1871, 1902 and 1923, have been suggested by Carey (1971), because of the severe pains in the joints, to have been due to chikungunya virus.

possible that the same origin, the slave trade out of Zanzibar, carried the infection to the Red Sea ports and thence to the Mediterranean for the first time, the previous epidemics having been due to the type-B virus WN (West Nile). Dengue spread to the Black Sea ports in 1889 and to Chile and Argentina in 1914. In 1895, dengue reached

1635	Caribbean	1870	Zanzibar, Tanzania
1780	Java, India ports	1873	Indo-China, China
1818	Peru	1889	Black Sea ports
1826	U.S. ports	1895	Australia
1828	India interior	1914	Argentina, Chile
1845	Brazil, Senegal, Hawaii	1927	Natal
1850	U.S. interior	1942	Japan, South-West Pacific
1851	Mascarenes, Tahiti	1972	Samoa, Niue

Table 12.3 Dates of first epidemics of dengue in various areas of the world.

Queensland and in 1942 it struck the ports of Japan and subsequently most of the islands of the South-West Pacific, an infection process which was nearing completion in 1973. Although dengue is typically a disease of seaports and coastal areas, it has at one time or another penetrated inland for 200 km in Australia, for 300 km in the southern U.S.A. and for 800 km up the Mississippi valley; antibodies to dengue 1 have been found 2000 km up the Amazon. In West Africa, epidemics of dengue have been recorded from the Senegalese towns of Gorée in 1845, 1865 and 1878, Saint Louis in 1845 and 1926 and Dakar in 1899 and 1926 (usually preceding a yellow-fever outbreak in the subsequent year) and in the Upper Volta town of Ouagadougou in 1926; dengue has been recognized as a non-fatal fever liable to attack Europeans entering the area.

By the first decade of the 20th century, dengue had become endemic in India, South-East Asia and the Philippines, epidemics being chiefly among immigrant groups; no haemorrhagic symptoms were reported during the period preceding and including the Second World War. In the Caribbean, dengue remained intermittently active after 1912; in 1919 and 1920, it spread to the southern U.S.A. There followed the vast epidemic of 1922, which started in Galveston and infected some 600 000 people in the coastal areas of Texas. Activity was also high in Louisiana, the southern Atlantic states and the Caribbean. This 1922 epidemic may have involved 2 million people. In 1925–26, an epidemic in Queensland and New South Wales infected an estimated 500 000 people. In 1927, an outbreak at Durban, South Africa involved some 50 000 persons. This was followed by the great Mediterranean epidemic of 1927–29 which started in the Athens area, Euboea and the Gulf of Aegina and finished on the Turkish coast from Izmir south to Rhodes, affecting at least one million people.

Smaller epidemics occurred in the 1930s, namely Taiwan in 1931, Townsville, Queensland in 1934 and Egypt in 1937. Dengue struck Miami, Tampa and other cities of Florida in 1934 and remained epidemic in the Caribbean area until 1938.

The coming of the Second World War brought dengue into prominence in East Africa. Between 1941 and 1944, epidemics developed among military personnel based on the following stations: Dire Dawa and Harar, Ethiopia; Mogadishu, Berbera, Hargeisa and Kismayu, Somalia; Mombasa, Kenya; Dzaoudzi, Comores Islands; Diego Suarez, Madagascar; Mauritius. In the Pacific theatre, a pandemic raged in the ports of southern Japan (particularly Nagasaki, Kobe and Osaka) from 1942 to 1945, affecting a total of 1–2 million persons during the period. In 1943–45, an estimated 560 000 cases were infected in Australia and epidemics occurred in New Guinea, the Solomon Islands, New Hebrides, New Caledonia, Fiji, the Society Islands, Tahiti, Guam, Fanning Island and Hawaii. During 1941–46, dengue was also pandemic in the Caribbean area and around the Gulf of Mexico.

After the Second World War small epidemics in Tunis in 1945 and in Beirut and Palestine in 1946 brought dengue to a close in the Mediterranean area, where the vector *Aedes aegypti* was becoming eliminated. Ever since a small rural outbreak in Louisiana in 1945, traceable to a returnee from the Pacific war theatre, no dengue epidemics have occurred in the southern U.S.A. despite the persistence of the vector there and the frequent return of infected tourists from the Caribbean area. The last epidemics in Australia were sporadic ones between 1953 and 1955, although dengue remained endemic in a zone across the north and east of the continent from Broome to Sydney.

In eastern India and South-East Asia, however, dengue had become so strongly endemic in the rural areas that a 1955 survey in Selangor state, where the principal vector was *A. albopictus*, revealed that virtually all of the human population over 30 years of age were

	1963	1964	1965	1966	1967	1968	1969	1970	1971	1972	1973
Dominican Republic	350	407	527	0	0	0	16	0	3	0	—
Puerto Rico	25 737	2440	93	2	1	0	16 665	136	15	85	658
Jamaica	1578	156	36	6	6	367	545	31	14	4	3
Lesser Antilles	2	1008	8	0	0	220	81	15	29	2	—
Venezuela	0	18 306	4040	7750	1330	383	3917	405	5	25	0

Table 12.4 Number of cases of dengue reported from the Caribbean area, 1963–69.

positive for dengue antibodies. The epidemics, confined mainly to the cities, were of a variant, dengue haemorrhagic fever, which will be discussed later in a separate section. In the Caribbean area, where in 1952 virtually all the over-30 population in rural Trinidad were found positive for dengue-2 antibodies, epidemics have become almost continuous since 1961, although no cases of haemorrhage or shock have been observed until very recently. In the South Pacific area, dengue has recently reappeared in epidemic form, first on Tahiti in 1964 and then in 1971 on the neighbouring Society Islands (5619 cases), in Fiji (2952 cases), at Rabaul, New Guinea (1058 cases) and on New Caledonia. In 1972, epidemics developed in Western Samoa, the New Hebrides, Tonga, Nauru and Niue. A few of the Society Islands' cases showed minor haemorrhagic symptoms but a considerable percentage of the Niue cases were fatal and were suggestive of dengue haemorrhagic fever. Symptoms of DHF were also observed in the 1974 outbreaks on Nauru and in Tonga, as well as among c. 100 000 cases on the Fiji archipelago in 1975.

In the Caribbean area, the dengue epidemics of the last decade have involved thousands of cases (Fig. 12.16). A severe outbreak commenced in the Greater Antilles in 1963 and extended to the Lesser Antilles and Venezuela in 1964. In 1966–7, the infections moved to western Venezuela, which had not been involved in the 1964 epidemic, while the Caribbean islands were silent. The next epidemic in 1969 involved the entire Caribbean area, having started the previous year in Jamaica and the Lesser Antilles (Table 12.4). In 1971, following extensive reinfestation of northern Colombia by *Aedes aegypti*, an extensive epidemic of dengue in that area involved an estimated 416 000 persons (Fig. 12.17). By 1945, the vector and the disease had extended south to Neiva in the Upper Magdalena valley. An outbreak of dengue developed in late 1975 in Puerto Rico, with three cases suggestive of DHF.

Of the four serotypes of the virus, dengue 1 was predominant in the Pacific area during the Second World War, having been isolated in Hawaii in 1944, and later in Japan, with serological evidence from Tahiti and Australia; this serotype evidently had been active in the Caribbean area and in the Amazon valley during this period, and in Greece and Durban in 1927; it was incriminated in 1975 epidemics in Nauru, Tahiti and the Fiji archipelago. Dengue 2, first isolated in Japan in 1943 and New Guinea in 1945, was found in Trinidad in

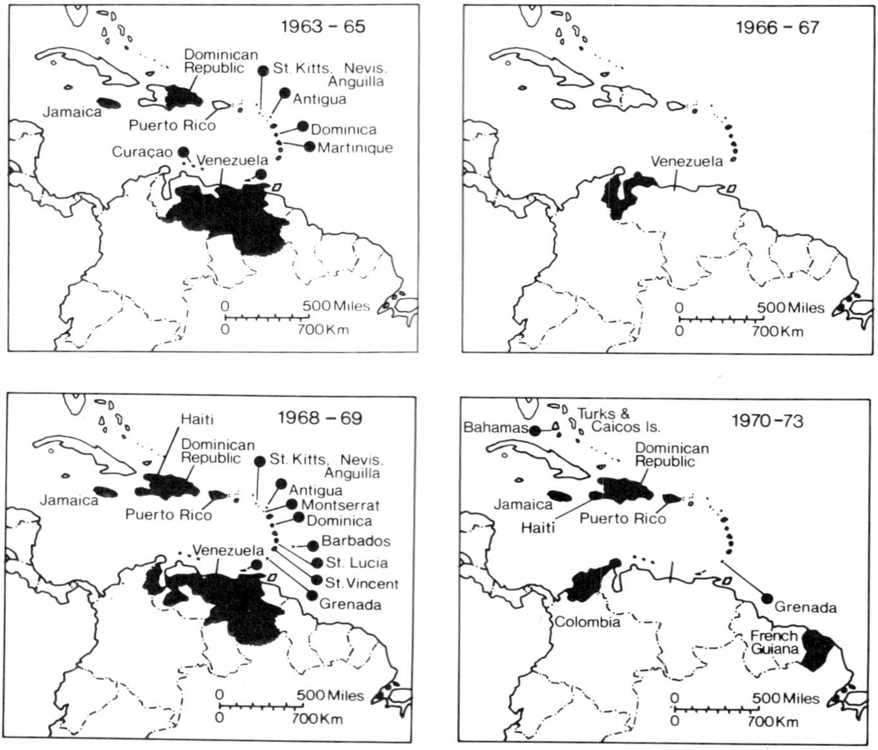

Fig. 12.16 Occurrence of dengue in the Caribbean area, 1963–73. (From Pan American Health Organization, 1970 and Colombia University of Health, 1973.)

1953 and was mainly responsible for the Caribbean epidemic of 1969, the Colombian epidemic of 1971 and the Fiji and Society Islands' epidemics of 1971, besides being implicated by serological evidence in the Australian epidemic of 1943–45. Dengue 3, isolated in the Philippines in 1956 caused the 1964 Tahiti epidemic and was evidently responsible for the 1963 and 1964 Caribbean epidemics.* Serological evidence for dengue 4, also isolated in the Philippines in 1960, was obtained from people who were resident in Japan and New Guinea during the 1943–45 period; similar evidence was obtained for dengues 1, 2 and 3 in these areas. In Africa, isolations of dengue 1 and 2 have been made in Nigeria, and of dengue 2 in Senegal.

* Although the strain isolated in Puerto Rico in 1963–64 showed differences from the South-East Asian strain.

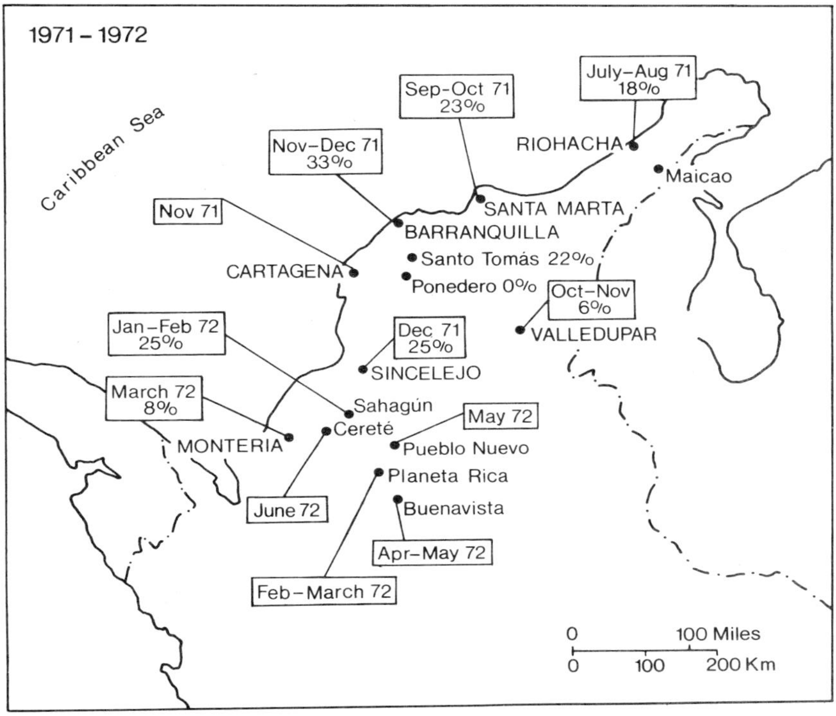

Fig. 12.17 Progression of the dengue epidemic in northern Colombia, 1971–72.

Aedes aegypti is the principal vector of the dengue viruses, all four serotypes having been isolated from it. It is the sole known vector in the Americas and Australia. *A. albopictus* has also yielded all four serotypes; it was the sole vector in the Japan epidemic of 1942–45 and the principal vector in the Taiwan epidemic of 1931 and the Chefoo (China) epidemic of 1918. *A. scutellaris* was demonstrated to be a vector in New Guinea in 1946, and a Samoan strain of *A. polynesiensis* to be a vector in the laboratory in 1954. In the South-West Pacific, epidemics are most pronounced where *A. aegypti* is present, but there are frequent instances where members of the *scutellaris* complex such as *A. polynesiensis* must be the principal or only vector despite their more sylvan habits.

With regard to mammalian reservoirs evidence for "jungle dengue" has not been obtained in the Americas although the negative findings in Panama monkeys were made at a time when dengue was silent there. Dengue antibodies were detected in more than 50% of the Malayan monkeys and slow lorises tested 20 years ago. Recently, an isolation of dengue virus has been made from a sentinel monkey placed in the Malayan forest. Investigations made 40 years ago had found monkeys in the vicinity of Manila to be immune to dengue while those from up-country non-endemic areas were not. Antibodies for dengue 1 were present 15 years ago in flying foxes (*Pteropus*) and even gulls and migratory sandpipers on the Queensland coast; later, dengue-2 antibodies appeared in *Pteropus*. Very recently, antibodies for dengue 2 have been found in about one third of the green and mona monkeys examined in western Nigeria. Since dengue-1 and dengue-2 antibodies have also been isolated from man in Nigeria, it is reasonable to conclude that dengue is endemic in West Africa and the source of much of the general group-B immunity in that region. Thus, the apparent origin and history of dengue comes to resemble that of yellow fever, except that the dengue viruses have evidently been present in tropical Asia also, possibly maintained in *Macacus* monkeys to which dengue, unlike yellow fever, was not fatal.

DENGUE HAEMORRHAGIC FEVER

In 1954, an epidemic occurred among children in Manila characterized by fever and haemorrhages, in some cases accompanied by shock and not infrequently fatal; this syndrome had been observed sporadically since 1950. A second epidemic of this Philippine haemorrhagic fever occurred in 1956, with 1207 hospitalized cases showing a mortality of 6% yielding dengue-2 virus and two new serotypes dengue 3 and 4. Cases became general throughout the Philippine Islands in 1958 with an epidemic in 1961 and a severe outbreak in 1966 (Table 12.5).

In 1958 a major epidemic of haemorrhagic fever, with 2500 hospitalized cases, occurred in Bangkok and Thonburi; smaller epidemics had occurred since 1954 and cases had been observed since 1950. A similar outbreak occurred in 1960, and by 1962 the disease had spread inland from the Gulf of Thailand and caused 6000 hospitalized cases. By 1964, it had spread to the north and northeast of the country, since when it has been causing an increasing number of reported cases and deaths. From these cases of Thai haemorrhagic

	Philippines			Philippines		Thailand		South Vietnam		Indonesia	
Year	Cases	Deaths	Year	Cases	Deaths	Cases	Deaths	Cases	Deaths	Cases	Deaths
1960	551	40	1966	9384	250	5844	131				
1961	1459	33	1967	1371	105	2060	64				
1962	134	62	1968	1116	115	6052	65				
1963	189	74	1969	1336	103	8673	101	2813	87	101	23
1964	759	169	1970	922	80	2766	46	242	38	253	56
1965	652	109	1971	438	34	11 522	299	196	36	129	22
			1972	1570	83	23 786	682	763	215	970	25
			1973	591	62	8280	315	14 320	986	9947	454
			1974	300	?	8160	328	4261	438	3667	188

Table 12.5 Numbers of cases and deaths of dengue haemorrhagic fever reported from the Philippines, Thailand, South Vietnam and Indonesia, 1960–71.

fever, dengue 1, 2, 3 and 4 have been isolated along with the type-A chikungunya virus.

In 1960 mild haemorrhagic symptoms occurred in adults during an epidemic of dengue in Singapore, dengue 1 and 2 being isolated. In 1961 cases of haemorrhagic fever started to appear among children and epidemics in 1962, 1963, 1964 and 1966 yielded a total of 897 hospitalized cases of Singapore haemorrhagic fever from which dengue 3 and 4 were isolated.

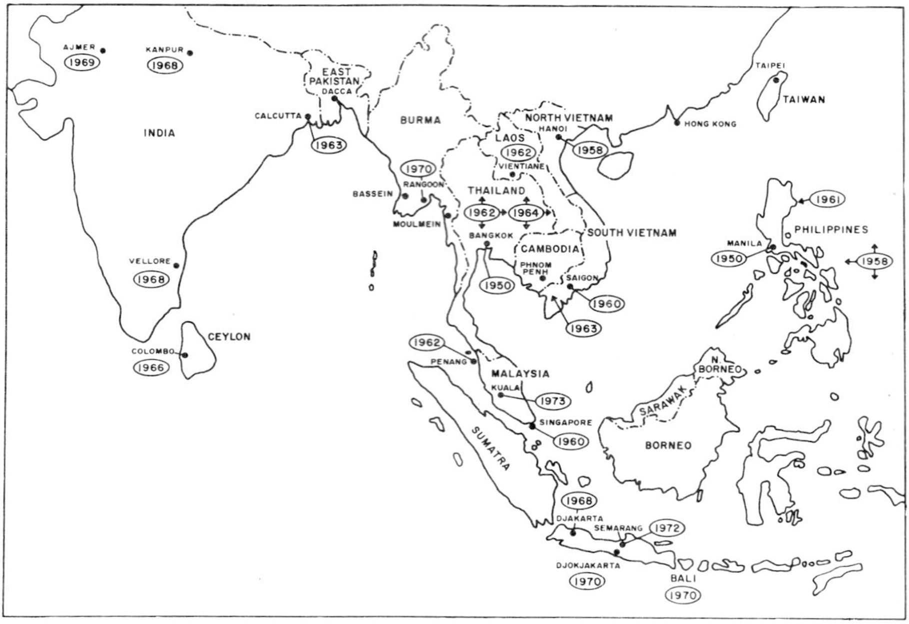

Fig. 12.18 Dengue haemorrhagic fever in South-East Asia: dates of first recorded occurrence.

In all three areas (Fig. 12.18), the symptoms were characterized by (a) the absence of the joint pains typical of classical dengue fever, (b) the presence of haemorrhagia escalating from petechial rash to internal bleeding in the lungs and (c) the frequent occurrence of a shock syndrome (fall in blood pressure, collapse and semicoma). This new disease entity is termed dengue haemorrhagic fever (DHF) and is characteristic of the indigenous Asian children; adults and

Europeans usually show only classical dengue symptoms. Occasional cases of haemorrhagia, shock and death had occurred in the dengue epidemics of 1931 in Taiwan, 1928 in Greece, 1927 in Durban, 1922 in Texas, 1904 in Brisbane and 1897 at Charters Towers, Queensland. It is now concluded by many experts that the DHF syndrome, derived from damage to the capillaries, is a hypersensitivity reaction to simultaneous or sequential infection by more than one dengue serotype.

An epidemic which occurred in Hanoi in 1958, involving many hundreds of cases and a 7% mortality among the 68 hospitalized, was evidently DHF. The disease appeared in Saigon in 1960 and by 1963 it had involved the entire Mekong delta with 116 cases among the 331 cases recorded in that year; all four serotypes of dengue and also chikungunya were isolated. DHF was recognized in Penang in 1962 and by 1965 a total of 67 cases had been diagnosed; dengue 2 was again isolated.

In 1963, an epidemic of DHF with severe haemorrhagic symptoms caused at least 158 deaths in Calcutta, dengue 2 being isolated. This was followed in 1964 by a wave of typical dengue fever from which chikungunya virus was isolated. In Colombo, a similar dengue epidemic, at this time involving chikungunya and some dengue virus, was followed in 1966 by the appearance of DHF (12 cases, two deaths). In Vellore, Madras, an endemic dengue area where dengue 1, 2 and 4 were isolated in 1960–63 and chikungunya had occurred in epidemic form in 1964, haemorrhagic symptoms appeared in 1968, when dengue 3 was first isolated there. In the same year (1968), haemorrhagic symptoms and mortality occurred in an epidemic of dengue at Kanpur, Uttar Pradesh involving 200 000 persons. In 1969, a similar epidemic struck Ajmer, Rajasthan yielding 55 cases with haemorrhagic symptoms from which dengue 3 was isolated as well as dengue 1.

In Rangoon, Burma, an outbreak of dengue-type fever in 1963, due primarily to chikungunya virus, was followed in 1970 by an epidemic of DHF, with 1974 cases and 87 deaths; dengue 1 and 3 were isolated among the predominant chikungunya infections. The 1970 epidemic spread to Bassein and Moulmein, and was followed by a 1971 Rangoon epidemic yielding 685 cases and 34 deaths. In 1971 also, 17 cases of DHF were reported from Vientiane, Laos, where similar cases had been noted in 1962 and 1968. In South Vietnam, 1969 was a major epidemic year with nearly 300 reported DHF cases and 87 deaths (Table 12.5).

By 1971, the number of DHF cases occurring annually in Thailand reached the 10 000 mark, with more than 23 000 cases in 1973 and 17 000 cases in 1975. In neighbouring South Vietnam nearly 1000 deaths were reported in the 1973 epidemic. DHF was first recognized in Jakarta, Indonesia in 1968, and 2 years later in Jogjakarta, other parts of Java and also in Bali, with a total of 253 cases and 56 deaths. An epidemic in Semarang in 1972–73 caused 949 cases and 24 deaths in a 3-month period. In an 8-month period in 1973, an epidemic on the Malayan peninsula caused 586 cases and 37 deaths, more particularly in Kuala Lumpur but also in Penang and Johore.

REFERENCES

Ash, J. E. and Spitz, S. (1945). "Pathology of Human Diseases: An Atlas". W. B. Saunders, Philadelphia and London.

Bres, P. (1972). Recent epidemics of yellow fever in Africa. *Pan. Amer. Hlth Org. (Washington) Sci. Publ.* **238**, 17–19.

Brown, A. W. A. (1973). Surveillance system for *Aedes aegypti* and related Stegomyia mosquitos in terms of density. W.H.O./VBC/73.464, 32pp. mimeo.

Carey, D. E. (1971). Chikungunya and dengue: a case of mistaken identity? *J. History Med. Allied Sci.* **26**, 243–262.

Cartron, A. (1929). Note sur une épidémie de dengue à Saint-Louis (Sénégal) en 1926. *Bull. Soc. Pathol. Exot.* **22**, 228–229.

Chambon, L. *et al.* (1967). Une épidémie de fièvre jaune au Senegal en 1965. *Bull. W.H.O.* **36**, 113–150.

Chan, Y. C., Chan, K. L. and Ho, B. C. (1971). *Aedes aegypti* and *Aedes albopictus* in Singapore city. *Bull. W.H.O.* **44**, 617–657.

Clarke, D. H. and Casals, J. (1965). Arboviruses: Group B. *In* "Viral and Rickettsial Diseases of Man" (Eds F. L. Horsfall and I. Tamm) (4th edn), pp. 606–658. J. B. Lippincott, Philadelphia.

Colombia Ministry of Public Health (1973). Report on dengue, 1971–1972. *Bol. Ofic. San. Panam.* (English edn) 7, 97–104.

Ehrenkranz, N. J., Ventura, A. K., Cuadrado, P. R., Pond, W. L. and Porter, J. E. (1971). Pandemic dengue in Caribbean countries and the southern United States; past, present and potential problems. *New Engl. J. Med.* **285**, 1460–1469.

Grzimek, B. (1967). "Tierleben: Enzyklopädie des Tierreiches", Vol. X, Saugetiere I. Kindler Verlag, Zurich.

Halstead, S. B. (1966). Mosquito-borne haemorrhagic fever of South and South-East Asia. *Bull. W.H.O.* **35**, 3–15.

Hamon, J., Pichon, G. and Cornet, M. (1971). La transmission du virus amaril en Afrique occidentale. Cah. ORSTOM, *Ser. Ent. Med. Parasit.* **9**, 3–60.

Hayes, G. R., Scheppf, P. P. and Johnson, E. B. (1971). An historical review of the last continental U.S. epidemic of dengue. *Mosquito News* **31**, 422–427.

Metselaar, D., Henderson, B. E., Kirya, G. B. and Timms, G. L. (1970). Recent research on yellow fever in Kenya. *E. Afr. Med. J.* **47**, 130–137.

Monath, T. P. and Kemp, G. E. (1973). Importance of non-human primates in yellow-fever epidemiology in Nigeria. *Trop. Geogr. Med.* **35**, 28–38.

O.M.S./OCCGE (1972). Informal consultations on yellow fever in tropical Africa: collected papers. Cah. ORSTOM. *Ser. Ent. Med. Parasit.* **10** 2, 188 pp.

Pan American Health Organization (1970). Report of the Study Group on the Prevention of *Aedes aegypti*-borne Diseases. Washington, 24 pp. (mimeo).

Pichon, G., Hamon, J. and Mouchet, J. (1969). Groupes ethniques et foyers potentiels de fièvre jaune dans les états francophones d'Afrique occidentale. Cah. ORSTOM, *Sér. Ent. Méd. Parasit.* **7**, 39–50.

Reeves, W. C. (1972). Recrudescence of arthropod-borne virus diseases in the Americas. *Pan. Am. Hlth Org. (Washington) Sci. Publ.* **238**, 3–14.

Serie, C., Lindrec, A., Poirier, A., Andral, L. and Neri, P. (1968). Etudes sur la fievre jaune en Ethiopie. *Bull. W.H.O.* **38**, 835–884.

Smith, C. E. G. (1952). The history of dengue in tropical Asia and its probable relationship to the mosquito *Aedes aegypti. J. Trop. Med. Hyg.* **59**, 243–251.

Smith, H. H. (1951). *In* "Yellow Fever" (Ed. G. K. Strode). McGraw-Hill, New York.

Strode, G. K. (1951). "Yellow Fever". McGraw-Hill, New York; after Biraud, Y. (1935). *Epidem. Rep. Hlth Sect. League of Nations* **179**, 103–173.

Taufflieb, R., Robin, Y. and Cornet, M. (1971). Le virus amaril et la faune sauvage en Afrique. Cah. ORSTOM. *Sér. Ent. Méd. Parasit.* **9**, 351–371.

Theiler, M. and Downs, W. G. (1973). "The Arthropod-Borne Viruses of Vertebrates". Yale University Press, New Haven.

Venzon, E. L., Rudnick, A., Marchette, N. J., Fabie, A. E. and Dukellis, E. (1972). The Greater Manila dengue haemorrhagic fever epidemic of 1966. *J. Philippine Med. Assoc.* **48**, 297–313.

Wisseman, C. L. and Sweet, B. H. (1961). The Ecology of Dengue. *In* "Studies in Disease Ecology" (Ed. J. M. May), pp. 15–40. Hafner, New York.

W.H.O. (1971). Third Report, Expert Committee on yellow fever. *W.H.O. Techn. Rep. Ser.* **479**, 56 pp.

W.H.O. (1973a). "Vaccination Certificate Requirements for International Travel". Geneva.

W.H.O. (1973b). Computer Survey of Stegomyia Mosquitos, 1973. VBC/73.11. 50 maps (mimeo).

W.H.O. Regional Office for the Western Pacific (1969). Report on Regional Seminar on Mosquito-Borne Virus Diseases, Manila, 58 pp. (mimeo).

13. Bronchitis

J. C. Young

During the 19th century, the disease patterns of the rapidly industrializing countries of Europe were dominated by respiratory tuberculosis, or, as it was more commonly known, by "consumption". On account of this preoccupation with the "white plague", concerted medical attention and enquiry could scarcely be diverted to apparently less significant chronic ailments such as bronchitis. Consequently, it was not until the middle of the present century, when at last the scourge of tuberculosis had been successfully reduced to manageable levels, that any considerable concern was expressed over the human misery and suffering of chronic bronchitics and attention paid to the social and economic costs to the community at large.

In England and Wales alone, it is calculated that, quite apart from the 30 000 deaths each year which are directly attributable to chronic bronchitis, well over 30 million working days are lost as a result of sickness from this cause. Moreover, it should be stressed that these statistics do not take into account the tens of thousands of workers who have had to accept lighter work, often at a substantially reduced wage, as a direct result of the disability inflicted by their bronchitic condition.

With rapid urbanization and industrialization occurring in many areas of the world, the incidence of the chronic form of the disease appears to be increasing at an alarming rate. At the present time, there is still no known simple cure for chronic bronchitis: all that can be done is to relieve and to reduce the suffering of the patient with the aid of a wide range of inhalents, expectorants and cough suppressants.

The term "bronchitis", introduced by Charles Badham in 1808, is used to describe a condition in which there is an abnormally high secretion of bronchial mucous, often initiated by the catalytic effect of the presence of a bacteriological or viral pathogen. An isolated bout of this type of bronchial abnormality, particularly in childhood, represents the simple or acute form of bronchitis which may often be conveniently cured by modern antibiotics. When, in later life, the bouts of bronchitis become prolonged and recurrent, the condition is redefined as chronic. The precise W.H.O. definition of "chronic or recurrent" is given as being "present on most days during at least 3 months in each of 2 successive years". In its mildest form, the clinical manifestation of bronchitis may be restricted to bouts of coughing and expectoration. However, as the chronic stage of the disease advances, the airways of the lungs and bronchus become impeded by a build-up of excessive mucous secretions, thereby progressively impairing the respiratory efficiency of the patient. Moreover, each succeeding bout is liable to promote irreversible damage to the tissue of the lungs. Ultimately, the individual becomes so breathless that he finds that he is unable to continue his normal pattern of activity, and his clinical condition passes from "simple chronic" to "disabling chronic" bronchitis. As Capel and Caplin (1964) comment "the tragedy of bronchitis is not the passing illness, it is the probability that each attack damages the lungs still further and that a succession of attacks ruins them and life as well".

In the developing areas of the world, the occurrence of bronchitis is, as yet, largely restricted to the simple or acute form of the disease. In this case, the true significance of the disease is reflected in its impact upon mortality patterns and, in particular, upon the infant mortality rates (viz. deaths under 1 year). In contrast, the developed and industrialized world is characterized by a marked excess of the chronic forms of the disease (Fig. 13.1). Despite the fact that bronchitis may account for a significant proportion of deaths from all causes—approximately 5% in England and Wales—the morbidity effects of the disease have an even more dramatic impact upon the social and economic life of the community. By virtue of the insidious nature of the disease, a chronic bronchitic may often become a substantial burden not only to himself but also to his family and

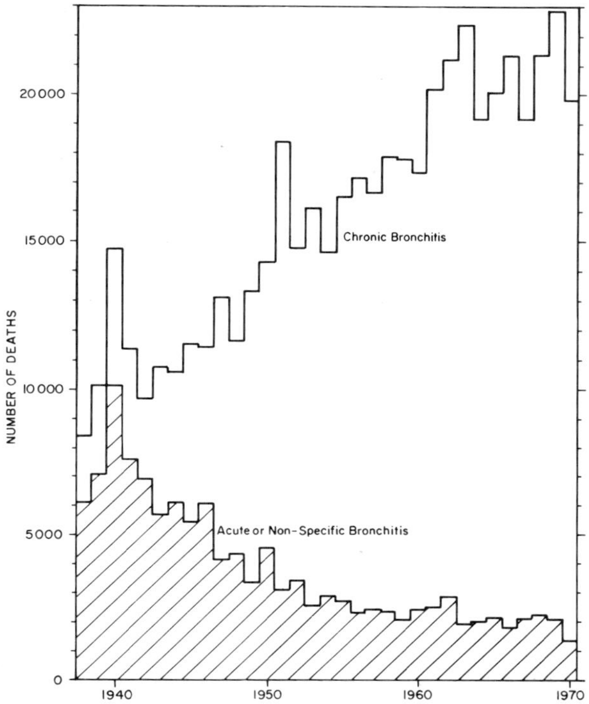

Fig. 13.1 Annual number of male deaths from bronchitis for England and Wales, 1938–70 (Registrar General's Statistical Reviews of England and Wales).

society for a period of 5–30 years. In addition, chronic bronchitis may very often be implicated as an important predisposing factor for the onset of a number of other degenerative disorders, such as lung cancer, pneumonia and cardiovascular diseases. As such, the true significance of bronchitis in its effect upon the mortality experience of a community often remains unappreciated by virtue of its influential or contributory role in the causation of death.

When considering the spatial distribution of the disease at a global scale, the very considerable variations in diagnostic procedures and standards between countries must not be overlooked. In parts of Latin America, for example, the mere suggestion of a cough prior to the death of a child may be sufficient justification for recording bronchitis as the substantive cause of death, even though the underlying cause may have been related to nutritional factors or infectious disease. Under these circumstances, a "convenient" or

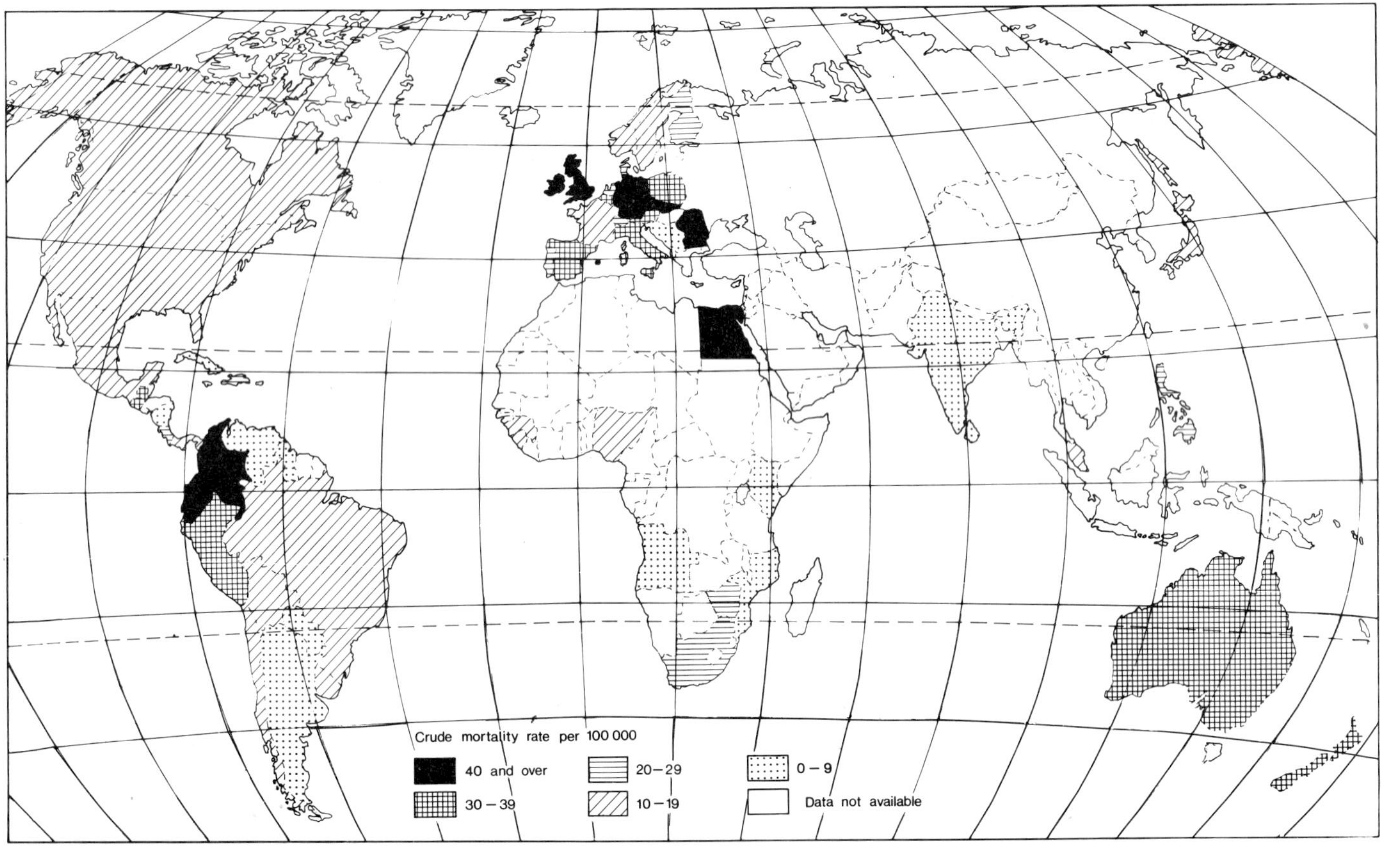

Fig. 13.2 Crude mortality rates from bronchitis (both sexes), 1970. (Data from U.N. Demographic Yearbook, 1970.)

"fashionable" classification of death suffices, particularly where medical services are totally inadequate in relation to the population at risk. However, even in the developed world, considerable mis-registration of bronchitis mortality occurs. For example, Anderson (1968) reports a substantial confusion of bronchitis with emphysema, a related though distinct cause of death, in particular provinces of Canada. This situation was eventually traced to basic differences in diagnostic procedures adopted by the major teaching hospitals.

A further severe limitation in considering the distribution of the disease at the global scale is the lack of reliable data for much of the developing world, even in respect of total number of deaths. As a result, crude mortality rates must inevitably be relied upon to provide the only available indicator of geographical distribution. This is a far from satisfactory measure of comparative disease incidence, particularly for a disease category such as bronchitis which is both age- and sex-selective.

WORLD DISTRIBUTION

The world distribution of crude mortality rates for bronchitis for the period 1969–70 is given in Fig. 13.2. As may be seen, statistics were not available for several countries in Africa and Asia, including the Soviet Union and China. However, interpolation from available sample points, together with additional evidence drawn from secondary source material tends to suggest relatively low mortality from bronchitis in these areas (viz. less than 20 per 100 000 per annum).

The most significant area of high mortality rates is located in western Europe with seven nations recording rates in excess of 40 per 100 000. These are the United Kingdom (62)*, Ireland (68), West Germany (44), East Germany (71), Czechoslovakia (56), Bulgaria (45) and Rumania (69). In such cases it is the chronic form of bronchitis which is responsible for the high mortality experience. It is interesting to note, however, that for Europe as a whole, the pattern is far from uniform. A number of countries, particularly those which are less urbanized and industrialized, record only moderate to low

* Crude mortality rates per 100 000.

mortality from the disease, e.g. France (10), Yugoslavia (9), Sweden (13) and Norway (14).

A second area of particularly high incidence occurs in the three Latin-American countries of Colombia (48), Ecuador (92) and Peru (31). Here there appears to be a predominance of the acute form of the disease amongst infants, rather than the chronic forms (Fig. 13.3). As already stated, part of this apparently excessive mortality experience may well be explained simply in terms of mis-registration and diagnosis. However, it seems not unlikely that aspects of the physical environment in these Andean states, possibly associated with unfavourable socio-economic conditions and malnutriton, promote a substantive increase in childhood respiratory disorders, and more particularly bronchitis (Townsend, 1973).

A third area of exceptionally high bronchitis mortality rates occurs in Egypt (172). Here again it is the acute form of the disease, affecting principally the younger age groups, which appear to dominate.

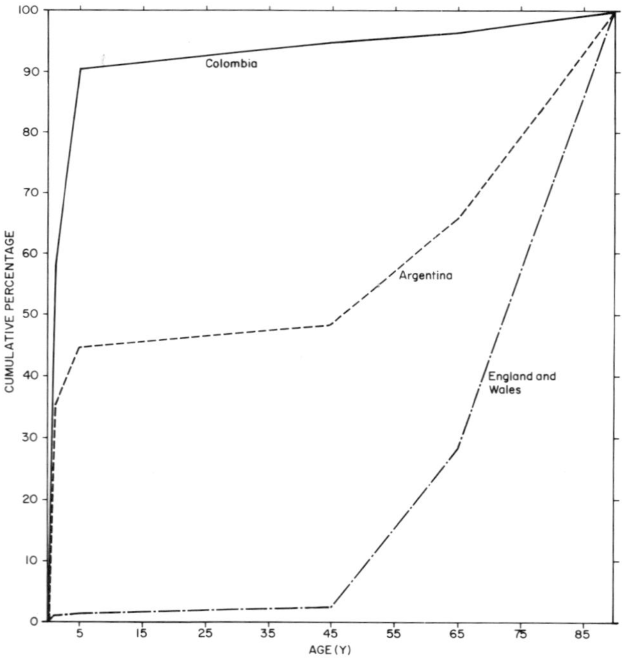

Fig. 13.3 Cumulative age distribution of male mortality from bronchitis for selected countries. (Data from U.N. Demographic Yearbook, 1967.)

Australia and New Zealand display surprisingly high mortality rates. They are between 30 and 39 per 100 000, and relate more especially to the chronic form of the disease. Such rates may be associated with the high degree of urbanization and increasing industrialization of these countries. The white population of South Africa and Rhodesia also experience moderately high death rates. Such rates contrast markedly with the particularly low prevalence of bronchitis among the coloured population of these two countries, and those in the adjacent territories of Angola, Mozambique and Kenya.

In addition to the Andean states of Colombia, Ecuador and Peru considered above, the remainder of Latin America, together with the islands of the Caribbean, display a very complex pattern of generally high mortality rates from bronchitis. Such spatial variation in mortality experience is to be explained, at least in part, in terms of differences in diagnostic procedures. Even so, urbanization appears to be playing a role in promoting rapidly increasing rates for bronchitis, not least in association with the immense social and economic dislocation brought about by the spawning of shanty-town development at the urban fringes of many Latin-American cities. This has had far-reaching consequences on the health of the population. Fox (1972), commenting on morbidity and mortality patterns in Mexico City, attributed over half of the appallingly high mortality of children under 5 years old to respiratory disorders linked to poor housing and low nutritional standards. In particular, he recognized a strong positive correlation between respiratory disease and poorly ventilated dwellings. In addition, the physical situation of Mexico City tends to exacerbate these conditions, since atmospheric pollutants tend to accumulate in the depression within which the city is largely located.

Canada and the U.S.A. exhibit remarkably low crude mortality rates for bronchitis, viz. 15 and 14 per 100 000 respectively. Even when the rates have been standardized for differences in age and sex structure and for life-time cigarette consumption, Reid (1964) discovered that bronchitis prevalence in the U.S.A. as a whole remained significantly less than for the rural areas of the United Kingdom. Moreover, Colley and Reid (1970) demonstrated that when people move from the United Kingdom, "particularly in childhood, to more favourable conditions in the U.S.A., they smoke no less, but the death rates from chronic lung disease among them fall remarkably." Obviously there are additional and, as yet, unexplained factors accounting for this significant differential between the European and American experience.

The lack of available mortality statistics for most of the countries of Asia makes an analysis of the spatial distribution of bronchitis virtually impossible. It is worthy of note, however, that Japan records only a modest rate, viz. 14 per 100 000. This is far less than might be expected for such an urbanized and industrialized society. Nevertheless, the trend in mortality from bronchitis over the last decade reveals a two- to three-fold increase in the annual deaths from the disease.

AETIOLOGICAL FACTORS

A wide range of factors have been cited in the aetiology of bronchitis. No single factor is readily identifiable as the predominant influence in promoting the disease; combinations of factors are rather implicated in causation. Three main groups of factors, biological, physical and social, are recognized. They incorporate both predisposing and causative elements, all of which contribute to the patterns of bronchitis morbidity and mortality outlined above.

Biological factors

The biological influences are concerned primarily with the predisposition of the individual to the disease. It has been suggested that there are certain genetic or constitutional factors which make certain individuals or, indeed, whole populations inherently more susceptible to the disease than others. On the other hand, a certain proportion of a given population may be immune to the disease by virtue of its particular genetic make-up (Capel and Caplin, 1964). Reid (1964), for example, has posed the question "Are the British more bronchitic than anyone else?" bearing in mind the excessively high mortality rates in Britain compared with those for America and Norway. Massaro *et al.* (1964) undertook a statistical comparison of bronchitis morbidity between the negro and the white populations of the U.S.A. Making due allowance for differences in smoking habits, findings indicated a very significant excess of the disease in the white population and for all age groups. Stanek *et al.* (1966) on the other hand found no evidence to suggest that heredity factors were significant in predisposing individuals to the disease. Instead they stressed the role of external factors.

The two most important biological determinants of morbidity and mortality rates for bronchitis are age and sex although, in both cases, very considerable global variations in influence were recorded. Table 13.1 reveals significant sex differentials in bronchitis mortality experience. They range from Australia, with over five times more male deaths than female deaths from bronchitis, to Hong Kong where the number of female deaths from the disease is considerably more than for males. By and large, the countries which exhibit an excess of bronchitis mortality for males are located in the developed world and are characterized by a predominance of the chronic form of the disease.

Superimposed upon the sex differential is an appreciable variation in both disease incidence and prevalence between the several age-groups. For acute or non-specific bronchitis, deaths of infants under 5 years predominate. Where the chronic form of the disease is the more common, mortality occurs principally in the late-middle and old-age range, usually following a prolonged period of chronic disablement. This would account for the marked difference between the mortality regime of Colombia, which recorded over 90% of its

Country	Crude mortality rates per 100 000		Ratio
	Males	Females	
Australia	37.8	6.8	5.56
England and Wales	98.8	35.4	2.80
France	5.7	3.7	1.54
Ecuador	113.3	104.6	1.08
Japan	7.0	6.8	1.03
Jordan	39.4	47.4	0.83
Hong Kong	6.4	9.6	0.67

Table 13.1 Bronchitis: a comparison of crude mortality rates for males and females in selected countries (U.N. Demographic Yearbook).

male mortality from bronchitis in the 0–4 year age group, and that for England and Wales with over 70% of the male mortality occurring in the over-65 year age category (Fig. 13.3). Argentina exhibits an intermediate position with almost 45% of the male bronchitis mortality occurring in the 0–4 year age group, and a further 35% in the over-65 year category.

Apart from its direct effect upon mortality levels, the age factor has a further indirect influence on the insidious progress of the chronic form of the disease. A previous history of respiratory disorders, including bouts of non-specific bronchitis during the early years of life, may well predispose to the incursion of the chronic form of bronchitis in later life. Consequently, when the influence of other non-biological aetiological factors in chronic bronchitis are being considered, an individual's respiratory history and previous environmental circumstances cannot be overlooked.

Physical environmental factors

The second major group of factors implicated in the aetiology of bronchitis is associated with the physical environment. In this respect, the influence of climate is particularly important. Figure 13.4 demonstrates the significance of seasonality in the regime of male mortality from acute bronchitis in England and Wales. The winter months, characterized by cool to humid conditions, exhibit a mortality rate some five times greater than that recorded for the warmer summer period with the lower relative humidities. The regime for chronic bronchitis is similar (Fig. 13.5) although the difference between winter and summer is not quite so large. It is generally agreed that there is a substantive relationship between the incidence of bronchitis and certain climatic factors but the linkage is, in many cases, indirect. For instance, an attack of bronchitis may result not from prevailing environmental circumstances *per se* but as a secondary complication of a primary respiratory conditions such as influenza.

Associated with the influence of seasonality is the factor of atmospheric pollution. This is held by most authorities to be one of the two most important causative agents of bronchitis. Ashley (1967) obtained a highly significant positive correlation between levels of particulate air pollution and standardized mortality rates for

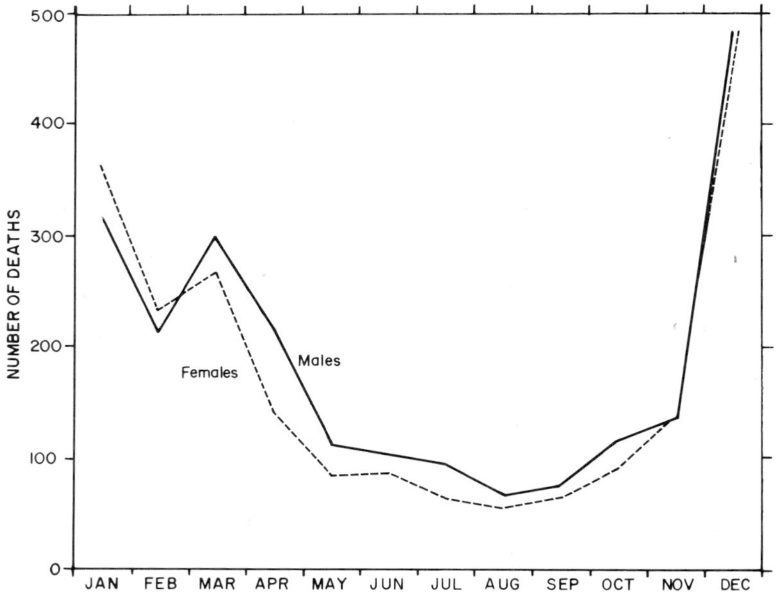

Fig. 13.4 Deaths from acute or non-specific bronchitis in England and Wales, 1969 (Registrar General's Statistical Review of England and Wales).

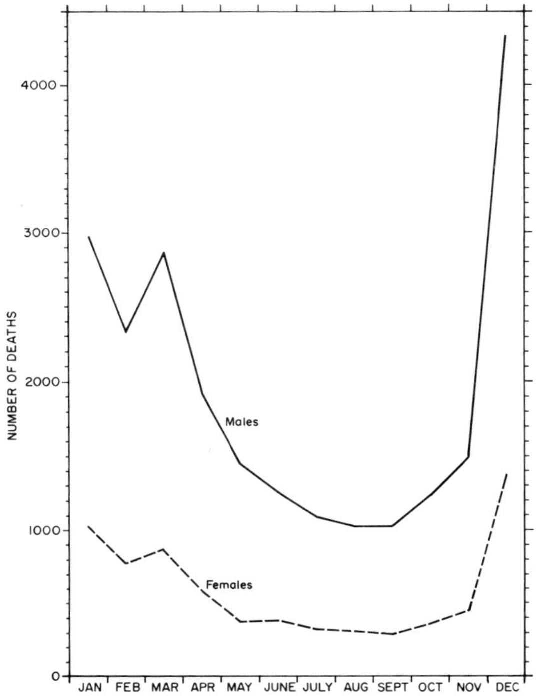

Fig. 13.5 Deaths from chronic bronchitis in England and Wales, 1969. (Data from Registrar General's Statistical Review for England and Wales.)

bronchitis for the 83 county boroughs of England and Wales. In particular, pollutants derived from domestic rather than industrial sources were primarily implicated. At the local level, Young (1972), working in County Durham, observed a similar relationship between the levels of atmospheric pollution and mortality patterns from chronic bronchitis. The high mortality rates of the heavily polluted areas of South Tyneside contrasted sharply with the substantially lower mortality rates of the central and southern areas of the county.

It is possible that the association between air pollution and bronchitis, and more particularly with the chronic form of the disease, is the main determinant of its global pattern of distribution (Fig. 13.1) and especially the high mortality rates recorded for most West-European countries. Available evidence suggests that rapidly rising pollution levels throughout the world associated with

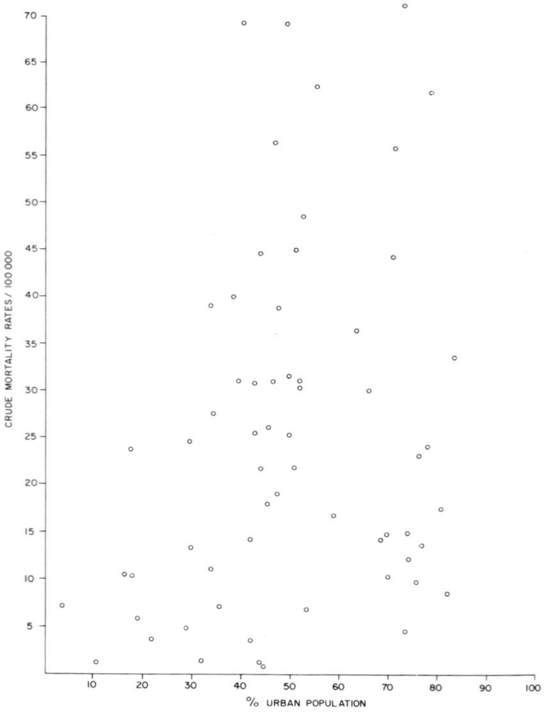

Fig. 13.6 Relationship of crude mortality rates for bronchitis and percentage of population classified as urban (based on a sample of 62 countries). (Data from U.N. Demographic and Statistical Yearbooks.)

accelerated consumption of fuels, especially since the Second World War, has been matched by an equally alarming increase in the number of deaths from bronchitis. Despite attempts to reduce levels of atmospheric pollution by the setting up of smoke-free zones in many major urban areas, the disease appears to be on the increase. It is a matter of regret that continuing industrialization and urbanization appears to negate any advantages accruing from concerted remedial action.

Figure 13.6 demonstrates, for a sample of 62 countries, the relationship of crude mortality rates for bronchitis and the percentage of the population classified as urban. A strong positive correlation emerges ($R = 0.77$); statistically this is highly significant. It must be appreciated, however, that there are basic statistical limitations inherent in the data. These limitations relate to diagnostic differentials and the complete lack of mortality standardization, and as such, have not been taken into account. Nevertheless, the relationship may provide a useful indicator to the very much higher levels of chronic bronchitis morbidity and mortality which will seemingly be experienced over much of the Third World in the wake of continued and rapid urbanization. Appropriate counter measures need to be instituted to combat the insidious side effects of the process of urbanization, and more particularly the increasing levels of atmospheric pollution.

At national and local levels, the urban-rural differential in

	No. of Deaths	Rates per million	
		Males	Females
Conurbations	13 112	1197.3	418.8
Urban areas with over 100 000 persons	4965	1166.8	376.8
Urban areas with 50 000 − 100 000 persons	3278	1052.4	340.8
Urban areas under 50 000 persons	7235	1064.1	329.2
Rural districts	5367	784.6	246.7

Table 13.2 Bronchitis and asthma: deaths in England and Wales, 1969, by selected population aggregates. (Ministry of Health and Social Security figures published in the *Brit. Med. J.* (1971) **1**, 616.)

bronchitis incidence emerges. In England and Wales in 1968, the Ministry of Health and Social Security issued a statement of deaths from bronchitis and asthma which indicated that mortality rates for rural districts were almost 35% lower than those for conurbations (Table 13.2).

Social environmental factors

The third and final group of aetiological factors relate to aspects of the socio-economic environment. Chief among these is the habit of smoking, particularly of cigarettes. This may be regarded as the single most significant contributory factor in the causation of bronchitis. An investigation conducted at the end of the 1960s estimated that chain smokers had a probability of dying from chronic bronchitis which was some 12 times greater than that for non-smokers (*Brit. Med. J.* 1970, **1**, 312). A comparative study of 20 selected countries (Stocks, 1967) demonstrated that there was a strong positive correlation between annual average cigarette consumption per person and the 1960–61 bronchitis mortality rates for males aged 55–65 years. At the local level, Neilson and Crofton (1965), studying the social effects of chronic bronchitis in Scotland, found in a sample of 500 chronic bronchitics that 62.6% were smokers, 34.8% were ex-smokers and only 2.6% had never smoked in their lives. On the other hand, there are many life-time smokers who apparently remain totally unaffected by the disease. Nevertheless, the fact remains that by smoking an individual increases considerably his chances of contracting chronic bronchitis. An example of one of the most tragic follies of contemporary consumer-orientated society is that of the Government of the United Kingdom which recovers over £1125 millions in duty on tobacco annually and yet spends a mere £110 000 or less than one ten-thousandth part of the tax revenue on warnings to people of the inherent health risks involved in smoking.

In addition to the recognized health hazard associated with cigarette smoking, there is also the increased risk of contracting bronchitis in certain occupational groups. The evidence for this is still contradictory (Lane, 1964), but there is a limited number of industries in which operatives exposed to moderate to high levels of dust and gaseous contaminants suffer an excess morbidity from bronchitis. This aetiological linkage may represent but an additional contributory influence in causation superimposed upon the more important effects of general atmospheric pollution and smoking. Nevertheless, a significant excess of bronchitis morbidity and mortality has been recorded amongst coalminers, foundry workers and operatives in certain sectors of the chemical industry. Added support for the occupation link is provided by the socio-economic differentials in bronchitis mortality noted by Capel and Caplin (1964) and other workers. A comparison of standardized mortality ratios suggests that the chances of unskilled manual workers and their wives (socio-economic group 5) dying from bronchitis is five times greater than their counterparts in the professions (socio-economic group 1). Similar results have been quoted by Colley and Reid (1970) in a study of age-adjusted morbidity ratios for chronic cough (Table 13.3). In this case, ratios for individuals in socio-economic groups 4 and 5 were two to three times greater than those for groups 1 and 2. It is of interest to note that this class differential was larger in the more highly industrialized towns of Newcastle and Bolton, where presumably the pollution gradients between social areas within the town were greater.

	Socio-economic class		
	1 and 2	3	4 and 5
Newcastle and Bolton	56	105	149
Bristol and Reading	69	104	126
English rural	48	89	96

Table 13.3 Chronic cough: age-adjusted morbidity ratios for males and females by social class for selected English areas (after Colley and Reid, 1970).

DISCUSSION AND CONCLUSION

In England and Wales alone, approximately 20 000 men and 8000 women die each year from chronic bronchitis. Whilst it is true that this disease category accounts for fewer deaths than such other mortality categories as lung cancer and coronary heart disease, the fact remains that annual deaths from bronchitis in England and Wales comprise over 7.5% of the total male mortality and 3% of female mortality. What is perhaps more significant is that these percentages appear to be increasing. Bronchitis is continuing to take an ever greater share of overall mortality, a trend which appears to be common to most other developed countries of the world.

Levels of morbidity and mortality of the acute or non-specific form of bronchitis tend to reflect in part the social and economic status of communities or nations. In the developing areas of the world, the acute form of the disease constitutes a significant fraction of the moderate to high levels of mortality in the infant age range, themselves a reflection of poor standards of nutrition and housing, inadequate provision for sanitation and hygiene, together with a lack or scarcity of adequate medical facilities. It is to be hoped that in the future the economic development process in these countries will be able to make very substantial inroads into the problem of the excessively high levels of mortality amongst infants. This in turn should lead to a marked reduction in acute bronchitis deaths in these areas. Unfortunately, as noted above, it would appear likely that advances on this front will be more than compensated for by an increase in the chronic form of the disease as a greater proportion of the population survive to an age when the disease is more commonly contracted. Moreover, this process will be aided by the action of certain deleterious environmental side-effects of continuing industrialization and urbanization.

It is, of course, all too easy to reduce the study of disease to glib statistical comparison and the contrite analysis of spatial distributions derived therefrom. The far-reaching human and social implications of such a disease as chronic bronchitis can so easily become forgotten. Very few have any concept of the prolonged period of misery and hardship that invariably precedes death resulting from this insidious cause. Nor does the statement of simple statistical fact convey the enormous cost to the community purely in financial terms. Lost working days from bronchitis mean not only lost production and efficiency, particularly in industry, but also increased sickness and social-security payments. There is also the additional cost of expensive medical care and attention particularly during the more advanced stages of the disease, when hospitalization may become necessary. Well over 30 million working days a year are lost through bronchitis in England and Wales alone. This is equivalemt to giving the entire labour force of the country one day's public holiday. Put another way, at any one time, upwards of 100 000 persons are receiving sickness benefit for some form of bronchitis while one in 10 of all new sickness benefit claims from male employees mentions the disease as the certified diagnosis.

Apart from the immense personal suffering endured by the bronchitic, his progressive disability inevitably has a considerable effect upon the quality and style of life not only of himself but also other members of his immediate family. Once the disease has progressed past the initial stages, an individual may find that he is no longer able, by virtue of his increasing breathlessness and bouts of coughing, to continue in his former occupation, particularly where this involves strenuous manual work. In consequence, he may be obliged to seek alternative lighter employment, which invariably involves a commensurate drop in real earnings. Eventually, the disablement becomes so severe that the bronchitic has to stop working altogether, accompanied by a further reduction in income. At both these stages, the individual suffers not only a loss of personal status and dignity but also has to try to adapt to a drastic fall in living standards. This latter situation often leads to the bronchitic patient being unable to afford to maintain his original home. He is then forced to move to more modest and cheaper housing. The irony of this situation is that in the majority of cases this transfer of residence often means a move to less desirable areas within a town or city. Here the environment is often such as to be pathologically inimical to the bronchitis sufferer by virtue of the higher levels of atmospheric pollution often coupled with cold and damp housing conditions. Unlike his American counterpart who appears to migrate to the surrounding rural districts to escape the hazards of the urban environment, the British bronchitic is unwittingly attracted by force of circumstance to just those areas that will intensify or aggravate his clinical condition.

Chronic bronchitis, perhaps more than any other disease category, can lay claim to the well-worn adage "prevention is better than cure". It may be argued that there is, in fact, still no absolute cure for the disease; all that can be done is to arrest and to alleviate the symptoms. Consequently, the solution to the urgent problem of rapidly increasing morbidity and mortality rates for many countries of the world must inevitably lie in finding ways of reducing the risk of contracting the initial stages of the disease. First, smoking should no longer be regarded primarily as a necessary or convenient source of governmental revenue. Strenuous efforts, involving the expenditure of large sums of governmental money, should be made in an effort to educate the population, particularly the younger generation, to the extremely severe health risks involved in cigarette smoking. Second, the number of urban areas with designated smoke-free zones should be increased, together with the areal extension of already existing smoke-free zones. At the same time, industrialists must be subject to much more stringent legislation not only in respect of the prohibition of the emission of noxious or harmful substances into the atmosphere but also with the improvement of working conditions. The latter should apply more particularly in those industries that have been shown to experience excessively high rates of morbidity and mortality from bronchitis. Only then will it prove possible to break down the vicious circle existing between environmental hazards, chronic bronchitis and poor social conditions, so that progress can be made towards the gradual alleviation of the severe burden that the disease imposes on the individual and on society in general.

REFERENCES

Ashley, D. J. B. (1967). The distribution of lung cancer and bronchitis in England and Wales. *Brit. J. Cancer.* **21**, 245–259.

Anderson, D. O. (1968). Geographic variations in deaths due to emphysema and bronchitis in Canada. *Canad. Med. Assoc. J.* **98**, 231–241.

Badham, C. (1818). "Observations on the Inflammatory Affections of the Mucous Membranes of the Bronchiae". J. Callow, London.

Capel, L. H. and Caplin, M. (1964). "Chronic Bronchitis in Great Britain". The Chest and Heart Association, London.

Colley, J. R. T. and Reid, D. D. (1970). Urban and social origins of childhood bronchitis in England and Wales. *Brit. Med. J.* **2**, 213–217.

Fox, D. J. (1972). Patterns of morbidity and mortality in Mexico City. *Geog. Rev.* **62**, 151–185.

General Register Office. *The Registrar General's Statistical Reviews for England and Wales*, London.

Lane, R. E. (1964). Chronic bronchitis and occupation. *In* "Some Aspects of Chronic Bronchitis" (Eds F. A. H. Simmonds and L. B. Hunt). Proc. Roy. Soc. Med. Symp., London.

Massaro, D., Cusick, A. and Katz, S. (1964). Racial differences in incidence of chronic bronchitis. *Amer. Rev. Respirat. Dis.* 92, 91–101.

Neilson, M. G. C. and Crofton, E. (1965). "The Social Effects of Chronic Bronchitis". The Chest and Heart Association, London.

Reid, D. D. (1964). Chronic bronchitis—a British disease? *In* "Some Aspects of Chronic Bronchitis" (Eds F. A. H. Simmonds, and L. B. Hunt). Proc. Roy. Soc. Med. Symp., London.

Stanek, V., Fodor, J., Hejl, Z., Widimsky, J., Charvat, P., Santrucek, M., Zaffic, F. and Vavrik, M. (1966). A contribution to the epidemiology of chronic bronchitis. *Acta Med. Scand.* **179**, 737–746.

Stocks, P. (1967). Lung cancer and bronchitis in relation to cigarette smoking and fuel consumption in twenty countries. *Brit. Prev. Soc. Med.* **21**, 181–185.

Townsend, J. G. (1973). Personal Communication.

United Nations, Statistical Yearbooks, New York.

United Nations, Demographic Yearbooks, New York.

Walker, D. D., Archibald, R. M. and Attfield, M. D. (1971). Bronchitis in men employed in the coke industry. *Brit. J. Ind. Med.* **28**, 358–363.

Young, J. C. (1972). Some aspects of the medical geography of County Durham. Unpublished Ph.D. Thesis, University of Durham.

14. Influenza

G. C. Schild

There is little doubt that for the past several hundred years, and probably during earlier times also, influenza has exerted an enormous impact in all areas of the world in terms of morbidity and mortality. In countries with developed economies, economic loss is a further important factor. Kavet (1972) has estimated that in the U.S.A. the cost of influenza is some $3500 million annually. In the United Kingdom sickness-benefit claims during the Hong Kong influenza epidemic of 1969–70 cost over £30 million in direct payment to insured persons and involved the loss of approximately 25 million working days in the period December 1969 to March 1970. The number of lost working days due to industrial disputes was approximately one third of that number for the whole year. As an infectious agent of man influenza is unique in its ability to produce outbreaks of worldwide dimensions (pandemics) and has been justifiably called the "last great plague". Although many previous causes of epidemic diseases of major significance such as smallpox and poliomyelitis have now been eliminated or reduced to insignificant proportions in many countries of the world, the influenza virus continues to produce repeated, almost annual, outbreaks of the disease. The biological success of the virus and our current inability to prevent the disease by vaccination are due largely to its intrinsic antigenic mutability.

Although techniques for the isolation of the influenza virus have been established since 1933 and laboratory characterization of virus strains is now a routine procedure, surveillance of the disease and the virus has in the past been largely fragmentary and our knowledge of its epidemiological behaviour and impact in most areas of the world is sadly incomplete. Through the W.H.O. influenza surveillance programme, detailed epidemiological information is now being continuously collected and, with the accomplishment of meaningful levels of surveillance in a larger number of countries, it is likely that the future will bring increased levels of understanding of the epidemiology of influenza and improved insight into methods of controlling and preventing epidemics.

This chapter reviews the biological nature of the causative agent, its clinical manifestations and the early and recent epidemiological behaviour of the virus in different areas of the world.

THE INFLUENZA VIRUSES: BIOLOGY AND ANTIGENIC VARIATION

Human influenza viruses

Influenza viruses are classified as Orthomyxoviruses (Melnick, 1973). These are lipid-containing, "enveloped" viruses which possess the property of haemagglutination of erythrocytes, a useful characteristic in their laboratory detection and bioassay, and which contain the enzyme neuraminidase. Figure 14.1 illustrates diagramatically the structure of the virus and its main antigenic components. The virions are roughly spherical in shape and some 75 nm in diameter. The surface antigens haemagglutinin (HA) and neuraminidase (NA) are present as radial projections from the lipid membrane of the virus particle which internally possesses a coiled nucleocapsid containing the virus genome. The virus genome consists of single stranded RNA present in the virus as eight distinct species of RNA and the virus particle contains RNA-dependent RNA polymerase. The fact that the genome of the influenza virus is fragmented has important implications for the understanding of the antigenic variability of the virus and epidemiological relationships between human and animal influenza viruses. For details of the structure and antigenic composition of influenza viruses see Stuart-Harris and Schild (1976a). Since antigenic variation is a factor essential to the biological success of the influenza viruses as human pathogens, some comment on the antigenic features of the virus is not

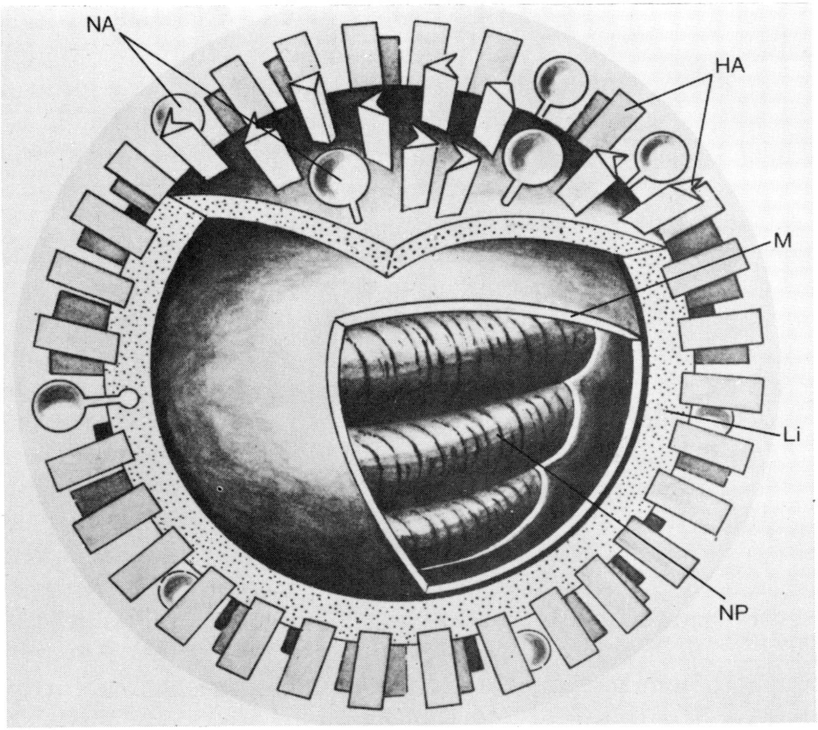

Fig. 14.1 Antigenic structure of the influenza virus particle. The influenza virus particle is roughly spherical or sometimes filamentous in shape and some 75 nm in diameter. Four major protein antigens (and two or three minor protein) constitute the particle. Two major proteins are on the virus surface, the haemagglutinin (HA) and the neuraminidase (NA), and are inserted in the lipid bilayer (Li) which bounds the particle. Internally there are two major proteins the matrix protein (M) and the nucleoprotein (NP). The genome of the influenza virus is in the form of single-stranded RNA but is fragmented, each virus particle containing molecules of eight distinct RNA species, each species being unique in its capacity to code for a specific virus protein.

out of place here. Antibodies to each of the two surface antigens of the virus particle, HA and NA, provide the basis for immunity in individuals possessing them. Internally, the virus possesses two other antigens, the nucleoprotein and matrix protein. The internal proteins are antigenically invariable and antibody to them does not confer immunity. These antigens do, however, provide the basis for the classification of influenza viruses into types A and B (for system of classification of influenza viruses see W.H.O., 1971).

The surface antigens of the virus, HA and NA, are antigenically variable for influenza viruses types A and B and from time to time undergo independent antigenic changes. At unpredictable intervals of 10–39 years, complete antigenic changes have occurred in the antigenic character of the haemagglutinin and, in 1957, simultaneously in the neuraminidase antigen of the prevalent influenza A viruses. Such changes are known as antigenic "shift" and strains of virus bearing novel surface antigens may spread rapidly since there is little or no immunity in the population to these new pandemics of disease. Pandemics are caused only by the influenza A virus. At more frequent intervals, minor changes termed antigenic "drift" take place in the HA and NA antigens. Although each of these changes is minor their effects are additive and, over a period of several years, result in a virus showing a considerable degree of antigenic difference from the parent strain. Antigenic "drift" gives the viruses possessing it a selective advantage in the interpandemic period and "drifted" strains of virus usually, but not always, gain international prevalence, the formerly prevalent strains being replaced over a period of several months. Influenza A viruses undergo both "shift" and "drift", whilst influenza B viruses undergo only "drift". Antigenic "drift" is thought to be due to the selection of spontaneously occurring mutants under pressure of increasing immunity in the population. The mechanism of antigenic "shift" remains a mystery. It seens unlikely, however, that antigenic shift can be due to mutation of the previous strain. Recent hypotheses are that new "shifted" strains may arise from reservoirs of influenza A viruses in animals or birds. Indeed influenza A viruses occur in nature in swine, horse and many avian species. Alternatively, it is possible that genetic recombination between human and animal influenza A virus, resulting in re-assortment of their RNA components may be the cause of antigenic "shift". The mechanisms of antigenic variation of influenza virus have been reviewed in detail by Webster and Laver (1975).

Since the isolation of the first human influenza A virus in 1933, antigenic "shift" has occurred in 1957, resulting in the appearance of the Asian influenza virus and in 1968 resulting in the Hong Kong virus. The antigenic subtypes of human influenza viruses isolated from 1933 to the present are shown in Table 14.1.

The 1957 "shift" involved both the HA and NA antigen whilst in 1968 only the HA antigen "shifted". Both "shifts" were associated

Period of prevalence of subtype	Reference strain	HA and NA subtypes	Variants showing antigenic "drift"	Type of antigenic variation	and pandemic periods
				"SHIFT"	
1918–20 + 1933–57	A/Swine/15/30* A/PR/8/34 A/FM1/47	Hsw1N1† HoH1† H1N1†	A/Weiss/43(HoN1) A/England/1/51(H1N1) A/Denver/1/57(H1N1)	"drift"	great pandemic of 1918–20 probably caused by swine/30 virus
				"SHIFT"	
1957–68	A/Singapore/57	H2N2	A/England/12/64(H2N2) A/Tokyo/3/67(H2N2)	"drift"	Asian pandemic 1957–58
				"SHIFT"	
1968–?	A/Hong Kong/68	H3N2	A/England/42/72(H3N2) A/Port Chalmers/1/73(H3N2) A/Victoria/3/75(H3N2)	"drift"	Hong Kong pandemic 1968–69
				"SHIFT"?	
1976	A/New Jersey/76	Hsw1N1			Possible future pandemic virus

* Viruses antigenically close to the swine influenza virus (A/Swine/Iowa/1930(Hsw1N1) are thought to have caused the 1918 pandemic on the basis of indirect evidence since virus isolation from man was not achieved before 1933.

† Although designated Hsw1, Ho and H1 the haemagglutins of strains isolated from man 1933–57 and of A/Swine/Iowa/1930 are of a single antigenic subtype.

Table 14.1 Antigenic subtypes of haemagglutinin and neuraminidase of influenza of man.

with pandemics of influenza; the mortality associated with the 1957 pandemic was, however, greater than that encountered in 1968 due probably to the protective effect of antibody to the unchanged NA antigen in the case of the 1968 epidemics. The enormous impact of the pandemics which occurred in 1918–20 is now legendary. It seems likely that the onset of the outbreaks in 1918 coincided with an antigenic "shift" in the influenza A virus and that this subtype virus persisted from 1918 until 1956, undergoing only antigenic drift during this period (Table 14.1). There is indirect circumstantial evidence based on studies of the sera of persons alive before 1918, that the 1918 pandemic virus is closely related to influenza A viruses of swine, and the recent events in the U.S.A., involving the isolation of swine-like influenza A viruses from military recruits in a New Jersey military camp (see below), has lead to considerable, but probably unfounded, speculation on the possibility of a return of pandemics of a severity not seen since 1918.

It is remarkable that on the appearance of completely new antigenic variants (antigenic "shift") in 1957 and 1968, the formerly prevalent strains rapidly disappeared from most of the world over the period of a few months persisting only in a few isolated foci. There is currently no explanation for this dramatic disappearance of former epidemic viruses from man. There is, however, evidence mentioned elsewhere in this chapter that former human strains may persist in animal hosts possibly emerging after several decades as new pandemic viruses.

Animal influenza and its possible association with human disease

Influenza A viruses produce outbreaks of disease in swine, horses and many species of wild and domestic birds. Influenza B viruses, in contrast, infect only man. It is possible that the fact that influenza B does not undergo antigenic "shift" is related to the apparent absence of animal reservoirs of this virus. The antigenic subtypes of influenza A viruses from swine, equine and avian sources are shown in Tables 14.2, 14.3 and 14.4. The ecology antigenic spectrum and biology of animal influenza viruses have been recently reviewed (Easterday, 1975; Stuart-Harris and Schild, 1976b). Classical swine influenza

HA subtype	NA subtype	Strains
Hswl	N1	*A/swine/Iowa/15/30 (Hswl N1)
Hswl	N1	*A/swine/Manitoba/ /67 (Hswl N1)
Hswl	N1	A/swine/Hong Kong/1/74 (Hswl N1)
H3	N2	A/swine/Taiwan/70 (H3N2)

* Strains isolated from swine fall into two distinct subtypes HswlN1 and H3N2. The "classical" swine influenza viruses produce epidemics of clinical influenza in swine herds and are all antigenically closely related (Hswl N1). The reference strain (*) of this subtype is the 1930 isolate of Shope. Note that the neuraminidase N1 of classical influenza viruses is antigenically related to that of human strains isolated between 1932 and 1956 (A0 and A1 strains). In addition the haemagglutinin antigen (Hswl) shows some degree of antigenic relationship to the (H0) of the human strains isolated from 1932 to 1946 (A0 strain). In contrast, A/Hong Kong/1/68-like strains of subtype H3N2 have been isolated from sporadic, asymptomatic infections in swine.

Table 14.2 Antigenic classification of influenza A viruses of swine origin; haemaglutinin and neuraminidase strains.

viruses exist as a single antigenic subtype (Hsw1N1). Viruses of this type are endemic in swine herds over the U.S.A. but have been only sporadically isolated elsewhere (Central Europe, Hong Kong, Italy and Sweden). The swine populations in the United Kingdom and Ireland have apparently been free of swine influenza infection since the 1940s when the last evidence of infection was detected.

Two subtypes of equine influenza virus (Heq1 Neq1 and Heq2 Neq2) exist and appear to be of wide international distribution.

Numerous antigenic varieties of avian virus have been isolated already and new subtypes are still being identified. Such viruses have been found in each country where they have been seriously sought. These viruses are known to be prevalent in domestic poultry and more recently have been found in wild birds including several species of duck, tern (*Sterna* sp), shearwater (*Puffinus pacificus*), puffin

HA subtype	NA subtype	Reference strains
Heq1	Neq1	A/equine/Prague/1/56 (Heq1 Neq1)
Heq2	Neq2	A/equine/Miami/1/63 (Heq2 Neq2)

Table 14.3 Antigenic classification of influenza A viruses of equine origin; haemaglutinin and neuraminidase subtypes.

HA subtype	Reference strains	NA subtype	Reference strains
Hav1	A/FPV/Dutch/27 (Hav1Neq1)*	N1	A/chicken/Brescia/1902 (Hav1N1)
Hav2	A/chicken/Germany'N'/49 (Hav2Neq1)	N1	A/chicken/Scotland/59 (Hav5N1)
Hav3	A/duck/England/56 (Hav3Nav1)	N2	A/turkey/Massachusetts/65 (Hav6N2)
Hav4	A/duck/Czech/56 (Hav4Nav1)	Neq1	A/chicken/Germany'N'/49 (Hav2Neq1)
Hav5	A/tern/S.Africa/61 (Hav5Nav2)	Neq1	A/FPV/Dutch/27 (Hav1Neq1)
Hav6	A/turkey/Mass/65 (Hav6N2)	Neq2	duck/Ukraine/1/63 (Hav7Neq2)
Hav7	A/duck/Ukraine/1/63 (Hav7Neq2)	Nav1	A/duck/England/56 (Hav3Nav1)
Hav8	A/turkey/Ontario/6118/68 (Hav8Nav4)	Nav2	A/tern/S.Africa/61 (Hav5Nav2)
Hav9	A/turkey/Wisconsin/66 Hav9N2)	Nav3	A/turkey/England/63 (Hav1Nav3)
		Nav4	A/turkey/Ontario/6118/68 (Hav8Nav4)
		Nav5	A/shearwater/Australia/72 (Hav6Nav5)

Table 14.4 Antigenic subtypes of haemagglutinin and neuraminidase of avian influenza A viruses.

(*Fratercula artica*) and wagtail (*Motacilla* sp). Infection in wild birds has been detected frequently in the U.S.A., U.S.S.R. and several European countries (reviewed by Easterday, 1975) and in South Africa. It should be emphasized that the ecological investigation of influenza in birds and mammals has been fragmentary. However, there is now renewed interest in this field and the W.H.O. is co-ordinating an expanded programme of animal influenza surveillance. Frequent isolations of virus are now being made from several species, in particular from wild birds and knowledge of the ecology of the virus in non-human hosts is increasing rapidly on an international scale.

Influenza A viruses from non-human sources have rarely been antigenically identical to those isolated from man but amongst them are commonly found strains containing HA or NA antigens, or both, showing clear antigenic relationships to those of human viruses (Table 14.5; see also Stuart-Harris and Schild, 1976b). The only exception to the above is the Hong Kong virus which, after it appeared in man in 1968, was found to be capable of crossing species barriers to infect swine and domestic chickens, though without producing symptoms in these hosts, and the swine (Hsw1 N1) viruses.

The earliest recognition of epidemic swine influenza in the U.S.A. in 1918 is worthy of special comment. At the time of the onset of the severe pandemics in the human population in the U.S.A., a vetenarian in the Midwest, Dr. J. Koen, noted the sudden appearance of an influenza-like illness amongst swine herds. According to Koen, this was hitherto an unrecognized disease in swine and its temporal co-incidence with the human disease was emphasized. Since 1918, outbreaks of swine influenza have occurred annually in the fall in the Midwest area of the U.S.A. The aetiological agent of swine influenza was identified as a virus by Drs Shope and Lewis at the Rockerfeller Institute, Princeton, New Jersey in 1930 (Shope, 1931), even before the isolation of influenza from man, and subsequently the virus was identified as an influenza A strain. The swine influenza viruses isolated in recent years are antigenically close to the original isolate of 1930. Recent studies have shown that, although it possesses some minor antigenic differences from them, the swine influenza virus belongs to the same subtypes of HA and NA antigen as the human influenza virus strains which were isolated from 1933 until 1956, i.e. H0N1 and H1N1 (Table 14.1). The earliest

Human: type A influenza viruses		Swine origin		Equine origin				Avian origin													
Human epidemic era and period of prevalence of antigen	H and N antigen subtype or group	A/swine/Iowa/15/30		A/equine/Prague/1/56		A/equine/Miami/1/63		A/chicken/Scotland/59		A/tern/S.Africa/1/61		A/duck/Germany/1215/73		A/Fowl Plague/ Rostock/34		A/duck/Germany/1868/68		A/turkey/Mass/65		A/duck/Italy/574/66	
		Hsw1	N1	Heq1	Neq1	Heq2	Neq2	Hav5	N1	Hav5	Nav2	H2	Nav2	Hav1	N1	Hav6	N1	Hav6	N2	Hav2	N2
Haemagglutinin antigens																					
A0–A1																					
1933–56	H0–H1	+		0		0		+		+		0		0		0		0		0	
Asian (or A2)																					
1957–68	H2	0		0		0		0		0		+		0		0		0		0	
Hong Kong																					
1968– ?	H3	0		0		+		0		0		0		0		0		0		0	
Neuraminidase antigens																					
A0–A1	N1		+		0		0		+		0		0		+		+		0		0
Asian and Hong Kong																					
1963– ?	N2		0		0		0		0		0		0		0		0		+		+

*Indicates evidence of antigenic relationship demonstrated by haemagglutination–inhibition tests (for H antigens), neuraminidase–inhibition tests (for N antigens) or by immunodiffusion tests.

Table 14.5 The major antigenic relationships between human type A influenza viruses and those of lower animals and birds.

suspicion that swine influenza virus may have had an epidemiological association with the pandemic of 1918 was based on the early work of Laidlaw and his colleagues (Andrewes *et al.*, 1935). It was found that persons who, in 1935, were old enough to have experience of infection in the 1918 pandemic possessed antibody to the swine virus; younger persons did not. This finding has been confirmed in recent studies and, in 1976 essentially, persons of 50 years or older possess such antibodies, representing a cohort of the population who, even half a century afterward, still appear to retain the immunological memory of their earliest experiences with influenza. The term "original antigen sin" has been used to describe this phenomenon.

Swine influenza remained of only speculative significance for man until 1976. In mid January of that year, an outbreak of influenza occurred amongst young military recruits who were recently enrolled at the Fort Dix army camp, New Jersey (W.H.O., 1976). Twelve isolates of influenza virus were made of which six were antigenically identical to the A/Victoria/75 virus which was currently predominant in many areas of the U.S.A. and in Europe. The remaining six strains were identified as being swine influenza virus. The outbreak at Fort Dix, which ended some 6 weeks later, appeared therefore to be of mixed aetiology involving two distinct influenza A viruses. An immediate serological survey indicated that in all, some 500 recruits in the camp were infected with the swine influenza virus. Intensive surveillance outside the camp had not detected evidence of spread of the outbreak in general up to the end of June 1976. Nevertheless, the isolation of swine influenza-like viruses was considered to be of great potential significance by health authorities and virologists in the U.S.A. as a possible beginning of a new pandemic era and preparations were made to carry out mass vaccination against swine influenza in the entire population of the U.S.A. during the autumn and winter of 1976–77. Some 150 million doses of inactivated swine influenza vaccine were manufactured in the U.S.A. and, during the large scale vaccination programme of 1976–77, some 39 million doses were administered to healthy adults and "high risk" patients between October 1976 and January 1977 when the programme was terminated prematurely. This was due to finding of an increased incidence of neurological illness (Guillain Barre Syndrome) on vaccinees (approx 1 case per 130 000 vaccinees). Vaccination with swine vaccine has not been planned for the winter 1977–78 in the U.S.A. or most other countries including the United Kingdom. Since the Fort Dix outbreak, up to July 1977, only very few sporadic cases of swine influenza infection in man have been detected in the U.S.A. and none elsewhere.

As will be described below, there is evidence, based on the distribution of antibody in the sera of older persons, that the Asian (H2N2) virus which appeared in 1957 had produced widespread outbreaks some 67 years previously, in 1890. Similarly, the Hong Kong (H3N2) virus may have circulated around 1900 before its re-emergence in 1968. Based on the acceptance of this historical evidence, cyclical re-emergence of influenza A viruses with a 60–70 year periodicity, it might be expected that the swine (Hsw1N1) virus would become the prevalent influenza A virus at the end of the present decade or in the 1980s. This hypothesis is of interest in regard to the significance of the outbreak at Fort Dix.

CLINICAL MANIFESTATIONS OF INFLUENZA

Although the influenza virus is constantly changing in its antigenic characteristics, the clinical disease it produces may have remained relatively constant over several centuries according to some of the earliest descriptions of the disease. Thus, influenza has been described as "an unchanging disease due to a changing virus" (Kilbourne, 1975). The most detailed information on the clinical aspects of influenza is derived from accounts in developed western countries.

Detailed comparisons of the clinical aspects of the disease in the populations of geographically different areas or countries have not been carried out and the extent of the geographic variability of the disease is unknown. Clinical aspects of influenza have been reviewed by Douglas (1975) and Stuart-Harris and Schild (1976).

In uncomplicated influenza the commencement of symptoms occurs some 2–4 days after infection. The first symptoms are headache, shivering and a dry cough accompanied by a sudden onset of fever. Malaise and aching of the limb muscles and back may occur especially in the adult patient. There may be nasal irritation or discharge and loss of sleep and dizziness may occur. In some patients, the symptoms may subside rapidly after the first 24 hours of illness. In others, the disease takes a more prolonged course, the temperature remaining high for 2–5 days, and the patient may have residual weakness and a cough for some days. In the absence of complications, the patient is usually sufficiently recovered to return to work within 7–10 days from the onset of illness. In a proportion of cases, persistent weakness or mental depression following the illness may require a longer convalescence. Amongst the clinical features of influenza the fever, 38–40°C (100–104°F), is the one which most characteristically distinguishes the disease from the common cold (an infection caused by the rhinoviruses, a group of agents unrelated to the influenza virus).

There are few physical signs in the patient enabling the clinician to make a hard diagnosis of influenza. Indeed the disease has no unique signs clearly distinguishing it from infections with other respiratory viruses. The diagnosis of influenza is made largely on the basis of the patient's symptoms in association with knowledge of epidemiological features of the outbreak in the community. Unequivocal identification of the disease is entirely dependent upon virus isolation or the detection of a diagnostic rise in specific influenza antibodies between serum samples taken in the acute and convalescent stages of the illness, respectively.

Influenza in children varies according to the age group. In general, childhood attack rates are high. In the very young, under 4 years of age, convulsions, croup and vomitting and neck stiffness may occur accompanied sometimes by a prolonged high fever and influenza is undoubtedly an important cause of severe clinical illness in these age groups. Though it occurs, mortality is uncommon in the healthy child. In older children, the prevalent symptoms may be coughing and the onset of a croup-like illness. Muscular aching is a more prevalent feature of the disease in older children and adults.

In major outbreaks, such as occurred in 1957 due to the Asian (H2N2) virus, a number of deaths have occured in previously healthy pregnant women, particularly those in the last trimester. There is no clear evidence that the virus has teratogenic effects resulting in the development of congenital defects in the babies of mothers infected during pregnancy. However, there is some evidence of increased rate of perinatal mortality in babies born to affected mothers. A number of studies, notably from Finland and Britain, suggest an enhanced frequency of leukaemia (1.5 times normal) in children whose mothers developed clinical influenza during pregnancy. Other studies in the U.S.A. do not support this finding. The statistical validity of these findings is uncertain but even if they are valid, it is still not established whether the increased incidence of leukaemia is an influenza virus-specific phenomenon, due to non-specific manifestations of infection as fever, or due to other associated factors such as medication which may accompany influenza infections.

The major complications of influenza involve the lower respiratory tract and the circulatory and nervous systems. Complications of the lower respiratory tract may be due directly to the virus, as for example in primary viral pneumonia, or may involve secondary bacterial infections. Bronchitis, bronchiolitis or pneumonia may occur in some 10% of all adult influenza patients and the frequency of these complications is also higher in patients with a previous history of a chronic pulmonary or heart disorder. Complications of influenza in the elderly contribute the major part of the considerable mortality attributed to the disease in major epidemics. Most bacterial complications of influenza are due to the pneumococcus, though staphylococcal influenzal pneumonia does occur during epidemics and may, if untreated, result in extremely rapid death. Bacterial complications may frequently be amenable to treatment with antibiotics, whilst there is currently no routinely used specific anti-viral drug to prevent or treat the primary viral infection. The lack of bacterial antibiotics in the times of earlier pandemics, e.g. 1918, may contribute to their much higher mortality rates in contrast to those of epidemics which occurred in the present era of routine use of antibiotics.

Chronic heart disease itself is a predisposing factor in the development of severe complications of influenza but also the influenza infection may produce various cardiac complications from temporary changes in electrocardiogram patterns to inflammatory changes in the heart muscles, myocarditis. The pathogenesis of these phenomena is unknown. Neurological illness such as encephalitis or encephalopathy may follow influenza, particularly in children but the frequency of such cases is low. Again, the exact pathological association of such complications with the influenza virus is unknown. Reye's syndrome is an encephalopathy associated with liver degeneration which is thought to be associated with influenza B infection in children. This disease is usually fatal though fortunately rare. Diabetics who suffer from influenza usually exhibit a worsening of their metabolic state, and influenza deaths amongst diabetic patients are not uncommon.

Although, as stated above, detailed comparisons of the clinical differences between the features of the disease in different countries have not been made, there is evidence in some areas that exceptionally high mortality rates are associated with influenza. For example during August 1975, an outbreak in Papua and New Guinea caused by A/Victoria/3/75 (H3N2) virus resulted in 400 deaths (W.H.O., 1975).

MECHANISMS OF INFLUENZA SURVEILLANCE

For influenza, international surveillance is of particular importance because of the constantly changing antigenic character of the prevalent virus and the association of major changes (antigenic "shifts") with pandemics of disease. Continuous international surveillance is conducted under the auspices of the W.H.O. In some countries, intensive local surveillance programmes are in operation.

International surveillance, W.H.O. programme

In 1947, worldwide surveillance of influenza was initiated by W.H.O. as part of the organization's influenza programme. At first, surveillance was on a modest scale with one international influenza centre in London and a few regional centres in other countries. The system has now grown into an extensive network of laboratories. The main purpose of the programme is the early detection and isolation of new antigenic variants of influenza virus and the collection of epidemiological data leading to a fuller understanding of the eidemiology and natural history of the disease. The early and accurate information available to the W.H.O. on the behaviour of the virus provides the basis for recommendations to be given to national authorities enabling the preparation of appropriate public health and prophylactic measures for combating with the disease (Schild and Dowdle, 1975). The activities of the programme are coordinated by the W.H.O. in Geneva. There are two international influenza laboratories, the W.H.O. Collaborating Centre for Reference and Research on Influenza in London and the W.H.O. Collaborating Centre for Influenza for the Americas in Atlanta, Georgia together with 97 national influenza laboratories in 69 different countries (Table 14.6).

When new influenza virus isolates showing significant antigenic change are detected, they are made available by the international centres to competent laboratories, including organizations producing influenza vaccines. The characterization of new viruses is carried out in the two international centres in London and Atlanta. The national centres are provided annually with a kit of reagents enabling them to identify current subtypes. Isolates not readily identifiable by reference reagents are of interest as possible variants, and national

African region	
Central African Republic	Bangui
Kenya	Nairobi
Nigeria	Ibadan
Senegal	Dakar
South Africa	Cape Province; Johannesburg
Uganda	Entebbe
Region of the Americas	
Argentina	Buenos Aires; Cordoba
Brazil	Rio de Janeiro; Sao Paulo
Canada	Ontario
Chile	Santiago
Cuba	Havana
Ecuador	Guayaquil
Jamaica	Kingston
Mexico	Mexico City
Peru	Lima
Trinidad and Tobago	Port of Spain
U.S.A.	Berkeley, California, Boston, Massachusetts, Ann Arbor, Michigan, Albany, New York, San Juan, Puerto Rico
Uruguay	Montevideo
Venezuela	Caracas
South-East Asia region	
India	Bombay, Nilgiris
Indonesia	Jakarta
Sri Lanka	Colombo
Thailand	Bangkok
European region	
Austria	Vienna
Belgium	Brussels
Bulgaria	Sofia
Czechoslovakia	Prague
Denmark	Copenhagen
England	London
Federal Republic of Germany	Berlin, Frankfurt, Hamburg, Hanover, Marburg/Lahn
Finland	Helsinki
France	Lyons, Paris
German Democratic Republic	Berlin, Niederschoneweide
Greece	Athens
Hungary	Budapest
Iceland	Reykjavik
Ireland	Dublin
Italy	Rome
Luxembourg	
Netherlands	Rotterdam
Northern Ireland	Belfast
Norway	Oslo
Poland	Warsaw
Portugal	Lisbon

Romania	Bucharest (2) Iassy
Scotland	Aberdeen, Edinburgh, Glasgow
Spain	Barcelona, Madrid
Sweden	Stockholm
Switzerland	Bern, Geneva
Turkey	Ankara
U.S.S.R.	Leningrad, Moscow
Yugoslavia	Belgrade, Novi Sad, Zagreb
Eastern Mediterranean region	
Algeria	Algiers
Egypt	Cairo
Sudan	Khartoum
Israel	Tel Aviv
Lebanon	Beirut
Morocco	Rabbat
Western Pacific region	
Australia	Melbourne, New South Wales, Perth, Victoria
Fiji	Suva
Hong Kong	
Japan	Tokyo
Malaysia	Kuala Lumpur (2)
New Zealand	Auckland, Dunedin, Wellington
Philippines	Manila
Democratic People's Republic of Korea	Pyongyang
Republic of Korea	Seoul
Singapore	

Table 14.6 National centres participating within the W.H.O. influenza surveillance programme, as of June 1, 1975.

influenza centres isolating such viruses submit them immediately to one of the international centres for rapid identification. The W.H.O. programme involves the collection and distribution of epidemiological information from national authorities. This comes variously from national influenza centres, national epidemiological services or the Ministries of Health of different collaborating countries. During the influenza season in the part of the world concerned, a report is sent weekly to the W.H.O. virus unit in Geneva, where the information is collected and published in the W.H.O. Weekly Epidemiological Record.

A summary of the functions of the W.H.O. influenza programme is illustrated in Figure 14.2.

Although the programme has attained a considerable degree of success in meeting its objectives, influenza epidemics remain largely unpredictable.

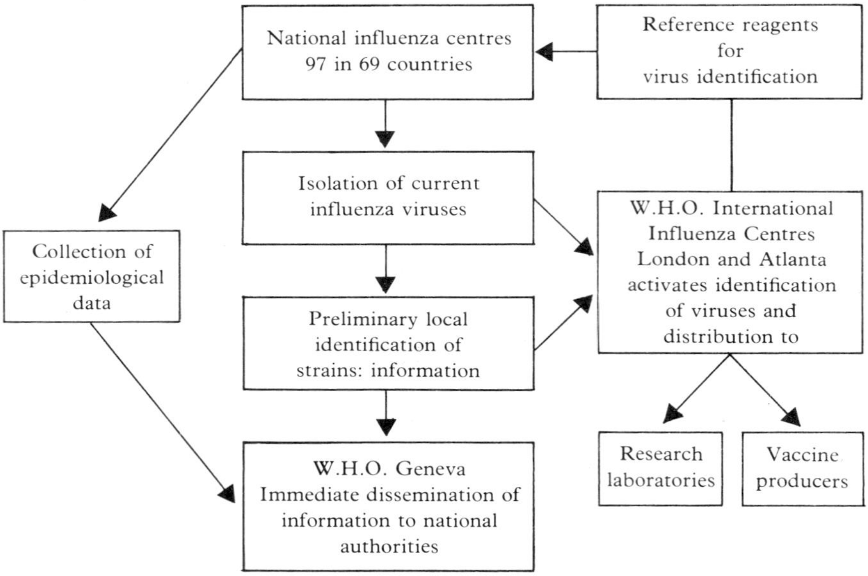

Fig. 14.2 W.H.O. influenza surveillance

The W.H.O., in recognition of the possibility that animal sources of influenza may play a role in the emergence of new human epidemic viruses, also co-ordinates ecological studies of animal influenza in various countries, notably U.S.A., U.S.S.R. and several European countries. Two W.H.O. collaborating centres of studies of animal influenza have been set up in the U.S.A.

National surveillance

The basis of national surveillance is the existence of a laboratory service able to diagnose influenza infection and isolate the causative viruses. In many countries, there are already entirely adequate laboratories for this purpose. In some countries, there is also a system of notification which, in co-operation with the laboratory, provides information on the incidence and severity of influenza. A method which has proved useful in some countries is to set up a network of "spotter physicians" sending specimens to the diagnostic laboratory from suspected clinical cases. In many countries, however, plans for regular and uniform collection and dissemination of epidemiological information on influenza are yet to be developed.

Epidemiological data, from which useful indication of the prevalence of influenza can be obtained in the country concerned, are as follows.

Mortality rates These are the weekly number of deaths from influenza and its complications from all causes in the whole country (or in selected areas). Excess mortality due to influenza or pneumonia and influenza (Assaad *et al.*, 1973; Langmuir and Housworth, 1969) is assessed by comparison of mortality rates during epidemics with those which occur in the same population and at the same period of the year in non-influenza years. The strikingly different mortality impacts of influenza epidemics in different countries during the same years has been emphasized by Assaad *et al.*, (1973) who compared excess mortality data from 13 different countries. Data for the United Kingdom, U.S.A. and U.S.S.R. from 1963–1973 are shown in Fig. 14.3.

Morbidity rates These are the weekly number of cases of influenza, or of acute respiratory disease including influenza from national sources or from selected practices or hospitals, the weekly number of absentees due to acute respiratory disease, or to all causes from sickness benefit claims or from reports from selected groups, factories, administrative services, military units, schools, universities, and the weekly number of emergency hospital admissions.

In case of an outbreak, the clinical features of the illness, estimated attack rates in various age groups of the population and an account of locations involved and duration of illness and its age distributions should be reported on.

The basis of the collection of epidemiological information in the United Kingdom and U.S.A. are described below in the next two subsections.

United Kingdom

Indirect methods for the detection of influenza (Smith, 1975; Pereira, 1976) in the United Kingdom can be summarized as follows: (a) sickness benefit claims are assessed and cover the whole of the adult working populations; (b) total mortality and mortality due to

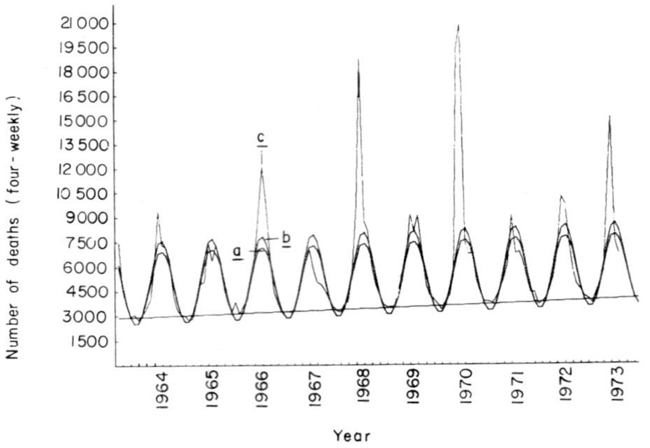

(a) (England and Wales)

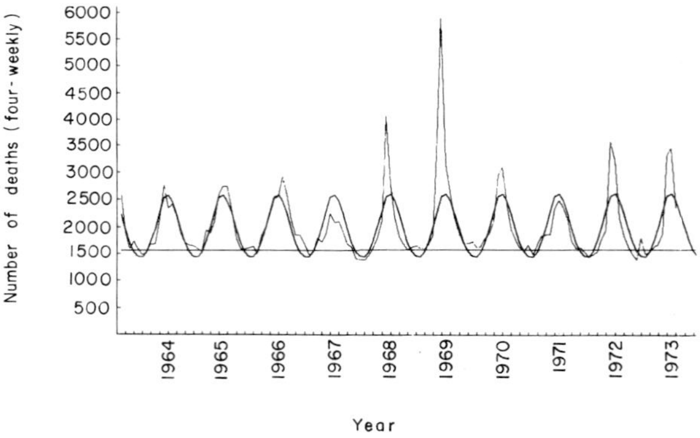

(b) (USA)

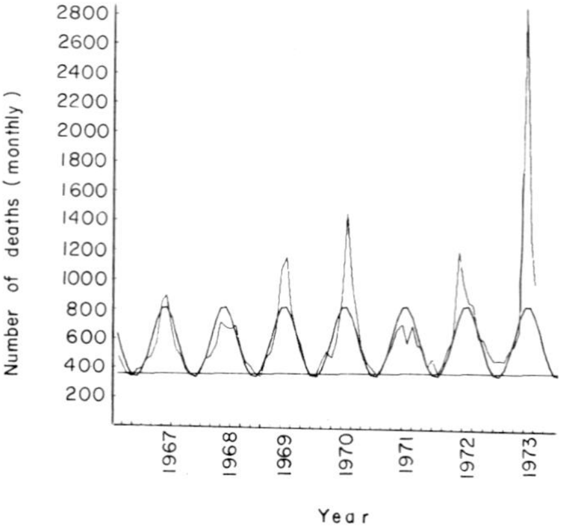

(c) (USSR)

respiratory diseases and their complications are determined on the basis of an examination of death certificates sent to the Registrar General; (c) rates of emergency admissions to hospitals are recorded weekly; (d) industrial and school absenteeism give valuable information; (e) returns of new consultations for acute respiratory infection from general practitioners in 100 practices under the auspices of the Royal College of General Practitioners are particularly useful in that they reflect experience in all ages of the population; (f) some 44 regional public health laboratory service virological units in the United Kingdom routinely return laboratory evidence of influenza isolation to the Central Public Health Laboratory Service or the Communicable Diseases Unit in Scotland (Pereira, 1976); (g) excess mortality is used as an index.

The most informative sources of information are total deaths and excess mortality estimates, sickness-benefit claims, general-practitioner consultation rates and virus isolations. The use of such surveillance provides immediate and reliable information, locally and nationally, of exactly how epidemics are progressing and permits the measurement of the size, impact and attack rates of epidemics.

U.S.A. (See review Dowdle *et al.*, 1974).

In the U.S.A., influenza surveillance activities are co-ordinated by the Centre for Disease Control (C.D.C.) at Atlanta, Georgia. The C.D.C. collects current epidemiological data and disseminates information to state health officers, evaluates it and facilitates the exchange of information with the W.H.O.

In the U.S.A., as in the United Kingdom, influenza is not a

Fig. 14.3 Deaths and excess mortality from influenza, pneumonia and bronchitis (England and Wales) and from influenza and pneumonia (U.S.A. and U.S.S.R.).

(a) England and Wales (1963–64 to 1972–73). The three curves, plotted by computer, represent during periods of 4 weeks, (*a*) the expected seasonal curve constructed from deaths in the years of low mortality when no sizeable outbreaks of influenza occurred, (*b*) the expected seasonal curve based on deaths in all the years under study except those in which very high peaks occurred, and (*c*) the curve of actual numbers of deaths.

(b) U.S.A. (1963–64 to 1973–74) and (c) U.S.S.R. (1966–67 to 1972–73). Curves plotted by computer on figures for actual and expected seasonal numbers of deaths due to influenza and pneumonia. (From Assaad *et al.*, 1973.)

nationally notifiable disease. Although data on the incidence of influenza and influenza-like illness are collected in about half of the states in the U.S.A., the uncertainty of clinical diagnosis, the presence of many of mild or unreported cases and variations in reporting criteria where such activities are carried on limit the value of such data and impair their comparability.

The major emphasis of the CDC has been on the concept of mortality as an index of the presence of influenza. The level of observed influenza-pneumonia mortality relative to the expected level for a given time period seems to be the most sensitive, uniform and readily available indicator of the presence and impact of influenza activity. It is clear that excess influenza-pneumonia mortality is accompanied by excess mortality due to other causes, and that taken together they present a broader and more complete picture of the impact of epidemic influenza. Weekly mortality reports, stating the total number of deaths as well as deaths due to influenza and pneumonia, are submitted to the C.D.C. by 122 large cities across the U.S.A. (Serfling *et al.*, 1967). Reports of school closures, industrial absenteeism, virus isolations, increased utilization of medical services and facilities provide additional information and are also of importance since they may precede discernable elevations in mortality levels. Peak mortality tends to lag behind morbidity by about 4 weeks.

Although several developed countries have evolved local systems for influenza surveillance, these may differ somewhat from those used in the United Kingdom and U.S.A. in the mechanisms of surveillance employed. There is little doubt that the use of "spotter" clinics or medical practitioners in differing areas of the country backed up by the availability of a national influenza centre provides a sensitive system for the early detection of epidemics and new variant influenza viruses. Such systems are in use in several European countries and elsewhere. In only a few countries, e.g. U.S.S.R., is influenza an officially notifiable disease.

ENVIRONMENTAL AND NON-SPECIFIC HOST FACTORS IN INFLUENZA

It is notable that influenza epidemics occur in the colder half of the year in both the northern and southern hemispheres and, essentially between December and April in the northern hemisphere and May to September in the south. Thus the disease appears to be under climatological influence. However, exceptions to the winter prevalence of epidemics in the northern temperate zone may occur with the emergence of new pandemic strains. Such an occasion was in 1957 when summer and early autumn outbreaks due to the Asian virus occurred. In tropical areas, influenza may co-incide with the wet season. Schild and McGregor (1976) noted widespread outbreaks of Hong Kong influenza in tropical West Africa (The Gambia) in autumn 1968 and again in autumn 1971. In equatorial areas, outbreaks may not be of clear-cut seasonal occurrence: in Singapore the influenza A virus may be isolated the whole year round but typically with a peak incidence of isolations and disease in June and July.

The way in which climatological conditions effect the epidemiological behaviour of the virus is not clearly established. An analysis of the situation must take into consideration that certain factors may influence the susceptibility of the host to become infected, to develop disease and to shed virus whilst others may influence the virus itself. Hope-Simpson (1958) and Davey and Reid (1972) found a positive correlation in successive winters between the incidence of acute respiratory disease and various parameters of influenza activity respectively and the coldness of the winter. Later studies (Reid, 1975) suggested that rapid fluctuation in temperature values may be more important than actual values. Similarly the effect of humidity is not well established. Hemmes *et al.*, (1960) found that the influenza virus itself survives best in aerosols at low relative humidities. The effects of temperature and humidity on aspects of human physiology which may influence virus replication are unknown. It is of interest, however, that in experimental mice (Schulman and Kilbourne, 1963), which were maintained under even conditions of temperature and humidity in winter and summer, transmission of influenza was significantly higher in winter possibly suggesting that other unidentified factors are involved. However, it must be emphasized that severe influenza epidemics are truly global in distribution and environmental effects must therefore have a relative rather than absolute controlling influence on influenza epidemiology.

Other factors which may be involved are concerned with population distribution at different seasons. At certain times of the year, the requirement for heating in the temperate zones cause relative crowding of persons in heated areas. The school year also has an effect on local population density. Possibly the efficient spread of the virus in the winter of temperate countries is as a result of a combination of several of the above factors (low exterior temperature, low interior humidity and high local population density). There is evidence that spread of infection is generally more efficient in densely populated urban areas than rural or remote areas of low population density. A low socio-economic status contributes to high population density and may thus influence the impact of influenza epidemics. Assaad and Reid (1971) found that the lower socio-economic groups in Glasgow suffered a higher mortality risk from influenza than higher groups. Other, non-specific factors may be the distribution in the population of non-influenzal microbial factors such as organisms which produce secondary bacterial pneumonia (*Pneumococcus*, *Staphylococcus*, *Haemophilus*). Such organisms may themselves have a season-dependent distribution in the population. A more detailed review of non-specific factors in influenza epidemics is given by Kilbourne (1975).

THE HISTORY OF INFLUENZA EPIDEMICS AND PANDEMICS

The unpredictability of the disease in mediaeval times, as now, is emphasized by the fact that its name is derived from the Italian *influenza* suggesting that the disease appeared under the influence of extra-terrestrial forces. During outbreaks of disease in the Court of Mary Queen of Scots in 1562, the disease earned the title of the "Newe Acquayantance" (Francis, 1953) with a similar significance. Although the influenza virus was not isolated until 1933 there is circumstantial evidence, discussed below, as to the causative influenza viruses of major outbreaks which occurred in 1889–90, 1898–1900 and 1918–19. The isolation and characterization of the influenza virus (Smith *et. al.*, 1933) lead to rapid progress in the identification of viruses and the study of their epidemiological behaviour thereby putting the epidemiological study of the disease on a sound scientific basis. Since 1933, recurrent epidemics of influenza A or influenza B infection have been identified in all countries where virological investigations have been carried out.

In countries from which epidemiological information is available, years in which no influenza outbreaks are recorded are rare. Most outbreaks of influenza and all pandemics are due to the influenza A virus. Influenza A, although most characteristically an infection of children and young adults does affect all age groups of the population. The major impact on mortality is, however, in the older age groups of the population, 70 years and above, and in the medically debilitated. In contrast, influenza B outbreaks are 4–6 times less frequent than those caused by influenza A virus, are relatively localized, producing their major impact in children. Whilst influenza A outbreaks are frequently accompanied by increased mortality rates, raised mortality is not a constant feature of influenza B epidemics, probably because of the relatively young age group affected. Figure 14.4 shows the relatively frequent occurrence of influenza A outbreaks in the U.S.A. from 1934–70 and the lower frequency of influenza B epidemics. Excess mortality associated with influenza A epidemics was of a considerably higher order than for influenza B, with the exception of, in 1935–36, when high mortality rates were apparently associated with influenza B epidemics. Data on the mortality associated with influenza outbreaks in England and Wales from 1940–71 is shown in Fig. 14.5 and also indicates the higher frequency of influenza A outbreaks and their association with raised mortality levels.

Early epidemics

It is difficult to establish with certainty the past history of influenza epidemics even in the developed areas of the world. It is important that, in the interpretation of historical accounts of influenza-like diseases, caution be exercised because of the abundance of epidemics of disease of diverse aetiology in mediaeval times, some of which may have a clinical resemblance to influenza. From as early as the 12th century onwards (Hirsch, 1883), descriptions of extensive outbreaks of disease appear in the literature which apparently showed close clinical and epidemiological similarities to present day outbreaks and were reportedly associated with high mortality rates. Severe outbreaks of influenza-like illness reportedly occurred in Europe in

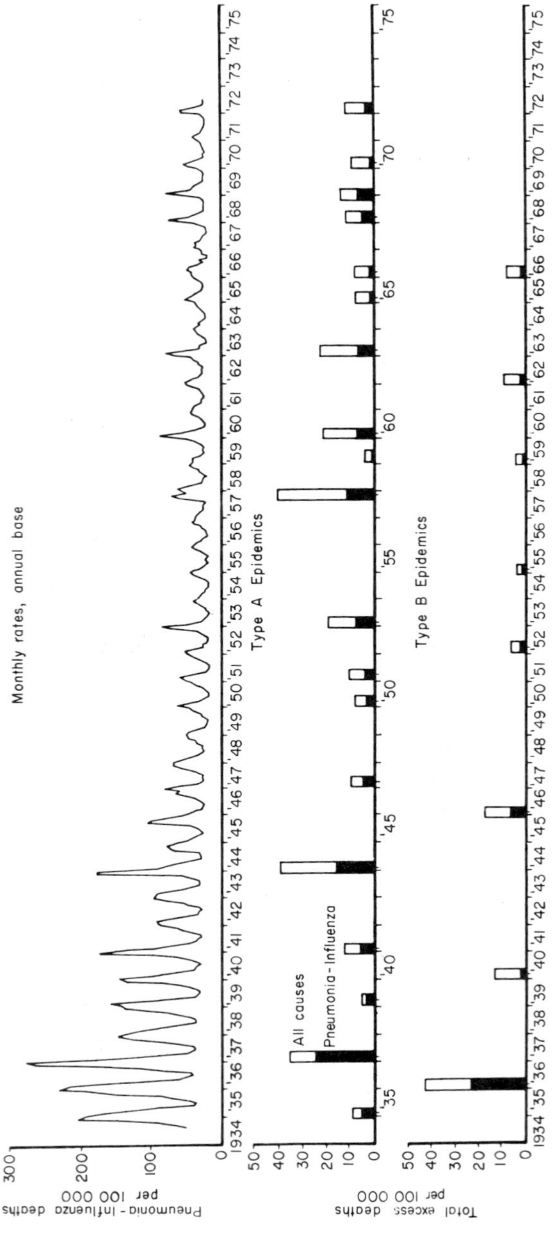

Fig. 14.4 Pneumonia and influenza death rates and excess mortality during epidemic periods in the U.S.A., 1934–70 (Dowdle *et al.*, 1974).

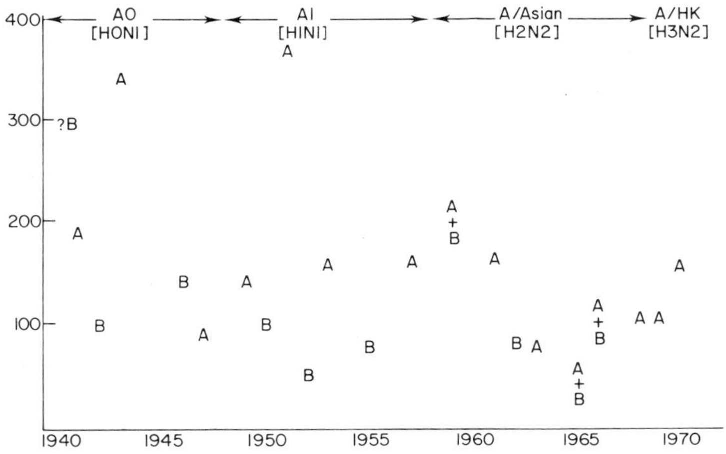

Fig. 14.5 Influenza death rate per million inhabitants in England and Wales, 1940–71 (returns of Registrar General and Office of Population Censuses and Surveys). The periods of prevalence of successive antigenic variety of influenza A virus are indicated thus—HON1, H1N1, H2N2 and H3N2. (From Stuart-Harris and Schild, 1976.)

1510, 1693 and 1729 but it is difficult to obtain evidence of their worldwide distribution. Later outbreaks of widespread nature occurred in 1781–82, 1803, 1833, 1837, 1847–48, 1889–90, 1898–1900 and 1918–19. Of these outbreaks, there is little doubt that those of 1847–48 and 1889–90 were pandemic in nature as were the subsequent outbreaks of 1918–19, 1957–58 and 1968–70.

Available information on the earlier outbreaks of influenza-like illnesses have been reviewed by Hirsch (1883), Creighton (1891, 1894) and Burnet and White (1972).

The 1781 outbreak appeared in Asia and spread west to Europe by 1782. This outbreak was reported to have affected persons of middle age rather than the young or elderly but the mortality rate was not high. The 1847 pandemic spread from the East through Russia reaching the United Kingdom in the winter of 1847–48. This pandemic was reported to have been associated with high rates of mortality in the elderly. The 1889–90 pandemic also spread from the east through Russia to Europe and subsequently to the U.S.A. during the autumn and winter producing outbreaks with high mortality levels. The following 4 years in Europe were also marked by waves of severe influenza, possibly caused by the same pandemic virus.

The 1918–19 pandemic

The years 1918–19 saw the most severe pandemic of influenza yet recorded, the so-called "Spanish influenza" pandemic. Although much anecdotal information is available on the distribution and severity of this pandemic (see Collier, 1974), the place of its origin is uncertain (Burnet and Clarke, 1942). However, it seems probable that the infection spread from Asia to Europe. The pandemic occurred in several waves during a period of little over a year. The first, in spring of 1918, was relatively mild, the attack rate being 20–40% in those aged up to 50 years but with a considerably lower rate in the aged. The second wave in the autumn of 1918 was exceptionally severe, producing enormous mortality in the 20–40 year age groups. A less severe wave occurred in early 1919. The total mortality for the pandemic is estimated at 15–50 million deaths for all countries, closer estimates being impossible to ascertain. Estimates of the mortality by continents are shown in Table 14.7. In the U.S.A., over 500 000 deaths occurred and the estimate for the United Kingdom was some 200 000. In India, which recorded the highest mortality rate of any country from which data is available, an estimated 5 million persons died. Amongst Alaskan Eskimos, some settlements were reported to have suffered 100% mortality of the

Continent	Influenza mortality 1918–19
North and Central America	100 000
South America	300 000
Europe	2 200 000
Australia and Oceana	900 000
Africa	1 300 000
Total for all Continents	21 500 000

Table 14.7 Estimated mortality during the 1918–19 pandemic. (From Jordan, 1927, cited in Collier, 1974.)

adult population. It should be emphasized that the causative virus of the 1918 pandemic was not identified since virus isolation techniques for influenza were not then available. However, as described earlier in this article (section on animal influenza), there is circumstantial information suggesting that this pandemic was caused by the classical swine influenza virus (Hsw1N1) or a virus antigenically close to it. First, the initial appearance of swine influenza in pigs in the U.S.A. coincided with the onset of human pandemics. Second, antibody to the swine virus is present in a high proportion of individuals who were alive in 1918. It thus seems likely that the swine influenza virus isolated by Shope in 1930 was transmitted from man to pigs in 1918 and has remained since then as an endemic infection of swine in the U.S.A. The recent, 1976, isolation of swine influenza virus from man in the U.S.A. described above is of considerable potential importance possibly, but not necessarily, signalling the early stages of a new Hsw1N1 pandemic era.

The "Asian" influenza pandemic and the period 1957–68

The "Asian" (H2N2) influenza virus first appeared in Central China in February 1957 (Jensen, 1957). This virus possessed haemagglutinin and neuraminidase antigens showing complete antigenic differences (antigenic "shift") from the formerly prevalent H1N1 strain and probably represented the first antigenic shift in the influenza A virus since the pandemic of 1918 (Table 14.1). The new virus spread rapidly to other areas in Asia including Hong Kong, Taiwan and Singapore producing severe outbreaks. As early as June 1956, outbreaks occurred in several European countries (Czechoslovakia, the Netherlands, the United Kingdom), the Middle East and the U.S.A. In the Southern Hemisphere, epidemics reached South Africa and South America by July. By August, the epidemics in the Far East had subsided but, by late September, the U.S.A., northern areas of South America and the whole of Europe suffered rapidly evolving outbreaks associated with high rates of morbidity and mortality. The peak of the epidemic in the U.S.A. and Europe was in October 1957. Virtually every country of the world had been infected by the end of November 1957 (Dunn, 1958). The virus had thus behaved in a truly pandemic manner. Some countries, notably Japan and the U.S.S.R. in September 1957 and the United Kingdom

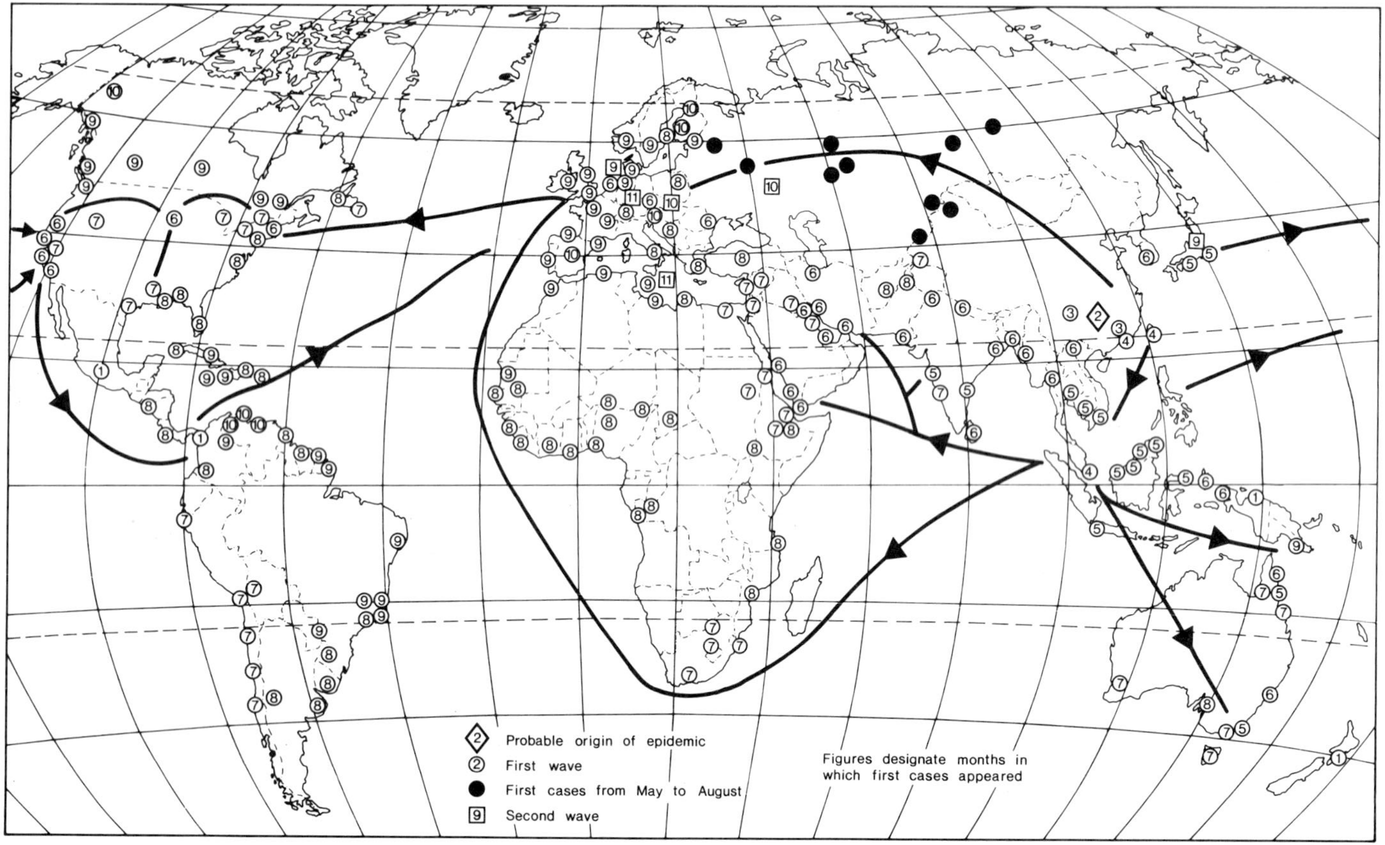

Fig. 14.6 Spread of "Asian" influenza, February 1957 to January 1958 (after Langmuir, No. 2, pt 2, p. 2).

and U.S.S.R. in early 1958, experienced second waves of infection. The early spread of the Asian virus is illustrated in Fig. 14.6.

The "Asian" virus produced high attack rates during the 1957–58 pandemic period which varied from 20–80% in different countries. Highest rates of attack were in the younger age groups of the populations and in areas of high population density (reviewed by Stuart-Harris and Schild, 1976). In the United Kingdom and U.S.A. (Woodall *et al.*, 1958; Langmuir, 1961), approximately 50% attack rates were recorded in the 5–15 age group.

It is of considerable interest that in 1957, before the circulation of the "Asian" virus, some 30% of serum samples from the aged persons (75–85 age group) were found to contain antibody to the "Asian" strain. This has been taken to indicate that the "Asian" virus of 1957 represented a reappearance of a virus which had circulated some 68–70 years previously. As already mentioned, pandemics occurred in the period 1889–90 which might therefore have been produced by an earlier emergence of the "Asian" virus.

During the following 10 years 1958–68, many influenza outbreaks due to the influenza A (H2N2) virus occurred. In general these had a small impact on mortality and morbidity in comparison to the first waves of the "Asian' epidemic. In the U.S.S.R., significant outbreaks occurred in 1959 but not elsewhere. In 1960 and 1963 widespread influenza occurred in many countries. Again, in 1965, widespread outbreaks occurred in Europe and the U.S.S.R. During the next 2 years, outbreaks were mild and sporadic but, in the winter of 1967–68, major influenza epidemics were documented in the United Kingdom and other European countries and in Taiwan and Australia. During this period, progressive antigenic "drift" occurred in the HA and NA antigens of the prevalent strains. These were typified by the A/England/12/64 (H2N2) strains which caused the 1965 outbreak and the A/Tokyo/3/67 (H2N2) strain which was involved in the outbreak during the winter 1967–68.

The "Hong Kong" pandemic and the period 1968–76

Although its true geographical origin is not known, the "Hong Kong" (H2N2) virus was first isolated during influenza outbreaks in Hong Kong in July 1968 (Chang, 1969). It has been suggested that outbreaks of respiratory disease on the Chinese mainland some weeks earlier were caused by the same virus but so far no confirmation of this has been reported from China. The virus spread rapidly in the Far and Mid-East regions, to India, Japan and Australia by the early autumn (Cockburn *et al.*, 1969). However, only the U.S.A. suffered major outbreaks with increased mortality during the winter 1969–70 (Sharrer, 1969). In other countries, although it was present in the population, the strain produced a relatively mild epidemiological impact. The full-blown effect of the Hong Kong pandemic did not occur until the next winter 1969–70 in Europe, Asia and most other areas of the world.

In the U.S.A., Hong Kong influenza produced more than 51 million illnesses during the epidemic of 1968–69, an incidence of 25% (Kavet, 1972). The disruptive effect of the epidemic is evident in that it caused excessive school absenteeism or closure in 24 states and elevated industrial absenteeism in 32 states. School-aged children (6–16 years) missed almost 35 million days from school (16% of the total number of days of school missed by all school children during the entire school year). Currently employed persons missed more than 66 million days from work, a figure which represented 22% of total annual days lost from work due to all acute conditions. An estimated 27 495 excess deaths were attributed to the epidemic. Roughly 37% of this total was attributed to influenzal-pneumonia. The mortality rate in the population at large was 14.0 per 100 000 population, the case fatality rate was 53.7 per 100 000 cases. Excess mortality increased with age, only 7% of the mortality occurred in the under 45 age group and 58% in age group 65 years and older. Approximately 42% of the cases of influenza reported to the National Health Survey received medical attention. This involved some 21 million medical consultations for patients not requiring hospitalization. Hospitalization was required for 640 000 persons who spent approximately 5.76 million days in hospital.

The differing chronology of the outbreaks in the U.S.A. and the United Kingdom is shown by the excess mortality data for these countries in the successive winters of 1968–69 and 1969–70 (Fig. 14.7) but is completely unexplained.

Table 14.8 shows the claims for sickness benefit due to influenza amongst insured persons in the United Kingdom. The Hong Kong outbreak of 1968–70 produced some 25 million lost working days during the period December 1969 to March 1970; this was

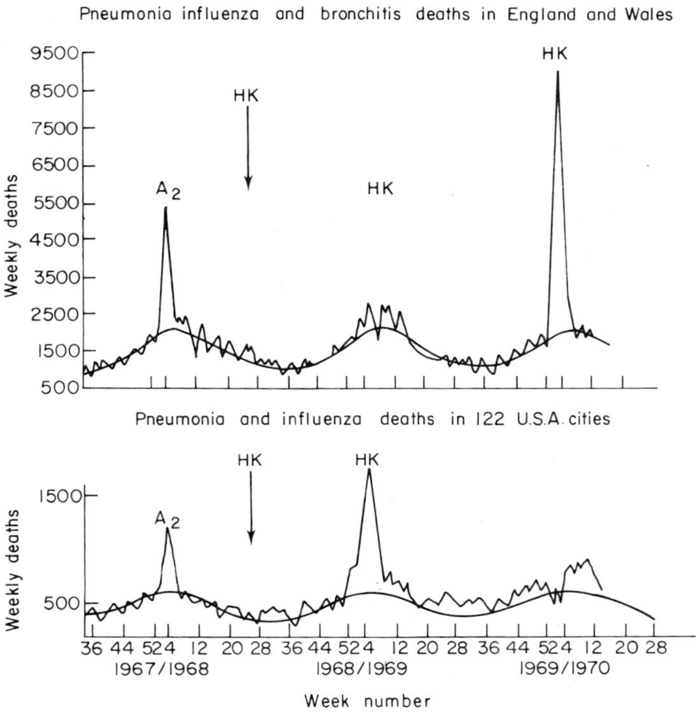

Fig. 14.7 Comparative mortality patterns in the United Kingdom and the U.S.A. from influenza and associated diseases, 1967–70. The first isolations of A/Hong Kong/68 virus in each country is marked thus $\overset{\downarrow}{\text{HK}}$. The mortality peak marked A2 was produced by outbreaks of "Asian" (A/Tokyo/3/67 (H2N2)) virus and those marked HK by A/Hong Kong/1/68 (H3N2) virus.

approximately 7% of the total lost working days for all causes during the whole year. In general, the Hong Kong pandemic was of less severity in terms of mortality and morbidity than was the Asian pandemic in 1957. The antigenic changes in the virus may provide a clue to its epidemiological behaviour. Whilst the HA antigen (H3) was completely different from that of the Asian virus (H2) the neuraminidase was of the same antigenic subtype (N2). Thus the Hong Kong virus showed only partial antigenic "shift". The common NA antigen of the Asian and Hong Kong virus may thus have contributed to a cross-immunity between these strains.

From 1970, recurrent influenza outbreaks have been associated with H3N2 viruses. Only the period of 1970–71 being free of influenza activity. Successive antigenic variants of the Hong Kong virus typified by the strains A/England/42/72 (H3N2), A/Port Chalmers/73 (H3N2), A/Scotland/42/72 (H3N2) and A/Victoria/3/75 (H3N2) have produced outbreaks of almost annual incidence in many countries. The most recent variant A/Victoria/75, first isolated in Papua and New Guinea in outbreaks associated with high mortality in autumn 1975 (W.H.O., 1975), produced severe outbreaks of disease in both Europe, including the United Kingdom,

Period June–May	Days claimed (millions) All causes	Influenza
1962–63	289	13.9
1963–64	287	9.4
1964–65	299	9.6
1965–66	312	16.7
1966–67	301	6.8
1967–68	328	15.5
1968–69	329	15.7
1969–70	342	25.7*
1970–71	314	6.6
1971–72	307	10.4
1972–73	320	13.6
Mean	312	13.8

* Hong Kong/68(H3N3) pandemic period.

Table 14.8 Sickness benefit claims due to influenza and all causes amongst insured persons in the United Kingdom (data from official U.K. statistics).

and in the U.S.A. during the winter 1975–76 which were associated with excess mortality rates higher than any since the 1968–70 pandemic period. The incidence of influenza in the season 1976–77 was low in almost all countries. Where viruses were isolated these often were A/Victoria/3/75-like. However several variants (A/Texas/1/77, A/England/321/77, A/England/932/77) were also isolated.

The extremely high rate of antigenic "drift" of the Hong Kong virus which for the past four years has produced variant strains at annual frequency is worthy of note (Schild *et al.*, 1974) and is in contrast to the relatively low frequency of antigenic "drift" of the Asian virus from 1957–68.

Influenza B epidemics since 1940

The first successful isolations of influenza B virus were made in 1940 in the U.S.A., although undoubtedly influenza B viruses had circulated before this time. Since 1940, the influenza B virus has been shown to produce outbreaks of disease in a number of countries. In the United Kingdom, these have occurred notably in 1946, 1950, 1962, 1965 and 1966. Outbreaks of influenza B in the U.S.A. in 1962 and 1966 were associated with increased mortality rates (Fig. 14.4). As mentioned above, excess mortality is not frequently associated with influenza B in contrast to the situation for influenza A viruses. Influenza B outbreaks may follow influenza A epidemics in the same community or may occur simultaneously with influenza A. It is infrequently that influenza B precedes influenza A outbreaks during the same season. However, this did occur in the United Kingdom in the winter of 1974–75. The influenza B virus typically causes localized outbreaks in children and sporadic cases in adults. In school populations, attack rates may be as high as 80% (Stuart-Harris and Schild, 1976) and school closures may frequently result from influenza B outbreaks. Influenza B undergoes progressive antigenic "drifts" but not "shifts". The most recent variant was first isolated in Hong Kong in 1972 (B/Hong Kong/5/72; Schild *et al.*, 1973). After 1972, this strain became the prevalent influenza B strain in the world replacing the former variant in a matter of 1–2 years in different countries and was the prevalent influenza B strain in 1976. The relatively infrequent periods of influenza B epidemic activity may be associated with the rather long time intervals between the appearance of antigenic variants of this virus.

IMMUNOPROPHYLAXIS OF INFLUENZA

Inactivated influenza vaccines for injection prepared from influenza antigens grown in fertile eggs and also live, attenuated vaccines for intranasal administration have been available for several years. The past few years have seen considerable technical improvement in the design and production of such vaccines. Modern inactivated vaccines have a somewhat variable protective efficacy which has been estimated at between 60–80% (Stuart-Harris and Schild, 1976), but considerably lower values have also been recorded. High rates of protection are dependent on the virus strain in the vaccine being antigenically identical or closely related to the prevalent epidemic strain(s) of virus against which it is required to protect. Modern vaccines of both types are well tolerated in adults but less so in children.

Vaccination programmes have not been shown in any country so far to prevent epidemics. However, it should be emphasized that routine vaccination in most countries has involved only a small proportion of the populations, usually the elderly, those at high risk and essential public service workers. Outstanding problems which have hindered the mounting of mass vaccination campaigns, even in developed countries of the world, are (a) the need for annual reformulation of vaccines so as to include up-to-date variants of influenza A and influenza B virus. This prevents preparation of large vaccine stocks in advance of requirements and means that only limited time is available for vaccine manufacture, especially in a pandemic situation, and (b) the need for annual reimmunization of individuals if immunity is to be maintained.

The current mass vaccination, employing inactivated vaccines, against swine influenza in the U.S.A. has established the technical feasibility of mass vaccination with inactivated vaccines. The success of this campaign will be viewed with interest and may prompt future extensive vaccination campaigns amongst other developed countries. Inactivated vaccines are expensive and are unlikely to be employed on a large scale by the poorer nations. It would seem likely that prevention of influenza on a world wide scale will have to await further developments with live attenuated influenza vaccines which may be prepared more rapidly and cheaply than inactivated vaccines.

REFERENCES

Andrewes, C. H., Laidlaw, P. P. and Smith, W. (1935). Influenza: observations on the recovery of virus from man and on the antibody content of human sera. *Brit. J. Exp. Path.* **16**, 566.

Assaad, F. and Reid, D. (1971). *Bull. W.H.O.* **45**, 113.

Assaad, F., Cockburn, W. C. and Sundaresan, T. K. (1973). Use of excess mortality from respiratory diseases in the study of influenza. *Bull. W.H.O.* **49**, 219.

Burnet, F. M. and White, D. O. (1972). National History of Infectious Disease (4th edn) pp. 202–212. Cambridge Univ. Press, London and New York.

Burnet, F. M. and Clarke, E. (1942). "Influenza". Monogr. No. 4, Walter and Ely Hall Institute, Melbourne, Australia.

Chang, W. K. (1969). National influenza experience in Hong Kong, 1968. *Bull. W.H.O.* **41**, 349–351.

Cockburn, W. C., Delon, P. J. and Pereira, W. (1969). Origin and process of the 1968–69 Hong Kong influenza epidemic. *Bull. W.H.O.* **41**, 345–348.

Collier, R. (1974). "The Plague of the Spanish Lady". Macmillan, London.

Creighton, C. (1891). "A History of Epidemics in Britain", Vol. 1. Cambridge University Press, London and New York.

Creighton, C. (1894). "A History of Epidemics in Britain", Vol. 2. Cambridge University Press, London and New York.

Davey, M. L. and Reid, D. (1972). *Brit. J. Prev. Soc. Med.* **26**, 28.

Douglas, G. R. (1975). "The Influenza Viruses and Influenza" (Ed. E. D. Milbourne) pp. 395–443. Academic Press, New York and London.

Dowdle, W. R., Coleman, M. T. and Gregg, M. B. (1974). National history of influenza type A in the United States. 1957–72. *Prog. Med. Viol.* **17**, 91–135.

Dunn, F. L. (1958). Pandemic influenza in 1957—a review of international spread of the new Asian strain *J. Amer. Med. Ass.* **166**, 1140–1148.

Easterday, B. C. (1975). "Animal Influenza in the Influenza viruses and Influenza" (Ed. E. D. Milbourne), pp. 449–478. Academic Press, New York and London.

Francis, T. J. (1953). Influenza: The newe acquayantance. *Ann. Atern. Med.* **39**, 203.

Hemmes, J. H., Wiulderke and Kool, S. M. (1960). *Nature, Lond.* **188**, 430.

Hirsch, A. (1883). "Handbook of Geographical and Historical Pathology", Vol. 1, p. 7. New Sydenham Society, London.

Hope-Simpson, R. E. (1958). *Proc. Roy. Soc. Med.* **51**, 267.

Jensen, N. E. (1957). New set of type A influenza viruses. *J. Amer. Med. Ass.* **164**, 2025–2029.

Jordan, E. A. (1927). *In* "Epidemic Influenza", cited in Collier, 1974.

Kavet, J. (1972). Influenza and public policy. Doctorate thesis, Harvard Sch. Publ Hlth, Cambridge, U.S.A.

Kilbourne, E. D. (1975). *In* "The Influenza Viruses and Influenza" (Ed. E. D. Kilbourne) pp. 483–539. Academic Press, New York and London.

Langmuir, A. D. (1961). Epidemiology of Asian influenza. International Conference of Asian Influenza. *Amer. Rev. Resp. Dis.* **83**, 2.

Langmuir, A. D. and Housworth, J. A. (1969). A critical evaluation of influenza surveillance. *Bull. W.H.O.* **41**, 393.

Melnick, J. (1973). Classification and nomenclature of viruses. *Prog. Med. Virol.* **15**, 380.

Pereira, M. S. (1976). The role of epidemiological surveillance in the immunoprophylaxis of influenza. *Postgrad. Med. J.* **52**, 323–326.

Reid, D. (1975). Personal communication.

Schild, G. C. and Dowdle, W. R. (1975)."The Influenza Viruses and Influenza" (Ed. E. D. Kilbourne), pp. 316–368. Academic Press, New York and London.

Schild, G. C. and McGregor, I. (1976). *W.H.O. Weekly Epidemiological Record* **6**, 46.

Schild, G. C., Pereira, M. S., Chakraverty, P., Coleman, M. T., Dowdle, W. R. and

Chang, W. K. (1973). Antigenic variants of influenza B virus. *Brit. Med. J.* **4**, 127.

Schild, G. C., Oxford, J. S., Dowdle, W. R., Coleman, M., Pereira, M. S. and Chakraverty, P. (1974). Antigenic variation in current influenza A viruses: evidence for a high frequency of antigenic drift for the Hong Kong virus. *Bull. W.H.O.* **51**, 1.

Schulman, J. L. and Kilbourne, E. D. (1963). *J. Exp. Med.* **118**, 267.

Serfling, R. W., Sherman, I. L. and Housworth, W. J. (1967). Excess pneumonia—influenza of age and sex in three major influenza epidemics in the U.S.A. *Amer. J. Epidem.* **86**, 433–441.

Sharrer, R. G. (1969). National influenza experience in the U.S.A. 1968–69. *Bull. W.H.O.* **41**, 361–366.

Shope, R. E. (1931). Swine influenza III filtration experiments and aetiology. J. Exp. Med. **54**, 373.

Smith, J. W. G. (1977). Surveillance of influenza. Public Health Laboratory Service, London. Unpublished report.

Smith, W., Andrews, C. H. and Laidlaw, P. P. (1933). A virus obtained from influenza patients. *Lancet* **ii**, 66.

Stuart-Harris, C. H. and Schild, G. C. (1976a). "Influenza—the Viruses and the Disease", pp. 22–75. Edward Arnold, London.

Stuart-Harris, C. H. and Schild, G. C. (1976b). "Influenza—the Viruses and the Disease", pp. 77–95. Edward Arnold, London.

Webster, R. G. and Laver, W. G. (1975). Antigenic variation of influenza viruses. *In* "The Influenza Viruses and Influenza" (Ed. E. D. Kilbourne), pp. 270–314. Academic Press, New York and London.

Woodall, J., Rowson, K. E. K. and McDonald, J. C. (1958). Age and Asian influenza. *Brit. Med. J.* **2**, 1316.

W.H.O. (1971). A revised system of nomenclature for influenza viruses. *Bull. W.H.O.* **45**, 119.

W.H.O. (1975). *W.H.O. Weekly Epidemiological Report* **43**, 366.

W.H.O. (1976). *W.H.O. Weekly Epidemiological Report* **14**, 108.

Part Two

15. Industrial Lung Disease

G. E. Ffrench

Man is not born to solve the problems of the universe but to find out where the problem lies and then to keep within the limits of what he can comprehend.

(Geothe, "Conversations with Eckermann").

HISTORICAL REVIEW

The tools of food-gathering Palaeolithic man were crudely fashioned in contrast to the wonderful naturalistic and mystical cave paintings which symbolized his understanding of life. About ten-thousand years ago, his successor, Neolithic man, started a revolution in tool-making and took the first steps in agriculture which were to lead, without interruption, through the Copper, Bronze and Iron Ages to the time when recorded history began, some five-thousand years ago in Egypt, Mesopotamia, India and China. These Neolithic tools, often finely polished, of remarkable quality and functional design, must have been created in physical conditions which were often unsavoury. There is archaeological evidence in Suffolk, England that industrial specialization began during this early Neolithic period. It was here that flint, a quartz of almost a hundred percent silica, was chipped and shaped: it continued to be worked there in the traditional manner known as "knapping" until less than 50 years ago. From the evidence of silicosis and tuberculosis in these latter day flint workers, it can be surmised that silicosis has a fair claim to be the oldest industrial disease.

The flint knappers generated by their hammering a large amount of fine dust. Middleton took samples of atmospheric dust at breathing level of two men knapping flints. The counts gave up to 1313 particles per milli-litre, with two per cent of particles over two microns in diameter. They worked in ill-ventilated sheds and undoubtedly had silicosis and suffered a high mortality from phthisis. (Hunter, 1957.)

The coincidental improvements in tool-making and the introduction of metals undoubtedly led to the developments in agriculture which succeeded in producing food, fuel and fibre. Animal husbandry required the production of fodder and clothing the invention of the primitive loom. Flax was the staple fibre from which ropes, mats, nets and cloth were made. From our present knowledge of allergic respiratory conditions associated with the storage of hay, cotton, flax and coarser fibres, it is reasonable to suppose that some of these illnesses may have been experienced by prehistoric man (Fig. 15.1).

The subsequent five-thousand years of written history suggest that dust deposition in the lung continued to plague man in the pursuit of tool-making and fashioned articles, large and small: among the earliest were the temples and pyramids of Egypt, built principally of hewn granite blocks, sometimes faced with limestone. Sigerist (1951) records the hardships of the stone masons of four-thousand years ago. The cutting, shaping and polishing of granite, which gives rise to quantities of silica-containing dust, must have taken its toll although there is no remaining evidence of this; not until many centuries later was the mummification of the common man practised.

Hippocrates, in the 5th century B.C. was in no doubt that those who dug for metal and smelted the ore suffered severely for their trouble. They were ravaged by consumptive disease, a product of the dust and the ever-present tuberculosis. Four centuries later, in the Egypt of the Ptolemies, Diodorus Siculus recounts the conditions in the gold mines of Nubia: here again the silica-containing dust of the gold-bearing quartz would have been the offender. He describes

... streaks and veins of a remarkable whiteness, the lustre of which surpasses the most brilliant natural products. From this earth, those who have charge of the mining operations obtain the gold by means of a large number of workers, for the kings of Egypt collect condemned prisoners, prisoners of war and others who, beset by false accusations, have been in a fit of anger thrown into prison; these, sometimes alone, sometimes with their entire families, they send to the gold mines . . . the hardest of the earth that contains the gold is exposed to fierce fire, so that it cracks and then they apply hand labour to it; the rock that is soft and can be reduced by a moderate effort is worked by thousands of the luckless creatures with iron tools that are ordinarily used for cutting stone. Of those who are condemned to this disastrous life such as excel in strength of body pound the shining rock with iron hammers, applying not by skill but by sheer force to the work, and they drive galleries, though not in a straight line, but in the direction taken naturally by the glistening stone.

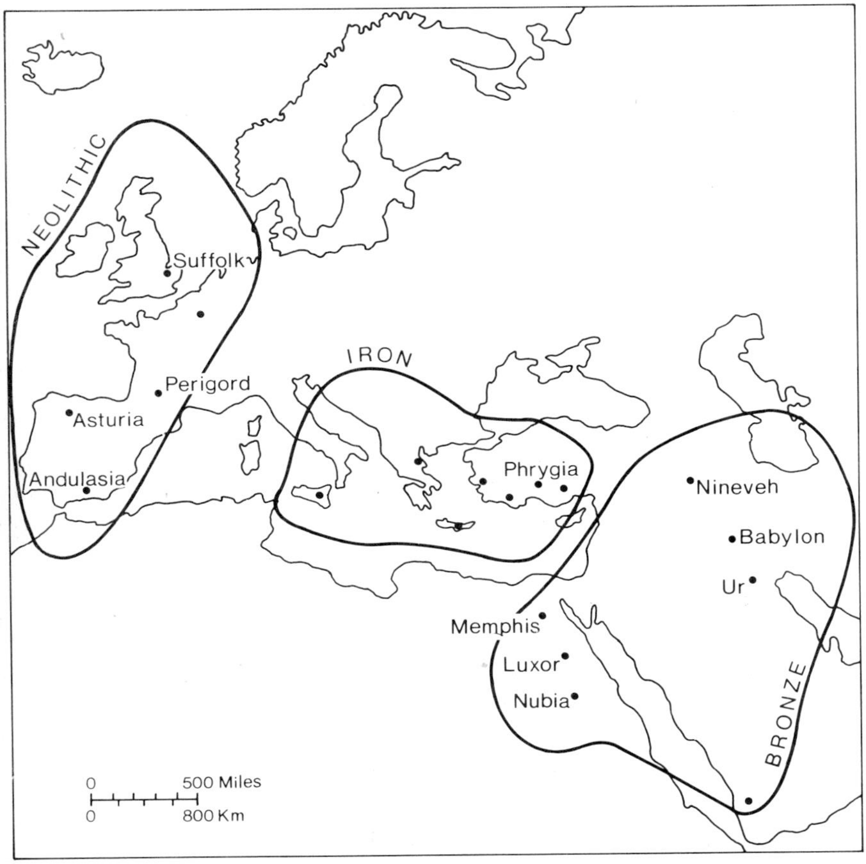

Fig. 15.1 Geographical areas in the Western World where Neolithic, Bronze and Iron Age man ran the risk of industrial lung disease.

These quartz streaks or lodes within the country rock are characteristic of the mining of gold.

Sigerist (1951) chides us that

> we like the reliefs and paintings that adorned the interior of tombs and temples and give such a vivid picture of Egyptian life. But we often forget that these creations, great and small, are the result of the labours of millions of anonymous people, slaves and serfs and small freemen who toiled for a bare living, who often sacrificed their health and their life for the enjoyment of a small upper class.

Impressed labour of this kind has continued to be used to this day in different parts of the world but seldom are we made aware of any industrial diseases that may be suffered by these latter-day slaves.

A century later, Pliny the Elder (A.D. 23–79) provides the first description of efforts to prevent the damage caused by breathing asbestos dust during mining operations by the use of crude pumps and protective masks. Asbestos was then a very precious substance out of which sacred cloth and shrouds were made. By the 15th century, the crafts and metal industries throughout Europe had developed a distinctive pattern. Their noxious effects, however, stimulated a number of observant and curious physicians, imbued with the Galenic tradition but eager to describe their experience. First came Ulrich Ellinbog in 1473, followed shortly by Paracelsus (Theophrastus Bombastus von Hohenheim, 1493–1541) and Agricola (George Bauer, 1494–1555), all with experience in the mining and industrial centres of Bohemia during the Middle Ages. Agricola was the first to recognize the true nature of miners' diseases and made the greatest contributions towards prevention up to that time. His descriptions of mining methods, ventilation practices and dust suppression are models of graphic and technical precision. Another century was to elapse before the first unequivocal demonstration of the pathological effects of dust on the lungs was made by Isbrand van Diemerbroeck (1609–1674) of Utrecht in his postmortem studies of men who had died with the "stone-cutters' disease". The pace was quickening: within 50 years the "father of occupational medicine", Bernadino Ramazzini (1633–1714), Professor of Medicine at the Universities of Modena and Padua in

Italy, had published his classic "De Morbis Artificum". This unusual man took the trouble to see for himself the conditions of the lowliest worker over a broad range of the industries of his day, from mining to the measuring of grain and from cheesemakers to corpse carriers. These were then, and indeed still are, occupational lung hazards. He pleaded that particular attention should be given to workers in the dusty trades and made recommendations that could not be faulted today. The study of occupational lung diseases received further encouragement from Linnaeus in 1741, on the occasion of his inaugral lecture as Professor of Medicine at the University of Upsaala. He asked the question and demanded an answer, "Why do all the men of Orsa die of grindstone phthisis before they are thirty?" (Hendschen, 1967).

Among the early workers in this lethal field was Charles Turner Thackrah (1795–1833). This young physician devoted his life to the study and prevention of disease in the dusty trades in the West Riding of Yorkshire, England. He made a particular study of the cutlery grinders of Sheffield. His work was cut short by tuberculosis but remains an object lesson to those who explore the fascination of occupational medicine (Thackrah, 1831).

This brief historical review is completed by two London physicians, T. B. Peacock and E. H. Greenhow who, in 1861, differentiated the specific dust diseases of miners from the frequently accompanying tuberculosis. Ten years later the Italian physician, Visconti (1870) coined the term "silicosis". This, by its sonorous yet sombre implication, immediately suggests the nature of the poison and the fate of the victim. It is rather ironic that a century later efforts continue to be made to complete their work, the emphasis now being directed to a definition of the fair and legal position of chronic bronchitis.

Until recently, these historical associations have tended to restrict industrial lung disease to mining and metallurgy. Today there is an infinitely wider range of industrial activities with which it is linked, some of them seemingly far removed from the environments of traditional "industry". They exert their effects through physical and biological action dependent upon the nature of the agent itself, the atmospheric conditions in which it exists or is activated and the prevailing situation in the lungs.

CLINICAL CONDITIONS

The agent occurs in the form of dust, fume, smoke, gas and aerosol droplets. Strictly speaking, it is only dust which causes pneumonconiosis (Greek, *pneuma* breath, *konia* dust), silicosis being but one example, although the most grievous. The dusts and aerosols can be of mineral, vegetable, synthetic, chemical and biological origin (Fig. 15.2): in addition certain mineral dusts may be radio-active. Their molecular construction, particle size, shape, aerodynamic qualities, concentration and total mass reaching the lungs over a working life are the important criteria (Beadle, 1971).

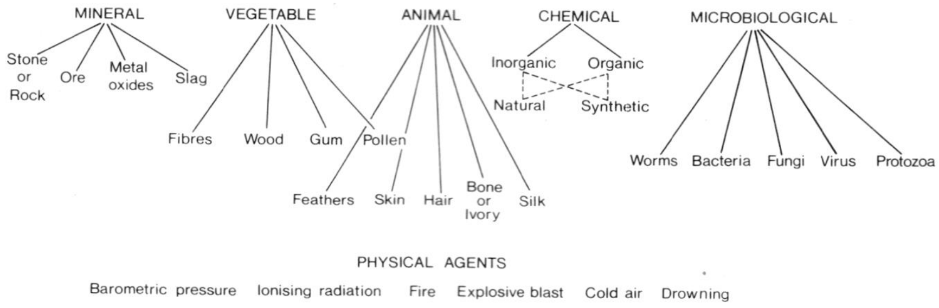

Fig. 15.2 Agents known to be implicated in industrial lung disease.

Local atmospheric conditions.

These relate principally to those associated with the environment in which the job is being done. Temperature and humidity, particularly the absolute humidity, are the main governing factors. Air movement can be paramount in blasting operations and in forced air ventilation and in those situations where minute amounts of irritating or sensitizing material, such as epoxyresins or isocyanates, are all that are needed to provoke acute symptoms. Of these materials, certain wood dusts are perhaps the most frequent, though mild, offenders. Peculiarities of the occupation sometimes provoke a significant increase in the incidence of a disease: the predominance of byssinosis in certain groups of card-room workers in cotton mills is related to the excessive dustiness when the carding machines are being cleaned in contrast to when they are in use.

There has been little practical outcome from the work which has been done on the effects of atmospheric ionization and the influence of magnetic fields: it would seem that dust diseases offer a challenging field here. Again changes in barometric pressure of the atmosphere in mining, while sometimes not inconsiderable, have received little attention. In Peru, there is an institute which studies the health of miners who work at heights up to 3900 m. In Brazil, India and Africa, there are mines which descend to nearly that depth. In the case of underwater diving and other situations in the occupational field where barotrauma is a hazard, e.g. in hospitals where operations and treatment may be given in high pressure chambers, the danger of explosive decompression has to be anticipated. Again, high explosive blast and the very hot air of fires may severely damage lungs. In contrast, the very cold dry air of either great heights or the polar regions may precipitate acute disease of the lung.

Within the past 40 years, evidence has accumulated that radon gas and its daughters are responsible for ionizing damage to the lungs of miners. Cancer of the lung has long been observed in the metal mines of Schneeburg in Germany and Joachimstal in Czechoslovakia. More recently, the danger has been observed and the hazard measured in uranium and other metal mines and in the flourspar mines in Newfoundland, Canada. In Newfoundland, the problem has been well studied because of the static nature of the work force. Elsewhere, because of the mobile nature of the mining population, this has proved difficult, particularly so in the case of Africa.

In less developed countries, where primary ore production is not infrequently the major industry and where social and living conditions may dictate a communal living and sleeping pattern, the constant breathing of stale and smoke-laden air, together with the increased chance of tuberculosis from close human proximity, may provoke both acute and chronic forms of lung disease. These have special relevance to industrial lung disease but, until the emergence of the Third World as a secondary industrial producer, such observations that were made were of little general interest. The earlier exploitation of the world's mineral wealth, often located in remote and inaccessible places, together with the growing of food and fibre in the plantation industry, preceded the now widespread public, economic and moral concern.

The ill effects of poor working conditions in the mines, so characteristic of Europe until well into the 20th century, were repeated among populations previously remote from such insults. Many of these peoples became migrant and intermittent workers, showing little resistance to disease, of which the occupational component may not have been recognized sufficiently early. The definite but still imperfect control under which many of these diseases now come, together with the recognition of the various component factors and specific clinical and pathological effects, justifies a short description of those processes which operate inside the lungs and contained bronchi following exposure to industrial pollutants.

Prevailing situation in the lungs

The constitution and susceptibility of the individual worker have assumed a growing importance following the identification of a number of features which may govern the response to disease-provoking agents. The predisposition of the lung will depend very much on the insults it has already had to suffer, particularly infection in youth and irritation from cigarette smoking. The importance of cigarette smoking in the overall picture of industrial lung disease has been recognized for only a comparatively short time. It complicates the assessment of specific causes, potentiates their effects and plays some part in the different geographical patterns and prevalence of disease. Little data is available to do more than speculate, except in those conditions associated with an increased prevalence of lung cancer. Asbestos and uranium mining are well-documented examples (Selikoff *et al.*, 1968; Lundin *et al.*, 1969). Consumption of cigarettes throughout the world has escalated. In 1900, only 12% of tobacco in the United Kingdom was used for cigarette making; by 1970 this figure had reached 80%. During this period, the Virginian-type tobacco used in cigarettes gained in popularity at the expense of Egyptian, Turkish and other local oriental tobaccos. Cigarette import and manufacture figure prominently in the priority lists of developing countries and certainly march with the improvement in the standard of living. The problem is further compounded by those Governments which have encouraged the replacement of food crops with cash crops.

Previous lung infection and chronic irritation may interfere with intrinsic defence mechanisms. When there is also an inbuilt cellular failure, such as genetically-controlled enzyme (alpha anti-trysin) deficiency, the lung may be especially at risk. To date no useful geographical studies of its distribution have been reported. The presence of the enzyme is essential for the gas exchange surface of the lung tissue to resist expansion and ballooning (Kueppers and Donhardt, 1974). It is convenient to illustrate the functioning units of the respiratory system diagrammatically (Fig. 15.3). Areas 1 and 2 in Fig. 15.3 comprise the conducting system and areas 3 and 4 represent the gas-exchange unit together with the lung coverings or pleura.

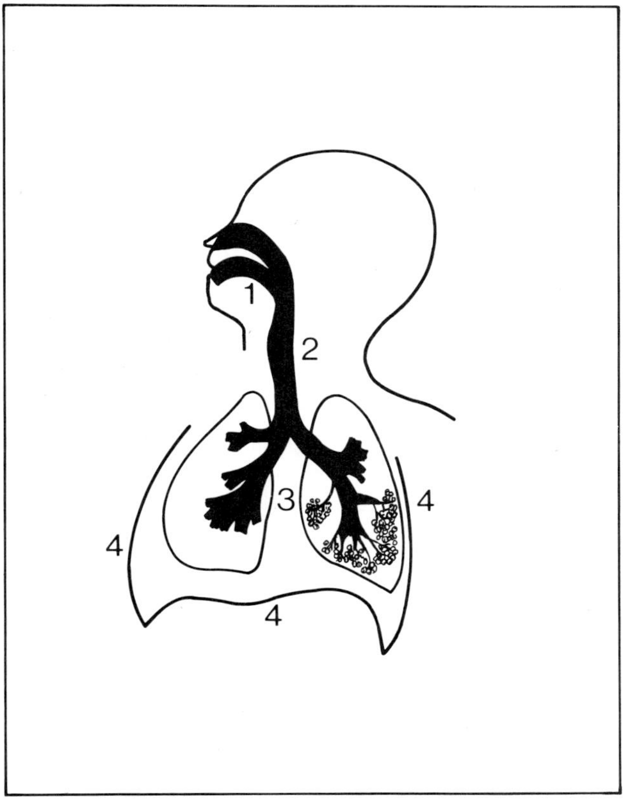

Fig. 15.3 The functioning respiratory system. 1. Oro-pharynx and larynx; 2. trachea and main bronchi; 3. intra-pulmonary bronchi and gas-exchange unit (alveolus); 4. lung covering or pleura.

The principal events that occur in industrial lung disease are, in order of frequency rather than importance, irritation, dust deposition and blockage of fine drainage channels, hypersensitivity reactions and immune response and malignant change. These events may arise severally or together.

Irritation

This causes inflammation of the lining membrane of the bronchi with destruction of the fine brush-like, dust-removing cilia, increased secretion of mucus, contraction of smooth muscle in the walls of the smaller bronchi and disruption of the lace-like walls of the air spaces with ballooning of the lung leading to a reduction of the capacity for gas exchange. These effects are known respectively as bronchitis, asthma and emphysema which together create the clinical picture of obstructive lung disease.

Dust deposition and blockage of drainage channels

The smaller dust particles in the range 0.5–10.0 μm, which can remain suspended in air for relatively long periods, are breathed in and reach the interstices of the lung where they may aggregate as they come to rest. This may happen with remarkably little tissue reaction as exemplified by miner's candle soot, tin and fibre-glass. Most dusts stimulate the tissue to try and remove them. This is accomplished in the main by special scavenger cells which take up the particles and penetrate deep into the lung, moving along channels which eventually lead to lymph nodes. Depending on the reactionary quality of the dust, these may become replaced by scar tissue. Their *raison d'etre* is the containment of foreign matter and the maintenance of an efficient immunity state. Certain dusts may gradually dissolve in the tissue fluids but the solutes continue to irritate. Other dusts such as the long fibres characteristic of the various forms of asbestos (a fibrous silicate) may penetrate far into the lung. They may reach its covering and cause considerable damage to blood vessels and the production of scar tissue thereby restricting the lung's elasticity or compliance. Malignant change is their final weapon, either within the lung itself or its covering, the pleura, the dreaded mesothelioma (Tables 15.1 and 15.2).

Year	Ontario	Quebec	Other Provinces	Canada
1960	—	6	9	15
1961	1	6	3	10
1962	4	4	5	13
1963	9	3	7	19
1964	6	8	3	17
1965	7	7	5	19
1966	8	14	9	31
1967	6	13	6	25
1968 (1st half)	5	9	2	16
	46	70	49	165
Incidence/ Million/Year 1960–67	0.8	1.5	0.9	1.0

Table 15.1 Primary malignant mesothelial tumours in Canada.

Sometimes there appears to be a reduced prevalence of cancer of the lung tissues in those dust diseases associated with a large amount of scar tissue. This has been observed in miners who have developed their silicosis in South Wales, and may be due to the restriction of the growth of cancer cells in a medium with very poor blood supply. This, however, is no more than supposition.

Asbestos mine mill	3
Textile manufacture	4
Brakeline installation	2
Insulation	5
Other occupations but contact with insulation material	5
Hardware store (handling asbestos sheet and pipe)	1
Filled gas masks with asbestos textile	1

Table 15.2 Distribution of occupations classified under "definite" and "probable" in 21 men exposed to asbestos (McDonald *et al.*, 1970).

Hypersensitivity and immunity phenomena

Hypersensitivity or allergy is still incompletely understood. In its simpler forms, it is commonly experienced as "hives" or hay-fever. More severe effects, sometimes leading to sudden death, involve vital organs such as the brain, heart, lung and kidney. Hypersensitivity is closely related to the main defence mechanisms in the body, collectively known as immunity. The secrets of immunity are now being decoded at an exciting rate.

Whereas immunity was originally studied in relation to infectious, disease hypersensitivity has long been known to involve a wide range of substances ranging from highly complicated molecular structures to simple metal elements. Hypersensitivity creates a sudden chemical and cellular confusion which disrupts the tissue cells and, through interference with vital supply channels, causes local death.

Immunity is dependent on the ability of the body to recognize foreign substances and is now known not to be restricted to infectious agents. It produces an organized defence by mobilizing specific and non-specific pre- and newly-formed protein antibodies of intricate structure which lock-on to the foreign substance in an attempt to defuse it. The unceasing introduction of new substances into our living and working environment and our food and medicines, has kindled a widespread appreciation of the dangers. It is in this field of immunity response that recent work in industrial lung disease has produced encouraging results, particularly so in the agricultural, asbestos and coal industries (Blyth, 1973; Turner-Warwick, 1973; Wagner, 1971).

Cancer induction

The emotive tocsin of the word cancer may produce a paradoxical obliviousness of the long-term dangers of those few substances so far known to induce it: cigarette smoke, asbestos, certain metals, in particular nickel and chromium, and ionizing radiation. Recently, epidemiological evidence of the hazard of new chemical agents such as bischloro-methyl-ether has come to light. The manner in which these differing substances exert their effects still largely eludes the researcher. Opinion is hardening in the view that there occurs an interaction between immunologically and perhaps genetically-influenced tissue cells and a chemical or physical irritant or sensitiser of peculiar and insidious quality and intensity. Already geographical studies have contributed usefully towards the understanding of cancer (Cook and Burkitt, 1970).

ENVIRONMENTAL RELATIONSHIPS (SOCIAL, ECONOMIC, PHYSICAL)

Industrial lung disease has a fearful history and its reputation has taken longer to die than many of its unfortunate victims. Viewed against the social and industrial background of yesterday in Europe and North America and in the developing world today, it is surprising that so many people survived and continue to do so. The analogy with infectious disease will be noted. It is appreciated now that in the past many of the specific industrial lung diseases have been complicated by infective disease, the two most important being chronic bronchitis and tuberculosis. While tuberculosis has specific implications in certain occupations, principally medical, dental and nursing staff, together with human laboratory workers, chronic bronchitis, because of its proclivity for temperate climates, is not easily classified occupationally. Chronic bronchitis is high on the contemporary list of industrial lung diseases, although there is an awareness that important provoking factors lie outside the occupational environment.

Social, educational and literacy standards, cultural habits, nutrition and local disease provide the key as to whether or not industrial lung disease will strike sufficiently hard to be recognized (Fig. 15.4). The whole relevance of preventive medicine and occupational health education pivots on these factors, whether the deficiency is in the acrid smoke of the communal cooking fire or the ability to read and understand instructions given for safe working practice.

For centuries, certain kinds of industrial workers have either been imported from an exotic source *en masse* or migrated voluntarily in search of money and an improved standard of living. Today these migrant populations comprise a powerful industrial and political force. Nevertheless, there are still many industrial areas where local populations have not been diluted and where, for many years, whole

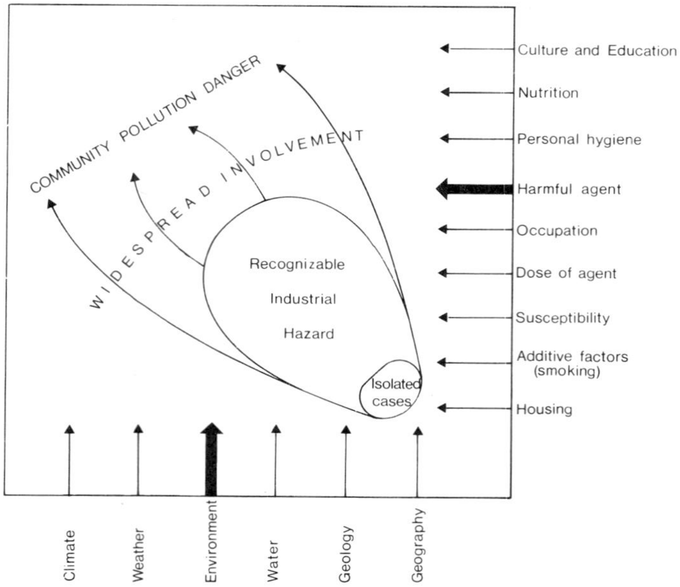

Fig. 15.4 Schematic presentation of the influence of geofactors (geogens) in industrial lung disease.

families have obtained their livelihood, sometimes at hard cost to their health. In the United Kingdom, the mill towns of Lancashire, the valleys of South Wales and the upland coal-mining villages of Durham attest to this.

Exactly what influence the different races and ethnic groups, indigenous and exogenous, may have on the disposition to overt lung disease is difficult to assess. It would seem more a question of social and cultural factors than any in-built susceptibility, apart from the case of acute pneumonia and tuberculosis. Experience has shown that most indigenous workers are better adapted to the local working environment, where this is above or below ground than are exogenous workers. Work patterns and rhythms differ markedly. This could be significant in lung disease since the total volume of air and mass of dust breathed over a working life is now considered to be important when measured against serial lung function studies. In making assessments for certain industries, the migrant worker and his occupational history constitute the main defeating element. During a working life he may have breathed a variety of dusts in different conditions and in different parts of the world. One classical example of this was that of the tin miners of Cornwall who went to work in the South-African gold mines for a number of years only to develop silicosis on their return to Cornwall (Fig. 15.5).

With the increasing longevity of western industrialized populations together with falling numbers employed in certain industries, the seeming contradiction of lower incidence (new cases) rates with increasing prevalence (number of cases at a given moment) rates appears confusing. It is however a classical feature of modern demography and one that complicates the picture of industrial lung disease (Amoudru, 1972). In addition, full employment in some countries has given partially disabled workers the opportunity to seek other employment. This has been seen in the cotton textile industry and in coal mining and has reduced the reliability of statistical studies, especially mortality rates (Schilling, 1960).

Certain races do exhibit specific differences in their reaction to injury and infection in addition to differences in cancer morbidity. Some of these differences seem to be sensitive to geographical as well as genetic and nutritional factors; studies in the U.S.A., Ireland and Japan have confirmed this. There is no doubt that the negro race has a disposition to develop bizarre tissue reactions during the defence and healing processes. This is shown by the incidence of keloid scarring of the skin and the granulomatous sarcoid reaction which may take place in the body tissues, particularly in the lungs (Young, 1971). Faced with particular meteorological and other environmental conditions, some industrial populations appear to be particularly prone to acute pneumococcal lobar pneumonia. This has been the experience among the migrant Bantu miners of the South-African gold fields and the stable Dravidian miners of the south-Indian gold

	Kolar Gold Field South India			Consolidated Main Reef South Africa		
Year	Underground	Surface	Total	Underground	Surface	Total
1948	18.4	11.9	16.07	19.5	8.5	17.5
1949	14.6	9.3	12.3	14.1	5.7	12.3
1950	17.8	13.4	16.3	12.4	6.06	11.9

Table 15.3 Lobar pneumonia. Incidence per 1000 in Dravidian miners of the South-Indian gold fields and Banta miners of South-African gold fields.

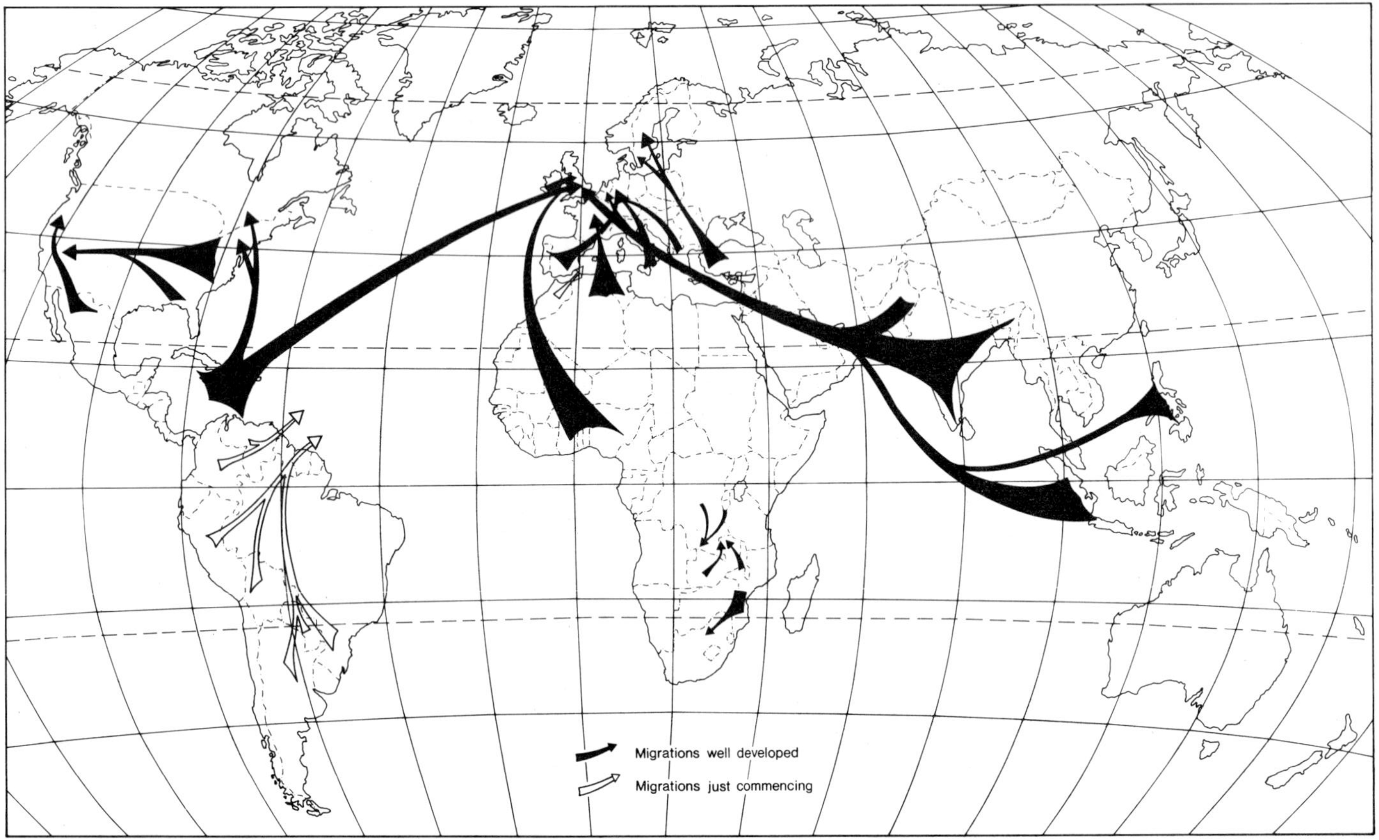

Fig. 15.5 Migrations of semi-skilled and unskilled labour, 1948–74.

fields: frequency here is nearly 20 times that of populations in temperate climates. At the time these observations were made, dust deposition in the lung was not considered to be a relevant factor.

Consideration of the social and organizational structure of industry itself is a prerequisite in any discussion. The nature of employment and whether it is regular or intermittent; the qualitative selection of the workers and the form of their training, particularly the understanding they are given about the hazards of manufacturing processes and the avoidance of risk. Then come the steps taken by industry to reduce those risks either by introducing good quality supervision of the control of environmental conditions or introducing alternative methods. This may be expensive and not immediately profitable where labour is transitory or prolific and remote from the public eye. Examples can be given where industries have been set up in developing countries either by private or government enterprise, only to find that within a few years a serious situation threatens. This has been particularly so in the case of asbestos products. Countries which publish their experience are to be commended (Chew *et al.*, 1973; Chevat and Mordish, 1964). Similar examples are found in older industrialized countries. The policy followed by some governments of gentle persuasion to adhere to factories acts and similar regulations, rather than a policy of coercion and strict enforcement, continues to allow unsafe practices and toxic materials to damage the health of workers. Newer countries have the opportunity to introduce stricter law enforcement and ideally should consider such a policy in preference to the opportunities for evasion under lighter control.

Statutory requirements to control industrial disease, which to a greater or lesser extent influence the prevalence within a country, are patterned either upon the experience of an older-established industrial country or upon a more standardized form of legislation. The International Labour Office in Geneva has for many years acted as advisor to a host of countries. On a more regional level, the E.E.C. countries have accepted the requirements of the Treaty of Rome (1957) in principle if not in practice. There is not, however, any international system for any world-wide collection and notification of industrial lung disease. Neither do safety standards command world-wide agreement. There are several puzzling discrepancies on toxic levels of airborne pollutants between Western-type industrialized countries and Eastern bloc countries. Such discrepancies may reflect the ability of the countries of the Eastern bloc to impose more stringent requirements rather than any formal disagreement. On occasions, the Western standard has been raised to conform with more "conservative" levels, but on the whole the Western countries follow the recommendations of the American Conference of Governmental Industrial Hygienists (1971).

Since the beryllium compound to which the patient is exposed as well as the character of the exposure tends to vary considerably from industry to industry, some distinctive histological pattern might be expected if this were a highly significant variable. As noted [Table 15.4] however, the distribution of histological patterns is essentially the same regardless of the source of the case. This is also true of the "neighbourhood" or non-worker cases, all but one of whom were exposed in the extraction and smelting industries. The results strongly suggest that dosage as measured by both intensity and duration of exposure may well be more significant than the exact nature of the active compound, and this is in agreement with clinical experience. It is also probable that the reactivity of the host plays a significant role, since not only do many workers equally fail to become ill, but the histological pattern of reaction varies widely even within the same industry. (Freiman and Hardy, 1970.)

Because of legal and other restrictions on the availability of important information, breakdowns in communication and even the non-acceptance of facts when they are received, there can sometimes be a failure to anticipate possibilities. This may well account for the almost explosive reappearance of coalminer's pneumoconiosis and silicosis towards the end of the last century, following the introduction of mechanical coal cutting machinery and pneumatic drilling equipment respectively. More recently, an abrupt increase of severe and progressive lung and other organ disease came shortly after the Second World War, when beryllium compounds began to be used in ever increasing quantities in the production of fluorescent and neon lighting. This was perhaps the first occasion when women workers became measurably affected by serious lung disease. Even so, the effects of beryllium in the extraction and smelting of the metal had been known for 25 years. Beryllium ceased to be used for these purposes in 1949, but its short history allowed an important clinical and pathological resemblance to sarcoidosis—a disordered reaction to infection with tuberculosis and possibly other agents—to be studied (Table 15.4).

The chances of such accidents persist. They demand a degree of alertness and anticipation which, in this specialized age, may sometime be wanting. In the geographical context, this may be illustrated by the problems of the respiratory fungal diseases (mycoses) and ionizing radiation. Throughout the New and the Old Worlds, the diffusion through, though not necessarily the disablement of, significant proportions of a population by certain soil fungi (which may be isolated from different animal habitats) is now recognized. Foremost among these fungi are the yeast-like *Histoplasma capsulatum* and the morular-like *Coccidiodes immitis*. The relation of infections by soil fungi to modern communications and industrial development has been reviewed by Campbell (1967) who emphasizes the fact that the respiratory mycoses, like certain (mostly tropical) other diseases are entities which follow in the wake

Industry	Group 1 Sub-group 1A	Group 1 Sub-group 1B	Group 2
Extraction smelting	21	15	5
Fluorescent lamp high phosphor	9	11	3
Low phosphor	5	6	7
Neon	6	3	0
Alloys	3	2	2
Machining metal	4	1	4
Ceramics	3	1	2
Cathode	0	2	2
Atomic	1	1	0
Research and development	2	2	0
Odd jobs in research areas	1	0	0
Total	55	44	25

Table 15.4 Histological classification of chronic beryllium disease in U.S.A. industry.

of expansion and progress in industry and medicine. The particular foci in which these potentially pathogenic organisms flourish become hazards to an incoming population only when the soil is broken up by ploughs, planes, cultivators, bulldozers, drills, tanks and trucks. Experience during the cutting of the Panama Canal illustrates this. Whereas the Canal itself was not opened for traffic until 1914, the ground had been dug and excavated intermittently since 1876 when the ill-fated French attempt under de Lesseps failed because of disease among the workers. Campbell (1967) makes the point that the first infection with *H. capasulatum* was diagnosed in 1906 in the Panama Canal Zone. It has subsequently become a well recognized infection among poultry raisers in the Ohio river valley in the U.S.A. and elsewhere and specifically among those who investigate caves where there are large accumulations of bat guano. *C. immitis*, on the other hand, has been reported frequently among citrus-fruit growers, particularly in south-western United States. It should be emphasized that in the infections cited and in others of a similar nature, the overt clinical cases are a small quantum of the much larger general population infection, which can be verified epidemiologically by skin and serological tests.

The exposure of miners to ionizing radiation has been mentioned earlier. The sources of the radiation are sometimes least expected and not necessarily related to the minerals being extracted. This was illustrated in the case of certain West-Newfoundland fluorspar mines, when a lung cancer mortality 21 times greater than that of the Province was discovered. The multicoloured nature of the fluorspars (calcium fluoride)—used mainly in the production of steel—was thought to be related to radioactivity. However, it transpired that the Newfoundland fluorspar contained only traces of uranium. Instead a heavy flow of ground water into the mines was responsible for conveying with it significant quantities of radon (Holaday, 1969).

Respiratory irritants, sensitizers and cancer-provoking agents conveyed into the home on the body and on clothing can cause disease among the family members. Together with such factors as the quality of housing, washing and smoking habits, and parasites and fomites which may respectively inhabit their bodies or litter their domestic environment, these agents may be provoked and potentiated to compound an already dangerous situation at work. The degree to which this risk is appreciated will be reflected in the efforts made to

Area	Range (WL)*
European mines	10–180
U.S. Uranium mines	2–200
Newfoundland	2.5–10
U.S. metal mines	0.5–1.5

These figures are estimates only. They represent conditions which probably continued for weeks; extreme values were not included. The American uranium mines show a much larger range than do other areas because of the much larger number of mines and much greater variation in ore bodies, types of host rock and mining practices.

* WL or working level is equivalent to any mixture of RaA, RaB, RaC and RaC in one litre of air which will release 1.3×10^5 MeV of alpha energy in their decay to RaD.

Table 15.5 Possible range of radon daughter concentrations.

educate and provide conditions which will prevent them. For this reason, an industry should be considered in relation to the social conditions in which its workers and families live. The study by Waddy (1952) of meningococcal infection among migrant crop gatherers in West Africa came sufficiently close to the clarification of the pattern of coal workers' pneumoconiosis throughout the United

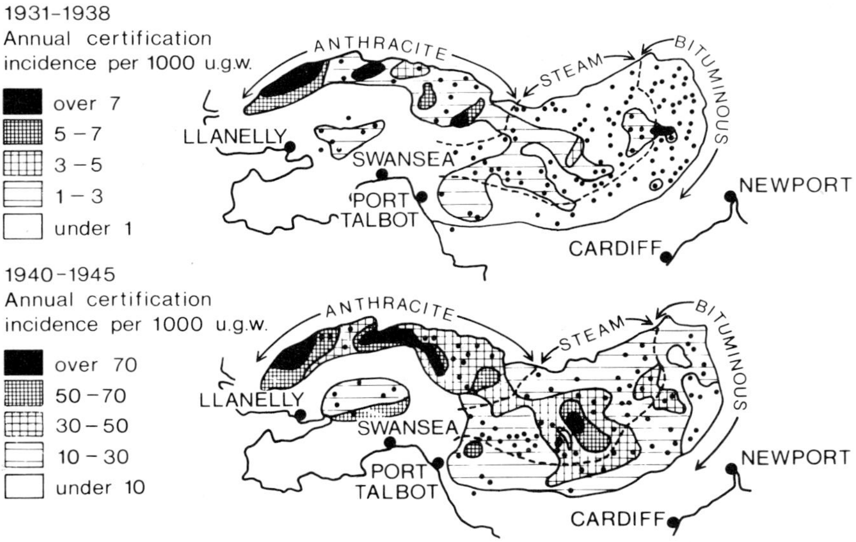

Fig. 15.6 Incidence of certified silicosis and pneumoconiosis in South Wales, 1931–38 and 1940–45.

Kingdom (Hart and Aslett, 1942; Fletcher, 1948) as to stimulate a re-appraisal of an old problem, i.e. the total conditions under which man lives and works. An early result was the suggestion that the incidence of coalworkers' pneumoconiosis was inversely proportional to the rank or percentage of volatile material in the coal. Anthracite and steam coal with a low percentage of volatile material had a higher incidence of pneumoconiosis than bituminous coal with its higher proportion of volatile material. Such findings have not stood the test of time neither in Britain nor elsewhere. Most recent opinion suggests that "this apparent effect is adequately comprehended by measuring the concentration of respirable dust in mass as opposed to particle count units" (Jacobsen *et al.*, 1971). It is necessary therefore to appreciate that the spatial relationship of disease and specific environmental factors do not, *per se*, imply a casual relationship.

DISCUSSION

The method of presenting this present study has raised a number of difficulties, not least being that of deciding the relationship of the geographical distribution and the factors which have been discussed. One major defect has been the absence of precise world-wide statistical data upon which comparisons may be based.

The use of a map with political or administrative divisions would seem to be the most sensible on which to superimpose distributions. The governing needs in searching out lung disease should be to find the answers to the questions, "what is done where and by whom?" A fair and reasonable corollary might be to add, ". . . and to whom go the profits?" No attempt will be made in the present study to answer this last question.

Distribution maps of industries known to provide the type of environment with which lung disease is associated answer the questions "what?" and "where?" An answer to the question "by whom?" requires a more discursive approach since the industrial worker of today is a relatively complex being, very often mobile or a migrant whose previous occupational history may not be available.

The main components of industry are (a) primary-producing enterprises such as mining, plantation, crude oil recovery, forestry and farming, and (b) secondary industries such as metal smelting, fabrication and assembly, plastics feedstock and hydrocarbon refining, sugar and molasses, wood pulping and paper production, together with a host of manufacturing undertakings in which raw or refined materials are subjected to a variety of physical, chemical and biological processes. Examples are motor vehicles, textiles, plastics, asbestos products, electronics and engineering. The plotting of industries has necessarily been somewhat crude, the information coming from a variety of sources. By no means all the industries mentioned have been reported to be associated with either nuisance or killing lung disease. The majority which have are of the primary group. Industrial processes are constantly changing. Dirty processes are being replaced with remote control or enclosed machinery, and new materials and products are being introduced which vastly improve the use to which the final article may be put. Some new products have proved insidiously harmful.

It is important, therefore, to discover beforehand whether people are likely to develop illness after exposure to industrial agents. Screening programmes are by no means universal and have been restricted in the main to large and wealthy organizations which have already experienced a major health problem and seek to avoid further repercussions. However, self-selection into various forms of work has been a feature throughout the western world and in some areas, until recently, it had been a tradition for the local industries to be worked by the local population as typified by coal-mining and cotton and wool textile industries in the United Kingdom. To date, there have been government requirements in certain countries only which stipulate that suitable people, in the sense that they are judged healthy as a result of their medical history and examination, should be employed in specific trades and industries. Some 10 years ago, a questionnaire was introduced in the United Kingdom by the British Medical Research Council which has served as a model for research and screening programmes in many parts of the world and has proved of great value in standardizing results (M.R.C., 1966). The effects of selective screening programmes must inevitably reflect on the distribution of lung disease over and above any "on the job" medical and engineering control. The paramount need is for a social conscience in industry and those who invest in it. Fortunately, there are many examples of the beneficial effects of an enlightened company health policy (Craw, 1964).

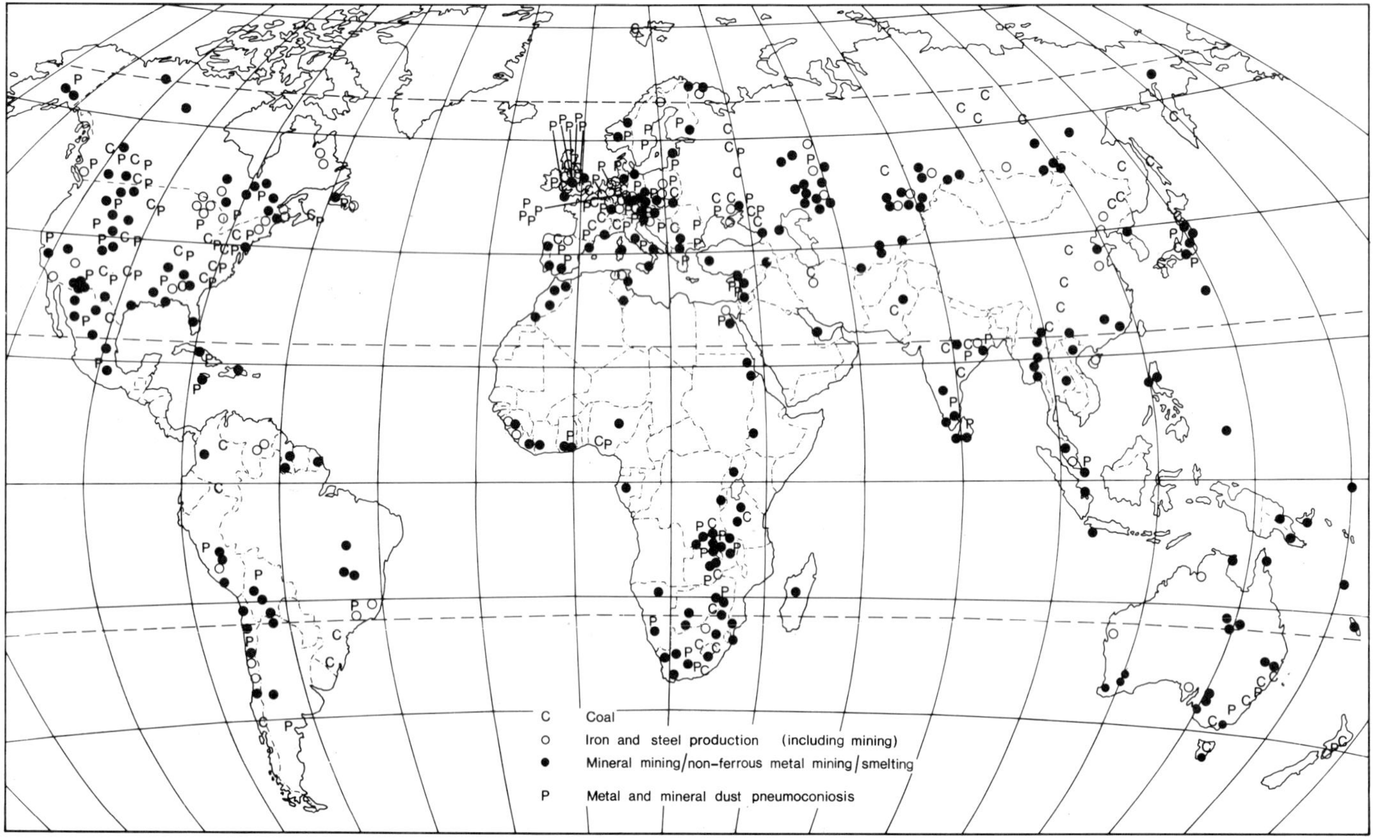

Fig. 15.7 Mining, steel production and related pneumoconiosis.

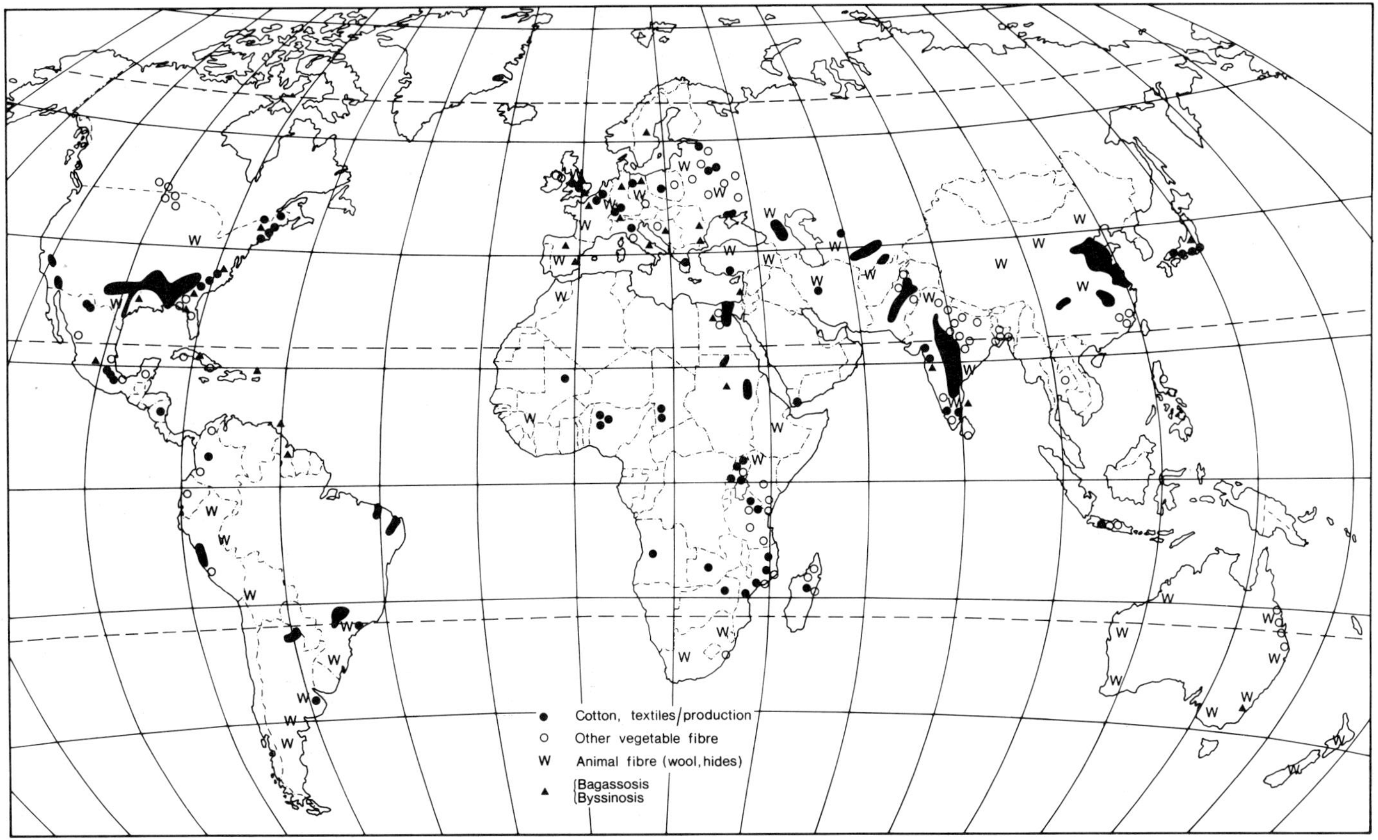

Fig. 15.8 Production of natural fibres and textiles and related diseases.

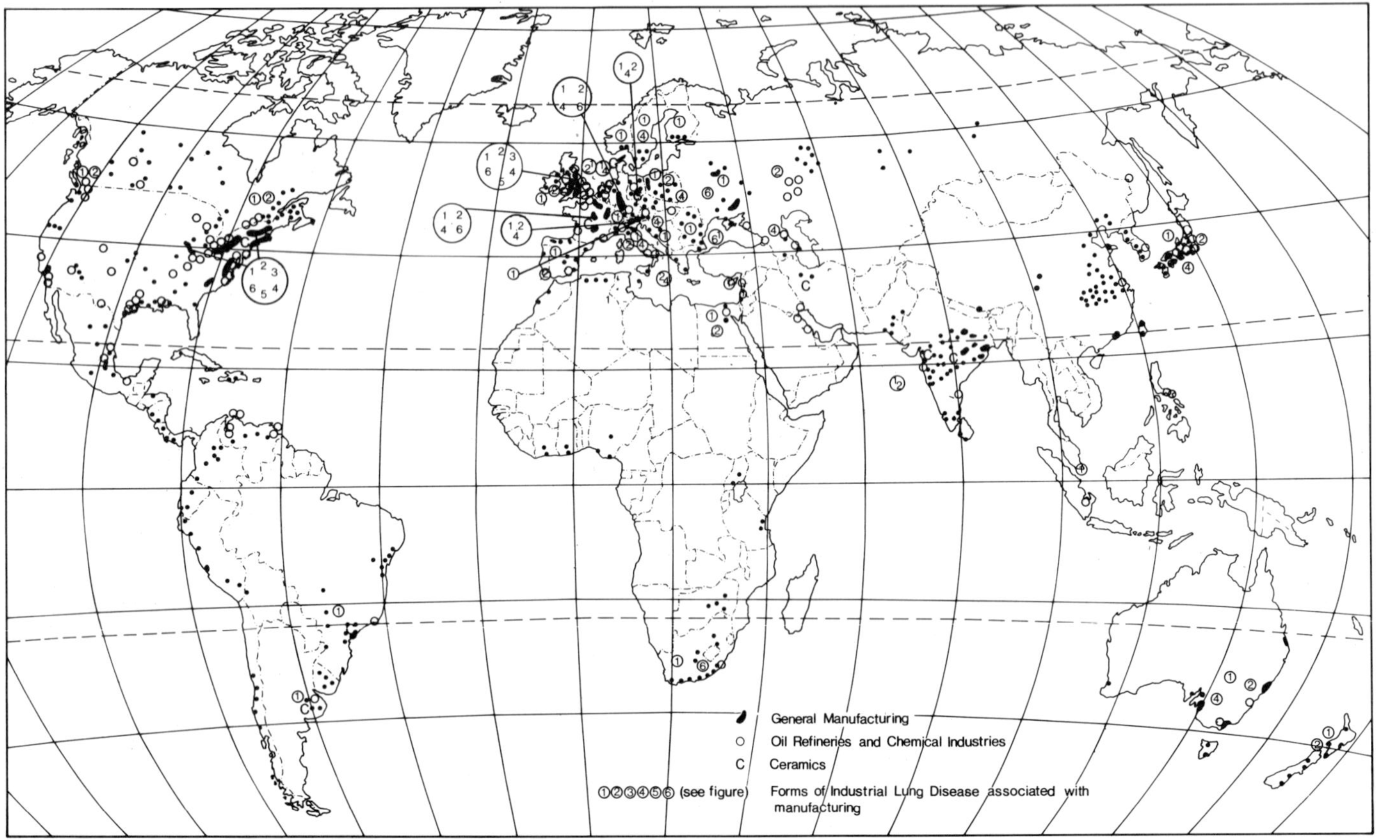

Fig. 15.9 General manufacturing, including crude-oil production and related diseases.

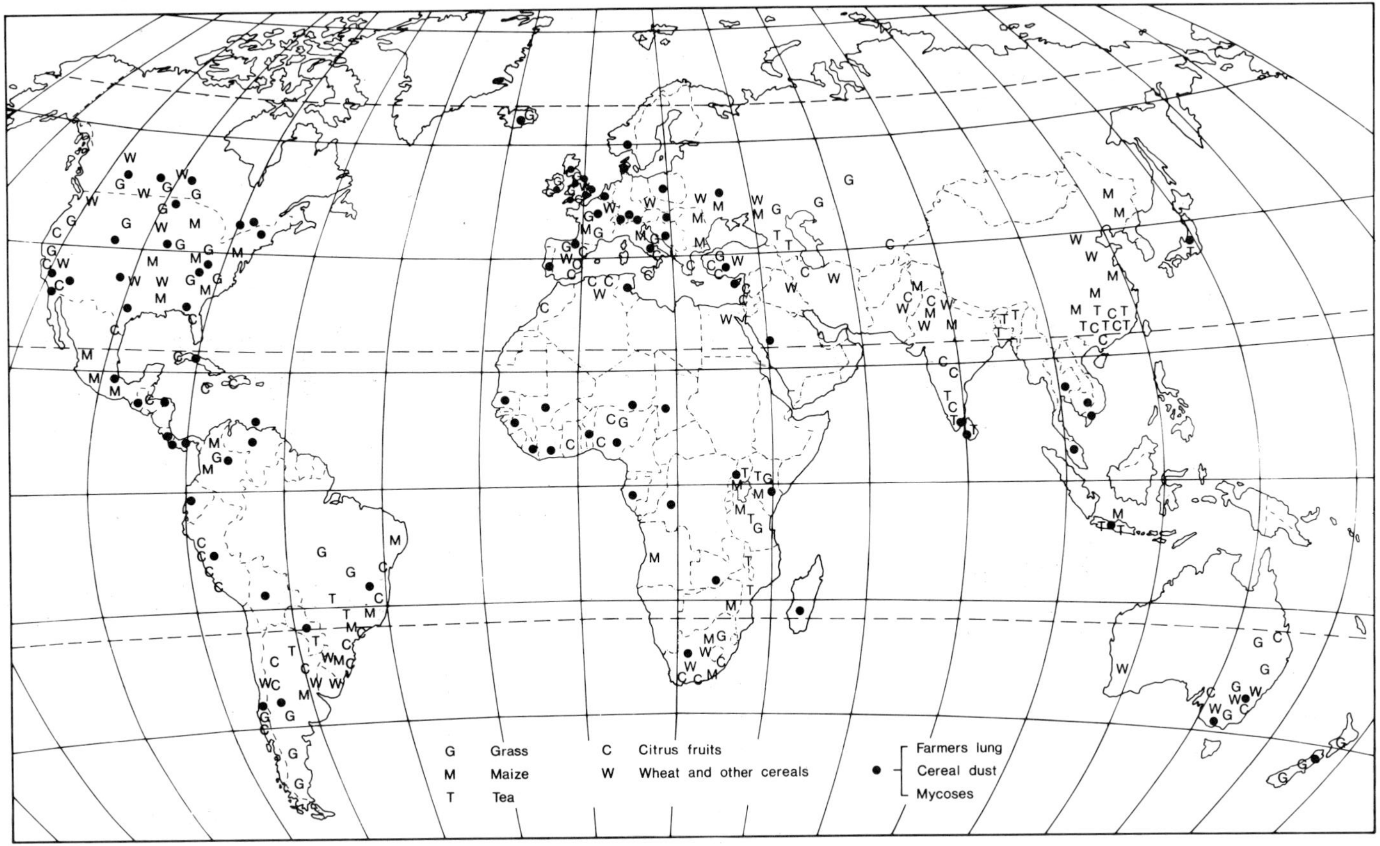

Fig. 15.10 Grass, cereal and citrus production and related diseases.

Schepers (1955), reviewing the situation on the South African gold mines at that time, said

> . . . the occupational disease problem . . . may be summed up as revealing overall favourable progress. Conquest is, however, by no means yet in sight. The fact that large numbers of extremely robust white miners nevertheless develop disabling disease within about 20 years indicates but one thing: there is still too much harmful dust being breathed by these men. Assuming that the generally "satisfactory" dust levels reported in official statistics are representative of mining conditions at all times, one is forced to the conclusion that the "ideal" dust level of 200 particles per cubic centimetre is not yet satisfactory. The engineers may have to adjust their sights once more. It is difficult to imagine precisely how this can be done having regard to the rigid precautions which are already enforced by government and the fabulous amounts already spent by the mine owners to meet the specified requirements.
>
> Pessimism concerning the increasing prevalence of these diseases among the negro labourers may be tempered with the thought that in the absence of existing engineering and medical control the situation would have been infinitely worse. It is rather obvious, however, that the occupational diseases among these employees need much more exhaustive study. This is logical but rather more easily proposed than carried into effect, having regard to the rapid personnel turnover, language and cultural barriers and the difficulty in obtaining technically qualified personnel for such an ambitious project.

Now, 20 years later some of the social and political scenes have changed little, and yet industrial disease continues to press. It is fundamental to any successful preventive programme that not only should the engineering and medical control be good but that there should be no administrative inadequacies. This is the point at which local, national and geographical traits may combine to deny success.

The pneumoconioses were first named because of their relation to the many varieties of hard and soft rock dusts and thus bore a geographical reference to the rock strata which was being worked. Today the pneumoconioses embrace a much wider range of materials, whose effects may be experienced in places far removed from their origin. This emphasizes the fallibility of applying geological map data uncritically. Again the potteries industry in the United Kingdom (North Staffordshire) provides an example of the operation of the distance or transport factor. Three hundred and fifty years ago when the industry was established, the raw materials, principally clay from Devon and Cornwall and flint from the chalk hills of the South of England, were carried, first by pack horse and mule and later in the 18th century by boat on the then new canals. A current instance is the condition known as byssinosis, a hypersensitivity disease due to some contaminant of the cotton dust which infects it somewhere along the journey from the cotton plant in the producing country to the card-room in the manufacturing country.

At the beginning of the recent spate of interest in human ecology Audy (1954), at that time a medical research scientist in Malaya, said

> in due course, there is always more or less urbanization of the community and at the same time more frequent traffic with other places. Many diseases, especially epidemic diseases, appear by introduction from areas which may be remote, to be added to a distinct urban pattern of disease. Traffic between urban centres leads to a dispersal of diseases and a tendency for urban patterns to be similar over very wide areas. Many urban epidemics tend to involve the rural population secondarily. Finally there may be industrialization which evokes its own elements in the disease-patterns. These individual diseases are, like the rural diseases, often very closely related to the geographical background: an example is the pneumoconioses, which are related to the geology.

As already noted, this situation is no longer wholly true but is now very much related to the dispersal and synthesis of materials of all kinds. Here lie perhaps the greatest dangers, because they may be unexpected and involve smaller and less protected groups of workers, particularly returning migrants. Audy's work at that time dealt with assemblages of parasites. "My object is to relate the parasite patterns of various communities to those elements of human existence and behaviour which themselves reflect the geographical background in one way or another." The biological action of many of the causative agents of the pneumoconioses may simulate that of a parasite for their continued existence and sequestration in the lungs is gained at the ultimate expense of the host and they contribute no benefit when in the particulate state. Audy, in his study of 20 000 animals and their parasites in Malaya, found that the parasite patterns of a community of animals differed among themselves in different communities, and that the parasite pattern is directly related to the environment and to the conditions of life experienced by the host. Here the analogy with the pneumoconioses is clearer, the inference being that the ecology must be examined. But whereas parasites are dependent upon a balanced ecology, the virulence and persistence of industrial agents in a community rely upon unsteady conditions, the occurrence of which may be intermittent.

With the exception of agriculture, climatic factors as distinct from weather play relatively little part in occupational lung disease. However, in arid countries where underground mining is undertaken, sufficient water to reduce and wet the dust may not be available. This has created appreciable problems in dust control in mines in the Sudan, Israel and Pakistan. On the other hand, the underground atmosphere of miners in humid climates can become very oppressive and limit the work output of even the most acclimatized miners. This may be accompanied by a significant reduction in the amount of air and mass of dust breathed. Local microclimates may thus be all-important, whether they arise and are maintained as a result of the industrial process itself or are man-made in order to facilitate that process. Occasionally, the weather plays a significant role, usually synergistically with specific occupational factors. In the coal mines of South Wales, bronchitis was thought in the past to have some relation to cold ventilation air causing severe chilling when the miners were leaving their work. Other factors may well have been responsible, not least the coal dust itself and cigarette smoking.*

The problem of acute lobar or pneumococcal pneumonia in gold miners in South Africa and India has been referred to above. The one significant variable appears to be the absolute humidity of the air at the time when miners reach the surface or during their passage from underground to the surface. In 1926, L. Rogers demonstrated this relationship in India with both lobar pneumonia and small-pox; low absolute humidities showed a close correlation to epidemics of both diseases among the general population. The positive influence of cold dry air on the incidence of influenza and respiratory disease has been discussed recently by Tromp (in Howe and Loraine, 1974).

Geographical data relating the density of the overall and occupational health services including post-graduate medical and nursing training and research, might be productive. The collection of material with a view to subsequent publication in the medical and scientific press is certainly stimulated by the presence within the country of doctors or others who have received training in this field,

* Cigarette smoking is of course forbidden in the mines themselves.

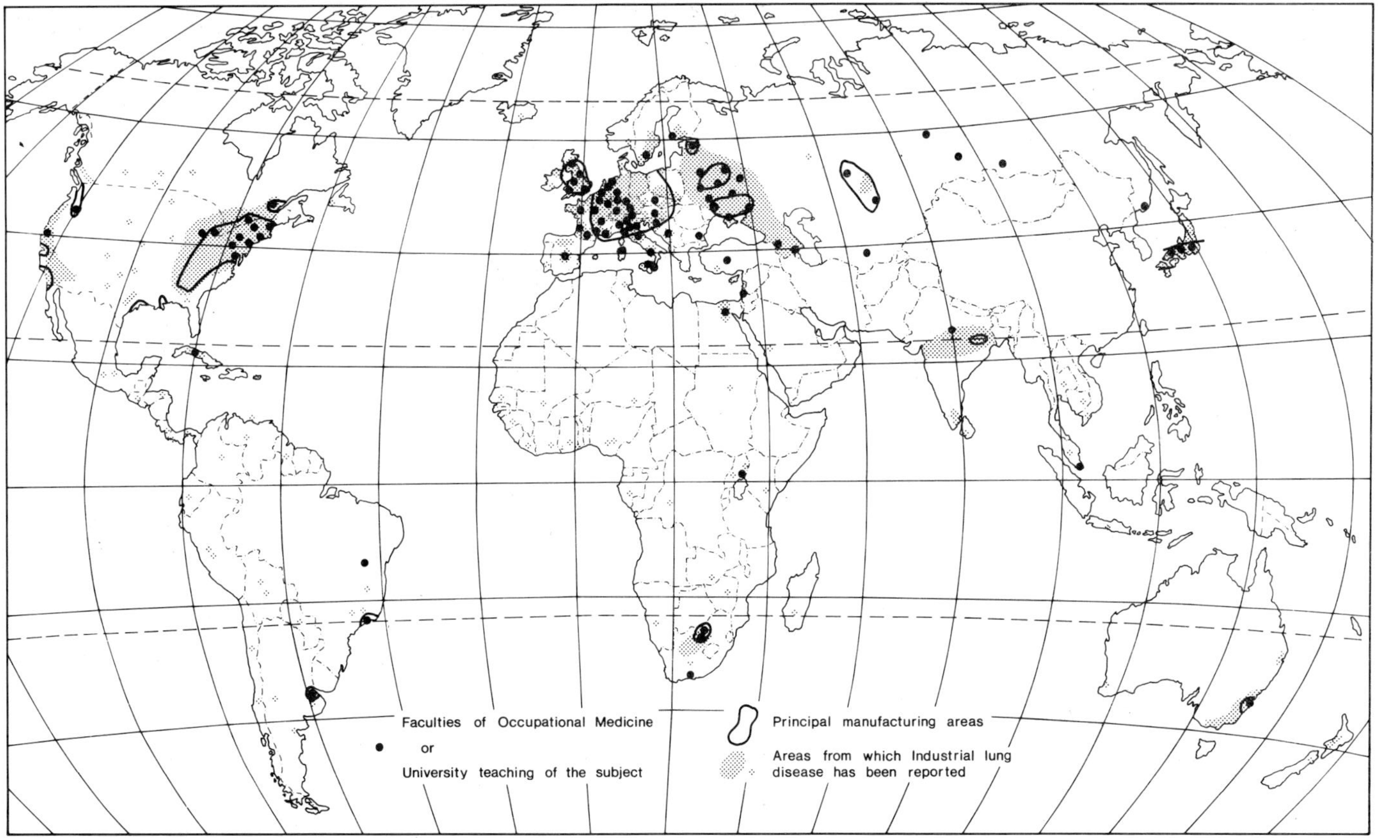

Fig. 15.11 Occupational health training.

e.g. Dar es Salaam Group Occupational Health Service. At present, the diagnosis and assessment of these conditions require technical facilities not always readily available and which may not be judged to have a priority in existing national-health services. In the United Kingdom for instance, preventive full-size chest screening of all exposed workers is not yet accepted as a charge on the public purse and has been left to individual industrial organizations, private and nationalized, and to government-backed research units whose responsibility rests in special fields.

The establishment of internationally-agreed criteria for diagnoses rests also upon these technical services which, in addition to good clinical units, must have the support of laboratory, radiological and autopsy studies. For a developing country, such studies can be a heavy commitment. Autopsy in particular may not be acceptable on cultural and religious grounds. The notification of industrial lung disease is a statutory policy in those countries with a pneumoconiosis compensation programme but terminology and classification are not universal. In Mexico for instance, the prevalence or otherwise of silicosis is uncertain because of the tendency for doctors to diagnose "fibrosis" from very slight X-ray changes which may or may not have been the result of dust exposure. In such cases, compensation is granted for the "fibrosis", the degree of disability being established by a compromise between a company physician and one representing the trade union. Approximately 4% of miners are said to be granted disability awards but the incidence of true silicosis is probably a small fraction of this (Nelson, 1967). This may be a problem elsewhere, as it has long been so in Italy. Certainly the definition of disability may be difficult since undue emphasis is given to radiological changes unsupported by functional measurements. Discrepancies in training and experience together with social and political motivation and intervention may obscure the picture.

A technical problem of mapping the relevant conditions lies as much in the complexity of symbols required to identify the factors ("geogens") as in the difficulty of collecting geographical data. The preparation of a map and its successful interpretation are not easy to equilibrate. To this end simplicity has been the guide. Political boundaries only have been used; demographic, geological and climatological influences are not indicated. Neither has any attempt been made to show what might be described as the dynamics of industrial lung disease, related as it must be to the establishment and growth of industry, the migration of workers and the evolvement of new techniques. Asbestos is perhaps a good example of the last of these, for with the control of the dust and lessening of the pulmonary fibrotic disease, increased longevity of workers has allowed for the development of specific forms of malignant disease.

The information presented is at best speculative and not amenable to statistical analysis or testing. It is selective in so far as the data is dependent on the information available in original published papers. Only broad categories of industrial lung disease are indicated in an endeavour to steer a path between the jargon of medicine and geography.

The material studied comes from several sources* some overlapping and necessarily restricted in time. Much of the older disease has been conquered and is no longer reported. The morbidity and mortality sequelae of earlier disease are, however, of current interest and continue to be studied. There must inevitably be, in a summary of this kind, numerous gaps for which apologies are made. A feature of many of the original reports from which information has been drawn has been the incompleteness of useful epidemiological, geographical and sociological data by which an integrated study, whether by computer graphics or more simply by "a piece of paper and a box of coloured pencils" could be assembled. If and when a wider study is contemplated, it might be possible, through a universal application of a standard questionnaire, to obtain this information. This would certainly constitute a grand design and industry would be well suited for this kind of exercise. It would certainly complement the type of pneumoconiosis register suggested

* These include the Proceedings of the 9th, 11th, 12th, 13th and 14th International Congress of Occupational Medicine (1948–63) and the Proceedings of the International Conference on Pneumoconiosis at Johannesburg 1969. The CIS cards of the International Labour Office Information Service have been scanned for the period 1964–73 together with the Excerpta Medica. A MEDLARS search for the period 1968–73 was also undertaken. The following publications of I.L.O., Geneva have been particularly helpful, viz. No. 16 International Directory of Occupational Safety and Health Services and Institutions, No. 19 International Directory of Occupational Safety and Health Courses, and No. 24 4me Rapport International sur La Prevention et la Suppression des Poussieres dans les Mines, Les Galeries and Les Carrieres. Finally, "The Nurse's contribution to the Health of the Worker" published by the Nursing sub-Committee of the Permanent Commission and International Association on Occupational Health in 1969 (obtainable from 42 Paternoster Close, Waltham Abbey, Essex) was consulted.

some years ago by Murray (1970). Throughout the world in the different government archives, doubtless statistical material is available but it has not been possible to use it in the present study. The W.H.O. through its Department of Occupational Health is hoping to develop a "programme aiming at the uniform collection of data on different occupational health problems from countries" (El Batawi, 1974).

For the purposes of this contribution, 116 countries and dependencies were surveyed; no information was available for 26: Afghanistan, Albania, Algeria, Angola, Barbados, Burma, China, Ethiopia, Fiji, Hong Kong, Jordan, North Korea, Libya, Malawi, Malta, Martinique, Mauritius, Mongolia, Morocco, Mozambique, Pakistan, Sierra Leone, South Korea, Syria, Taiwan (Formosa) and North Vietnam. Eight of these 26 countries are known to have experienced considerable industrial development during the 1955–73 period, viz. Algeria, China, Hong Kong, Malta, Pakistan, South Korea, Syria and Taiwan (Formosa). The nature of their industries known to the author are such that some forms of industrial lung disease might have been expected to occur: this may well have happened and been reported elsewhere other than in the media screened.

Of the 90 countries and dependencies for which information was available and from which at least one episode of an occupational lung disease was reported, 60 had government legislation and the means to support it and 27 maintained undergraduate and/or postgraduate training in occupational medicine. Fifty countries operated some form of field survey and research programme and 21 had national societies of occupational medicine: several also had similar organizations for occupational hygiene. In addition, 10 undertook occupational-health nursing training and one maintained a register of occupational-health nurses.

With the restricted means at our disposal, it can be said that, of all the countries surveyed, only 50% appear to have a government-backed organization to control occupational health in any of the main fields of industry, agriculture, fishing and marine, mining and manufacturing, transport and services and commerce. While 37 countries have some form of professional training, these are concentrated in the highly industrialized zones of the United Kingdom, West and Central Europe, Italy, the U.S.S.R. and the East

U.S.A. Egypt has two teaching units whose influence extends throughout North Africa and the Middle East, while in 1974 the University of the Witwatersrand, Johannesburg, instituted full time post-graduate teaching. Singapore has recently commenced teaching which should encourage the growth of studies in South-East Asia. France, with a relatively large concentration of teaching and research units in all fields of industry, extends her influence into the francophone countries of Africa and elsewhere, though most industry there is agricultural. The U.S.S.R. with over 20 teaching units reflects the relatively greater importance given to the health of the worker by eastern-bloc countries. The United Kingdom and U.S.A. contribute to the encouragement of occupational health in the anglophone countries and in the Spanish-speaking republics of South America. In addition, both now provide a triennial conference in London and Boston, respectively, on the problems of tropical industrial health. The paucity of information from South-American

---

Country..................Province or State..................City or Town........................

Type of industry.............................

Nature and source of materials used.............................

Nature of work force: Indigenous...........
Expatriate............If "Yes" from where?
Static/migrant. If "migrant" annual turnover rate

Government supervision of working environment: Yes/No

Provision of Occupational Health Service: Government/Company/Union

Health screening of employees: Yes/No

Regular occupational environment monitoring: Yes/No

Employees' washing facilities: Yes/No

Employees' work-clothes laundering facilities: Yes/No

Employees' housing: Government/Company/Private

Table 15.6 Tentative questionnaire for authors of papers on industrial lung disease.

countries may reflect the parochialism of their literature and research communications rather than a true deficiency. Nevertheless, it is regrettable that more information is not available.

The contribution which national organizations make to the study of industrial lung and other diseases could be further improved if facilities for certain professional advisory services were made available internationally to doctors and nurses in industry. Such people often work in isolation and would benefit from such a supporting service. The collection of international lung-disease data could be improved if authors of accepted papers were required to provide certain basic information about the industry which they were reporting: suggestions are made in Table 15.6. In the absence of information from the rapidly industrializing People's Republic of China and Hong Kong, we must speculate. In the case of the former, there may be language and other communication difficulties, combined with a natural reluctance governed by political and social factors. In the case of Hong Kong, such factors do not arise.

REFERENCES

American Conference of Government Industrial Hygientists (1971). Documentation of the TLV for substances in workroom air (3rd ed.) Cincinnati, Ohio.

Amoudru, C. (1972). Les pneumoconioses du houilleurs dans les mines de Charbon Francaises: Rappel Epidemiologique. *Lille Medical* **17**, 1078–1090.

Beadle, D. G. (1971). The relationship between the amount of dust breathed and the development or radiological signs of silicosis: an epidemiological study in South African gold miners. *In* "Inhaled Particles" (Ed. W. H. Walton), Vol. III, pp. 953–966. Unwin Bros, Surrey.

Blyth, W. (1973). Farmer's lung disease. *Soc. Appl. Bacteriol. Symp.* **2**, 261–276.

Campbell, C. C. (1967). Histoplasmosis and other respiratory mycoses in the tropics. *Ind. Trop. Hlth* **6**, 145–152.

Chew, P. K., Chia, M. and Chew, S. F. (1973). Asbestos workers in Singapore. *Arch. Environ. Hlth* **26**, 290–293.

Chevat, M. and Mordish, R. (1964). Byssinosis investigation in two cotton plants in Israel. *Proc. 14th Int. Congr. Occup. Hlth* Sept. 1963, Madrid, 572–573.

Cook, P. and Burkitt, D. (1970). "An Epidemiological Study of Seven Malignant Tumours in Africa". Medical Research Council, London.

Craw, J. (1964). The control and elimination of silicosis in the West Coast Haematite Ore Industry. *Proc. 14th Int. Congr. Occup. Hlth* Sept. 1963, Madrid.

El Batawi, M. A. (1974). Personal communication.

Great Britain: Foreign Office (1962). "Treaty Establishing the European Economic Community, Rome, March, 25 1957". H.M.S.O., London (Translation from the official and authentic text of the treaty).

Hendschen, F. (1967). "The History and Geography of Diseases". Translated by J. Tate, New York.

Holaday, D. A. (1969). History of exposure of miners to radon. *Hlth Phys.* **16**, 547–552.

Jacobsen, M., Rae, S., Walton, W. H. and Rogan, J. M. (1971). The relation between pneumoconiosis and dust exposure in British Coal Mines. *In* "Inhaled Particles" (Ed. W. H. Walton), Vol. III, pp. 903–917. Unwin Bros, Surrey.

Kueppers, F. and Donhardt, A. (1974). Obstructive Lung disease in heterozygotes for alpha-I antitrypsin deficiency. *Ann. Intern. Med.* **80**, 209–212.

Lundin, F. E. (Jnr), Lloyd, J. W., Smith, E. M., Archer, V. E. and Holaday, D. A. (1969). Mortality of uranium miners in relation to radiation exposure, hard rock mining and cigarette smoking—1950 through Sept. 1967. *Hlth Phys.* **16**, 571.

McDonald, A. D., Harper, A., El Attar, O. A. and McDonald, J. C. (1970). Epidemiology of primary malignant mesothelial tumours in Canada. *Cancer* **26**, 914–919.

M.R.C. (1966). Questionnaire on respiratory symptoms and instructions for its use. Printed and distributed by W. J. Holman, Dawlish, Devon.

Murray, R. (1970). An international view of coal workers pneumoconiosis. *J. Occup. Med.* **12**, 474–477.

Nelson, K. W. (1967). Environmental health problems associated with mining and smelting in tropical climates. *Ind. Trop. Hlth* **6**, 74–77.

Schilling, R. S. F. (1960). The epidemiology of byssinosis. *In* "Industrial pulmonary diseases" (Eds E. J. King and C. M. Fletcher), pp. 185–194. J. and A. Churchill, London.

Selikoff, I. J., Hammond, E. C. and Churg, J. (1968). Asbestos exposure, smoking and neoplasia. *J. Amer. Med. Assoc.* **204**, 106–112.

Tromp, S. W. (1974). The relationship of weather and climate to health and disease. *In* "Environmental medicine" (Eds G. M. Howe and J. A. Loraine). Heinemann, London.

Turner-Warwick, M. (1973). Immunology and asbestos. *Proc. Roy. Soc. Med.* **66**, 927.

Wagner, J. C. (1971). Immunological factors in coalworkers pneumoconiosis. *In* "Inhaled Particles" (Ed. W. H. Walton), Vol. III, pp. 573–575. Unwin Bros, Surrey.

Young, J. K. (1971). Pulmonary sarcoidosis in African mineworkers. *Proc. Min. Med, Off. Assoc.* **51**, 126–133.

16. Illness Associated with Drug Abuse

J. L. Reed

Almost contemporaneously with the first written accounts of the use of drugs came reports of the possibility that these drugs may be abused to the detriment of the individual or of the society in which he lived. In all the discussion that follows the word "drug" is taken to mean a chemical substance which, when taken by an individual, alters in some way his relationship with the reality of his environment. Although the term "drug dependence", implying a physical and/or psychological need for the continued administration of the drug, will be used, for the purpose of this chapter it is not necessary that the drug use which leads to illness is persistent.

"Drug" so defined does not, of course, limit the discussion solely to those drugs which are generally considered to be "drugs of abuse" e.g. heroin, cocaine, cannabis. These are the drugs of abuse which are also socially proscribed drugs. Of equal or greater importance are the drugs of abuse which are not socially proscribed (at least in most societies) e.g. tobacco, alcohol and the minor analgesics.

Much of the earlier literature concerning the ill-effects of drug usage is very difficult to interpret. Then, as now, cannabis, for instance, has been reported as a spiritually-fulfilling adjuvant, "the heavenly guide" to religious ceremonies, as "one of the most valuable medicines we possess" and as a certain recipe for insanity. What is clear, however, is that disease associated with drug use is no new phenomenon. The tremendous increase in drinking of cheap spirits in London between 1720 and 1751 was reflected in a greatly increased death rate for this period, and in 1894 the Indian Hemp Commission concluced that the excessive use of cannabis intensified mental instability.

ALCOHOL

The incidence of illness associated with excessive drinking has been one of the most widely studied in this field (see also Chapter 18, pp. 493–96). The physical damage of cirrhosis of the liver, polyneuropathy, dementia and cardiomyopathy and the personal and social damage of psychological dependence (with or without physical damage) have been both considered. The high morbidity of many types associated with excessive drinking is illustrated by reports from many different countries. Reports from America and Australia show that at least one in eight patients in general medical wards were alcoholics, while a report from Norway reveals a mortality rate in male alcoholics 113% in excess of the age-related rate for non-alcoholic population. Although most of these deaths are due to the physical consequences of alcoholism, researchers in England have found a 25% attempted suicide rate and a 7–8% suicide rate amongst alcoholics.

Another aspect of morbidity associated with alcohol usage is shown by the clear relationship between alcohol and traffic accidents. In 50% of fatal motor accidents in the U.S.A., alcohol has been considered to be an associated or contributory factor. In the United Kingdom, accidents most commonly occur within an hour of closing time of the bar in public houses. With a motor accident death rate (1966) of 27.1 per 100 000 population in the U.S.A. and 15.5 per 100 000 in the United Kingdom and with accidents being the fifth most common cause of death in the U.S.A. (1972), this morbidity arising, indirectly, from the use of alcohol is of considerable significance.

The figures quoted above represent but one instance of the very marked differences that may be found between one country and another in the degree to which they are affected by alcohol-related disease. The most widely studied condition has been cirrhosis of the liver. The death rate from alcoholic cirrhosis forms the basis of the

Jellinek formula for estimating the incidence of alcoholism (W.H.O., 1951). Although it has been widely criticized—not least by Jellinek himself—and the need for more field studies accepted, it does, in general, give figures for the incidence of alcohol closely corresponding to those reached by other methods. These studies (W.H.O., 1967, 1968) show a wide variation in incidence of alcoholism and of incidence of cirrhosis of the liver. Figure 16.1 shows figures for various countries relating the incidence of cirrhosis to the apparent consumption of alcohol per capita of the population, aged 15 years and over. Although the figures are for *apparent* alcohol consumption and are based on differing data (production, sales, etc.), there is a clear difference both in consumption and in the incidence of cirrhosis among differing countries (see also Fig. 18.8).

The cause of the differences between different countries and cultures has been much studied and some social and economic factors have become apparent which, it seems reasonable to believe, have a casual relationship to the degree of abuse (and of cirrhosis) in any culture. France, with no stigma attached to drinking, drunkenness or alcoholism, has a very high incidence of alcoholism and of cirrhosis. Regular drinking throughout the day is quite acceptable and there is considerable social pressure towards this. On the other hand in Italy, another major wine-producing and consuming country, drinking is largely limited to meal times. Drinking of alcohol is acceptable in

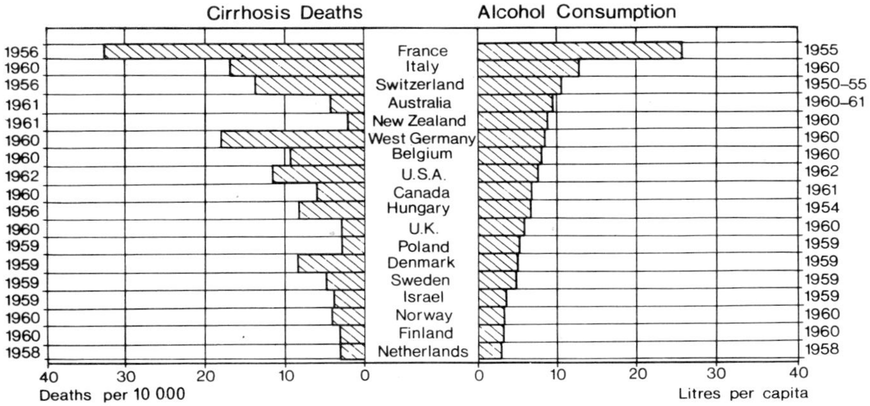

Fig. 16.1 Incidence of cirrhosis to apparent consumption of alcohol per capita, 15 years and over.

Italy but drunkenness is not. Such a cultural difference in attitudes towards drinking will clearly affect the total amount of alcohol consumed and hence the prevalence of alcohol-related diseases. It is difficult to generalize from such findings and then to draw inferences from them relating to alcohol-related disease in other countries. Other cultures and subcultures have been the subject of studies and, taken in conjunction, it is perhaps possible to determine some of the factors that relate to the development of disease. The influence of religion is shown by the work of Mulford (1964) and Snyder (1958) who find that, although 90% of adult Jews drink alcohol, there is a very low rate of alcoholism. This appears to be because among orthodox Jews drinking alcohol is part of strict religious observance and drinking is first seen by the young in a highly controlled family setting. In contrast to this can be taken the higher rate of alcoholism among emigrant Irish (Bates, 1946). The pattern of drinking as learned among the Irish is, in general, in a setting unrestricted either by religion or the family. Economic necessity often leads to a late marriage and religious factors contribute to drink being used as a substitute for sexuality. When the stresses and, at times, improved economic position resulting from emigration are added to these basic attitudes towards drink then a high incidence becomes understandable. Viewed as a world problem there would seem to be few areas exempt from alcohol-related diseases. Even in strictly Moslem countries, recent reports have suggested that the proscriptions against alcohol are breaking down and the use of alcohol is becoming more common.

Within any culture it seems that certain factors must be considered in assessing the likely degree to which alcohol-related disease will occur. The availability of alcohol is paramount. Countries where the production of alcoholic drinks is high are very much at risk, especially so when the production is of importance to the national economy. The attitude of a country to excessive drinking is also of prime importance and whether or not drinking occurs in a structured or unstructured setting. The third consideration is the economic state of the individual in relation to the cost of alcohol. Effective measures to control alcoholism and alcohol-related diseases can be taken on the basis of these factors. The gin-drinking "explosion" in London in the 18th century was rapidly controlled by limiting sources of supply and increasing the price of gin.

TOBACCO

Tobacco is perhaps the most widely misused of all drugs and one which has shown a speed of dissemination unrivalled by any other drug. The use of tobacco is now virtually world wide and is so common that the main cause for surprise is that there still remain some societies which have avoided its use.

Soon after its introduction into Europe, deleterious effects on health were reported and the use of tobacco came under a number of proscriptions varying from royal disapprobation in England to the death penalty in some Middle-Eastern countries. These reports of ill health were not confirmed and it is only within the last 25 years that strong evidence has been available linking tobacco with ill health. The relationship between tobacco and carcinoma of the lung, ischaemic heart disease and chronic bronchitis and emphysema now seems clear. The position of tobacco is of especial interest as it illustrates two points which at times make the recognition of drug-related diseases difficult. First, there is a very long period between starting to use the drug and the development of the drug-related conditions; a time lapse of 40 years not being exceptional. Second, it is clear that the incidence of the most common disease related to use of tobacco depends in large part on the presentation of the drug. It is only since the cigarette has increased in popularity over the pipe, cigar, or the chewing of tobacco that there has been a very marked increase in deaths from lung cancer and ischaemic heart disease.

This second factor leads to clear geographical differences in disease incidence which depends largely on the degree of development of a country. The United Nations has reported a 50% expansion in cigarette production in developing countries and only slightly lower in developed countries. Given the social status at present endowed on cigarette smoking and also the addictive nature of tobacco together with the economic benefits gained by countries from the production of tobacco and from the taxing of tobacco products, it seems all too likely that as countries continue to develop economically so they will experience a rise in the tobacco-related diseases.

Since, at present, the problem is confined mainly to the developed countries, statistics related to these illnesses come mainly from the U.S.A., Canada and the United Kingdom though there have been studies from most of the larger countries. Table 16.1 shows, that for

Type of smoking	Mortality ratio* British doctors (Doll and Hill, 1964)	U.S. Veterans (Kahn, 1966)	Canadian Veterans (Kahn, 1966)	U.S. Men (U.S. Dep. Hlth, 1964)
Cigarettes only	1.28	1.84	1.65	1.83
Cigarettes and others		1.51	1.23	1.54
Cigars only	1.01	1.10	1.11	0.97
Pipes only		1.07	1.10	0.86

* Mortality ratio: death-rate for current cigarette smokers divided by death-rate for those who never smoked regularly.

Table 16.1 Mortality ratios of men by current smoking habits from four large prospective studies (from Fletcher and Horn, 1971).

total mortality, that for cigarette smokers is approximately 30–80% greater than that for non-smokers. Studies of morbidity in the U.S.A. suggest that 28% of the man-days of disability in the 45–64 years age group were related to cigarette smoking. Reviewing the diseases where there appears to be a clear relationship between cigarette smoking and ill health, studies in more than 10 countries have shown that heavy cigarette smokers run a risk of lung cancer 15–30 times greater than for non-smokers. Although this is found as a general conclusion, it is clear that other environmental factors are of some importance. Higher rates of lung cancer are found in urban than in rural areas and it seems probable that exposure to general atmospheric pollution increases the risk of lung cancer. Even so, leaving aside other more specific pollutants such as asbestos and radioactive materials—exposure to which leads to an increased risk of lung cancer—atmospheric pollution is of minor importance in the causation of lung cancer when compared with cigarette smoking.

Similar reports from many countries confirm a greatly increased mortality from chronic bronchitis and emphysema and from ischaemic heart disease. In the case of the latter, cigarette smoking can be implicated both in the development of coronary artherosclerosis leading to occlusion and in factors such as liability to develop cardiac arrythmias, and increased levels of carboxy-haemoglobin which may increase the likelihood of a fatal outcome of the occlusion.

It has been said (Fletcher and Horn, 1971) that "the control of cigarette smoking would do more to improve health and prolong life ... than any other single action in the whole of preventative medicine." Since these are diseases currently mainly confined to the developed countries, there are important problems to be solved in relation to health education both in the developed and the underdeveloped countries. In the one, an existing problem needs to be dealt with, in the other, decisions must be reached as to whether steps should or could be taken to prevent such a problem developing. Fletcher and Horn propose a variety of means for controlling an existing problem involving education to prevent young people taking up smoking, education of and assistance to those already smoking (including the advertising of the health risks involved), control and abolition of advertising and the production of safer cigarettes. To these might be added, especially for countries where cigarette smoking is not yet widespread, the imposition of very much greater taxation on cigarettes as opposed to that on less harmful tobacco products.

MINOR ANALGESICS

Though geographically limited to developed countries and, numerically speaking, involving only relatively few people in severe illness, the part of the minor analgesics in the production of drug-related illness should not be overlooked. This is more especially the case since the general public take little account of the dangers of indiscriminate use of these drugs. The actual weight of simple analgesics (paracetamol and phenacetin) consumed in a year cannot possibly be accounted for in terms of the need to relieve physical pain. Several studies have shown that analgesic abusers show a high incidence of psychiatric disorder. Murray (1973) has shown that the basis of the abuse lies in the psychotropic effect of the analegesics and of the caffeine often present in compound tablets.

Persistent analgesic use can result in gastro-intestinal bleeding due to aspirin. For instance, 70% of people lose up to 10 ml of blood after a therapeutic dose of aspirin. Nephropathy is almost certainly due to phenacetin, e.g. 10% of all cases of renal failure occurring in one London hospital. More uncommonly, liver damage is due to aspirin.

As with other drugs, very encouraging improvements may be obtained by education and control. Marked reductions in the incidence of analgesic nephropathy have been reported from Scandinavia and Scotland following the withdrawal of phenacetin.

Apart from these unexpected for the patient effects of analgesics, it must be recalled that analgesics are the most commonly used method of self injury in cases of attempted suicide or para-suicide. These latter ones may occur in almost epidemic proportions in some areas, e.g. over 1000 cases of analgesic poisoning were admitted to the Edinburgh Regional Poisoning Centre in 1970.

CANNABIS

One of the prime centres of discussion in the drug abuse field over the last 100 or so years has been the liability of cannabis to produce disease. Unfortunately, because of legal restrictions on the experimental use of the drug and because of the high emotions that the subject has aroused, it is exceedingly difficult to state the facts of the case. Only in the last few years has scientifically controlled work been developed in this field. Lewis presents an admirable review of the current situation (Department of Health, 1970).

It seems clear that both physical and psychological disturbances can follow the use of cannabis. Physically rapid heart rate, gross incoordination, dyspnoea and temporary unconsciousness have been reported and death is said to have occurred due to cardiac failure. Severe psychological disturbances occurring acutely, usually after use of large doses, are typical acute organic reactions, with delirium, disorientation, and extreme anxiety followed by amnesia for the period of the reaction. In common with other acute organic reactions, persecutory delusions are common. There are, however, marked differences in reaction from individual to individual and possibly from country to country. This latter difference may be culturally determined or may reflect the differing sources of cannabis in the different countries. Whereas an euphoric, relaxed state is the usual effect, it has been reported, notably from South America, that overactivity and overemotionality are common.

There is also fairly general agreement that persistent and heavy use of cannabis over a period of years leads to a chronic state of inertia with inability to continue working. This is generally associated with progressive self neglect and malnutrition. Such a picture has been frequently reported from the North-African littoral, the Middle East and India. Estimates for the number of regular users have been as high as 50% of the population of Morocco or 80 000 regular users in Egypt. Such figures must be based inevitably and to a considerable extent on subjective guess work.

Areas of uncertainty concerning the effects of cannabis relate to whether the use of cannabis can produce persistent severe ("psychotic") psychological disturbance and to the effect of persistent moderate use of cannabis. Both of these areas await further investigation.

STIMULANTS

Synthetic

Since the end of the Second World War, several countries have experienced epidemic outbreaks of abuse of synthetic stimulants. In earlier outbreaks, amphetamine preparations such as dexamphetamine sulphate, methyl-amphetamine or amphetamine/barbiturate mixtures such as "Purple Hearts" predominated. Latterly, other synthetic stimulants such as methylphenidate and phenmetrazine have been widely used either in addition to or as a replacement for amphetamine. Major epidemics have occurred in Japan and Sweden, and abuse at a lower level of prevalence now presents a problem in most developed countries.

The principal problem of health associated with amphetamine abuse are acute intoxication, phycoses developing idiosyncratically during use and sepsis following injection.

Symptoms of acute intoxication include irritability, sleeplessness and overactivity. Psychotic reactions due to amphetamine have been reported since 1938 and the relationship between the illness and the drug clearly established by Connell (1958). The form of the illness is clinically indistinguishable from paranoid schizophrenia. There is no clear indication why one person taking amphetamine develops a psychotic illness while another does not. There is no relationship to dose, to length of drug misuse or previous personalities and the illness appears to be an idiosyncratic reaction which recovers with the withdrawal of the stimulant.

As with other injected drugs, either local sepsis (abscesses) or generalized infection (hepatitis, endocarditis and septicaemia) may occur.

Natural stimulants

This group of vegetable products includes tea, coffee, betel, kava and khat as well as coca and its product cocaine. *Tea* and *coffee* have been used very widely and for a long period of time with no serious medical problems arising besides insomnia and mild dyspepsia associated with excessive ingestion of excessively strong preparations.

Kava is widely drunk in Oceania and current opinion suggests that more medical problems have arisen from the substitution of alcohol for kava than from kava itself. Similarly the chewing of *betel* nut or leaf— widely practised from West Africa to Oceania—appears to present as little problem as do tea or coffee. However, opposition to the use of *khat* has grown over the years since, as with cannabis, its continued use is held to lead to self neglect.

The indigenous population of Peru have used the leaves of the *coca* plant as a stimulant and to allay pain, hunger and fatigue since time immemorial. A recent survey has shown that 12% of the population of a hill village regularly chewed the coca leaf, principally to relieve fatigue and hunger. Unfortunately, a vicious circle develops in the chewers of the leaf. Hunger and fatigue are allayed but this leads to loss of appetite, to further malnutrition, and to worse fatigue. Work performance declines and apathy about personal hygiene leads on to hookworm and other infestations. Those who are not regular chewers of coca recognize the dangers involved, and yet the poor physical and economic conditions of the indigenous population are such that, at times, use of the leaf is regarded as virtually inevitable.

The misuse of *cocaine*, often in conjunction with heroin or other narcotics, has occurred in spasmodic "epidemics" since its isolation in the 1850s. Medical complications have been similar to those of the synthetic stimulants but nasal ulceration from cocaine sniffing has also been reported.

Opiates and synthetic analogues

The eating or smoking of raw *opium* has a history of thousands of years in India and the Far East. In general, social attitudes have been of disapprobation of anything other than very moderate use and the pattern of ill health associated with opium use has been not unlike that of coca chewing and for very similar reasons. Occasional acute psychotic reactions are reported, but in general there is a slow deterioration of standards of self-care and hence of health. Like the changes in morbidity associated with the change to the use of cigarettes from tobacco in other forms, so the refining of opium and the production of *morphine* and *heroin* have dramatically altered the morbidity and mortality associated with opiate abuse. Problems of two types arise; first the direct toxic effects of the drug and second the infections which result from the method of administration. Since the active principle is now highly concentrated, the likelihood of overdosage is greatly increased. In a study of British addicts, Bewley *et al.* (1968) has shown that the mortality rate for non-therapeutic addicts is 27 per 1000, i.e. about 20 times the expected age specific rate. Although most victims died of the infective complications of injecting drugs, almost as many died from apparently unintentional overdoses. The suicide rate was also greatly increased with an age specific rate 50 times greater than that of non-addicted persons.

Since the study by Bewley *et al.*, legislation has regularized the ways in which heroin and other narcotics may be supplied to addicts in the United Kingdom. One result has been a very marked reduction in the suicide rate, presumably since some of the social pressures placed on an addict have been removed by placing him within the law. In the United Kingdom, the situation has been reached where the method of administration of the drug in narcotic use and the prevalence of the poly drug abuser causes more problems than the pharmacological actions of heroin itself.

BARBITURATES AND OTHER HYPNOTICS

Use and abuse of *barbiturates* and other hypnotics is extremely widepread in Western countries. Over 17 million prescriptions for barbiturates were in use in England and Wales in 1965 and the weight prescribed doubled between 1953 and 1959.

The problem of acute and chronic intoxication is very similar to that of alcohol and the intoxicated person can prove a serious threat to himself and to others through gross impairment of judgment, as, for example, when driving a vehicle. Death may occur from both the direct poisoning effect of hypnotics and also the trauma resulting from accidents due to intoxication. Chronic hypnotic addicts are also at serious risk if they are suddenly withdrawn from their drug since grand mal convulsions and status epilepticus commonly follow sudden falls in blood barbiturate level. Despite reports over the last three or four decades of withdrawal fits, this phenomenon still appears to be more widely known among drug abusers than among doctors.

Barbiturates present a further health problem in that they remain a principle method of lethal self-poisoning. In 1962, there were 1476 deaths in England and Wales due to barbiturate poisoning and of these 1083 were suicides. From the point of view of legislative control, the barbiturates present an extremely difficult problem. Despite the fact that W.H.O. has urged their stricter controls, barbiturates may have as many as 500 000 regular users in England and Wales alone and, with comparable numbers in other countries, they present so large a problem as not to lend readily to changes of legal status.

HALLUCINOGENS

The natural hallucinogens such as peyote, *Datura stramonium* and *Amanita muscaria* have a long history of use and present little problem of drug-related disease when used in their original, highly structured, usually mystical-religious, setting.

Both natural and synthetic hallucinogens such as lysergic acid diethylamide (LSD), dimethyltryptamine (DMT), dimethoxy-methamphetamine (DOM; STP) when used in an unstructured drug-orientated situation can result in serious adverse psychological reactions. Physical ill effects appear to be rare though fits and coma have been reported.

It is extremely difficult to assess the proportion of those taking hallucinogenic drugs who come to require medical attention. By the nature of the drug use, adverse reactions tend to be dealt with by fellow drug takers and there is, indeed, some evidence that they are better at dealing with a "bad trip" than most doctors. Some indication of the frequency of the problem is given by a series reported by psychiatrists working at the University of California at the Los Angeles Medical Centre. During an 8 month period, 12% of all attending as emergencies did so because of adverse reaction to LSD.

CONCLUSION

It is clear that drug use and abuse causes an enormous amount of ill health and, though the drugs themselves may differ from country to country, the problem is world-wide. Medicine cannot solve the problem alone. Indeed, alone, it can do little but repair such damage as it occurs in individuals. Although there appears to be an inate desire in man to experiment with substances which alter his relationship with reality, preventive measures for drug-associated diseases lie in fields which are controlled by government policy rather than by medicine. There seems little likelihood that drug use and abuse will be eliminated but the morbidity and mortality from abuse might be greatly reduced by any government prepared to take appropriate legal and fiscal measures to control the availability of drugs and to institute educational measures to attempt seriously to alter a population's attitude to drug taking. At present, in many countries, the emphasis lies on the individuals's right or freedom to chose to take a drug. There is perhaps an even greater freedom to emphasize, the right *not* to take a drug.

REFERENCES

Bales, R. F. (1946). Cultural differences in rates of alcoholism. *Q.J. Studies Alcohol* **6**, 480–499.

Bewley, T. H., Ben-arie, O. and James, I. P. (1968). Morbidity and mortality from heroin dependence 1: survey of heroin addicts known to the Home Office. *Brit. Med. J.* **1**, 725–732.

Connell, P. H. (1958). "Amphetamine Psychosis". Chapman, London.

Dept. of Health and Social Security (1970). "Amphetamines, Barbiturates, L.S.D. and Cannabis". H.M.S.O., London.

Fletcher, C. M. and Horn, D. (1971). "Smoking and Health". W.H.O., Geneva.
Mulford, H. A. (1964). Drinking and deviant drinking, U.S.A. 1963. *Q.J. Studies Alcohol* **25**, 634–650.
Murray, R. M. (1973). The origins of analgesic nephropathy. *Brit. J. Psychiat.* **123**, 99–106.
Office of Health Economics (1970). "Alcohol Abuse". O.H.E., London.
Synder, C. R. (1958). "Alcohol and the Jews". Thomas, New Haven.
W.H.O. (1951). *W.H.O. Techn. Rep. Ser.* **42**.
W.H.O. (1967). *W.H.O. Techn. Rep. Ser.* **363**.
W.H.O. (1968). *W.H.O. Statistic. Rep.* **11**.

17. Cardiovascular Disease

G. M. Howe, L. Burgess and P. Gatenby

The term "cardiovascular disease" embraces atherosclerosis of the coronary arteries and aorta, ischaemic heart disease, cerebrovascular disease (stroke), rheumatic fever and rheumatic heart disease and arterial hypertension. Taken as an entity, these diseases have a worldwide distribution. In the developed countries, and possibly even in all countries, they constitute the major cause of death and disability.

Though they relate to less than one-third of the world's population, data from W.H.O. reveal that in about 50 countries distributed throughout all continents, cardiovascular disease, in 1967, accounted on average for 37% of all deaths. Mortality from this cause was higher than that from cancer, accidents or communicable diseases. At present causing an annual increase of 30 million deaths, cardiovascular disease has assumed epidemic proportions and poses a major burden on, and one of the greatest threats to, modern urbanized and industrialized societies.

In presenting the analysis that follows, the term "cardiovascular disease" has been interpreted as including rubrics 390–438 inclusive of the W.H.O. International Statistical Classification of Diseases, Injuries and Causes of Death (ICD) (8th Revision, 1965), (ICD Nos 330–34 and 410–43 of the 7th Revision, 1955). Particular attention is being given to ischaemic heart disease, ICD Nos 410–414, ("arteriosclerotic heart disease including coronary disease" ICD No. 420–422 of the 7th Revision, 1955), to cerebrovascular disease, ICD Nos 430–438 ("vascular lesions affecting the central nervous system" ICD Nos 330–334 of the 7th Revision) and to hypertensive heart

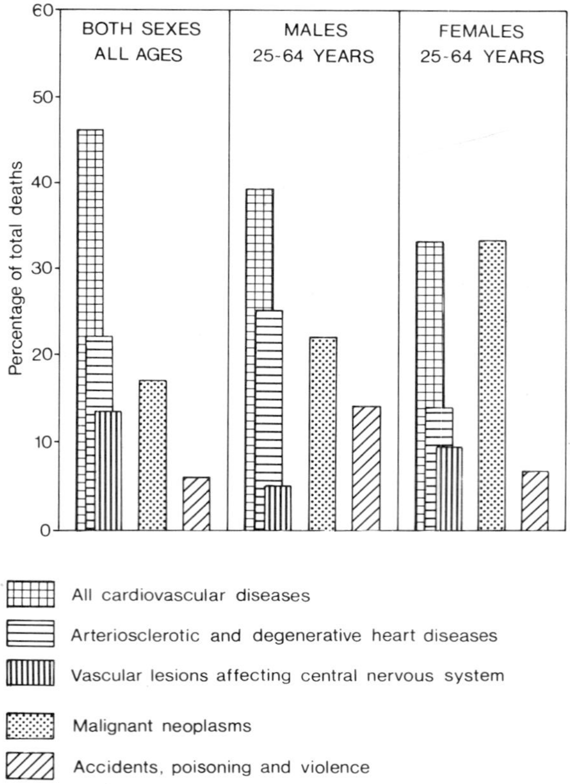

Fig. 17.1 Mortality from cardiovascular disease and malignant neoplasms and accidents, poisoning and violence, as percentages of deaths from all causes in 29 countries, 1967 (W.H.O. data).

disease, ICD Nos 400–404 (ICD Nos 440–443 of the 7th Revision). Hypertensive heart disease and cerebrovascular disease are thought to be world wide in their distribution, though there may be local differences in their clinical manifestations, aetiology and pathogenesis. On the other hand, ischaemic heart disease and cardiopathies of unknown origin seem to occur only in, or predominantly in, certain regions or in specific groups of people and at the same time demonstrate appreciable spatial variability.

Ischaemic heart disease occurs when there is a major reduction in the supply of blood to all or part of the heart. This may be brought on by various diseases and by various mechanisms. For example, a narrowing of the aortic orifice may interfere with the flow of blood to the coronary arteries which supply the heart walls and muscles. Alternatively, a syphilitic inflammation of the aorta may leave a fibrosed aortic plaque, a basis for thrombus formation. In almost 90% of cases however, ischaemic heart disease is due to arteriosclerosis combined with atheromatosis (atherosclerosis). These are conditions in which deposits of fatty substances resembling porridge in appearance (*athere*, porridge) form inside an artery and obstruct the flow of blood. When the blood supply to the heart is affected by these deposits (scars, lesions) the result is either a dramatic embolic myocardial infarct (heart attack) or else a slower, rather less dramatic coronary thrombosis, which, however, may produce infarction. Should the supply of blood to the brain be so affected, there is a stroke (apoplexy or cerebral accident).

The direct causes of atherosclerosis remain a mystery but an increasing number of facts about the disease are known. For instance, in developed countries such as the U.K. or U.S.A. coronary atherosclerosis is by far the most frequent cause of death. It is responsible for 50–60% of all deaths from cardiovascular disease, which itself accounts for more than half the total number of deaths. Coronary atherosclerosis kills three out of every thousand inhabitants in each of these two countries every year. In the U.S.A. alone, one million work days are lost annually and, as early as 1962, the President's Commission on Heart Disease, Cancer and Stroke stated that if all those people who had died that year of heart disease had lived one more year the nation's economy would have gained $2 billion in output.

Coronary atherosclerosis has been found to be far more common in men than in women. Almost all patients under the age of 40 years are men, though this ceases to be the case as people grow older. The death rate rises rapidly in men over 45 years and in post-menopausal women generally above the age of 55 years. From 60 years on, and more particularly after 70 years, the disease strikes equally at both sexes. Thus women are, in general, affected by coronary atherosclerosis later in life than men. In the case of cerebrovascular disease, there is no great difference in frequency between men and women but different rates of mortality and morbidity have been found in countries with varying physical and human environments.

Hypertension or high blood pressure is a rise in both maximum or systolic arterial pressure (i.e. when the heart contracts) and minimum or diastolic arterial pressure (i.e. when the heart relaxes) above the normal (see p. 452). Since coronary thrombosis and strokes are more common in people with high blood pressure, hypertension has come to be considered as a disease itself.

DISEASE INDICES

Various indices are used to measure disease frequency. The incidence rate, based on the number of new cases developing each year, is the most informative but is generally not available on a global basis. Neither is prevalence rate which provides a measure of the total number of people affected at a given point in time. Actual mortality is the most readily available statistic, since certified deaths are collected as a matter of routine by many governments. From this data, other indices may be calculated. Even so, the enormous differences that exist between the industrialized countries and the less developed areas of the world have a profound effect on the pattern and trends of the disease that occur in these regions. Differences in environment, stage and rate of social and economic development, methods of collecting data and, in particular, reliability and/or accuracy of diagnosis and certification are so different as to make valid comparisons extremely difficult.

There appears to be a tendency of over diagnosis of the cardiovascular diseases in the so-called developed world and under diagnosis in the less developed world. An editorial in the British journal, *Lancet* (Anon. 1966), commenting on the inaccuracy of death certificates in Britain, quoted over-certification of some neoplastic and cardiovascular diseases of the order of 100%. Under diagnosis in the less developed world is due to: (a) lack of adequate medical education of the certifying officer, and (b) lack of ante- and post-mortem diagnostic facilities. For reasons such as these, standards of diagnosis vary not only between countries but also between different sectors of the population in the same country. This, together with a general lack of basic demographic information for many of the less developed countries, particularly for areas outside the major urban centres, places major difficulties and constraints on any global examination of spatial variability of cardiovascular disease. For this reason, any comparisons offered must be accepted with caution.

ISCHAEMIC HEART DISEASE

Diagnosis of ischaemic heart disease is generally least good among the elderly where, without more detailed investigation, symptoms are often ascribed to "senility". Because the level of misdiagnosis varies from country to country, it is considered advisable to restrict comparisons of mortality to persons under the age of 65 years. Figures 17.2–17.5* have been drawn for the age group 35–64 years partly for this reason and partly because relatively few cases in adults occur under this lower age limit.

Data for ischaemic heart disease is available to the W.H.O. for only 65 countries; it is lacking for those other countries which together contain the greater part of the world's population. Despite the extensive blank areas shown on the maps for which data are not available, a number of trends or pointers emerge. The expected and generally accepted association between high mortality rates and the more industrially advanced countries is apparent in several countries, as for example in the case of the U.S.A. and the United Kingdom. However, such an association is not evident in France, Spain or Italy, nor in the countries of Eastern Europe, particularly in the Balkans. Neither is it evident in industrialized countries in Asia such as Japan, Hong Kong, Taiwan and Singapore. Despite the fact that the population of some countries is small and may produce large annual fluctuations, the distributional pattern for females is not unlike that for males.

Male rates (Figs 17.2 and 17.3) are higher than female rates (Figs 17.4 and 17.5). In the case of Finland, for example, female rates are only 19% of those for males. In relative terms, the difference between the rates for the two sexes is greatest in England and Wales, Scandinavia, the Netherlands, the Federal German Republic, Switzerland, Czechoslovakia, Italy, Austria and Spain. This difference is far less in Venezuela (where the female rate is 64% of the

* The world distributions of age-specific death rates from ischaemic heart disease mortality for males and females separately, are represented on both geographical and demographic base maps for 65 countries. In the case of the demographic base maps, the age-standard death rates are related to the populations of the countries "at risk" rather than to the geographical areas of the countries concerned. In such cases, the areas of the circles are in proportion to the populations "at risk". Where possible, the 1969, 1970 and 1971 data were averaged for each area and age-group, and expressed as an age standardized rate per 100 000.

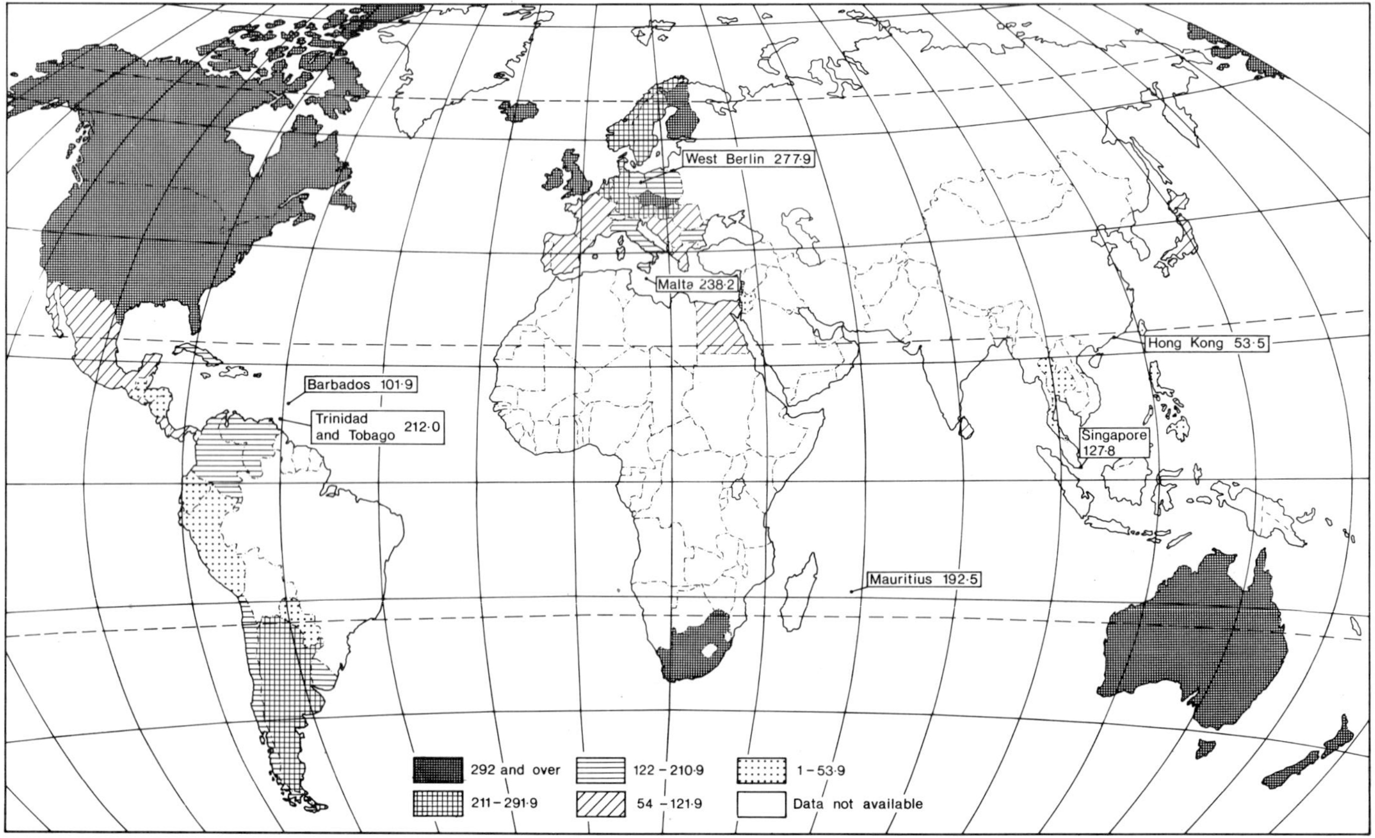

Fig. 17.2 Mortality from ischaemic heart disease for males aged 35–64 years per 100 000 in 1969–71 (based on W.H.O. data).

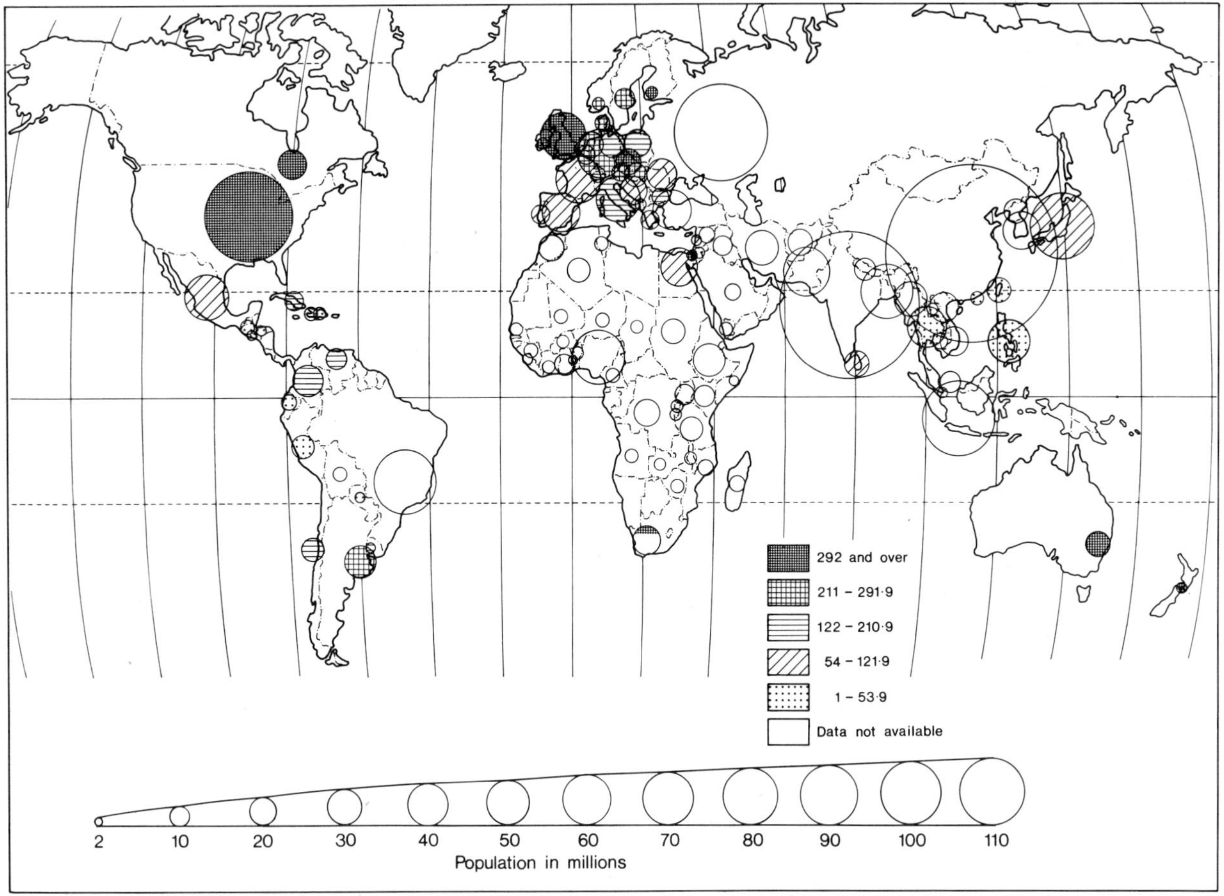

Fig. 17.3 Mortality from ischaemic heart disease for males aged 35–64 years per 100 000 in 1969–71 (based on W.H.O. data).

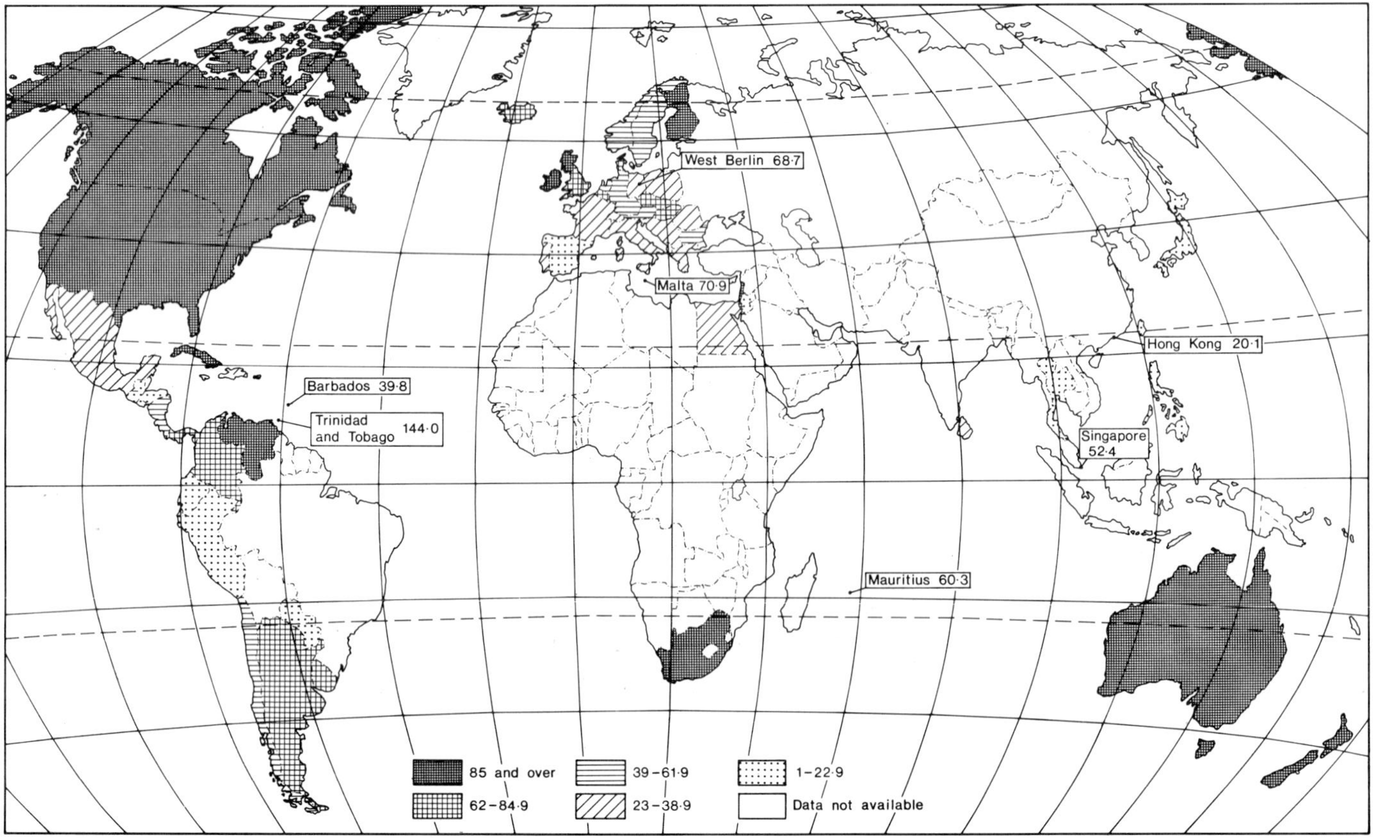

Fig. 17.4 Mortality from ischaemic heart disease for females aged 35–64 years per 100 000 in 1969–71 (based on W.H.O. data).

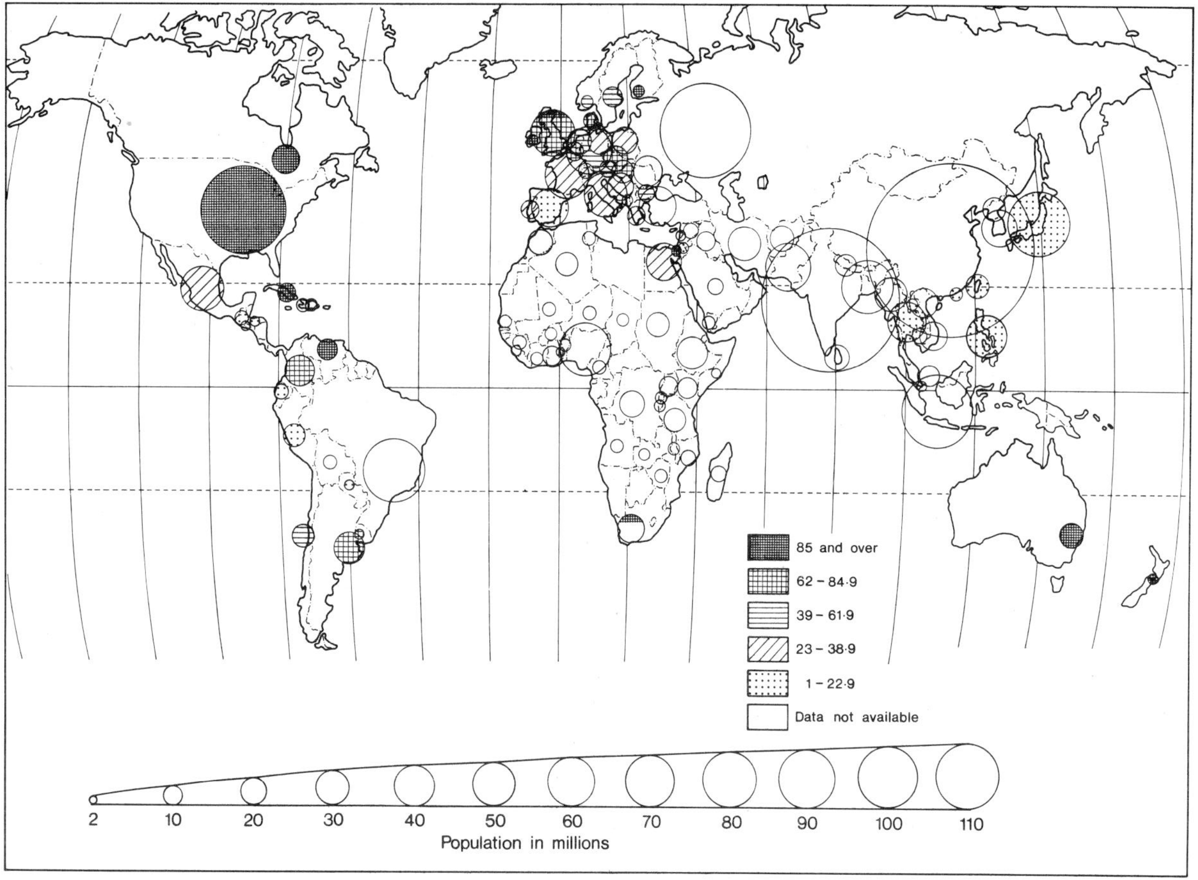

Fig. 17.5 Mortality from ischaemic heart disease for females aged 35–64 years per 100 000 in 1969–71 (based on W.H.O. data).

male rate), Cuba, Colombia, Panama, Costa Rica, Puerto Rico, Trinidad and Tobago, Uruguay and Israel.

For those countries for which data are available and relative to the populations "at risk", mortality from ischaemic heart disease for both sexes is highest in Finland, South Africa, the U.S.A., Scotland, Australia, Northern Ireland, New Zealand, Canada, Ireland and Israel. On the other hand, and in contrast, death rates from this cause are consistently low in Thailand, Honduras, Guatemala, El Salvador, Taiwan, Ecuador, Paraguay, Jordan, Peru, the Philippines and Hong Kong.

The variation in the mortality experience of Finland, the country with the highest male rate per 100 000 in the age group 35–64 years, and Thailand, the country with the lowest rate in the same age group, exceeds five hundred fold. The variation for females is similar.

As already mentioned, too much weight should not be given to the geographical differences noted because of the small number of countries for which data are available and also the different standards and fashions of diagnosis occurring in the various countries. Nevertheless, in a developed area, such as Europe, Rose (1973) suggests that different heart-disease mortality rates are chiefly the result of influences other than differences in interpreting the cause of death.

Table 17.1 lists death rates in the age group 45–54 years for a selection of 16 countries for which information was available to the W.H.O. This particular age group is significant because death is due mainly to atheroma and the factor of old age does not intervene. It shows that over the 15-year period 1955–70 mortality from ischaemic heart disease in Australia, Czechoslovakia, Finland, France, Hungary, Netherlands, Sweden and England-Wales was higher in 1970 than it was in 1955. In the case of Czechoslovakia, France, Netherlands and England-Wales, the death rates are continuing to rise, but in Hungary and Sweden peak rates were attained during the years 1967–68 and they are now showing a steady decline.

Of the countries for which information was available, mortality rates for men increased between 1955–70, but the rates for females for the same period showed a decrease, except in Australia, the U.S.A. and England-Wales. Death rates for men are, in general, about three times those for women.

In countries such as Hong Kong, Singapore and Papua and New

Country		Death rate per 100 000 inhabitants							% change
		1955	1960	1966	1967	1968	1969	1970	1955–70
	T	159.8	182.4	203.9	204.6	193.8	196.0	188.4	+18
Australia	M	247.0	287.0	324.4	325.0	311.9	314.7	297.4	+20
	F	65.2	71.9	81.3	82.1	73.9	75.1	76.9	+70
	T	72.4	83.3	80.8	88.6	82.4	77.9	68.8	−5
Austria	M	113.9	144.7	147.1	165.7	150.1	146.7	132.2	+18
	F	37.1	34.7	31.9	32.2	33.4	28.6	23.1	−38
	T	171.6	191.5	185.9	187.4	173.4	161.6	158.0	−8
Canada	M	277.0	307.6	312.0	314.7	293.8	273.1	270.1	−2
	F	59.0	69.0	59.3	60.5	54.4	51.9	48.4	−19
	T	74.1	76.8	93.9	101.3	103.7	113.3	117.0	+58
Czechoslovakia	M	114.1	127.2	159.7	178.1	181.0	194.2	204.4	+78
	F	36.5	29.3	32.3	29.7	31.7	38.2	35.7	−1
Federal Republic	T	90.0	97.3	107.6	102.3	76.4	75.9	77.2	−14
of Germany	M	134.2	159.5	186.5	179.7	148.9	146.4	147.7	+10
	F	51.9	48.5	49.7	46.0	24.1	24.8	25.9	−50
	T	173.8	186.1	226.1	244.7	240.4	220.3	212.8	+22
Finland	M	305.8	340.1	436.7	468.6	461.0	427.3	402.9	+32
	F	59.2	53.4	51.4	60.1	58.6	48.8	54.8	−9
	T	30.3	40.2	42.1	41.7	39.9	36.7	38.3	+28
France	M	49.2	67.8	73.3	72.4	70.5	63.2	65.8	+34
	F	12.0	13.5	12.2	12.2	10.5	11.2	11.6	−4
	T	84.5	91.7	104.1	111.2	119.3	84.6	88.4	+5
Hungary	M	109.2	119.2	148.5	160.7	181.9	142.8	145.7	+34
	F	61.9	67.2	65.3	67.9	64.5	33.3	37.6	−40
	T	69.7	75.7	78.0	78.9	65.8	65.4	61.8	−11
Italy	M	97.2	114.7	125.1	127.5	113.6	112.9	106.4	+10
	F	43.6	38.8	34.2	34.0	21.9	21.9	20.9	−51
	T	53.6	45.7	39.2	39.1	23.7	22.7	22.9	−57
Japan	M	58.3	52.9	51.5	50.4	36.4	34.4	34.2	−41
	F	49.0	39.1	28.9	29.9	13.4	13.2	13.6	−73
	T	69.9	73.3	98.0	106.9	102.6	106.0	111.2	+40
Netherlands	M	115.1	128.7	173.7	191.2	184.0	188.8	201.4	+74
	F	27.2	20.9	25.6	26.2	24.8	26.8	24.9	−7
	T	69.5	69.4	76.5	79.7	85.5	72.1	80.8	+17
Sweden	M	106.9	108.3	125.7	133.7	141.9	126.0	136.5	+28
	F	32.5	30.1	26.8	25.4	28.9	17.9	24.8	−22
	T	78.0	79.3	85.7	75.9	80.6	61.0	61.9	−21
Switzerland	M	117.1	124.7	135.8	126.2	129.3	103.4	107.2	−8
	F	41.8	33.9	37.1	27.3	38.3	19.7	17.8	−57
United Kingdom: England	T	109.1	121.2	144.5	140.9	141.9	148.1	149.4	+37
and Wales only	M	181.3	208.3	248.0	244.0	245.1	254.9	259.1	+42
	F	40.1	37.6	44.6	41.6	41.9	44.0	41.9	+4
	T	210.6	216.0	215.7	211.8	216.8	210.3	205.2	−3
United States	M	342.2	358.5	357.7	351.8	355.0	346.3	336.0	−2
	F	82.2	78.2	81.9	80.3	87.6	83.5	84.4	+1
	T	97.5	118.6	96.7	102.1	78.5	81.1	88.3	−9
Venezuela	M	127.3	158.1	126.8	139.6	108.6	110.6	121.2	−4
	F	65.1	75.1	65.2	61.7	46.3	49.4	52.9	−18

Table 17.1 Heart disease: death rates (45–54 years) per 100 000 population for selected countries, 1955–70 (W.H.O. data).

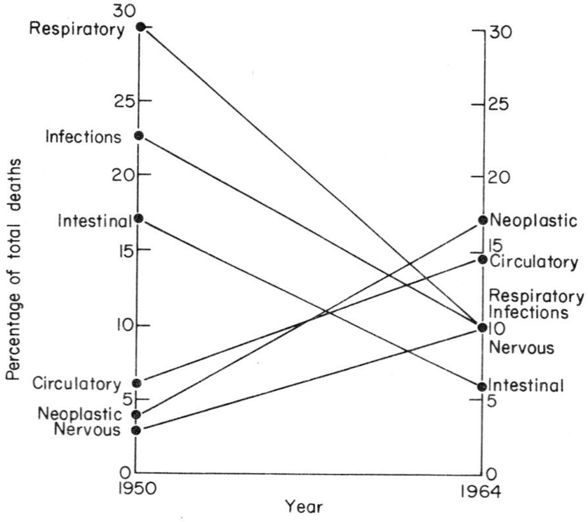

Fig. 17.6 Trends in the major causes of mortality in Hong Kong, 1950–64 (Fry and Farndale, 1972).

Guinea, which are becoming progressively more industrialized and where the western way of life is becoming increasingly adopted, there is a noticeable fall in the incidence of infectious, intestinal and respiratory diseases and a rise in degenerative (circulatory) and neoplastic diseases (cancer) (Figs 17.6 and 17.7).

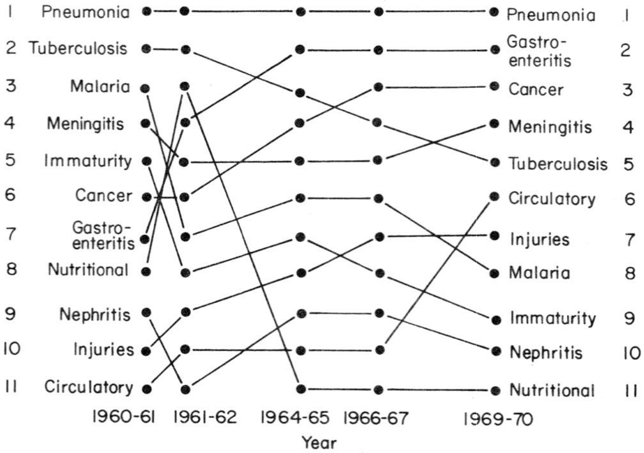

Fig. 17.7 Major causes of mortality in order of importance in Papua and New Guinea (Fry and Farndale, 1972).

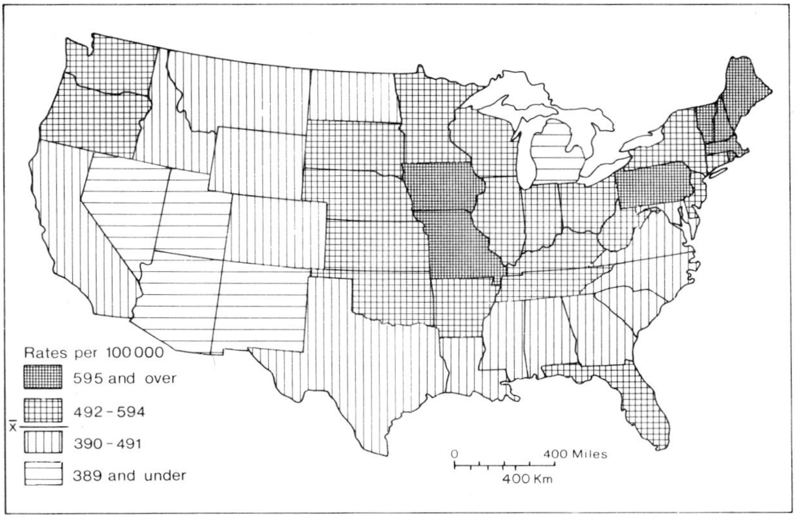

Fig. 17.8 Mortality from heart disease in the U.S.A. in 1967 (Pyle, 1971).

Crude mortality rates in the U.S.A. for heart disease (including vascular lesions), during 1967, for both sexes combined are shown in Fig. 17.8.

The heaviest concentration of high rates is in the main manufacturing belt of the country (especially in Pennsylvania, Vermont, New Hampshire, Iowa, Missouri) and the lowest rates are in the southwest (Nevada, Utah, Arizona, New Mexico). Apart from interstate differences in population structure, other factors such as hereditary background, level of physical activity and degree of urbanization, including perhaps atmospheric pollution, have been implicated as contributing to the observed spatial variations.

On a more limited city scale within the U.S.A., Figs 17.9 and 17.10 show, by trend surface analysis,* the patterns for heart disease mortality in Chicago for the years 1960 and 1967 respectively. For both periods, most of the inner suburbs and all of the City of Chicago demonstrate an incidence above the mean. Mortality decreases with distance from the centre of Chicago. The north-western part of the SMSA† shows a high incidence for both periods. In general the more youthful outer suburban fringe shows a lower incidence. This is not

* Trend surface analysis is a cartographic technique which facilitates extrapolation and smoothing of surfaces.

† Standard Metropolitan Statistical Area.

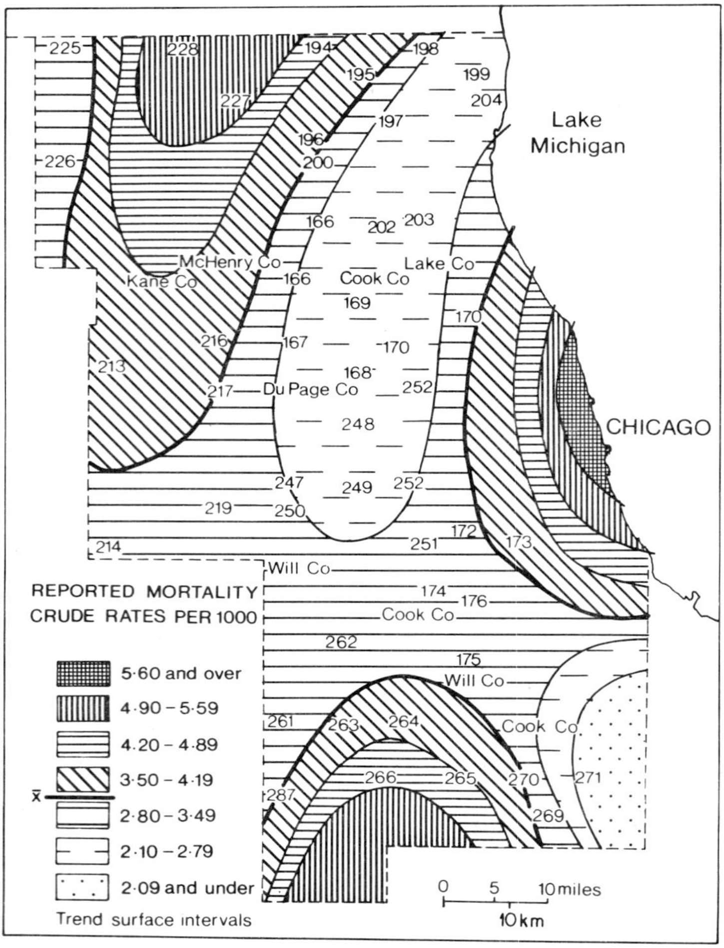

Fig. 17.9 Mortality from heart disease in Chicago, 1960 (Pyle, 1971).

altogether unexpected since the maps, as with the national map (Fig. 17.8), are based on crude, rather than age-specific, death rates. The incidence of heart disease mortality in most parts of the metropolis was similar for both periods (Pyle, 1971).

Ischaemic heart disease is the main cause of death in the United Kingdom, accounting for upwards of 25% of the total annual mortality. The spatial distribution of mortality, for males and females separately, is shown by means of standardized mortality ratios (SMR)* on a demographic base map† in Figs 17.11 and 17.12. The most obvious feature of the distributional pattern is the concentration of high mortality ratios in the north of the country and low mortalities in the south. For this purpose Northern Ireland may be classed with the north of Britain. The dividing line runs from the Mersey to the Humber. The only exceptions of this generalization are South Wales and a small number of London boroughs. The main areas of unfavourable mortality experience are Scotland, Tyneside, South Wales and Northern Ireland.

Britain's comprehensive National Health Service ensures that medical care and attention is available to all classes of society with a comparatively high degree of equality. Diagnostic fashions and practices undoubtedly vary but ischaemic heart disease is so common a cause of death that substantial diagnostic transfer to another cause of death category would have to produce a large excess in the alternative diagnosis. Since compensating variations of this kind are not apparent, the geographical patterns displayed in Figs 17.11 and 17.12 must be substantially real.

Internationally it is suggested that mortality from ischaemic heart disease correlates broadly with affluence. As already noted, the high rate of occurrence is a characteristic feature of many affluent societies and there are indications that the disease is on the increase in other societies that are moving rapidly towards the same type of civilization. Indeed, it is thought that ischaemic heart disease may well be an indicator of man's *maladaptation* to this kind of civilization and could prove an important limiting factor in the search for further technological and economic advances. In the United Kingdom, however, the pattern is, surprisingly, the reverse since SMRs are *lower* in the economically favoured South-East and high in the comparatively poor North and North-West.

* The Standardized Mortality Ratio allows for peculiarities of age structure in local populations. It is expressed in terms of the standard United Kingdom rate taken as 100 in each case. If the SMR for a local area is 100 then the area experiences, in the period under consideration, a mortality equal to that for the United Kingdom as a whole; if the SMR is 200 then the rate is twice as great as the United Kingdom average.

† The demographic maps relate the SMRs to the gross populations resident in each geographical area. The areas of the "squares" (representing urban areas) and "diamonds" (representing rural areas) are proportional to the populations at risk. Main centres of population thus assume increased proportions, while large counties with numerically small populations are reduced in area relative to the United Kingdom as a whole.

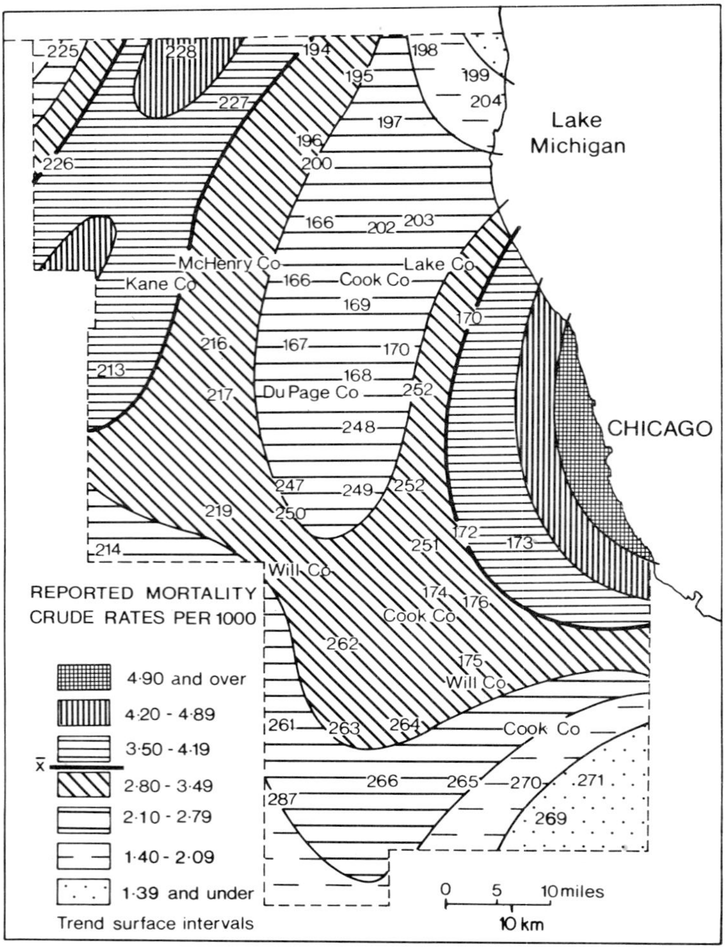

Fig. 17.10 Mortality from heart disease in Chicago, 1967 (Pyle, 1971).

London and Glasgow are representative of mortality experience in the favoured South-East and the less favoured North of Britain (Fig. 17.13).

Taking the cities as separate entities, Glasgow has a standardized mortality ratio 25% above the United Kingdom's average, whereas London approximates to the United Kingdom's average. However, each city displays unmistakable spatial or areal variations within its boundary. In Glasgow, there are several administrative wards where the mortality experience for ischaemic heart disease is below the United Kingdom average, while in London there are certain boroughs where the experience is above the national average. Mortality experience in the London boroughs of Hampstead and St. Marylebone is 16–18% above the United Kingdom's average. Such unfavourable ratios are paralleled in Glasgow by the wards of Pollokshaws, Cathcart, Parkhead, Shettleston, Tollcross, Ruchill, Whiteinch, Yoker and Knightswood. On the other hand, Glasgow contains eight wards— Cowlairs, Townhead, Exchange, Calton, Dalmarnock, Hutchesontown, Gorbals, Pollokshields—where the mortality experience is 15% or more below the national average whereas, in London, only the City borough comes into this same favourable category. Such considerable geographical variations in mortality experience at the local level serve to demonstrate the limitations accompanying generalization at the global and national levels and of the dangers inherent in assumptions that countrywide or even city environments and life styles are similar or homogeneous.

It is worth noting that, in Chicago (Figs 17.9 and 17.10), the mortality experience improves from the city centre to the outskirts, but, in both London and Glasgow, mortality patterns are irregular and no such gradation is evident. The value of this comparison is reduced because the Chicago maps are based on crude rates while the Glasgow and London maps show standardized mortality ratios.

The spatial variability in mortality from ischaemic heart disease within the city of Glasgow (Fig. 17.13) fails to support the widely held view that there is a negative correlation between cardiovascular mortality and the degree of hardness of the public water supply, since the whole of the city is provided with soft water from Loch Katrine.

Figures 17.14 and 17.15 show the distribution of standardized mortality ratios for ischaemic heart disease in Australia. The most noticeable high values occur in the south-east, in and around Melbourne, Sydney and the coastal divisions of New South Wales. For males, Adelaide also has a high standardized mortality ratio. Detailed local studies within Tasmania reveal striking spatial contrasts. Here, where ischaemic heart disease is responsible for 36% of all male deaths and 29% of the female deaths, mortality experience tends to be high in the west and south and low in the north (Fig. 17.16).

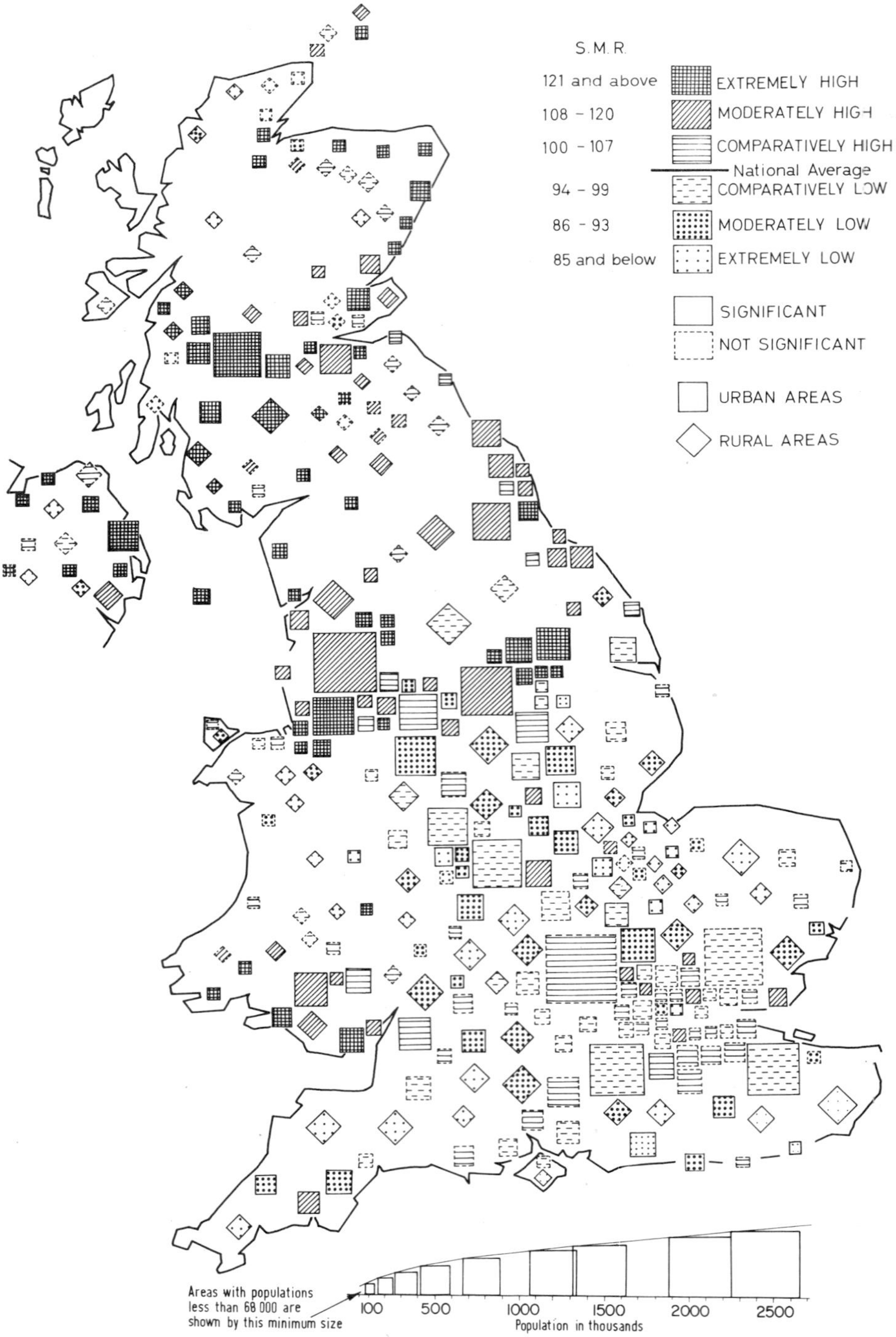

Fig. 17.11 Male mortality from ischaemic heart disease in the United Kingdom, 1959–63 (Howe, 1970).

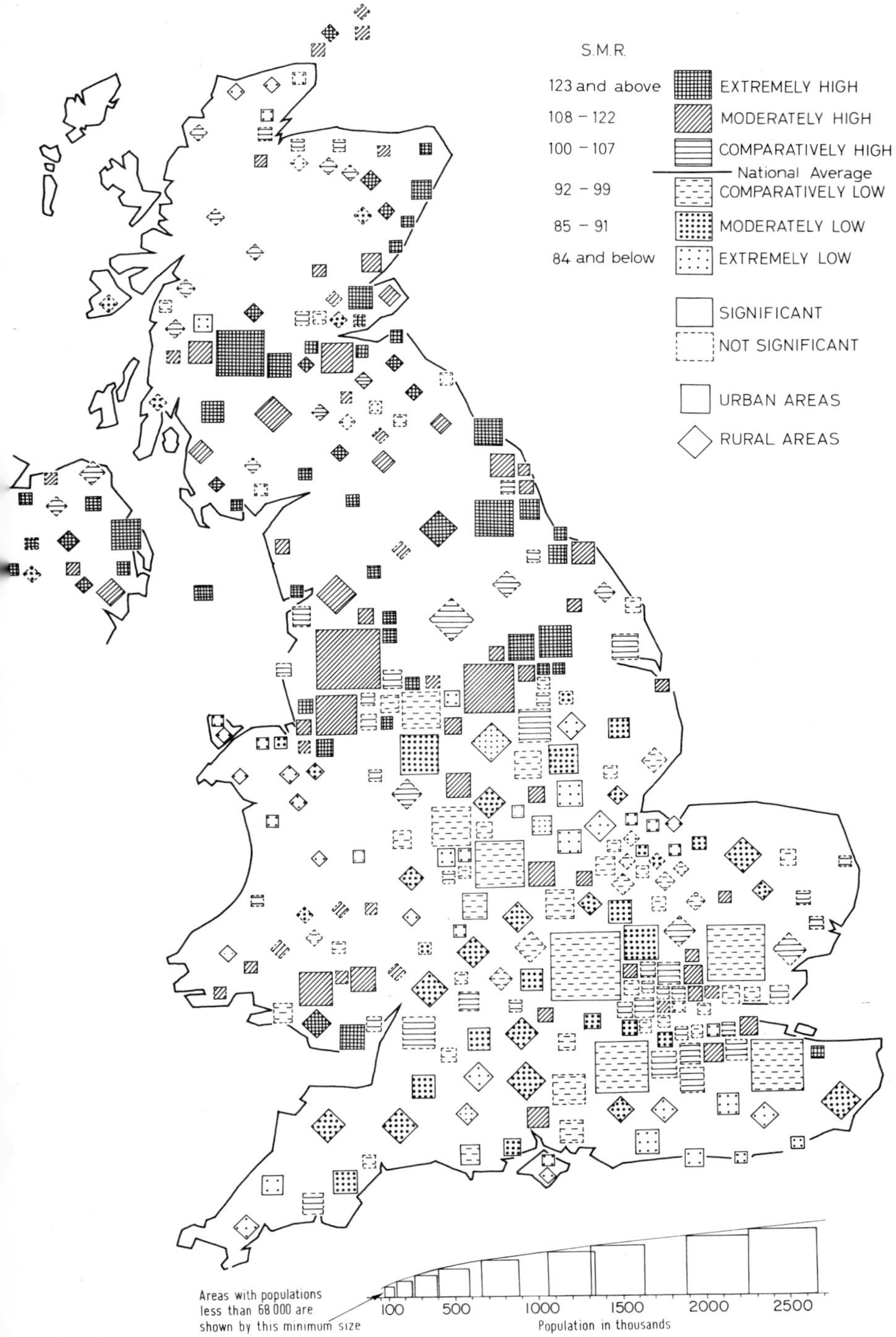

Fig. 17.12 Female mortality from ischaemic heart disease in the United Kingdom, 1959–63 (Howe, 1970).

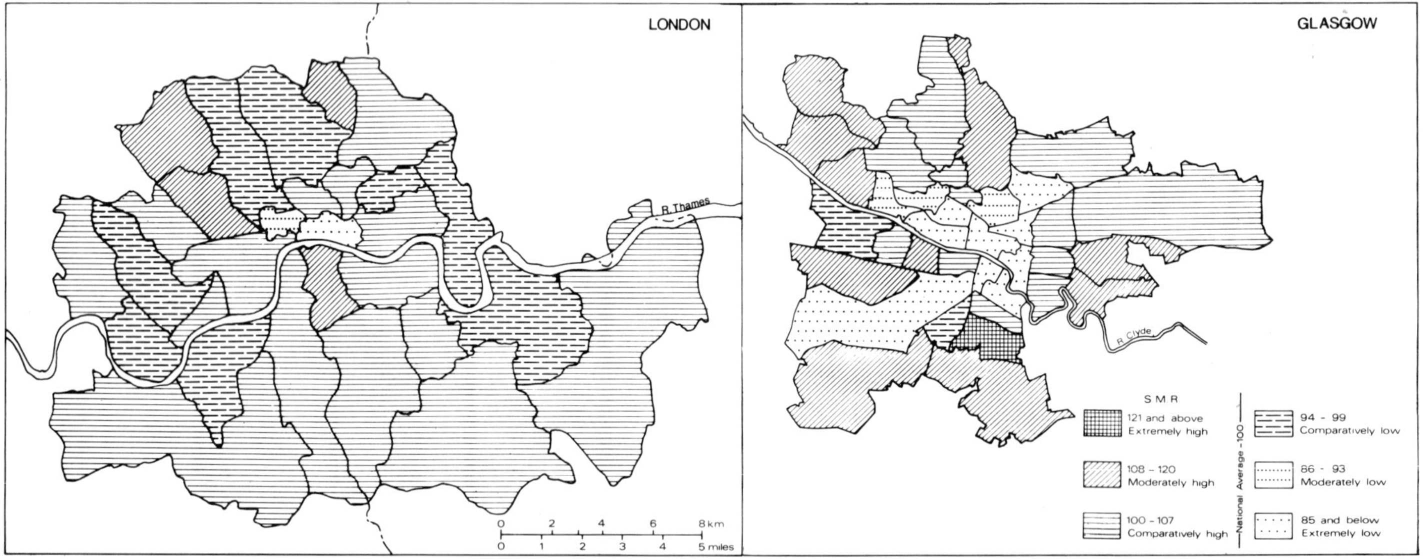

Fig. 17.13 Mortality from ischaemic heart disease for males in London and Glasgow, 1959–63 (Howe, 1972).

INVOICE

28

2 3 1974

Noah

...T. OF

Jordan Gallery.

Amsterdam House

Annie

McMullan 14.00

Paid

cook

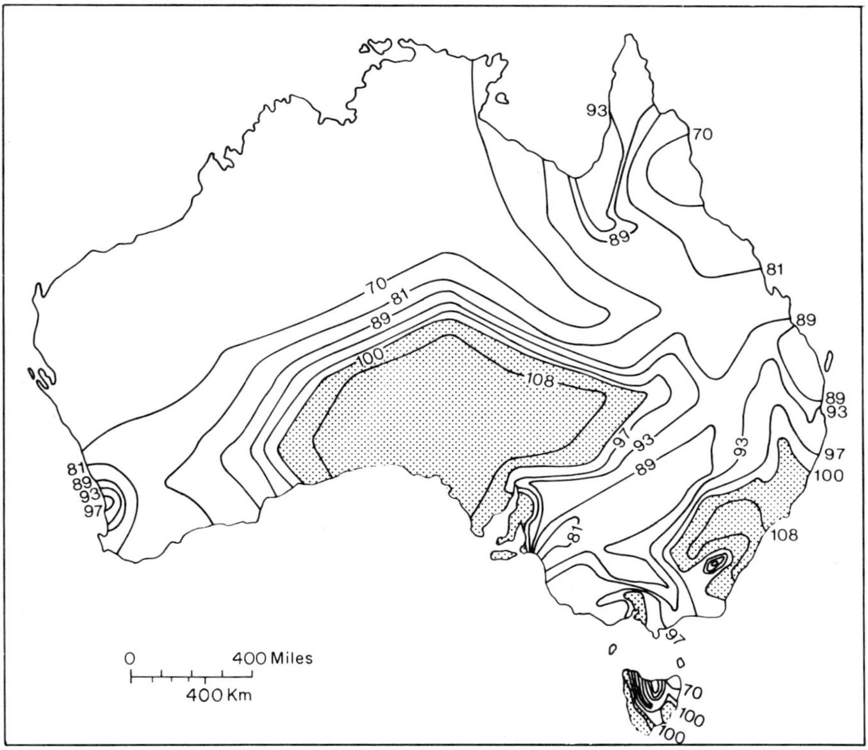

Fig. 17.14 Mortality from heart disease in Australia in males, 1965–66, based on standardized mortality ratios (Learmonth and Grau, 1969).

Reported risk factors in ischaemic heart disease

Ischaemic heart disease, resulting from atheresclerotic change, constitutes one of the principal unsolved problems of contemporary medicine. It is now generally accepted that this condition is not due to any one single factor or cause but rather to a combination of possibly related factors or stimuli. It is, in effect, a disease of multifactorial aetiology. Nevertheless in the case of ischaemic heart disease of atherosclerotic origin, the factors contributing to it are known to be already present in young people. Risk factors include hypertension, cigarette smoking, lack of physical exercise, obesity, high plasma lipoprotein, stress, diabetes, hereditary and soft drinking water.

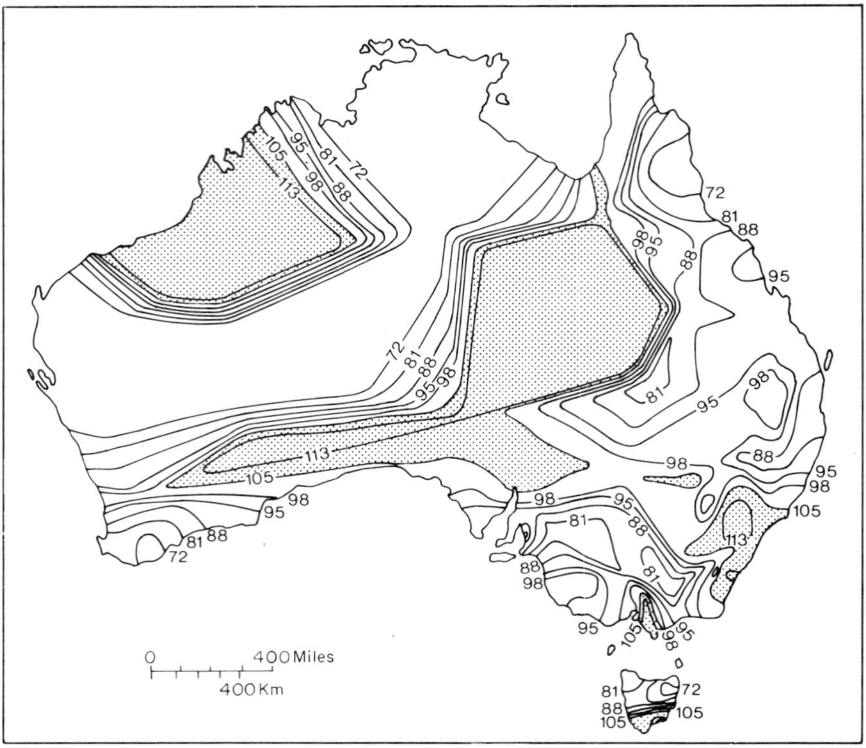

Fig. 17.15 **Mortality from heart disease in Australia in females, 1965–66, based on standardized mortality ratios (Learmonth and Grau, 1969).**

Hypertension

The previous existence of high blood pressure or hypertension is probably the most common single aetiological factor in the development of ischaemic heart disease as well as in hypertensive heart disease. Hypertension, the result of narrowing of the small arteries, is a condition that can produce heart failure by placing an abnormal strain on the heart and arteries when the blood pressure increases above the normal systolic pressure of 130–150 mm of mercury and a diastolic pressure of 70–80 mm. High blood pressure tends to increase with age and is found particularly in females over 50 years. Low prevalence rates of hypertension are found in Chinese, Puerto Ricans, African negroes, Australian natives and Indian peasants. However, North-American negroes have higher blood

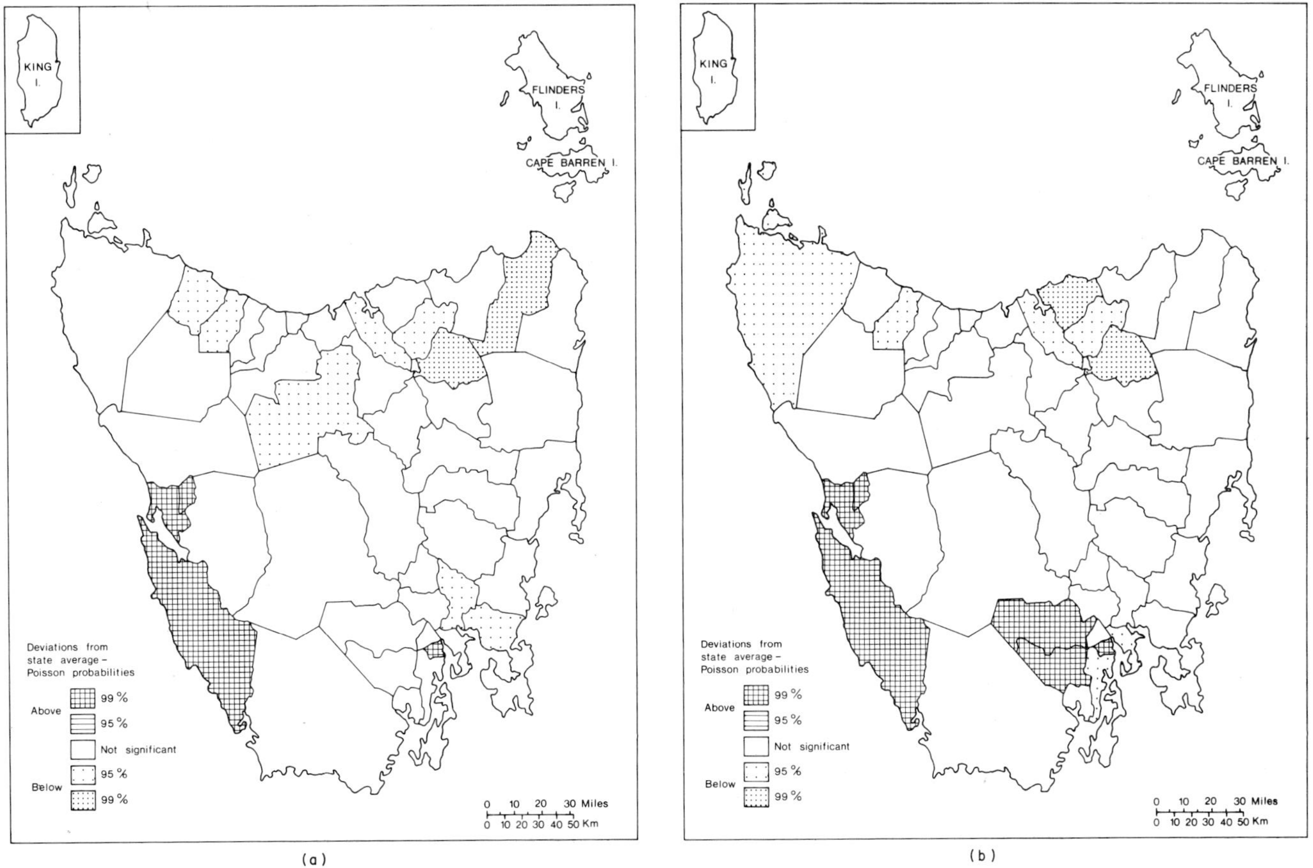

Fig. 17.16 Male (a) and female (b) mortality from ischaemic heart disease in Tasmania, 1958–73 (after McGlashan, 1974).

pressure levels, higher morbidity and mortality from hypertension, hypertensive heart disease and stroke than white Americans.

The Framingham Study conducted in the U.S.A. (Dauber *et al.*, 1962) showed that higher levels of blood pressure were related to higher rates of mortality from coronary heart disease and stroke. In men between the ages of 40 years and 59 years, the presence of hypertension increased the risk of future coronary disease almost threefold (Kannel *et al.*, 1961). Elevations of systolic and diastolic blood pressure were also accompanied by an increased risk of developing coronary heart disease in the Evans County (Georgia, U.S.A.) Long Term Study (Cassell *et al.*, 1971). Although there is a positive association between the existence of hypertension and cardiovascular disorders, not all people with high blood pressure develop cardiovascular disorders nor does heart disease occur only in those with hypertension. Research into the distinguishing characteristics of hypertensives who do not develop cardiovascular disorders has shown that low plasma renin concentration protects patients against stroke and heart attacks (Brunner *et al.*, 1972).

Cigarette smoking

There seems little doubt that cigarette smoking has a harmful effect on the lungs and is injurious to the general state of health of the individual. It is clearly related to cardiovascular disease in that it causes arterial constriction and has been shown to affect the development of atherosclerosis. Despite the acceptance of this assertion, numerous questions remain unanswered or only partially answered when attempting to define the precise link between the use of tobacco and morbidity and mortality from chronic illness. Among the questions are the variations in the effect of smoking a different number of cigarettes over a given period of time and the development and progress of heart disease and cerebrovascular disease. The differences involved when a person inhales smoke from a cigarette as opposed to one who does not habitually follow this practice, the influence on health in spending different lengths of time in the smoking of a cigarette, using different forms of tobacco, cigarette, cigar or pipe, the age when an individual commences smoking and the age when the habit was finally broken are all factors requiring precise inquiry. Of importance also is an understanding of which component of tobacco presents the greatest risk to health in relation to cardiovascular disease. The nicotine, tar and lead content of cigarettes and the carbon monoxide inhaled from them, separately or in aggregate, have been implicated in the development of chronic illness.

Attempts have been made and partial answers produced for some of these questions. Morris (1967) presents epidemiological data indicating the highest age-specific incidence of ischaemic heart disease as, in ascending order, non-smokers, ex-smokers, etc. Paul *et al.* (1963) report a high correlation between cigarette smoking and coronary heart disease, but no strong correlation between cigar and pipe smokers and this same condition (Friedberg, 1966).

Physical inactivity

A review of the relevant literature indicates strong support for the hypothesis that lack of physical exercise is linked with the development of cardiovascular disease. Nevertheless, the support is not unreserved since any possible relationship between chronic illness and physical inactivity is complicated by several factors. Morris (1967) found that there is a different incidence of ischaemic heart disease for different occupations. By associating different levels of physical activity with different occupations, he reached the conclusion that physical activity variations account for variations in ischaemic heart disease. Further research has supported the postulate that men in more sedentary occupations have more fatalities from coronary heart disease (Levy and Ernst, 1973). These findings are not entirely supported by Friedberg (1966) who suggests that factors other than physical activity may be involved.

Physical inactivity is implicated as an important risk factor in the Evans County (Georgia) Cardiovascular Disease Study (Cassel *et al.*, 1971). This research involved a study of non-white and white adult residents for cardiovascular disease for the period 1960–1962 and a follow-up study between 1967 and 1969. Consistently lower death rates among non-whites, the failure of other risk factors to account for this difference and the similarity of rates between share-croppers* of both ethnic groups supported an association between the occurrence of the disease and lack of exercise.

Any possible relationship between cardiovascular disease and

* Share croppers are tenant farmers of a specific kind. They are obliged to plant crops specified by the landowner and receive a share of the crop in lieu of wages.

physical activity—or lack of it—is complicated by measurement problems and associations with other risk factors. For example, those under stress are often those who take little exercise; obesity, exercise and diet are themselves all inter-related. This distinction must be made between occupational activity and leisure activity as both are important if total daily exercise is to be gauged. The question arises as to whether a direct link exists between physical inactivity and chronic disease or whether sedentary living is merely contributory to another risk factor.

Obesity

There is little concrete evidence that obesity itself bears a close relationship to either the incidence or prevalence of coronary heart disease. But the use of different criteria for the definition and measurement of obesity, the multifactorial aetiology of obesity and the inter-relationships between obesity and coronary heart disease complicate the issue. Clinical investigations have revealed strong relationships among and between obesity and hypertension and obesity and high blood lipid levels, while epidemiological surveys have shown the association between obesity and lack of physical exercise and overeating.*

Obesity and calorie intake are related in that serum cholesterol tends to fall on any reducing diet but, in the stable conditions of calorie equilibrium, there is little relationship between serum cholesterol and relative obesity. It would seem that, in the absence of these risk factors, the obese are at no greater risk to cardiovascular disease than people of average weight (Friedberg, 1966). This was shown in the study by Keys (1970) in which no relationship between an overweight condition and myocardial infarction was established and, in Epstein's study (Epstein *et al.*, 1956), a sample of 61 American Jews having coronary heart disease were found to be no heavier than their controls.

Plasma lipoprotein levels

The precise cause of atherosclerosis has yet to be discovered but key points on which almost all researchers agree are that fats and

* In the process of refining flour for white bread, which is a major item in the western diet, very little of the original nutritive value of the grain is left. This means that it may be necessary to eat too much to obtain adequate nutrition.

cholesterol occur in all atherosclerotic deposits and that at least some and possibly all of this cholesterol comes from the blood. Although much of it is manufactured by the liver, the amount of cholesterol which appears in the blood is influenced by the composition of the diet, and in particular the kind of fat consumed in the diet. Some foods such as egg yolks, cream, butter, lard and fatty meats produce a great deal more cholesterol in the blood than other foods such as vegetables and vegetable oils (e.g. sunflower-seed oil or corn oil—i.e. polyunsaturated fat). The modern western-type diet which is high in calories and high in animal (saturated) fats is thus associated with high-serum cholesterol levels.

Studies have shown a close statistical correlation between cholesterol levels in the blood and deaths from ischaemic heart disease among younger people. Men with blood cholesterol levels above 280 mg/100 ml are four times as likely to have a heart attack as those with a level below 200 mg/100 ml. As the blood cholesterol level rises, so does the risk of coronary heart disease.

Conclusive proof that fats and cholesterol cause heart disease in man is not available and unlikely to be obtained in the foreseeable future. However, several authorities are now advocating a change to diets low in saturated fat (with partial replacement of saturated or animal fat by vegetable oils with a high proportion of polyunsaturated fats), together with measures directed against cigarette smoking, obesity and high blood pressure.

Excessive consumption of sugar

Cleave (1956) was the first to point out that sugar excess and fibre depletion tend to be reciprocal to each other. Removal of unabsorbable fibre from natural carbohydrate foods results in a concentration of the starch and sugar with consequent over consumption. When food is diluted with fibre, satiety precedes over-consumption. Possibly the greatest change that has occurred in western diets since the last quarter of the 19th century, compared with those of the developing world include, in particular, a rise in sugar consumption, possibly up to 200% (Antar *et al.*, 1964; Walker, 1971). In the United Kingdom for example, consumption of sugar in pounds weight per head per annum was 64 in 1880, 96 between 1934–8, 111 between 1959–62 and 105 in 1974. Furthermore, carbohydrate as starch is digested to and absorbed as glucose in the body. Refined flour as used in the white bread of western style diets is almost pure starch, so adding to the refined sugar consumption. Dietary habits involving increased consumption of carbohydrates and refined sugar would appear to bear a relationship with increased incidence of ischaemic heart disease, but there is as yet no understanding of how glucose in excess of normal requirements can cause or contribute to the disease.

Stress

The concept of stress is not easy to apply to populations or sub-groups within a culture because of the variation in the individual's perception of what constitutes a stressful situation. A stress to one man is a challenge to another. In acute states possibly precipitated by a sense of time urgency and competitiveness, responses in individuals may take the form of hormonal and cardiovascular changes. For this reason, it has been suggested that, over a period of time, the repetition of such reactions might be an aggravating factor in cardiovascular disease. In one American study, interviews by a psychologist were used to classify individuals' behaviour patterns into Type A, with high levels of competitiveness and time urgency, and Type B, with low levels of competitiveness and time urgency. The subsequent incidence of coronary heart disease was reported to be approximately doubled in "Type A" individuals.

Diabetes mellitus

This disorder, in which the body is unable to control the use of sugars as a source of energy, is considered to be a risk factor in ischaemic heart disease. A study in Bedford (England) found that the age-adjusted prevalence of arterial disease was lowest in a control group of persons with normal blood sugar, intermediate in persons with "borderline" hyperglycaemia and highest among the diabetics (Keen *et al.*, 1965).

Water hardness

Substantial evidence has been produced to suggest a relationship between cardiovascular disease and hardness of water supplies. However, apart from a correlation between soft water (i.e. water deficient in calcium and magnesium ions) and a high incidence of cardiovascular disease, little is known of the possible preventive or pathological processes involved in this relationship. The initial work in this field was carried out by Schroeder (1960) who reported in a study in the U.S.A. that an association was clearly established between weighted average water hardness and average annual death rate from cardiovascular disease. Numerous other research workers have supported these findings. Morris *et al.*, (1961) working in England obtained a negative correlation of 0.54 between total hardness and cardiovascular mortality amongst males in age groups 46–64 years and 65–70 years. In an attempt at formalization, Muss (1962) established that the relationship followed a linear equation significant at the 99.9% level. A study carried out by Masironi considered water hardness and radioactivity. He concluded that areas supplied with water high in radioactivity and hardness showed lower death rates for diseases of the cardiovascular system. This relationship was strongest for hypertensive heart disease and suggests water hardness and radioactivity may be indicators of some unknown water factor (Masironi, 1970).

Not all the available evidence supports the findings of the above research. In the counties of Oklahoma state, Lindeman and Assenzo (1964) could not find any positive correlation between soft water and cardiovascular disease; neither could Howe (1970) in Glasgow (p. 447). Work by Roberts and Lloyd (1972) implied that a primary relationship existed between ischaemic heart disease and rainfall whereas the association between heart disease and hardness of water supplies was only of secondary importance.

CEREBROVASCULAR DISEASE

Cerebrovascular disease is the third leading cause of death in most countries for which national statistical data for international use are available through the W.H.O. It is surpassed only by ischaemic heart disease and cancer.

Different from ischaemic heart disease, cerebrovascular disease displays no great difference in mortality frequency between males and females though generally a slight preponderance of male deaths over female deaths is noted. On the other hand, different rates of mortality and morbidity have been found in countries with different physical and cultural environments. In the age group 55–64 years, its

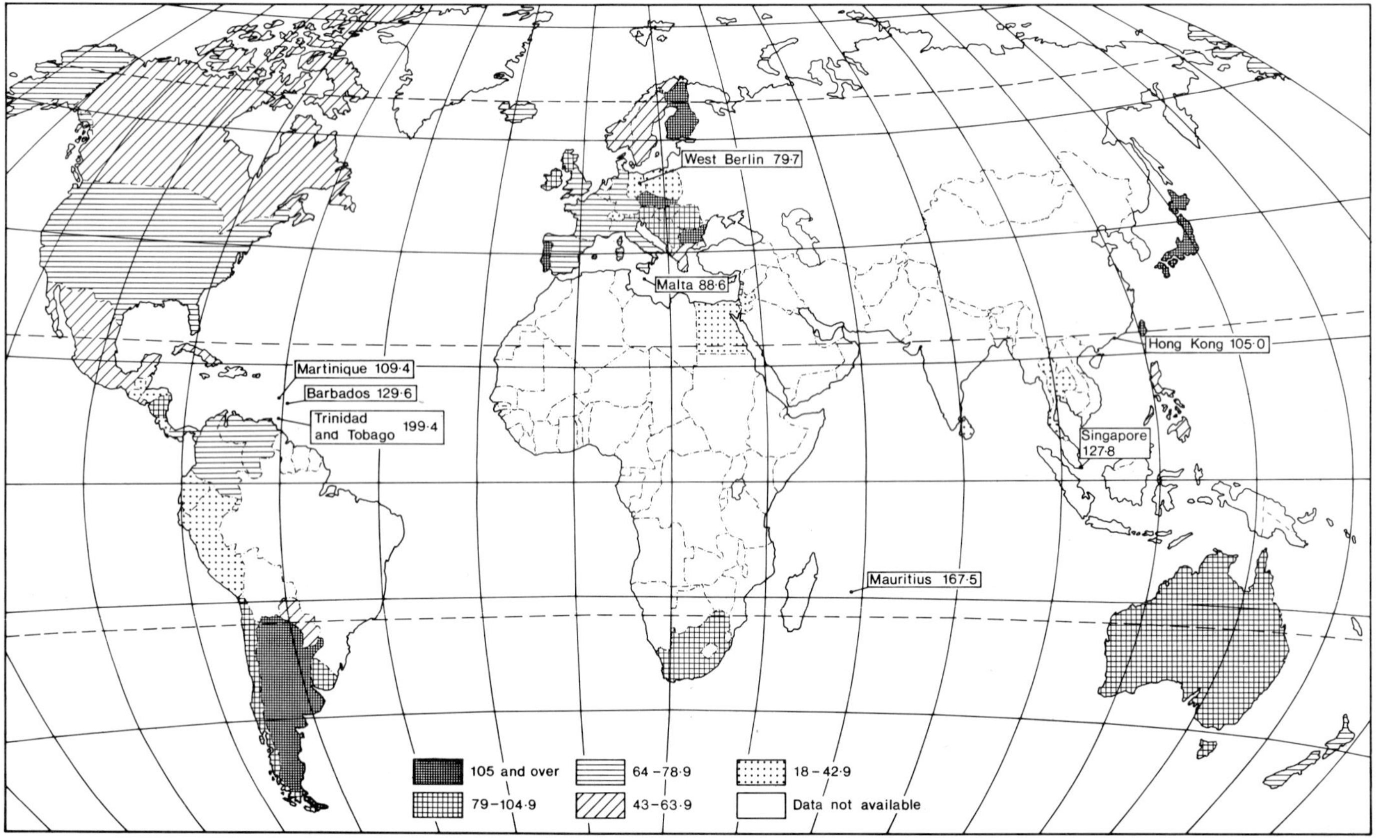

Fig. 17.17 Mortality from cerebrovascular disease for males aged 35–64 years per 100 000.

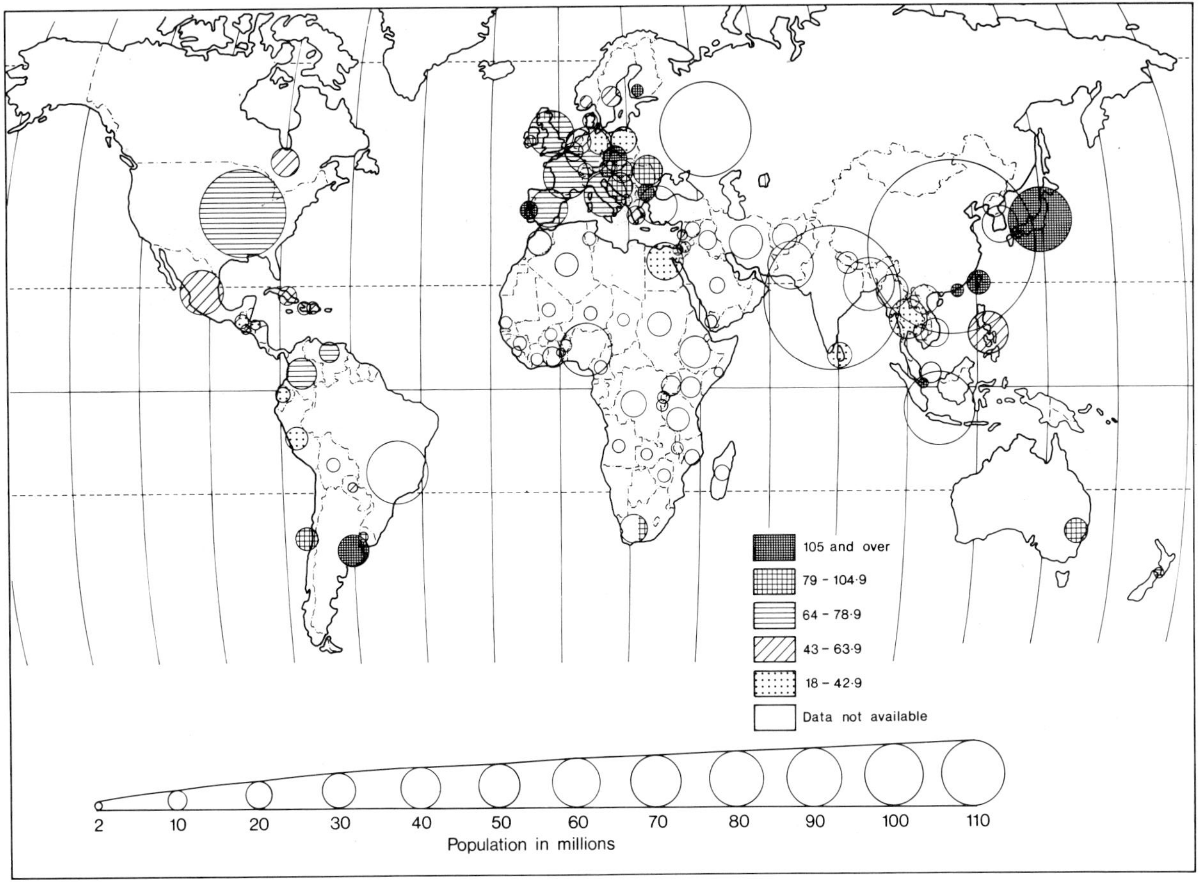

Fig. 17.18 Mortality from cerebrovascular disease for males aged 35–64 years per 100 000.

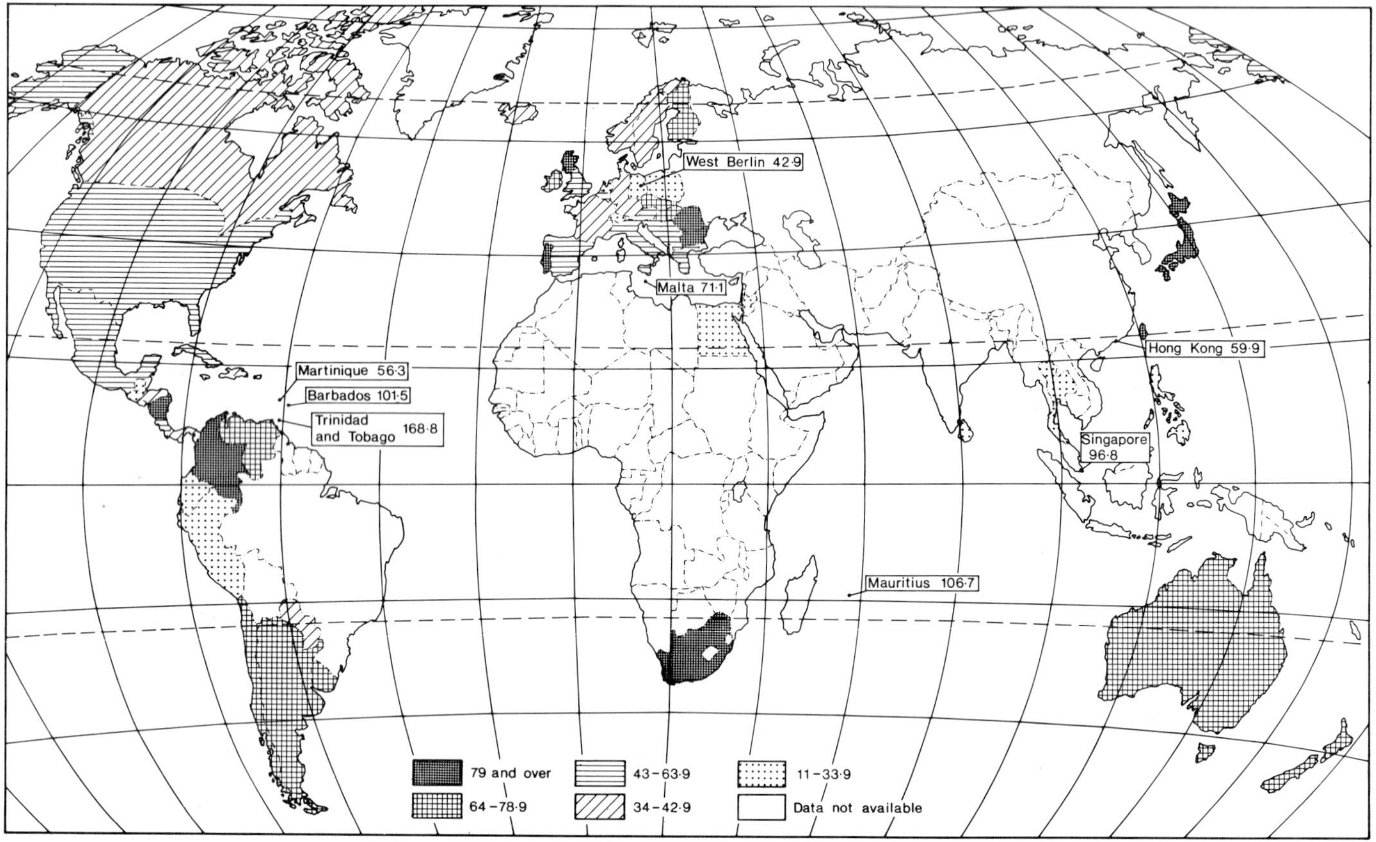

Fig. 17.19 Mortality from cerebrovascular disease for females aged 34–64 years per 100 000 in 1966–67 (based on W.H.O. data).

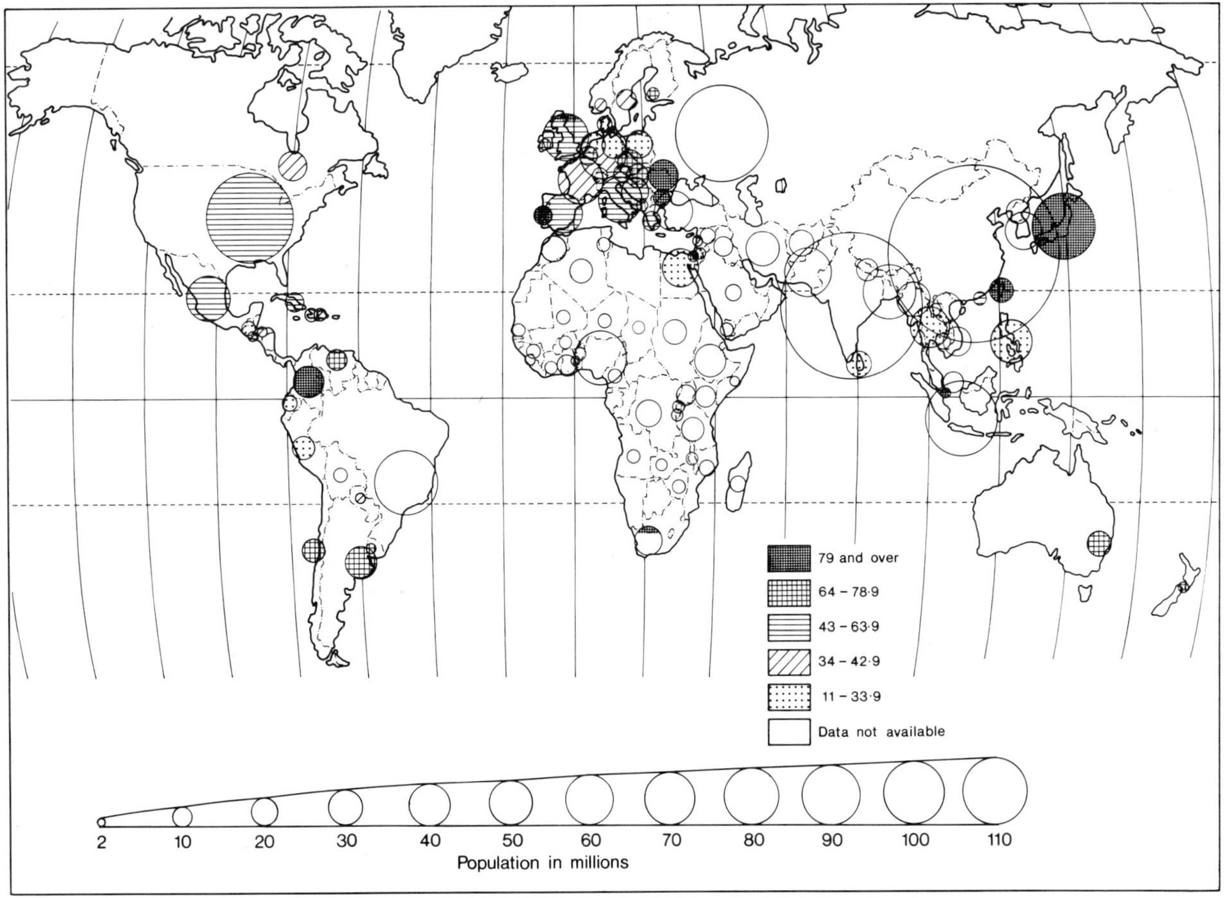

Fig. 17.20 Mortality from cerebrovascular disease for females aged 35–64 years per 100 000 in 1969–71 (based on W.H.O. data).

rate of frequency is higher in Japan, Taiwan, Mauritius, Trinidad and Tobago, Portugal, Bulgaria, Malta, Scotland and Chile than elsewhere: it is lowest in Central America, the Philippines and Thailand. Even within the same country, regional differences have been found. In Japan, for instance, it occurs most frequently in the northern part of Honshu Island, in the U.S.A. it appears mostly in the south-eastern states and is more frequent among negroes than among the white population. Cerebrovascular disease strikes more frequently among Japanese in Japan than among expatriate Japanese in Hawaii or in North America.

According to the W.H.O., the clinical diagnosis of stroke and therefore the mortality statistics relating to it seem reasonably accurate, but the accuracy of the differential diagnosis of *type* of stroke-cerebral embolism, cerebral haemorrhage, cerebral thrombosis-was found to be poor.

Figures 17.17–17.20 show the geographical distribution of death rates for males and females respectively for the countries for which statistical data are available. Although high mortality rates still broadly correspond with industrially advanced English-speaking countries, there is a change in the ranking of countries at the top of the

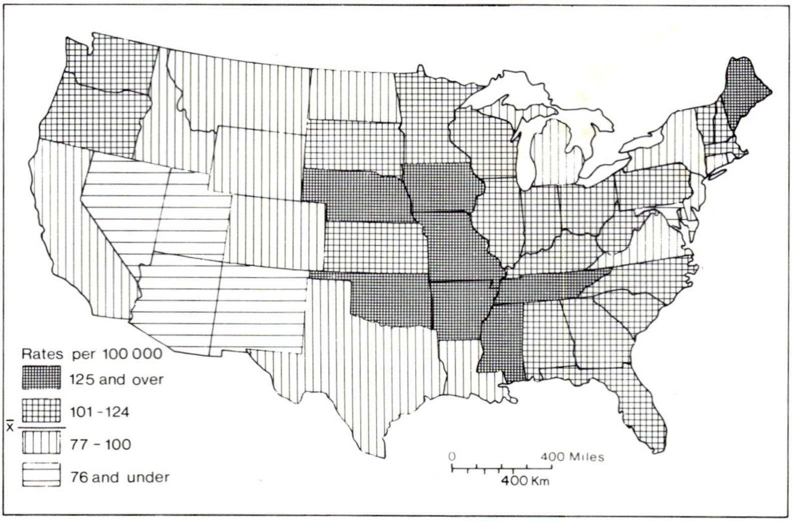

Fig. 17.21 Mortality from cerebrovascular disease in the U.S.A. in 1967 (Pyle, 1971).

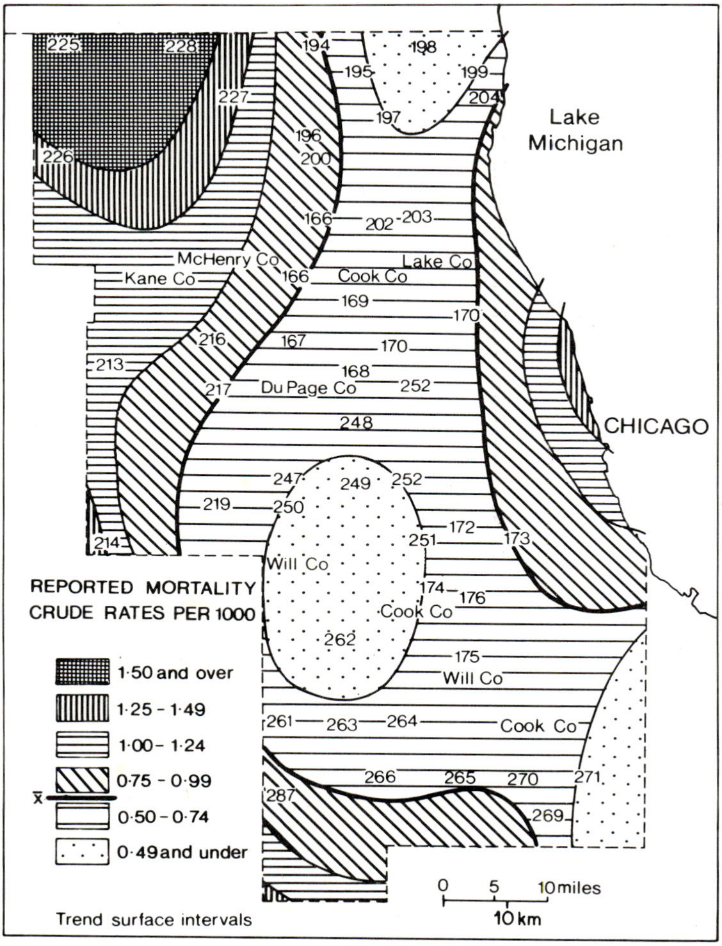

Fig. 17.22 Mortality from cerebrovascular disease in Chicago, 1960 (Pyle, 1971).

list. For the age group 35–64 years, Singapore, Taiwan, Japan, the Balkan states, Portugal, Mauritius and a number of West-Indian countries have noticeably increased mortality rates relative to other areas. Canada in particular, Ireland, England and Wales, the U.S.A., Australia, New Zealand, Israel and Scandinavian countries have decreased relative mortality rates. Consistently low mortality occurs in Egypt, Jordan, Thailand, certain European countries, Peru, Ecuador and Ceylon.

Table 17.2 presents mortality rates from cerebrovascular disease (stroke) for a selection of countries. The age group 45–54 years is selected because the factor of old age does not intervene. Nevertheless, extreme prudence is essential when making comparisons because of different habits and fashions in diagnosis.

Japan experiences exceptionally high rates from stroke. The male rate is twice the female rate but the latter is itself comparable with the

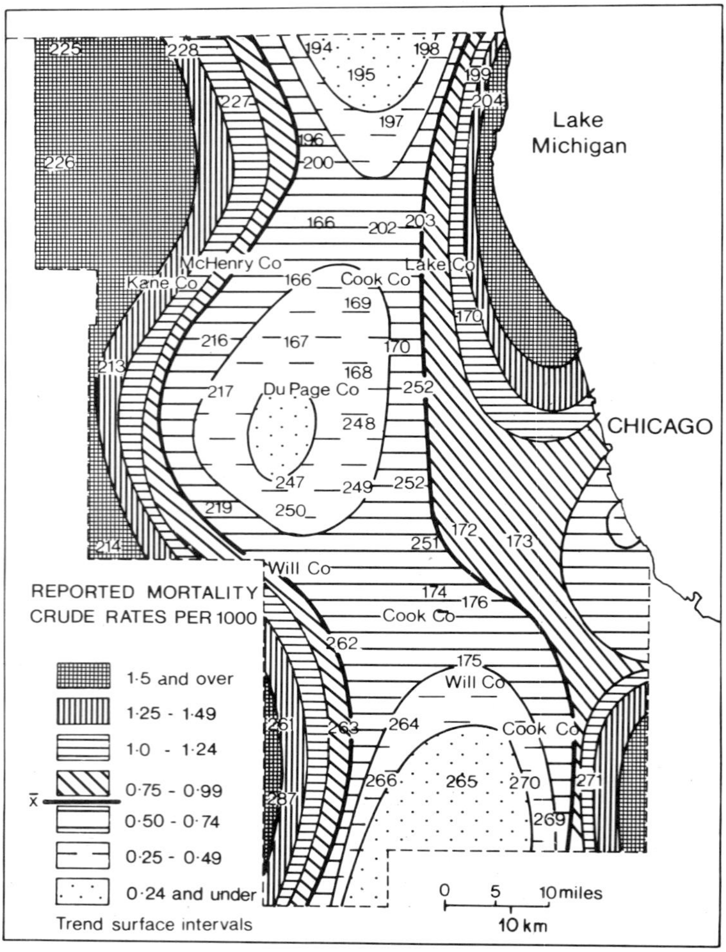

Fig. 17.23 Mortality from cerebrovascular disease in Chicago, 1967 (Pyle, 1971).

particularly high male rate in Finland. It is suggested that the high rates, especially in the north of the country, are related to the diet (which contains large amounts of salt) and to unheated, cold and draughty wooden houses. High salt intake and cold are regarded as important contributory factors in the development of hypertension which is itself considered to be the most frequent risk factor in stroke in most countries.

For the countries for which information is available and with the exception of Venezuela (both sexes), Czechoslovakia (males) and the Netherlands (males), deaths from cerebrovascular disease show a decline between 1955 and 1970. This noticeable improvement may be due, in part at least, to better control of hypertension.

The spatial variability of death rates from stroke in the U.S.A. in 1967 is shown in Fig. 17.21. The pattern of this, the "No. 5 killer of people in their most productive years in the U.S.A.," shows the highest rates in the mid-central part of the country and, as with ischaemic heart disease, lowest rates in the southwest states.

Figures 17.22 and 17.23 show, by means of trend surface analysis, the patterns of stroke mortality in Chicago in 1960 and 1967 respectively. There is a similarity in the patterns for death rates due to cardiovascular disease (Figs 17.9 and 17.10) and those due to cerebrovascular disease in that the higher rates occur in both the central city and rural fringe and the lower rates in the outer suburbs The exception is that, from 1960 to 1967, the area of highest stroke deaths "shifted" from the centre of Chicago City to a long band running up the North Shore, consistent with the new types of residential accommodation in that area (Pyle, 1971, p. 77).

In the United Kingdom, the regional differences in mortality from cerebrovascular disease (Figs 17.24 and 17.25) are strikingly correlated with those for ischaemic heart disease (Figs 17.11 and 17.12), i.e. high values in the North and West and low values in the South-East. This regional imbalance is not surprising since hypertension and atherosclerosis both play a part in each condition. It is perhaps remarkable that in a few areas, notably Northern Ireland (males), there are high rates for ischaemic heart disease and low rates for stroke; this is the reverse of the Japanese situation.

In Australia, areas with high standardized mortality ratios occur in South Australia, north and south of Adelaide and in the eastern parts of Victoria and New South Wales (Figs 17.26 and 17.27).

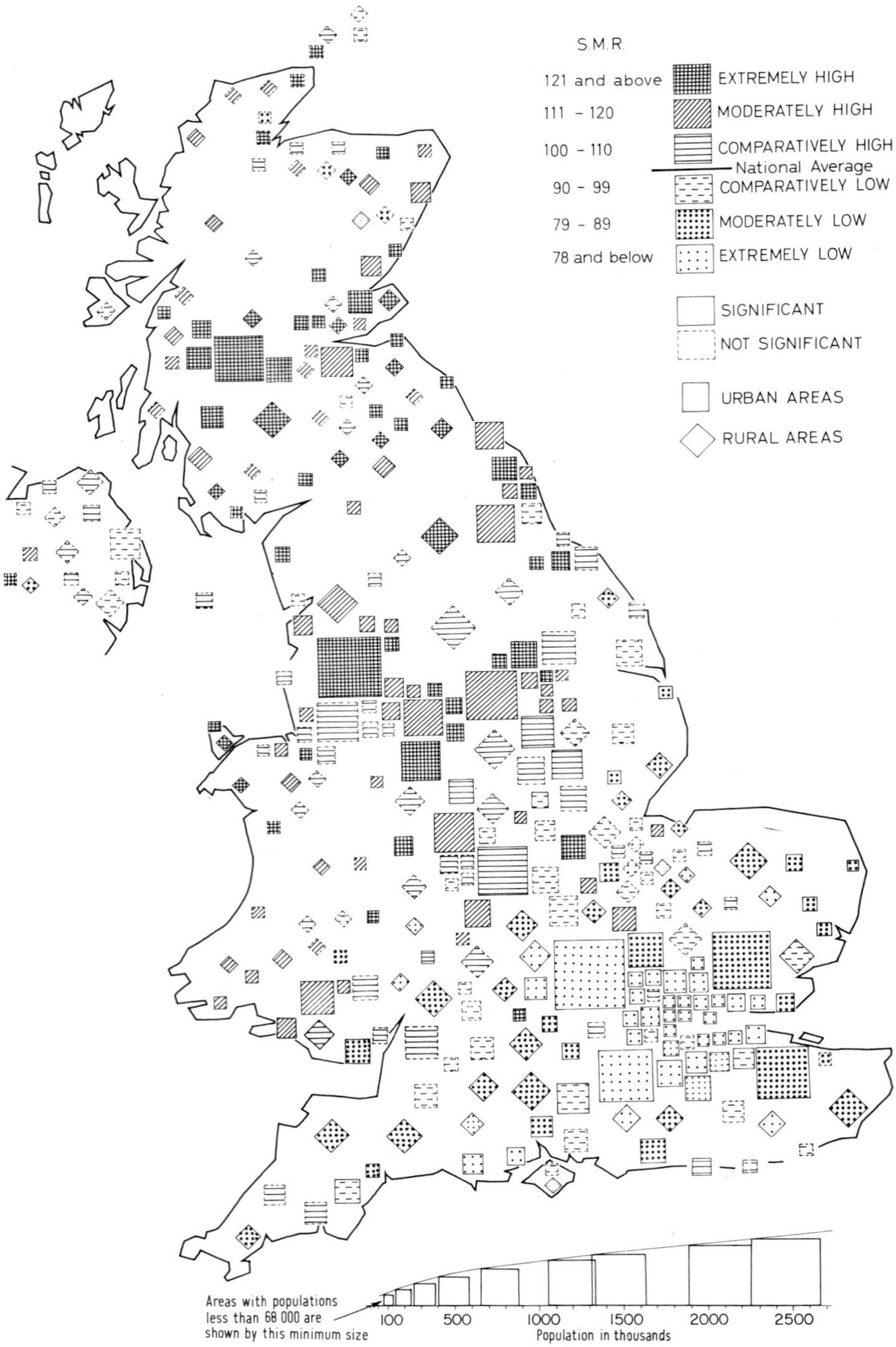

Fig. 17.24 Male mortality from cerebrovascular disease in the United Kingdom, 1959–63 (Howe, 1970).

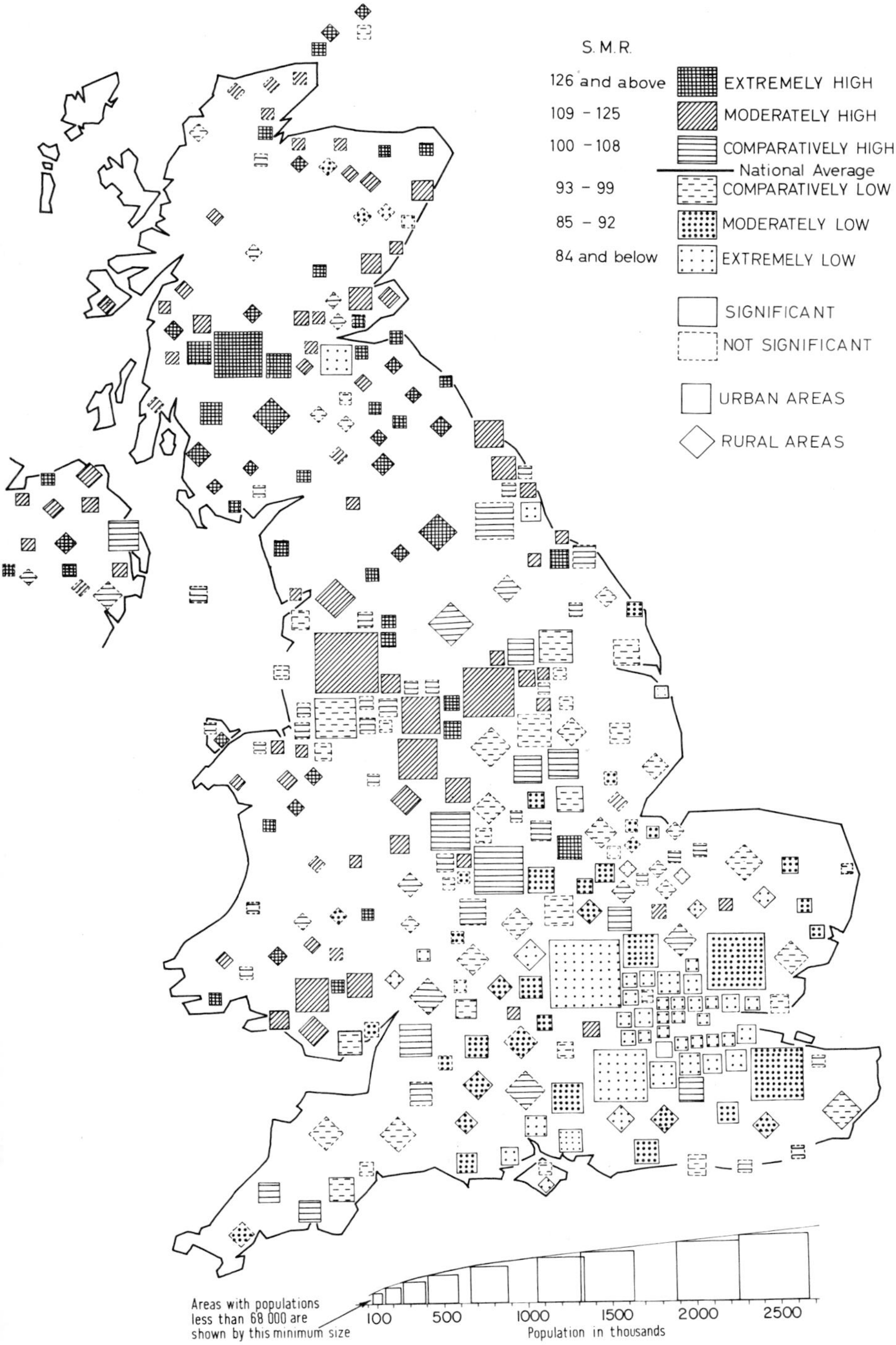

Fig. 17.25 Female mortality from cerebrovascular disease in the United Kingdom, 1959–63 (Howe, 1970).

County		Death Rate per 100,000 inhabitants 1955	1960	1966	1967	1968	1969	1970	% change 1955–70
Australia	T	77.5	62.5	55.7	57.9	56.8	55.3	52.9	−32
	M	71.3	59.2	51.9	58.0	58.1	56.6	50.7	−29
	F	84.2	66.1	59.7	57.8	55.5	53.9	55.2	−33
Austria	T	42.3	40.0	31.2	29.7	29.7	37.5	39.6	−18
	M	44.3	43.1	37.6	40.1	38.2	49.1	40.9	−8
	F	40.6	37.6	26.5	22.1	23.6	29.3	30.1	−25
Canada	T	42.8	34.4	29.5	31.1	30.2	30.4	27.9	−35
	M	39.9	34.9	30.4	32.9	33.3	31.7	29.1	−27
	F	45.9	34.0	28.7	29.4	27.1	29.2	26.8	−41
Czechoslovakia	T	43.7	30.1	27.4	28.4	37.8	41.5	44.4	+2
	M	44.7	32.9	33.7	32.4	44.7	54.0	49.9	+12
	F	42.7	27.4	21.5	24.8	31.4	29.8	39.3	−8
Federal Republic of Germany	T	38.9	34.2	30.2	27.2	28.2	27.2	25.4	−35
	M	40.1	37.1	35.5	33.6	35.3	34.3	31.4	−21
	F	37.8	32.0	26.3	22.5	23.0	22.1	21.0	−44
Finland	T	66.9	59.8	69.5	67.4	68.7	73.8	63.2	−6
	M	68.2	64.8	72.8	75.0	68.9	80.8	66.4	−2
	F	65.7	55.5	66.8	61.1	68.6	68.0	60.5	−8
France	T	55.7	43.8	34.8	33.0	34.8	36.4	33.3	−41
	M	64.7	49.7	43.7	40.4	44.9	47.9	41.4	−35
	F	47.0	38.1	26.2	25.9	25.1	25.3	25.4	−45
Hungary	T	63.2	51.1	43.6	40.0	40.2	43.3	44.1	−30
	M	60.0	49.8	42.9	44.2	48.0	50.6	50.1	−17
	F	66.2	52.2	44.2	36.4	33.4	36.9	38.7	−41
Italy	T	44.3	42.4	40.7	38.6	37.3	34.5	36.2	−18
	M	47.2	46.2	45.3	44.0	42.5	41.5	41.4	−12
	F	41.5	38.8	36.4	33.6	32.6	28.2	31.3	−24
Japan	T	152.2	140.3	113.2	104.6	101.4	97.3	91.6	−40
	M	168.8	168.0	145.9	135.7	136.2	128.7	121.8	−28
	F	136.1	115.0	86.0	79.0	73.1	71.6	66.6	−52
Netherlands	T	23.6	21.2	22.1	25.9	24.0	24.5	23.9	+2
	M	20.1	20.3	22.3	28.8	24.0	25.6	24.3	+20
	F	26.9	22.1	21.9	23.2	34.1	23.4	23.4	−13
Sweden	T	45.7	30.3	27.0	25.6	27.2	28.4	25.7	−44
	M	38.9	31.0	29.4	27.8	27.0	31.8	29.7	−47
	F	52.5	29.7	24.7	23.3	27.3	25.0	21.8	−59
Switzerland	T	39.6	25.9	21.5	22.6	20.3	20.0	20.3	−49
	M	38.1	24.9	22.3	24.9	24.5	25.5	20.6	−46
	F	41.0	26.9	20.8	20.3	16.2	14.7	20.1	−51
United Kingdom: England and Wales only	T	52.5	46.9	42.0	41.0	40.3	41.1	42.1	−19
	M	51.1	49.0	43.3	41.4	40.9	43.1	43.0	−15
	F	53.9	44.9	40.6	40.6	39.7	39.1	41.3	−24
U.S.A.	T	56.0	48.9	43.4	43.5	44.3	41.6	41.4	−26
	M	56.3	51.9	47.3	46.2	47.7	45.1	44.1	−22
	F	55.7	45.9	39.7	41.0	41.2	38.3	38.7	−31
Venezuela	T	36.8	48.9	45.3	44.4	43.4	45.3	43.7	+18
	M	33.9	53.9	48.6	44.0	47.6	43.9	44.3	+30
	F	40.0	43.3	42.0	44.8	38.9	46.8	43.0	+8

Table 17.2 Cerebrovascular disease: death rates (45–54 years) per 100 000 population for selected countries, 1955–70 (W.H.O. data).

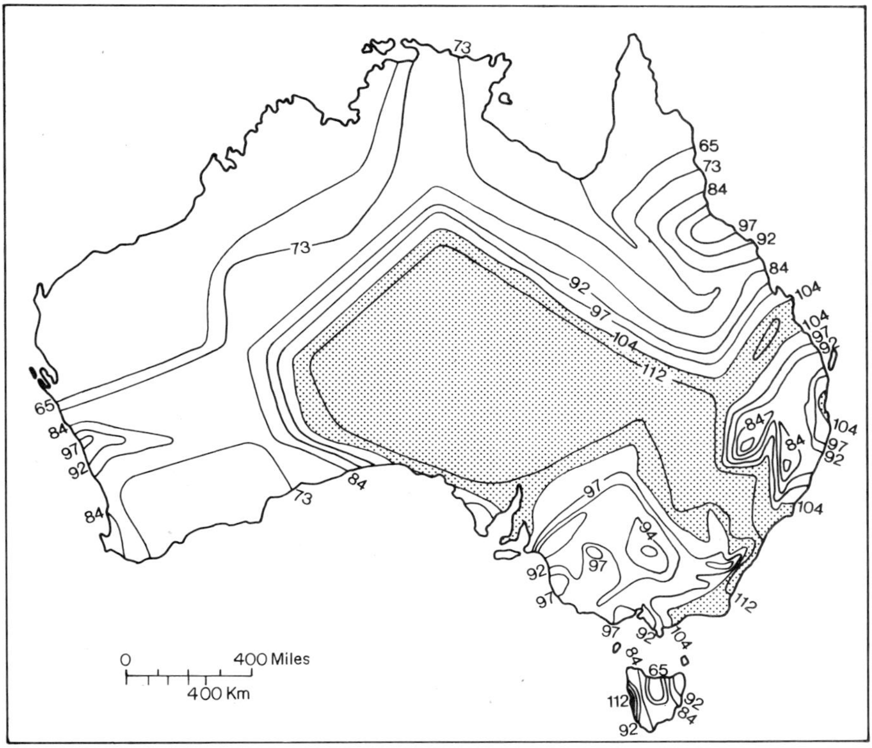

Fig. 17.26 Male mortality from cerebrovascular disease in Australia, 1965–66, based on standardized mortality ratios (after Learmonth and Grau, 1969).

HYPERTENSIVE HEART DISEASE

Population-based studies show that hypertension or high blood pressure is common in most parts of the world and its impact on health is great because of its direct complications in cerebrovascular disease, its accelerating effect on the progress of atherosclerosis and ischaemic heart disease, as well as in hypertensive heart disease itself. Phibbs (1967) explains hypertension essentially as a condition which can produce heart failure due to abnormal blood pressure. Normal blood pressure lies between 120–140 mm systolic and 70–80 mm diastolic but for reasons such as time of day, age, nervous tension and emotional stress "normal" pressure may vary appreciably. Only a few population groups, either living at high altitudes (e.g. indigenous

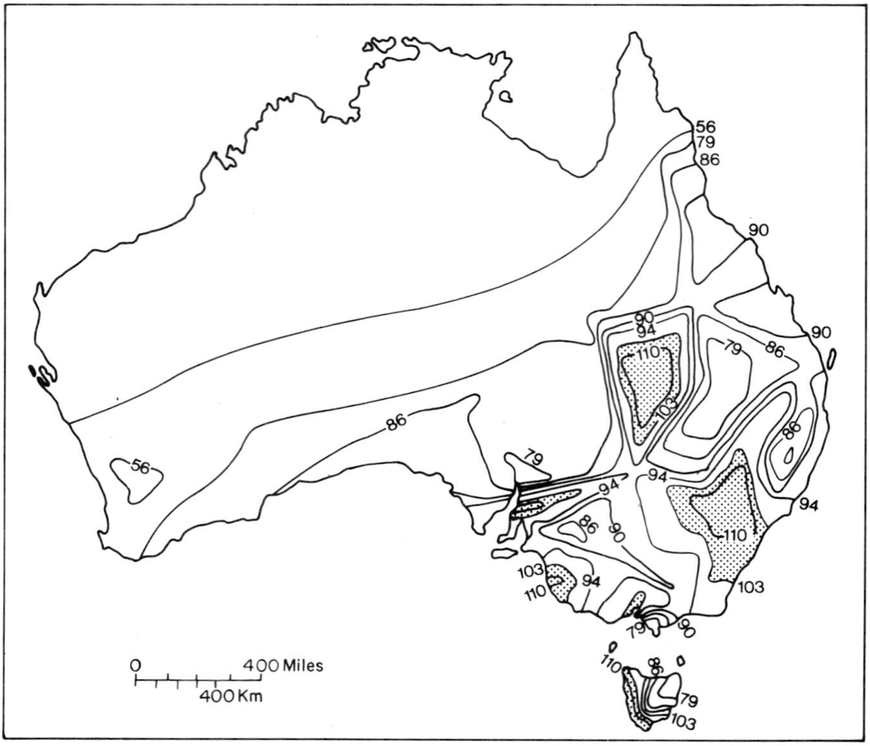

Fig. 17.27 Female mortality from cerebrovascular disease in Australia, 1965–66, based on standardized mortality ratios (after Learmonth and Grau, 1969).

peoples at over 14 000 feet in the Andes Mountains in Latin America or in the Caucasus Mountains in the Soviet Union) or belonging to primitive cultures, seem to have exceptionally low prevalence rates for hypertension. High blood pressure is thus one of the most common disorders. Strain is put on the heart and arteries when pressure increases and this can lead to heart failure, rupture of artery walls, stroke, haemorrhage and kidney failure.

In a study of the racial and regional distribution of average hypertension mortality in the U.S.A. for the period 1949–51, Rose (1962) reported that (a) there was not the large male excess of deaths as found with ischaemic heart disease; (b) the correlation between a measure of urbanization (U.S. Census: by State) and hypertension mortality was 0.490, though that for the "older" states were even higher and that for states similar to California were lower; and (c), when statistics for whites and non-whites were separated and mapped, the distributional patterns were similar even though the actual rates for the non-white population were higher. In general, the distributional patterns of mortality from hypertensive heart disease

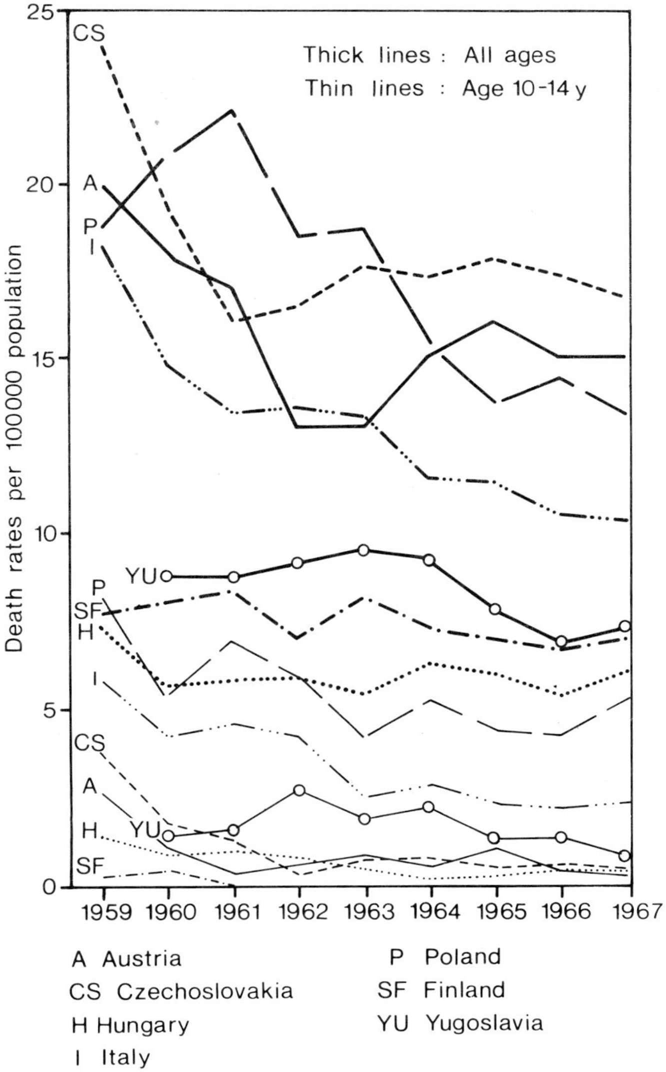

Fig. 17.28 Mortality from rheumatic fever and rheumatic heart disease in selected European countries, 1959–67 (W.H.O., 1974).

in the U.S.A. showed a high incidence in the south and in the east of the country.

RHEUMATIC FEVER AND RHEUMATIC HEART DISEASE

Rheumatic fever is a major human and medical problem in several countries scattered throughout the world. It is one of the leading causes of hospital admissions for cardiovascular disease of Morocco, Algeria, Nigeria, Egypt, Sudan, Iran, India, Mongolia and Chile. Mortality from rheumatic fever is decreasing in European countries but is still significant (Fig. 17.28). Rheumatic fever, a sequel to infection by Group A streptococci, usually begins with an acute attack in childhood. It may have a long-lasting course since the patient is liable to recurrences brought on by new streptococcal infections. Rheumatic heart disease results usually, though not exclusively, from rheumatic fever. Rheumatic fever has for long been recognized as a social disease and, though its incidence decreased in the more affluent countries as living conditions improved, there are still pockets of poverty in which rheumatic heart disease persists endemically.

REFERENCES

Anon. (1966). Accuracy of death certificates. *Lancet* (editorial) **ii**, 1349.

Antar, M. A., Ohlson, M. A. and Hodges, R. E. (1964). Perspectives in nutrition. Change in retail market food supplies in the U.S. in the last 70 years in relation to the incidence of coronary heart disease with special reference to dietary carbohydrates and essential fatty acids. *Amer. J. Clin. Nutr.* **14**, 169–178.

Brunner, H. R., Laragh, J. H. and Baer, L. (1972). Essential hypertension. Renin and aldosterone, heart attack and stroke. *N. Engl. J. Med.* **286**, 441–449.

Cassel, J. C. *et al.* (1971). Evans County cardiovascular studies. *Arch. Int. Med.* **28**, Dec.

Cleare, T. L. (1957). "Fat Consumption and Coronary Disease". Bristol-Wright, U.S.A.

Dawber *et al.* (1962). The epidemiology of coronary heart disease: The Framingham Inquiry. *Proc. Roy. Soc. Med.* **55**.

Epstein, F. H., Simpson, R. and Boas, E. P. (1956). Relations between diet and atherosclerosis among a working population of different ethnic origins. *Amer. J. Clin. Nutr.* **4**, 10–22.

Fejfar, Z., Strasser, T., Ikeme, A. and Masironi, R. (1974). Cardiovascular diseases: care and prevention. *W.H.O. Chronicle* **28**, Feb. (55–64), March (116–125), April (190–198).

Friedberg, C. K. (1966). "Diseases of the Heart". Saunders, London.

Fry, J. and Farndale, W. A. J. (1972). "International Medical Care: A Comparison and Evaluation of Medical Care Services throughout the World". M.T.P., Oxford.

Howe, G. M. (1970). "A National Atlas of Disease Mortality in the United Kingdom" (2nd edn). London.

Howe, G. M. (1972). London and Glasgow: a comparative study of mortality patterns. *Int. Geog. (I.G.U.)* **11**, 1214–17.

Kannel, W. B., Dawber, T. R., Kagan, A., Revotskie, N. and Stokes, J. (1961). Risk factors in the development of coronary heart disease. *Ann. Int. Med.* **54**, 1035.

Keen, H., Rose, G. and Pyke, D. A. (1965). Blood sugar and arterial disease. *Lancet* **ii**, 505–508.

Keys, A. (1970). "Coronary Heart Disease in Seven Countries". American Heart Association, Monogr. No. 29, New York.

Learmonth, A. T. A. and Grau, R. 1969. Maps of some standardised mortality ratios for Australia 1965–66 compared with 1959–63. Occasional Papers No. 8, Dept. Geog. Australian Nat. Univ. General Studies, Canberra.

Levy, R. I. and Ernst, N. (1973). Diet, hypertepidaemia and athesclerosis. *In* "Modern Nutrition in Health and Disease" (Eds R. S. Goodhart and M. E. Skils). Lea and Febiger, Philadelphia.

Lindeman, R. D. and Assenzo, J. R. (1964). Correlations between water hardness and cardiovascular deaths in Oklahoma Counties. *Amer. J. Publ. Hlth* **54** 7, 1071–1077.

McGlashan, N. D. and Chick, N. K. (1974). Assessing spatial variations in mortality: ischaemic heart disease in Tasmania. *Australian Geographical Studies* **12**, 190–206.

Masironi, R. (1970). Cardiovascular mortality in relation to radioactivity and hardness of local water supplies in U.S.A. *Bull. W.H.O.* **43**, 687–697.

Morris, J. N. (1967). "Uses of Epidemiology". Livingstone, London.

Morris, J. N., Crawford, M. D. and Head, J. A. (1961). Hardness of local water supplies and mortality from cardiovascular disease. *Lancet* **i**.

Muss, D. L. (1962), in Masironi, R. (1970). Cardiovascular mortality in relation to radioactivity and hardness of local water supply in the U.S.A. *Bull. W.H.O.* **43**, 1970.

Paul, O. *et al.* (1963). A longitudinal study of coronary heart disease. *Circulation* **28**, 20–31.

Phibbs, B. (1967). "The Human Heart". C.U. Mosby, St. Louis.

Pyle, G. F. (1971). Heart disease, cancer and stroke in Chicago. Research Paper No. 134, Dept. Geography, University of Chicago, Illinois.

Roberts, C. J. and Lloyd, S. (1972). Association between mortality from ischaemic heart disease and rainfall in South Wales and in county boroughs of England and Wales. *Lancet* **i**.

Robinson, D. A., Radford, A. J. and Rendall, N. R. E. (1974). Fallacies in comparing international disease trends. *J. Biosc. Sci.* **6** 2, 279–292.

Rose, G. (1962). The distribution of mortality from hypertension within the United States. *J. Chron. Dis.* **XV**, 1027–1034.

Rose, G. (1973). The epidemiology of coronary heart disease in Europe. "Chronic Diseases: Public Health in Europe", Vol. 2. W.H.O., Copenhagen.

Schroeder, H. A. (1960). Relations between hardness of water and death rates from certain chronic and degenerative diseases in the U.S.A. *J. Chron. Dis.* **XXII**, Dec.

Walker, A. R. (1971). Sugar intake and coronary heart disease. *Atherosclerosis* **XIV**, 137–152.

W.H.O. (1960). "International Classification of Diseases, Injuries and Causes of Death" (7th revision edn). Geneva; (8th revision edn). Geneva.

W.H.O. (1967). "International Classification of Disease 1965" (8th Revision). Geneva.

W.H.O. (1974). Cardiovascular disease: care and prevention. *W.H.O. Chronicle* **28, I** 2, 55–64; **II** 3, 116–125; **III** 4, 190–199.

18. Mental Disorders and Mental Subnormality

J. A. Giggs

INTRODUCTION

The study of international variations in the distributions of mental disorders and mental subnormality is a comparatively modern phenomenon. Since the Second World War, there has been a gradual swing from research into the epidemiology of infectious diseases to the growing public health problems of chronic, non-infectious diseases. This trend has been emphasized by the publication of a number of papers by the W.H.O. (1960, 1962, 1969) dealing with the epidemiology of mental disorders. The reasons for using epidemiological methods in this new field of study were effectively summarized in the report of a W.H.O. Expert Committee (1960), which averred that "the problems of studying personal susceptibility and the modifying effects of the environment or habit on the risks of attack were essentially similar in the communicable diseases and in other kinds of human illness. Consequently, the methods which had been used so successfully in uncovering the origin and mode of spread of diseases associated with microbial infection came to be increasingly applied to the study of mental disorders, and the use of the term "epidemiology", to imply the study of their distribution and behaviour in differing conditions of life in human communities, became widely accepted."

The use of epidemiological methods in the study of mental

disorders and mental subnormality has been restricted by a number of important problems.

Variations in case definition

A primary part of the epidemiological method is the identification of sick individuals. Unfortunately, recent experience has shown that it is difficult to differentiate clearly between "mentally ill" and "normal" persons or to classify particular categories of mental disorder in a uniform fashion. In a few narrowly defined behavioural states (e.g. alcoholism) and physical conditions (e.g. mongolism), a large measure of diagnostic accuracy and comparability between cases in different countries can be expected. On the other hand when broad diagnostic categories, such as schizophrenia, are employed, substantial margins of error appear and international comparisons become meaningless. Several international surveys have shown that the major variations in the incidence or prevalence of specific mental disorders are largely the products of national variations in the reliability of psychiatric diagnosis and the lack of agreement on the use of diagnostic terms. A recent survey published by the W.H.O. (1973) showed that some countries were seriously out of step with internationally accepted diagnoses of schizophrenia. Many of the patients who were classified as schizophrenics in their own countries were completely excluded from this category of mental illness when their case records were processed by the W.H.O. at Geneva. The disparities were greatest in the cases of the U.S.S.R. (50% of the sample) and the U.S.A. (40% of the sample).

Variations in classification

The specific process of classifying mental disorders is by no means complete. Few countries have identical classifications, since their concepts concerning the nature of mental illness and its correct mode of treatment tend to vary considerably. The appropriate sections of the W.H.O. "International Classification of Diseases" (I.C.D., 8th Revision, 1965) have been adopted as the standard model in the U.S.A. and the U.K. The main categories of this classification are presented in Table 18.1. Three broad categories of mental disorder are recognized: the psychoses, which are severe disorders, which often result in serious behaviour disturbance and in a break with reality; the neuroses and personality disorders; and mental deficiency or subnormality, i.e. retarded intellectual development. Twenty-six three-digit classes are recognized and each of these is further subdivided (.1, .2, etc.) to cover more specific conditions. The next revision of the I.C.D. was due in 1975.

Psychoses	
290	Senile and pre-senile dementia
291	Alcoholic psychoses
292	Psychoses associated with intercranial infection
293	Psychoses associated with cerebral conditions
294	Psychoses associated with physical conditions
295	Schizophrenia
296	Affective psychoses
297	Paranoid states
298	Other psychoses
299	Unspecified psychoses
Neuroses, Personality Disorders and Other Non-Psychotic Mental Disorders	
300	Neuroses
301	Personality disorders
302	Sexual deviation
303	Alcoholism
304	Drug dependence
305	Physical disorder of presumably psychogenic origin
306	Special symptoms not elsewhere classified
307	Transient situational disturbances
308	Behaviour disorders of childhood
309	Mental disorders not specified as psychotic associated with physical conditions
Mental Retardation	
310	Borderline mental retardation
311	Mild mental retardation
312	Moderate mental retardation
313	Severe mental retardation
314	Profound mental retardation
315	Unspecified mental retardation

Table 18.1 Major classes of mental disorders (W.H.O., 1967b).

Availability of morbidity and mortality data

Mental hospital statistics constitute the principal source of data on the incidence and prevalence of mental disorders. Their usefulness in this respect is limited by numerous selective factors which influence the probability of hospital admission. In both developing and developed countries, there are many mentally ill people who are not receiving psychiatric treatment. Many of these cases are never recorded because there is a chronic shortage of trained psychiatrists. A survey carried out by W.H.O. (1963), concerning the training of psychiatrists, revealed that there was no information for 24 countries (with an aggregate population of 191 million). Data were available for 85 countries and, in eight of these (with an aggregate population of 20 million), there were no trained psychiatrists. In 35 countries (aggregate population 890 million), the ratio of trained psychiatrists was less than one per 200 000 population. The fragmentary picture presented in Fig. 18.1 shows that most of the countries of the developing world have less than one trained psychiatrist per 100 000 population. In such countries, the true incidence and prevalence of mental disorders are therefore largely matters of conjecture.

Many of the mentally sick people in the countries of the developing world never visit psychiatrists or attend modern psychiatric hospitals, because these are often only found in the major cities. Thus in Latin America 28% of the psychiatrists live in but one city, Buenos Aires. In Colombia, in 1962, out of 836 towns and cities only 10 had psychiatrists and 171 had doctors. The mental health of the majority of the people living in developing countries is cared for by folk psychiatrists (e.g. witch doctors), rather than Western-trained psychiatrists.

Figure 18.2 reveals the extent of the differences which exist between industrial and developing nations in terms of patterns of mental-health care. Most of the nations of the tropical and sub-tropical latitudes have very low rates of hospital treatment, as indexed by the ratio of mental hospital beds to total population. Even in the developed countries, where psychiatric services have been operating for many years, the statistics concerning the incidence and prevalence of mental disorders are incomplete. A recent W.H.O. survey (1973) of the availability of statistics of patients admitted to psychiatric services revealed that the pattern of treatment in

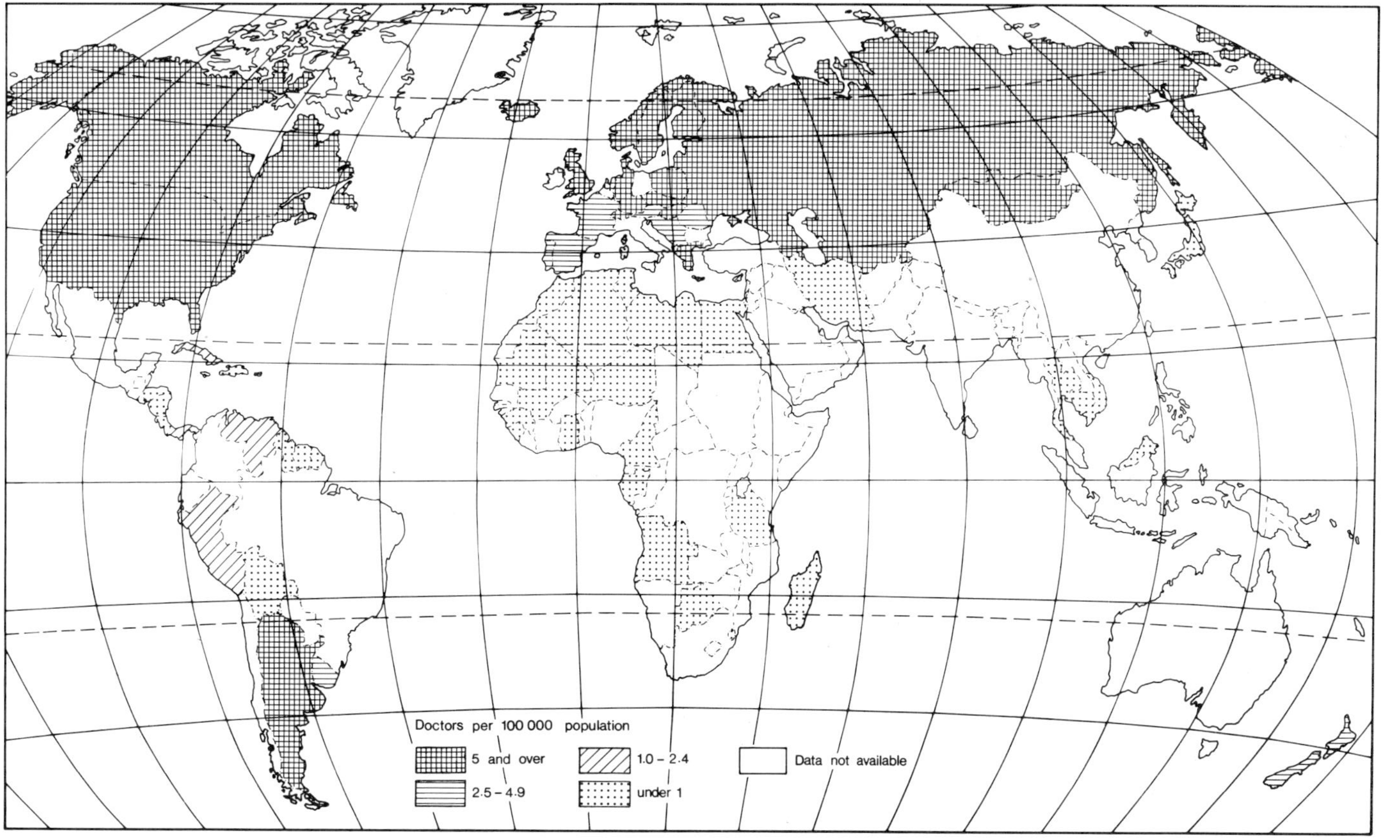

Fig. 18.1 Health personnel: neurologists and psychiatrists, 1963–69 inclusive (data from W.H.O., 1963–69).

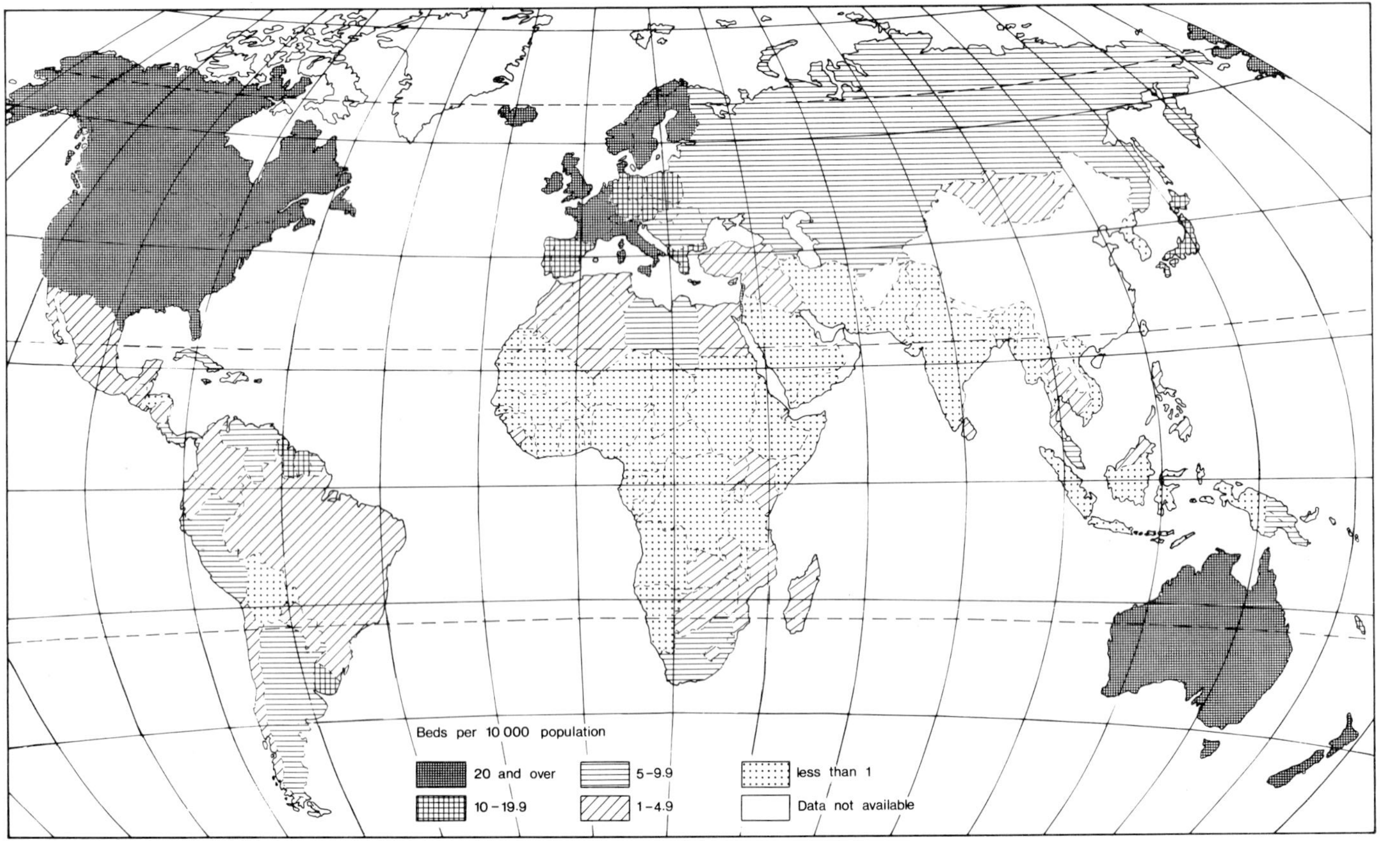

Fig. 18.2 Mental hospital beds, 1966–69 inclusive (data from W.H.O., 1963–69).

developed countries is changing. There has been a steady swing from the traditional in-patient treatment to an emphasis upon care in the community. Many developed countries have detailed statistics about the inpatients of psychiatric hospitals, but few have any information on a national scale about their outpatients.

The survey also revealed that many countries have distinct public and private health services and that, in 63 countries, only the data for the public health services is published. Similarly in some federated territories (e.g. Australia), the statistical reporting system does not cover the whole country. Out of 70 countries included in the survey, only 27 claimed to publish complete statistics classified by sex, only 19 countries published statistics classified by age and 21 by psychiatric diagnosis. Twenty-four countries publish complete statistics for mentally retarded patients.

For a variety of cogent reasons, therefore, the available statistics relating to the incidence and prevalence of mental disorders and subnormality have limited value for comparative purposes at the international level. Mortality statistics are useful in the small proportion of mental disorders which produce fatalities, particularly suicides, alcohol and drug addiction, congenital birth defects and diseases of the central nervous system. The numerically more important psychoses and neuroses, however, rarely provide the specific causes of death for most mentally sick people.

Availability of comparable demographic data

The comparison of mental disorders between different countries is also seriously hampered by the lack of accurate, comparable, demographic data. The incidence of many mental disorders varies considerably with such important variables as age, marital status, sex and occupation. Very few countries publish census data in a form which is suitable for calculating the appropriate accurate variable—specific rates.

At the present time, therefore, most serious research is still concerned with the fundamental problems of definition and method. Significant advances in the study of spatial variations in the distribution of mental disorders and of their underlying causal mechanisms lie some way in the future. Nevertheless, some modest beginnings have been made in some areas of the field and these are discussed below.

MENTAL SUBNORMALITY

Definitions of mental subnormality (also termed mental retardation and mental deficiency) tend to vary widely between countries. It is generally agreed, however, that low intelligence is an essential criterion. This attribute originates during pregnancy, birth or childhood and significantly and permanently impairs the abilities of those so affected to mature, learn and adapt to the demands of society. The term covers a wide range of degrees of intellectual deficit and social incompetence. Thus the W.H.O. Expert Committee (1968) suggested that, taken in conjunction with social factors, the mentally retarded could be broadly subdivided according to the following intelligence-quotient (I.Q.) ranges of standard deviations from a mean of 100, viz. mild: −2.0 to −3.3, i.e. I.Q. 50–70; moderate: −3.3 to −4.3, i.e. I.Q. 35–50; severe: −4.3 to −5.3, i.e. I.Q. 20–35; and profound: more than −5.3 standard deviations from the mean.

Mental retardation is not a single disease, but has many aetiological mechanisms. At least 200 have been identified to date and many of these are known to be mutually interacting. In the lower grades of retardation (i.e. severe–profound subnormality), the main causes are thought to be such pathological factors as trauma, infection or toxicity in the prenatal, perinatal or postnatal environments. The higher grades of subnormality, in contrast, are often the products of normal genetic variation. In addition, many of the milder cases are created by adverse sub-cultural and environmental factors.

Estimates of the prevalence of mental retardation range between 2 and 3% of the population in specific countries, chiefly as a result of variations in case definition. In the U.K., 75% of the cases are only mildly subnormal (i.e. having an I.Q. of between 50 and 70) and 5% are profoundly subnormal (i.e. I.Q. below 20). In the U.S.A. in 1970, 88% had an I.Q. of between 50 and 70 and 3.5% had an I.Q. below 25. Few investigations of spatial variations on the distribution of subnormality at the international level have been undertaken, mainly because very few statistics have been published in sufficient detail. The study of the spatial distribution of congenital malformations has attracted some attention, however, primarily because these extreme forms of mental retardation are so easily recognizable. Penrose (1958) has shown that there are wide variations in the reported incidence of anencephaly in different parts of Europe. This specific type of malformation, which is one of the commonest and most lethal, is characterized by a massive failure of development of the anterior part of the central nervous system and all cases are still-born or die within a few hours of birth. Penrose found that the incidence of anencephaly among infants born in hospital ranged between 0.12% in Lyon and 0.67% in Belfast.

Figure 18.3 shows that in Ireland, the western part of the United Kingdom and in Naples, the incidence exceeded 3.17 per 1000. Although the study raised the question of the relative significance of external (i.e. geographical) and internal (i.e. genetic) factors in the causation of anencephaly, no attempt was made to investigate this theme. Subsequent research has shown that anencephaly is strongly

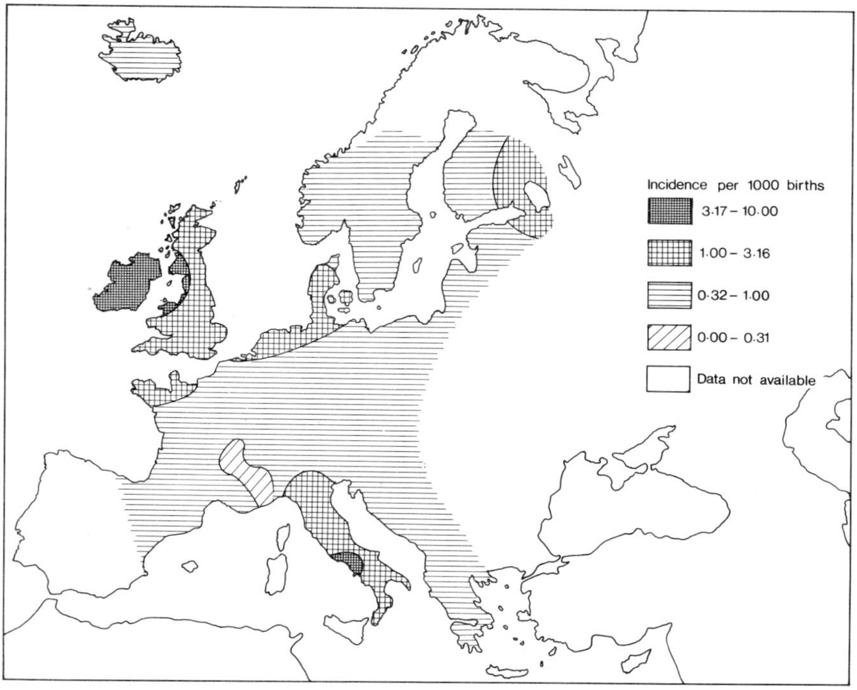

Fig. 18.3 Distribution of anencephaly in Europe based on births in hospital (Penrose, 1958).

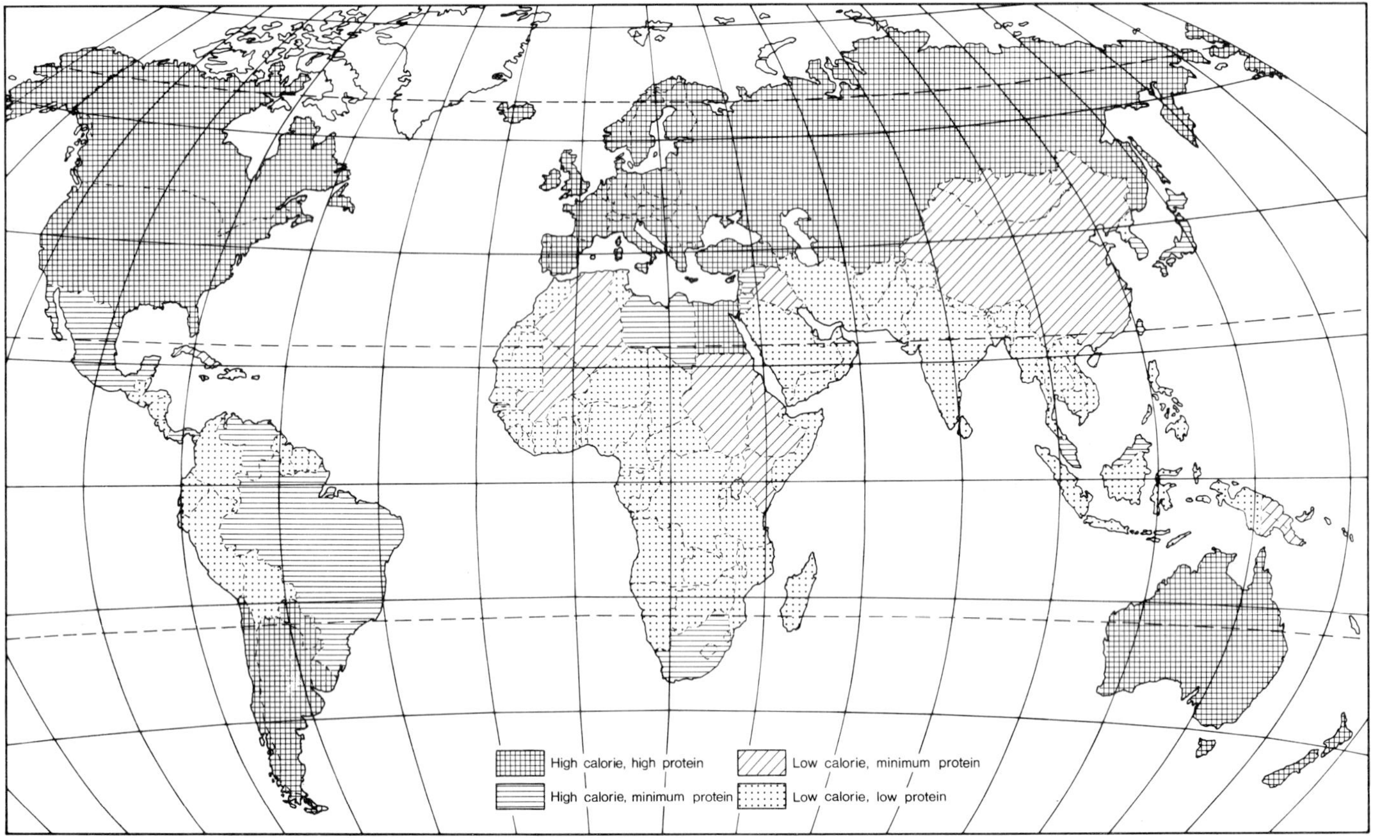

Fig. 18.4 The geography of hunger (based on Ehrlich *et al.*, 1973).

associated with several important environmental influences, notably a marked fluctuation with season. The condition is much more common in autumn and winter births than among births in spring and summer. There is also a pronounced association between incidence and the social class of the parents. In the United Kingdom, the incidence in the lowest social class (Class V) is four times higher than that in the highest social class (Class I). Although anencephaly has strong associations with such environmental influences, causal explanations have not been provided to date.

Many of the milder forms of mental subnormality are known to result from nutritional deficiencies and attendant infective processes and biochemical disturbances. Figure 18.4 shows that poor nutrition is still a major factor in ill health, especially in the developing countries. The incidence of malnutrition is highest in the developing countries of the tropics and sub-tropics, because protein-deficient diets are generally characteristic in these latitudes (see Chapter 20). The problem of severe malnutrition is particularly serious for certain physiologically vulnerable groups, notably pregnant and lactating mothers, infants and young children. This fact explains in large measure the very high infant mortality rates which are still common in these countries (Fig. 18.5). During these critical formative years the physical and mental development of many of the children who survive are permanently retarded by substantial nutritional deficiencies and attendant infections. The high infant mortality rates in the developing countries have, however, considerably reduced the number of severe cases of mental subnormality. Paradoxically, the problem will therefore become worse in these countries because, with advances in medical care similar to those obtaining in the developed nations, larger numbers of the severe cases will survive.

Among the nutritional disorders, iodine deficiencies have received much attention because of their causal roles in the development of mental abnormalities. There are still large areas throughout the world where iodine deficiencies are widespread because salt iodization programmes have not been implemented. The deficiency disturbs the relationship between thyroid functioning and the growth and maturation of the brain. Endemic goitre is the most frequent result of iodine deficiency and approximately 10% of the world's population lives in areas where goitre is common. The condition is known throughout the world (Fig. 18.6), but often

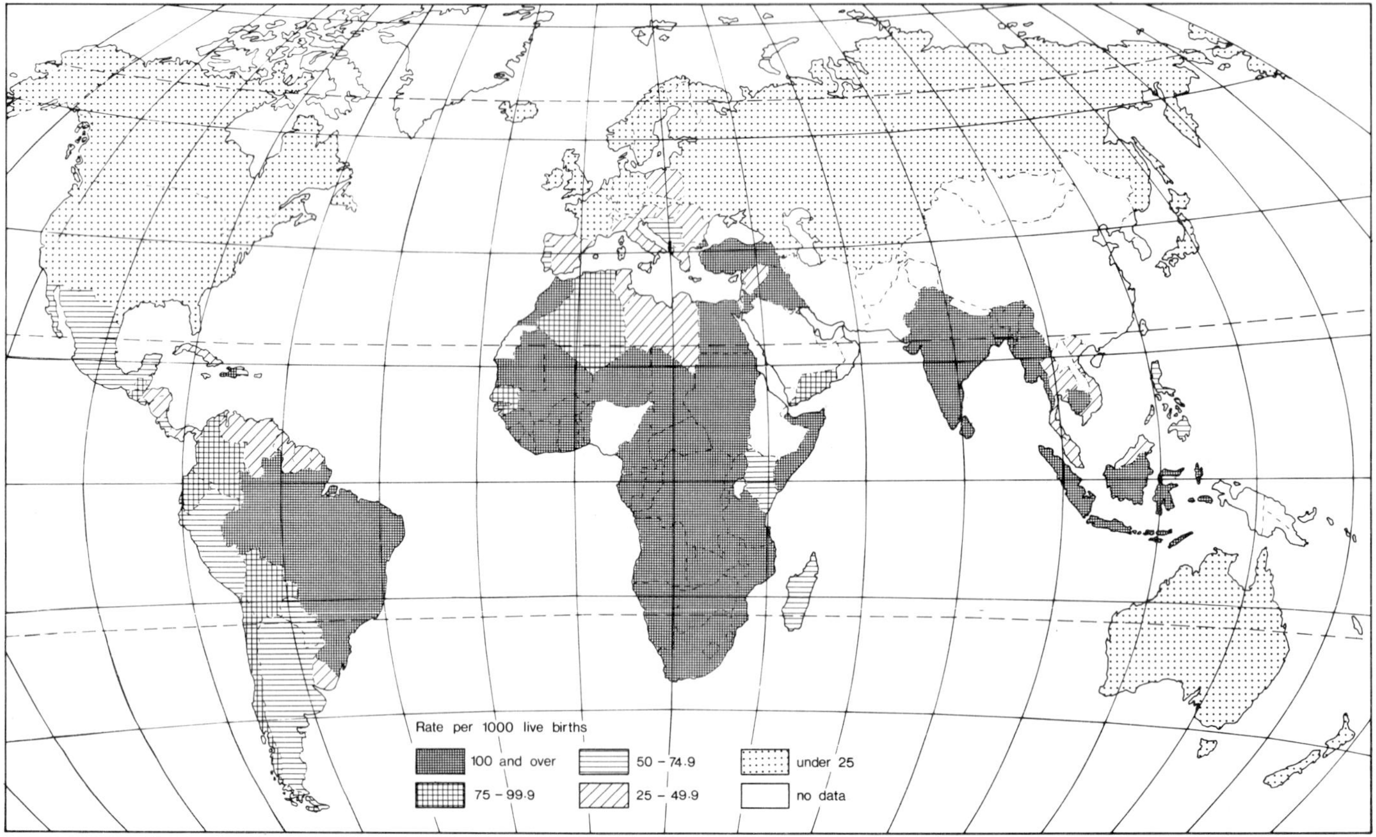

Fig. 18.5 Infant mortality (data from W.H.O. and U.N. in 1970).

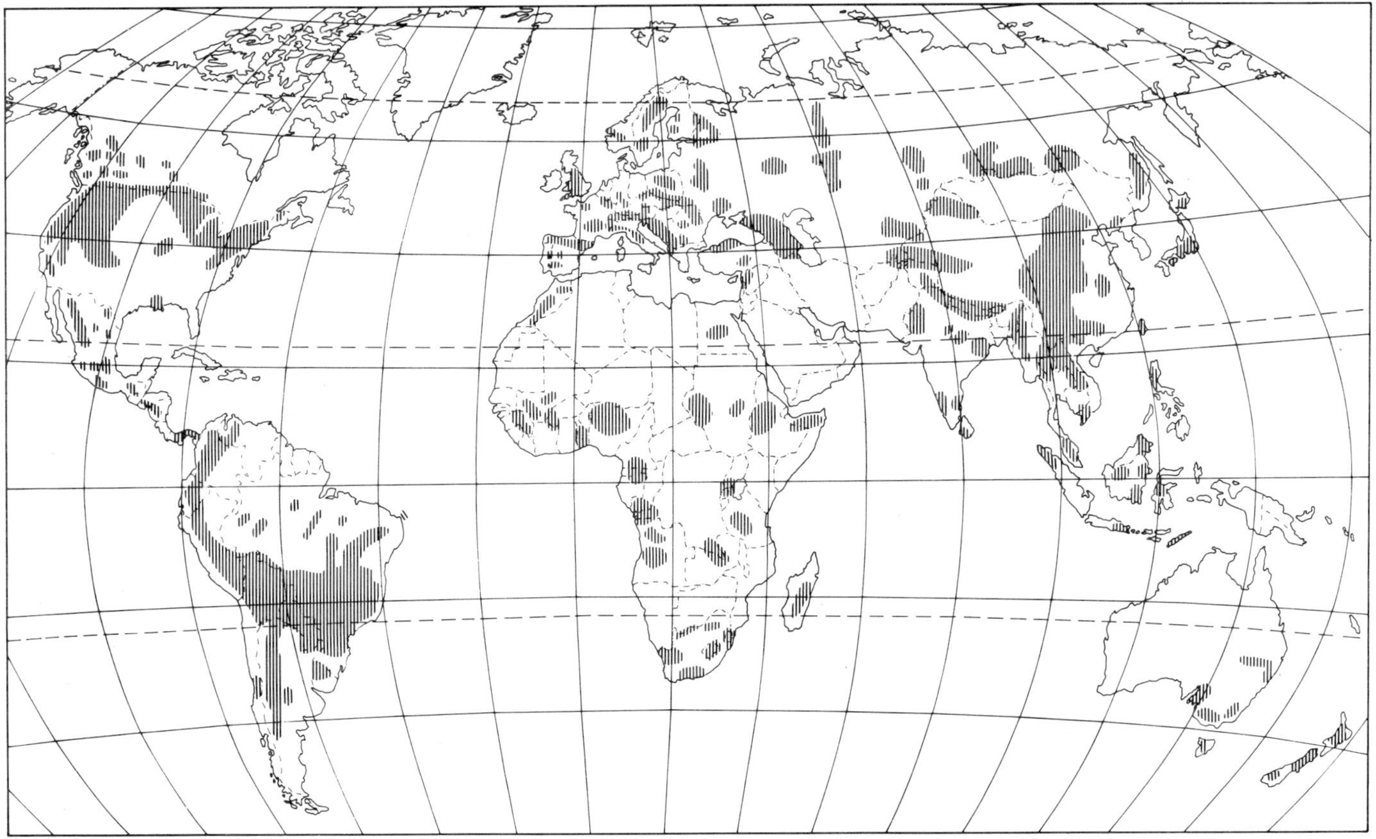

Fig. 18.6 Areas where endemic goitre has been found (W.H.O., 1970).

assumes endemic proportions in mountainous regions and other localities where the natural iodine content of the soil is extremely low. It has been estimated that there are nearly 200 million goitrous people in the world.

The most important aspect of endemic goitre is cretinism. This particular form of mental abnormality is probably the result of the physiological effects of goitre in the mothers of cretins rather than the direct result of iodine deficiency in the children. Many studies of the close geographical association of endemic goitre and congenital cretinism support the clinical view that both conditions are the results of iodine deficiency. Endemic goitre has also been associated with feeble-mindedness, lowered educational ability and deaf-mutism.

MENTAL DISORDERS AND OLD AGE

One of the most important demographic trends in almost every country in the world has been the progressive fall in the crude death rate and a concomitant change in the population age structure. In most of the developed countries, average life expectancy has steadily increased with the result that the number of old people has assumed considerable importance (Fig. 18.7). In England and Wales, the number of persons aged 65 years and over almost quadrupled between 1901 and 1971. They now constitute 13.2% of the population, numbering 7.1 million. Although the populations of the developing countries are still mainly concentrated in the younger age groups, the evidence provided by limited population censuses suggests that their population trends will gradually produce age structures similar to those in the developed countries. Thus in India, the proportion of the population aged 65 years and over rose from 1.8% in 1951 to 2.9% in 1961.

The rapidly growing numbers of old people have important repercussions for modern society. Several national and international surveys have shown that the incidence of mental disorders increases rapidly from middle age onwards. In the U.S.A., data published by the National Institute of Mental Health show that first admission rates to mental hospitals rose from 2.3 per 100 000 population aged under 15 years to 236.1 for those aged 65 years and over. In England

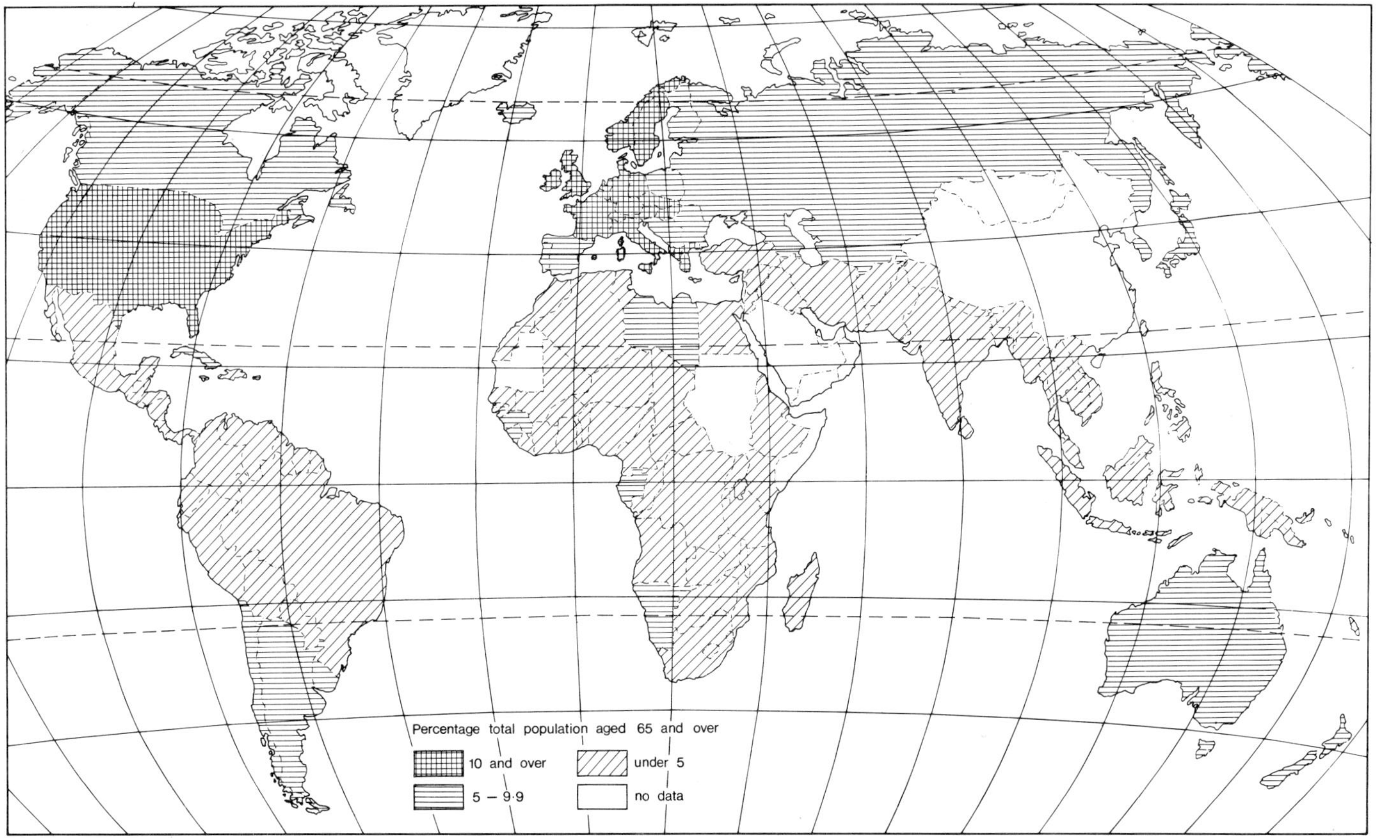

Fig. 18.7 Distribution of old people (based on data in the U.N. Demographic Year Book, 1970, U.N. World Population Prospects, 1965–85 and the U.N. Population Paper No. 30, 1969).

and Wales, the first admission rates for males and females aged 75 years and over in 1971 were 378 and 395 respectively per 100 000 compared with only 115 and 156 per 100 000 for those aged 15–19 years. The importance of greater life expectancy therefore lies in the fact that progressively more people are becoming vulnerable to the forms of mental illness which result from degenerative changes in the brain and its blood vessels. This fact is exemplified by the increasing rate of first (and subsequent) admissions of elderly people to mental hospitals in many countries. In England and Wales, the number of people aged 65 years and over increased by 1% between 1951 and 1960, but first admission rates rose by over 35%.

Hospital admission rates provide useful measures of the relative incidence of mental disorders in old age, compared with those earlier in life, but give a very limited picture of the total incidence. Detailed investigations of total populations or random samples in particular localities have shown that patients are admitted to hospital from only a small proportion of the total number of mentally disordered old people. In England and Wales, 3–5 per 1000 old people become inpatients every year, but this probably only represents 10% of the actual prevalence. Slater and Roth (1970) have estimated that the total prevalence rate for the main mental disorders of the aged is approximately 263 per 1000, compared with a rate of only 17 institutional cases per 1000. Intensive surveys in other countries (e.g. the U.S.A., Denmark, Poland and Israel) have shown broadly similar results. Between 20 and 30% of all persons aged 65 years and over suffer from some degree of mental disorder.

Slater and Roth estimate that 5% of old people in England and Wales suffer from functional (i.e. affective or psychotic) disorders. These are principally character disorders (including paranoid states), paraphrenia (late onset schizophrenia), chronic schizophrenia (excluding long-stay hospital cases) and manic depression. Neuroses and allied disorders affect an estimated 9% of the aged in England and Wales. Many of these conditions develop because the sufferer has been unable to adjust to the progressive physical handicaps, personal losses (e.g. the deaths of relatives and friends) and the reduced social and economic situation which follows compulsory retirement in industrialized countries. Many old people commit suicide and approximately half of them do so because of physical illness and/or depression.

Organic brain disorders are the most common set of mental illnesses found in the elderly. Slater and Roth estimate that 10–11% of the aged in England and Wales suffer from varying degrees of senile and arteriosclerotic dementia and other brain syndromes. These conditions develop as a result of brain damage created by degenerative diseases of the nervous system and of the cardiovascular system. In such cases, the usual processes of ageing appear to have been accelerated by genetic defects and unfavourable environmental factors. The search for risk factors in the aetiology of arteriosclerosis (or atherosclerosis) has revealed considerable international variations in the incidence of the disease (Chapter 17). Mortality data published by the W.H.O. confirm that there are immense variations in its impact. In 1967, the mortality rates for 47 countries ranged between 6.1 per 100 000 population in Salvador and 319.9 in Sweden. Figures 17.2–17.5 (Chapter 17) show that mortality rates are highest in the industrialized countries and lowest in the non-industrial nations. The evidence provided by detailed post-mortem work in many countries suggests that environmental factors are important in determining both the incidence and rate of progression of the disease. The variation in mortality rate between countries appears to be primarily a function of differing ways of life. Thus, in the developed nations, there is a rapid rate of progression with age and a high incidence in males, but not females. The western diet, which has high serum cholestrol and fat levels and sugar intake, is another important risk factor. Lack of regular exercise also plays an important role in the rate at which the disease develops. Racial and ethnic variations do not appear to constitute significant risk factors. Variations in culture and way of life thus appear to have significant influence upon this specific form of ageing process and contribute strongly to the high rates of organic mental illnesses in western countries.

ALCOHOLISM

Ethyl alcohol, in common with many other drugs, is beneficial to man when used in judicious quantities. In most societies, its moderate use has long been approved for various social and religious events, for the relief of anxiety and stress, and because of its nutritive and medicinal properties. Unfortunately, millions of people throughout the world have become addicted to alcohol in the sense that they have developed psychological, and more importantly, physical dependence upon the drug. This pathological dependence creates social disapproval, progressively impairs the efficiency of the economic and social functioning of the addicts and leads to a variety of harmful organic conditions and early death (see also Chapter 16, pp. 418–20). One authority has suggested that chronic alcoholism lowers average life expectancy by 10 years.

Reliable estimates of the extent and distribution of alcoholism are not available, since detailed morbidity surveys at national and international levels have never been undertaken. However, the approximate nature and magnitude of the problem can be gauged by using indirect measures of the prevalence of alcoholism. The most common procedure used to identify rate variations in the disease is to employ surrogate variables. Official statistics for per capita alcohol consumption have been employed in many studies, although the data are available for relatively few countries. Official mortality statistics for cirrhosis of the liver are more commonly used, however, since the condition is principally (but not exclusively) a consequence of nutritional deficiencies induced by alcohol consumption. More importantly, the appropriate statistics are available for a large number of countries and consequently the variable is very useful as an index of the prevalence of alcoholism throughout the world. In addition, the value of morbidity data has been confirmed by a number of national and international studies which have demonstrated that there are strong statistical relationships between spatial and temporal variations in the levels of alcohol consumption and mortality from liver cirrhosis.

Figure 18.8 presents the most recent available picture of the distribution of mortality from liver cirrhosis. Only 31% of the world's population is represented and no data are available for most of the countries of Africa, Asia and Oceania. Nevertheless, the limited available information reveals that there are substantial variations in the impact of alcoholism in different countries. Thus between 1964 and 1969, the average annual death rate from liver cirrhosis per 100 000 population ranged between 2.8 in New Zealand and 35.0 in France. In many countries the problem has assumed massive proportions, for data published by the W.H.O. for the period

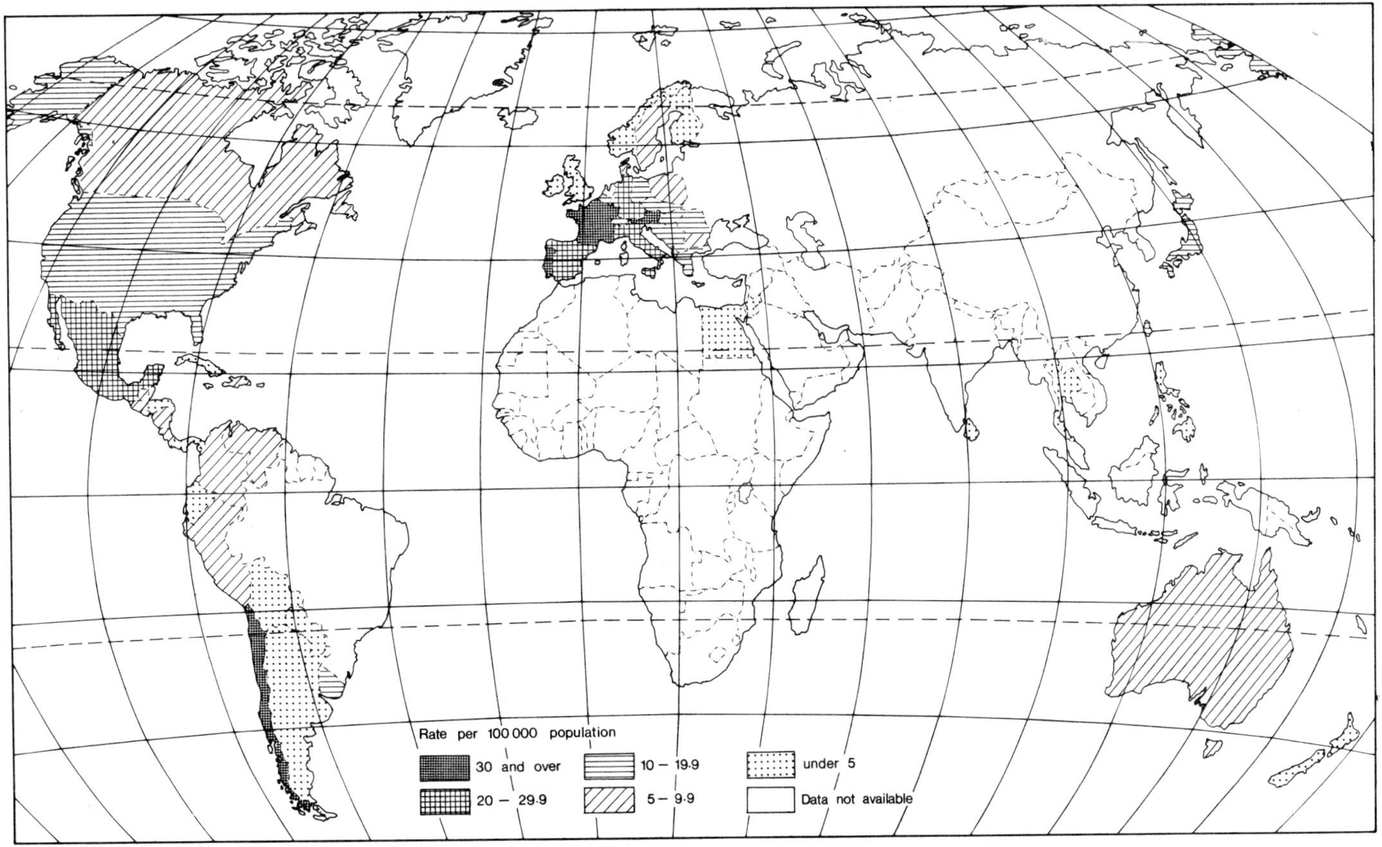

Fig. 18.8 Mortality for liver cirrhosis (data from W.H.O. Statistics Annual, 1970 and W.H.O., 1973).

1964–66 showed that in 13 countries mortality from liver cirrhosis was listed as one of the 10 leading causes of death for persons of all ages. The incidence of alcoholism (and hence of mortality from liver cirrhosis) tends to rise sharply with age and consequently, in 26 countries, the disease was one of the 10 leading causes of death for persons between 45 and 65 years of age.

Several authors have suggested that alcoholism is rare in underdeveloped countries and universal in highly developed and affluent societies. The evidence provided by the map, however, would appear to show that the problem of alcoholism is not simply a function of variations in national levels of industrialization and urbanization. Thus medium and high rates (i.e. 10–19.9 and 20 and over per 100 000) are found in both industrial and developing countries in Europe, the Americas and Asia. Similarly, some of the lowest mortality rates (i.e. less than 5 per 100 000) are evident in both highly industrialized countries (e.g. the United Kingdom and New Zealand) and less affluent countries (e.g. Sri Lanka and Thailand).

It is probable that the patterns and levels of alcohol consumption (and hence of alcoholism) are products of the socio-cultural environment which prevails in each country. The opportunity to become an alcoholic is clearly greater in some countries than in others because of variations in social attitudes towards the consumption of alcoholic beverages. Thus, in many of the countries with very high levels of liver cirrhosis mortality, the regular drinking of large quantities of alcohol (particularly wines and spirits) has traditionally played an important part in the life styles of their inhabitants. In other countries, by contrast, an array of social, religious and legal factors (e.g. government controls) reduces the opportunity for abuse.

It has been suggested that further evidence for the socio-environmental basis of this disease is provided by the difference between men and women in the prevalence of alcoholism. In almost every country, drunkenness among women arouses particular social disapproval and consequently the mortality rates from liver cirrhosis are invariably higher for men than for women. Thus, in 1969 the ratio of male to female deaths from liver cirrhosis ranged from 1:1 in some countries (e.g. Denmark) to more than 4:1 in others (e.g. Switzerland and Malta). These variations probably reflect the differing status of women in these countries.

SUICIDE

Suicide, the calculated act of self-destruction, is a specifically human behavioural attribute. Statistics published by the W.H.O. for 37 countries reveal that the average annual death rate from suicide has ranged around 10 per 100 000 population since 1960. Figure 18.9 shows that wide variations exist between the countries for which data are available. Thus in 1969 the suicide rate recorded for 37 countries ranged from 0.7 per 100 000 population in Mexico to 33.1 in Hungary. Between 1964 and 1966, suicide was included in the first 10 causes of death in 21 industrialized countries. The W.H.O. statistics show that in 1966 it was listed as one of the 10 leading causes of death in 33 countries for persons in the age group 15–44 years. In six European countries (Austria, Denmark, the Federal German Republic, Hungary, Sweden and Switzerland), suicide ranked third after cancer and coronary heart disease for this age group. These figures provide cause for concern, since suicide is generally considered to be the produce of social and psychological rather than physiological factors.

Many authors suggest that these great national variations are not easily explained since there is no international standard by which these deaths are identified, reported and recorded. Accordingly, some part of the variations can be attributed to contrasting definitions of suicide and to differing methods of certifying deaths. There is also powerful evidence that, even in countries where suicide mortality statistics have been recorded for a long time, the official published statistics tend to understate the true incidence of suicide. Thus detailed surveys of coroners' records in the U.S.A., the United Kingdom and parts of Ireland have produced rates which exceed the official figures by between 25 and 33%. The discrepancies probably arise because of the practical difficulties involved in determining suicidal intent and also because, in certain social settings (e.g. in countries where the stigma associated with suicide is high), it is considered preferable to substitute an alternative cause of death. However, Sainsbury and Barraclough (1968) studied suicide rates for 1959 among immigrants from 11 countries into the U.S.A. and discovered that they were virtually identical with those recorded in the countries from which they had emigrated. This evidence would

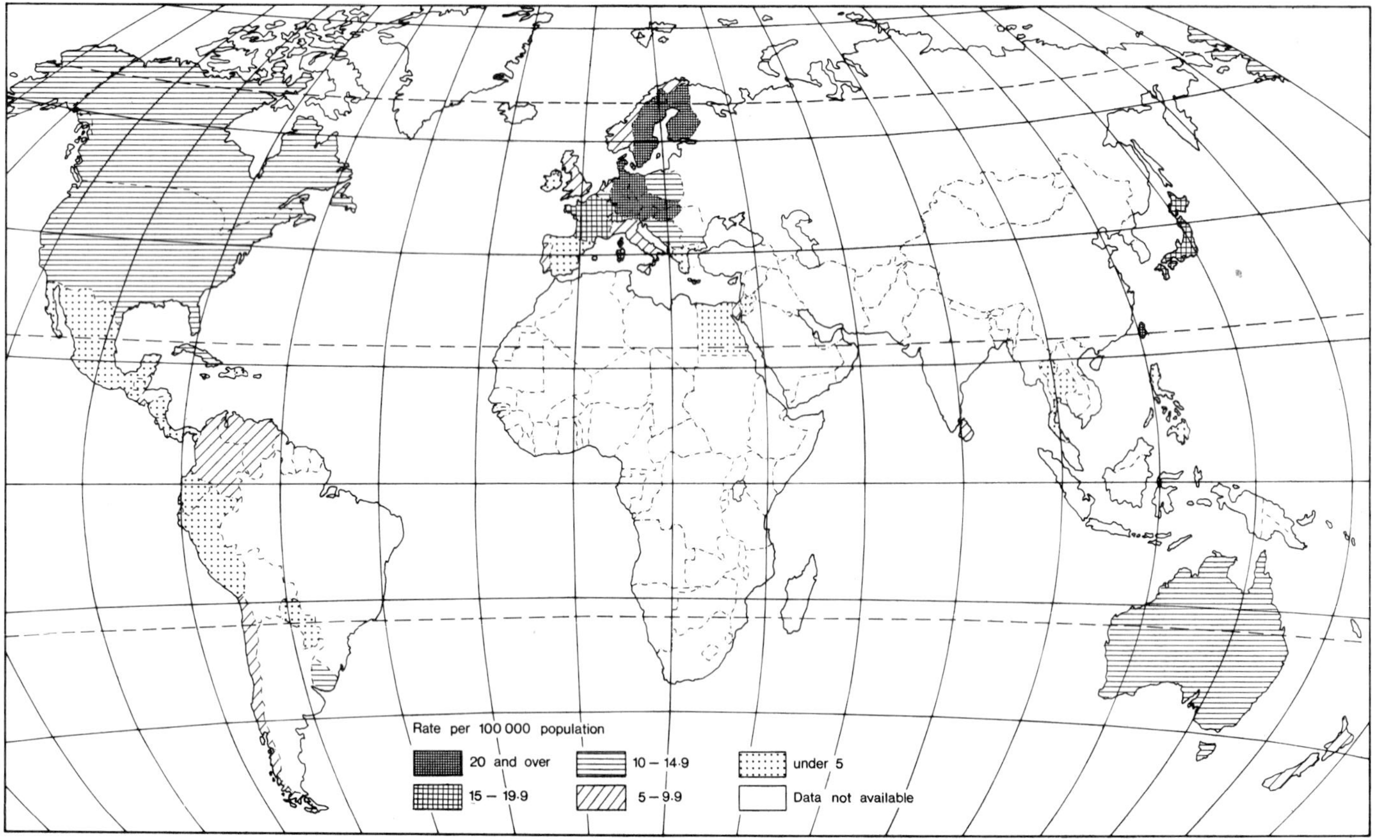

Fig. 18.9 Mortality for suicide (data from *Wld Hlth Stat. Rep.* **25** 11, 1972 and **26** 3, 1973).

suggest that national suicide rates do reflect significant variations in national characteristics.

The literature relating to the causes of suicide is immense. It is clear that the incidence of suicide is influenced by cultural, social and personality factors but it is not yet possible to identify the relative contributions of each of these precipitating factors. The findings provided by a limited number of comparative studies suggests that suicide rates tend to be lower in primitive and developing societies than in industrialized, affluent societies. In addition, it may be the case that some variations are race-specific or perhaps a function of the relative affluence of different population groups within countries. Thus in the U.S.A. in 1959, the suicide rates per 100 000 whites and negroes were 11.3 and 3.3 respectively. Similarly, in South Africa in 1960, the rates per 100 000 Europeans and Africans were 14.1 and 4.3 respectively. There are also several plausible hypotheses which suggest that variations in the incidence of suicide are due to contrasts in national character and are thus regarded as being culture-specific. None of these interesting suggestions have been firmly substantiated to date.

Religious affiliation has been invoked as an explanation for the rarity of suicide in some countries, notably Ireland, where the population is predominantly Roman Catholic. But the suicide rates in Roman Catholic Austria and Hungary (22.3 and 33.1 per 100 000, respectively) are among the five highest in the world. Low rates of suicide are therefore more probably a function of degrees of religious devoutness rather than specific religious affiliations.

In most of the developed countries, where suicide statistics have been collected for many years, several consistent social findings have emerged. In all countries, there is a sex difference in suicide, with males predominating over females. Figures published by the W.H.O. for 16 countries during the period 1965–69 show that the suicide rate for males averaged 12.8 per 100 000 population, whereas the average rate for females was only 6.0 per 100 000.

There is also a general tendency for suicide rates to rise with age, although several countries (and particularly the U.S.A.) have recently recorded a significant increase in the incidence of suicide among males aged 15–19 years. Thus the age-adjusted mortality rates for 16 countries during 1965–69 rose from 5.9 per 100 000 persons aged 15–24 years to 20.9 per 100 000 persons aged 75 years and over.

These figures support the findings of many authors within particular countries, namely, that most of the people who commit suicide are elderly and often physically or mentally ill. Clearly the relatively high incidence of suicide in industrialized countries compared with the low rates recorded in developing countries can be partly ascribed to the differing age structures of these two sets of nations. The industrialized countries have much higher proportions of aged persons than the developing countries and consequently generally higher rates of suicide could be expected.

Authors are generally agreed that there is a strong relationship between suicide and mental disorder. Stengel (1964) states that a third of the people who commit suicide have been suffering from some form of mental disorder and had received psychiatric treatment at some stage prior to their deaths. Retrospective enquiries also reveal that many suicides who had never received psychiatric treatment were also emotionally unstable. The incidence of suicide is particularly high among persons suffering from depressive illness (or melancholia), and among abnormal personalities, especially psychopaths and alcoholics. The strong positive correlation between the incidence of suicide and alcoholism among nations and small social groups has frequently been demonstrated. Alcoholism has, with considerable justification, been frequently described as "chronic suicide".

MENTAL DISORDER AND NATIONAL CHARACTER

It is generally recognized that the level of psychiatric services in specific countries is partly a function of national wealth. Thus the low level of admissions to mental hospitals, which is generally characteristic of the developing countries (Fig. 18.10), can mainly be attributed to their low national incomes. The substantial variations in the rate of hospitalization between the prosperous, developed nations, however, is less easily explained in these terms. Thus Lynn (1971) observed that in 1961 the national rates of hospitalized mental illness in selected European countries ranged between 7.3 per 1000 population in Ireland and only 1.7 in West Germany. He suggested that these variations can be interpreted as measures of national character.

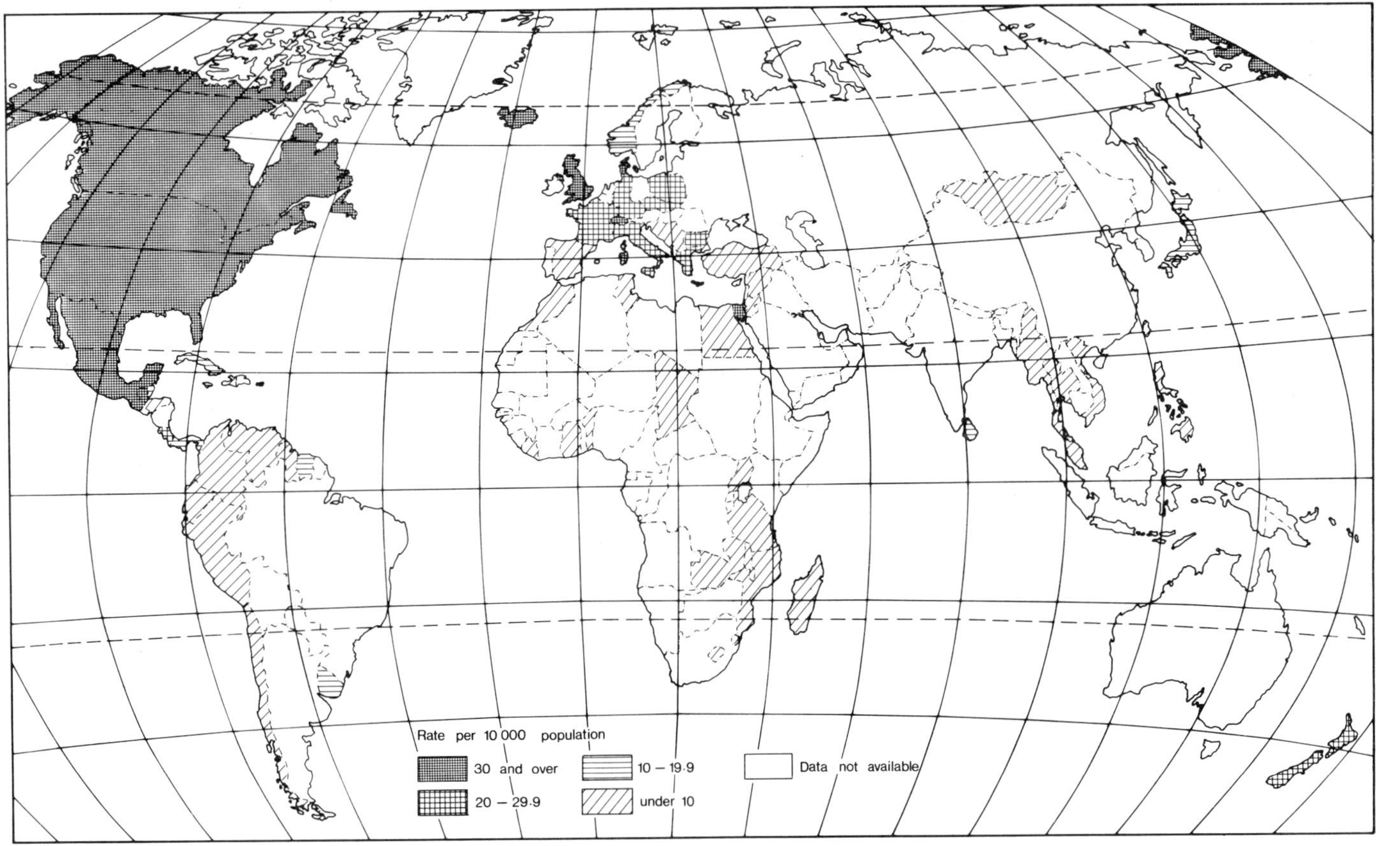

Fig. 18.10 Admissions to mental hospital (based on data from W.H.O., 1963–69).

In a carefully argued essay, Lynn attempted to analyse national character from the perspective of contemporary psychology. He demonstrated that psychologists have shown that anxiety (i.e. emotionality) is an important personality characteristic in individuals and suggested that there is a national personality characteristic, also termed anxiety, which distinguishes the peoples of some nations from those of others. In order to test this hypothesis, Lynn selected a homogeneous group of large and prosperous countries, thus reducing the effects of large variations of national wealth. Eighteen countries were included in the analysis and these consisted of the advanced nations in Western Europe (i.e. Austria, Belgium, Denmark, Finland, France, Ireland, Italy, the Netherlands, Norway, Sweden, Switzerland, West Germany and the United Kingdom), the old British Commonwealth (i.e. Australia, Canada and New Zealand), the U.S.A. and Japan.

Four key epidemiological variables were selected as measures of national anxiety levels in these countries, namely the rates of hospitalized mental illness, average per capita daily calorie intake, suicide and alcoholism (measured by liver cirrhosis mortality). Lynn suggested that hospitalized mental illness is virtually synonymous with psychosis and that physiological, Pavlovian, factor analytic and epidemiological sources provide evidence which shows that psychotics are lacking in anxiety. Similarly, a high per capita calorie intake is regarded by Lynn as a measure of low levels of anxiety, since emotionally stable people have good appetites, whereas among anxious people the appetite tends to be reduced. Suicide and alcoholism are commonly regarded as reactions to anxiety and consequently provide useful quantitative measures of anxiety levels among nations.

The theoretical justification for these four variables as functions of anxiety appears to be confirmed by their pattern of intercorrelation among the 18 countries. A rank order of the 18 countries, based upon these four variables (see Table 18.3), revealed that Ireland, the United Kingdom, New Zealand and Canada had low levels of anxiety, as indexed by high mental illness and high calorie intake associated with low suicide and low alcoholism. The reverse of this pattern is found in Austria, Japan, West Germany and France.

Further manifestations of national anxiety levels were then identified. The most important of these were accident-proneness and aggression. The positive association between anxiety and these two variables has been established in a number of psychological studies and Lynn demonstrated that there are strong positive correlations between the level of national anxiety and measures of accident-proneness (i.e. deaths from motor vehicle accidents) and aggression (i.e. deaths from homicide). Two further variables were found to correlate negatively with anxiety: cigarette consumption and mortality from heart disease (i.e. atherosclerosis and coronary heart disease). Several investigators have found that smoking is strongly correlated with extroversion rather than anxiety. The high incidence of atherosclerosis is influenced by a high calorie intake, to which low anxiety is a contributory cause.

Lynn argued that these manifestations of the anxiety level are associated together and form a pattern. The presence of this underlying pattern was confirmed by means of multivariate analysis. A principal components analysis of eleven variables for the 18 countries (Table 18.2) yielded four components with latent roots greater than unity. The first component accounted for 33.5% of the total variance and clearly represents the anxiety trait. The dimension is bipolar in character, with four variables loading negatively and

	Unrotated factor leadings			
Variables	I	II	III	IV
Mental illness	−0.87	−0.12	0.28	0.06
Coronary deaths	−0.84	−0.20	0.02	0.32
Vehicle deaths	0.82	0.32	−0.38	−0.07
Calorie intake	−0.79	0.26	−0.17	0.15
Suicides	0.60	0.22	0.18	−0.39
Alcoholism deaths	0.52	−0.24	0.43	−0.03
Cigarette consumption	−0.49	−0.72	−0.23	0.00
Ulcer deaths	0.19	0.72	−0.48	−0.18
Murders	0.07	0.59	0.63	−0.04
Celibacy	0.03	−0.23	−0.71	−0.37
Hypertension deaths	0.11	−0.27	0.33	−0.80
Eigen values	3.69	1.86	1.76	1.10
Variance (%)	33.5	16.9	16.0	10.1

Table 18.2 Factor loadings of international data (from Lynn, 1971, Table 20, p. 103).

indexing low anxiety traits (i.e. mental illness, coronary deaths, calorie intake and cigarette consumption). Conversely, three variables have high positive loadings which indicate high levels of national anxiety (i.e. vehicle deaths, suicide and alcoholism deaths).

Table 18.3 shows that the ranking of the nations on this component is broadly similar to that derived from the four original variables. Thus Ireland, the United Kingdom, New Zealand and the U.S.A. have low levels of anxiety, identified by high loadings for mental illness, coronary deaths, high calorie intake and cigarette consumption. Conversely, Japan, West Germany, Austria and Italy have high levels of anxiety, indexed by high loadings for vehicle deaths, suicides and alcoholism deaths.

In the second and more controversial section of his essay, Lynn discussed a number of influences which might be responsible for these observed variations in the national levels of anxiety. He suggested that they might be explained in terms of environmental

Rank order based on four original variables		Rank order based on component scores	
1.	Austria	1.	Japan
2.	Japan	2.	West Germany
3.	West Germany	3.	Austria
4.	France	4.	Italy
5.	Italy	5.	France
6.5	Belgium	6.	Belgium
6.5	Denmark	7.	Netherlands
8.	Switzerland	8.	Norway
9.	Norway	9.	Finland
10.	Finland	10.	Denmark
11.	Sweden	11.	Switzerland
12.	U.S.A.	12.	Sweden
13.	Australia	13.	Australia
14.	Netherlands	14.	Canada
15.	Canada	15.	U.S.A.
16.	New Zealand	16.	New Zealand
17.	United Kingdom	17.	United Kingdom
18.	Ireland	18.	Ireland

Table 18.3 Ranking orders of nations on "anxiety" on the basis of two different ranking methods (from Lynn, 1971, Table 20a, p. 104).

determinants and inherited factors. There is a substantial body of evidence which shows that there are pronounced seasonal variations in the incidence of anxiety, mental disorders and suicide and that these tend to peak in spring and early summer. Lynn raised the possibility that the national and seasonal variations in these phenomena are the result of such climatic factors as summer heat, solar radiation and storminess. Although the evidence is not yet sufficiently conclusive, it would appear that anxiety levels tend to be high in countries with warm and stormy climates.

Lynn also argued that there is a considerable body of evidence in the literature of psychology and psychiatry which shows that the differences in the incidence of psychoses and anxiety among individuals in western countries are determined to a considerable extent by genetic inheritance. This evidence is used to support a case for considering the view that there may be genetic (i.e. racial) determinants of national psychological differences. He advanced the hypothesis that the Nordic race is less anxious than the Alpine and the Mediterranean.

Although neither case is proven conclusively, it is clear that geographers have a potentially valuable contribution to make in this field. As new and more precise census information is published for the mental disorders in different countries, it will become feasible for geographers to use their developed statistical expertise and spatial perspective in determining whether these or other hypotheses have a substantive basis.

REFERENCES

Brocklehurst, J. C. (Ed.) (1973). "Textbook of Geriatric Medicine and Gerontology". Churchill Livingstone, London.

Clarke, A. M. and Clarke, A. D. B. (Eds) (1965). "Mental Deficiency: the Changing Outlook" (2nd edn). Methuen, London.

Cowley, R. W. (1973). "Economics of Mental Retardation". John Hopkins, Baltimore.

Farberow, N. W. and Shneidman, E. S. (Eds) (1961). "The Cry for Help". New York.

Israel, Y. and Mardones, J. (Eds) (1971). "Biological Basis of Alcoholism". Wiley-Interscience, New York.

Jones, R. J. (Ed.) (1970). "Atherosclerosis". Springer Verlag, New York.

Kramer, M. (1969). Applications of mental health statistics. W.H.O. Pamphlet No. 25, Geneva.

Lin, T. and Standley, C. C. (1962). The scope of epidemiology in psychiatry. *W.H.O. Publ. Hlth. Pap.* **16**.

Lynn, R. (1971). "Personality and National Character". Pergamon, Oxford.

Penrose, L. S. (1958). Genetics of anencephaly. *J. Ment. Defic. Res.* **1** 4, 4–15.

Popham, R. E. (Ed.) (1970). "Alcohol and Alcoholism". Univ. Toronto Press, Toronto.

Reid, D. D. (1960). Epidemiological methods in the study of mental disorders. *W.H.O. Publ. Hlth Pap.* **2**.

Sainsbury, P. and Barraclough, B. (1968). Differences between suicide rates. *Nature* **220**, 1252.

Skandia International Symposia (1972). "Suicide and Attempted Suicide". W.H.O., Stockholm.

Slater, E. and Roth, M. (1970). "Clinical Psychiatry" (3rd edn). Baillère, London.

Stanbury, J. B. (Ed.) (1969). "Endemic Goitre". Pan-American Health Organization, Scientific Pubn No. 193, Washington, D.C.

Stengel, E. (1964). "Suicide and Attempted Suicide". Penguin, London.

Tredgold, R. F. and Soddy, K. (1970). "Mental Retardation" (11th edn). Baillière, London.

Wissler, R. W. and Geer, J. C. (Eds) (1972). "The Pathogenesis of Atherosclerosis". Williams and Wilkins, Baltimore.

W.H.O. (1959). Mental health problems of ageing and the aged. *W.H.O. Tech. Rep. Ser.* **171**.

W.H.O. (1960). "Endemic Goitre". W.H.O. Monogr. Series No. 44.

W.H.O. (1963). Training of psychiatrists. *W.H.O. Tech. Rep. Ser.* **252**.

W.H.O. (1963–69). Health personnel and hospital establishments. "World Health Statistics Annual", Vol. III. W.H.O., Geneva.

W.H.O. (1967a). Services for the prevention and treatment of dependence on alcohol and other drugs. *W.H.O. Tech. Rep. Ser.* **363**.

W.H.O. (1967b). "Manual of the International Statistical Classifications of Diseases, Injuries and Causes of Death". W.H.O., Geneva.

W.H.O. (1968). Organization of services for the mentally retarded. *W.H.O. Tech. Rep. Ser.* **392**.

W.H.O. (1968). Prevention of suicide. *Publ. Hlth Pap.* **35**.

W.H.O. (1970). "Endemic Goitre". W.H.O. Monogr. Series No. 4, Geneva.

W.H.O. (1972). Psychogeriatrics. *W.H.O. Tech. Rep. Ser.* **507**.

W.H.O. (1973). Availability of statistics of patients admitted to psychiatric services, *Wld Hlth Stat. Rep.* **26** 1.

W.H.O. (1973). "The International Pilot Study of Schizophrenia". Geneva.

19. Malignant Neoplasms

C. R. Gillis

INTRODUCTION

The words "malignant neoplasms" may be defined thus—"malignant, which describes the tendency of a tumour to spread and to invade surrounding tissues, and neoplasm from the Greek *νεοσ* meaning new and *ήλασμα* meaning formation, thus a new formation of tissue in some part of the body; a tumour."

Not all tumours are malignant (non-malignant tumours are described as benign) and not all malignant tumours are fatal. Throughout the Western World, approximately 50% of malignant tumours actually cause death. Thus, cancer, a collective noun for a variety of different diseases which have particular features in common, should not always be considered as an irrevocably fatal group of diseases. Nevertheless, cancer is the second most common cause of death in most Western countries and thus presents an important challenge to both medical and social services. This is becoming as true in developing countries as in those countries already considered to be developed.

If population projections to the year A.D. 2000 for most Western countries are examined, and if present trends in the treatment of malignant neoplasms continue, then there will be considerably more cases in the year A.D. 2000 than at present.

The variety of malignant neoplasms has been referred to and thus some classification is required if order is to be brought to the study of cancer. Under the auspices of W.H.O. the International Statis-

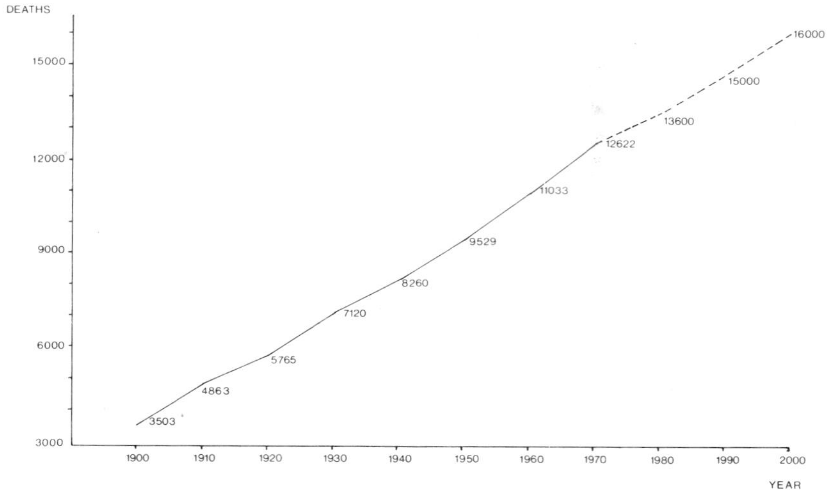

Fig. 19.1 Cancer deaths in Scotland, 1900–70 projected to 2000.

tical Classification, an internationally accepted classification for all kinds of cancer and other diseases, presently lists 100 different kinds of cancer in relation to their site within the body (W.H.O., 1967). Many of these cancers have wide sub-classifications, and with the advancement of knowledge more is being understood about their natural history. A separate classification for cancer has been developed by the W.H.O. (1975). This will be not only more comprehensive but will also be compatable with other classifications of disease in which cancer is included, notably the cancer classification used in the Systematized Nomenclature of Pathology issued by the American Cancer Society (1965).

Amongst the arguments for including a chapter on malignant neoplasms in a book concerned with the geographical distribution of disease, apart from the obvious one concerning cancer incidence, is the fact that cancer is a group of diseases whose study and treatment cross all boundaries in the medical and scientific fields. Inquiry into cancer and the treatment of cancer acts as a powerful unifying force for inter- and intra-disciplinary communication within the general field of science. A major aim of the present chapter is to illustrate the interface and some of the points of contact between the study of geography and the study of oncology;* it is written by a medical

* Oncology is yet another term for the study of cancer. It is derived from the Greek *ογκοο* meaning lump.

doctor responsible to local health authorities for the community care of cancer and interested in the practical considerations relating to collaboration with geographers.

A further argument for including a study of cancer in this book and perhaps the most important, is the likelihood that at least 80% of the cancers are diseases of our environment and that purely genetic factors play an insignificant part. Doll (1967) has expressed a major reason for this in his often quoted statement: "there is no cancer that occurs with even moderate frequency which occurs everywhere and always to the same extent." This statement is, of course, based on the ability to examine comparable data and the level of data recording exhibits considerable variation on a world scale even when it is available. The availability of geographical data about disease has been illustrated by Verhasselt (1975), and some indication of the size of the problem of data collection may be expressed by the fact that the W.H.O. possesses mortality data for only 27% of the total world population and that it has no mortality data from 132 countries out of

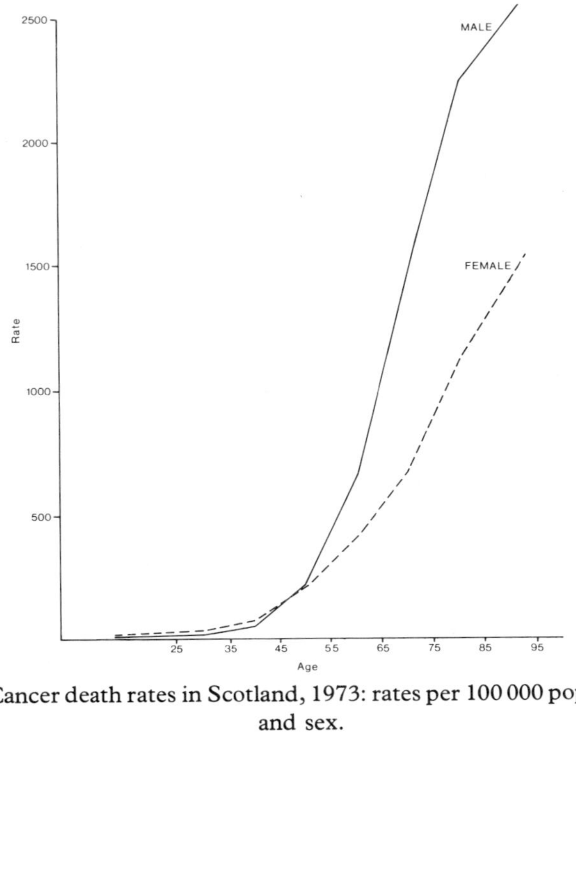

Fig. 19.2 Cancer death rates in Scotland, 1973: rates per 100 000 population by age and sex.

the 189 countries listed by the U.N. While these latter statements refer to data concerning all diseases, cancer is in a somewhat privileged position due to the existence in many countries of cancer registries. The major tasks of cancer registries are to monitor the incidence of cancer and its treatment, to trace inferences about the aetiology of cancer in different areas and to assist in the evaluation of health services in the areas concerned.

There are more registries for cancer than for other diseases because it is considered that at some stage most patients with cancer come into some form of contact with the medical profession; they are thus more likely to be documented. Figure 19.2 shows the age distribution of cancer in Scotland and it is clear that cancer has its major impact in the middle and older age groups in both sexes. Again this corresponds with the picture elsewhere. However, the old are traditionally less likely to come forward to receive medical attention. When they do present themselves, they are usually in the later stages of their disease when medical treatment may not only be less effective but when the situation may be complicated by the presence of other and sometimes more threatening diseases. It is for these reasons that those involved in the geographical and community study of cancer tend to study the age group 35–64 years. Experience has shown that this group not only present earlier in the course of the disease but are also more intensely investigated.

Children also suffer from cancer (Fig. 19.2) and, apart from accidents and congenital malformations, it is the commonest cause of death in childhood. Fortunately, the numbers affected are small and some of the most outstanding advances in the treatment of cancer have taken place in this poignant field. However, because of the statistical problem of comparatively small numbers, and, as with the old, the considerable variations in the completeness and accuracy of data concerning childhood cancer, both the very young and the old members of the population will be omitted from this discussion.

Ideally, cancer registries and other information services collecting data which relate to cancer should have access to the sources of data illustrated in Fig. 19.3. Very few registries have access to all the sources of data mentioned. Even if this were the case, the validity of the information would have to be monitored for quality-control to a degree which could only be rarely attainable within present and foreseeable resources.

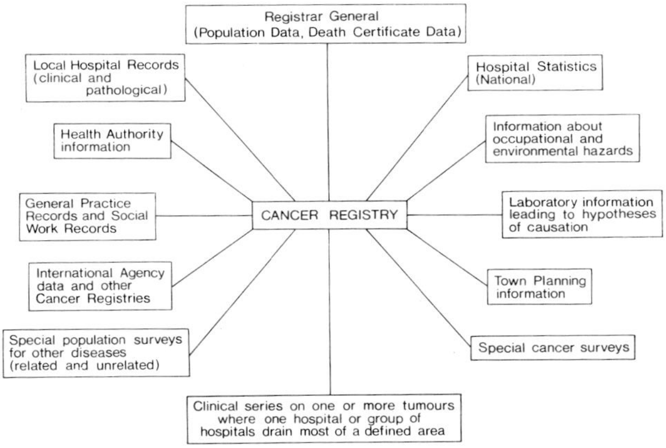

Fig. 19.3 Sources of cancer information in the ideal cancer registry.

If medical geography is to be of value in the study of cancer as a disease of the environment, it must be based on a discussion of comparable data. Such data may be found in Volumes II and III of "Cancer Incidence in Five Continents" (Doll *et al.*, 1970; Waterhouse *et al.*, 1976), though the extent of their coverage may be assessed by Table 19.1.

Figure 19.4 shows the important rise in mortality from lung cancer for males, which is still increasing. Most of the increase is due to people dying of cancer late in life. Another interesting feature is the fall in mortality from stomach cancer in males; this is even more marked for females (Fig. 19.5). It would seem from an examination of the results of treatment that the fall in mortality from gastric cancer is unrelated to advances in treatment. This is perhaps an indication of another important aspect which has been stressed by many investigators namely that cancer incidence varies both temporally

	Number of countries with cancer data	Number of cancer registries
"Cancer Incidence in Five Continents," Vol. II (Doll *et al.*, 1970)	24	48
"Cancer Incidence in Five Continents," Vol. III (Waterhouse *et al.*, 1976)	32	59

Table 19.1 Increased coverage of cancer registration data.

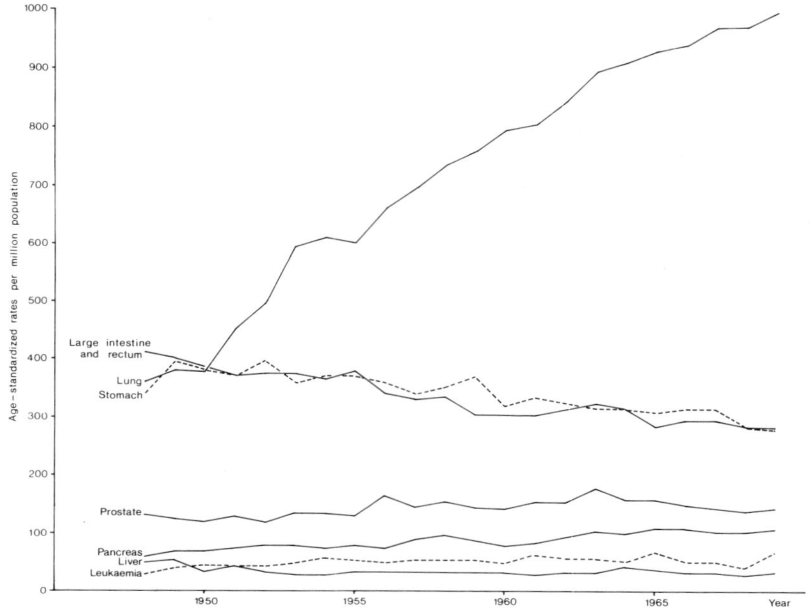

Fig. 19.4 Cancer mortality in Scotland, males, 1948–69.

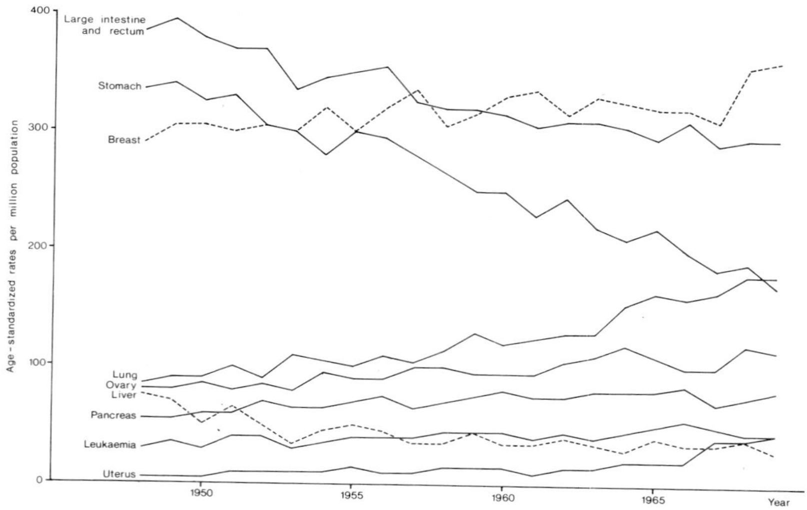

Fig. 19.5 Cancer mortality in Scotland, females, 1948–69.

and spatially. The opinion has been expressed that epidemics of cancer may be compared with the great plagues which swept through Europe in the Middle Ages and disappeared without obvious reason. Thus investigators in cancer are obliged to continuously monitor the behaviour of the various cancers in their different environments not only with reference to factors present in the contemporary environment but also to changes which may have occurred in these factors over time.

OESOPHAGEAL CANCER

Many consider that the most dramatic feature of oesophageal cancer (cancer of the gullet) is its geographical or spatial variation on a world scale (Fig. 19.6 and Table 19.2).

Place	Rate
Scotland	6.8
England (S.W. Metro)	5.2
Finland	8.1
California (Negro)	19.8
California (White)	7.2
South Africa—Natal (African)	93.1
Rhodesia—Bulawayo (African)	94.9
Nigeria—Ibadan	2.5

Iran, with probably the world's highest incidence of oesophageal cancer, is not included since data in comparable form were not included in "Cancer Incidence in Five Continents", Vol. II (1970).

Table 19.2 Oesophageal cancer: standardized morbidity rates per 100 000 population (after Doll *et al.*, 1970)

As more than 90% of these cancers are of the same type (i.e. when viewed in section, after surgical removal, they have the same microscopical appearance), it is clear that different factors must be operating in the areas of high incidence. In South-East Africa, the association has been with the use of maize in the preparation of certain alcoholic beverages; in the areas of highest incidence, maize has only been a staple crop since the beginning of this century.

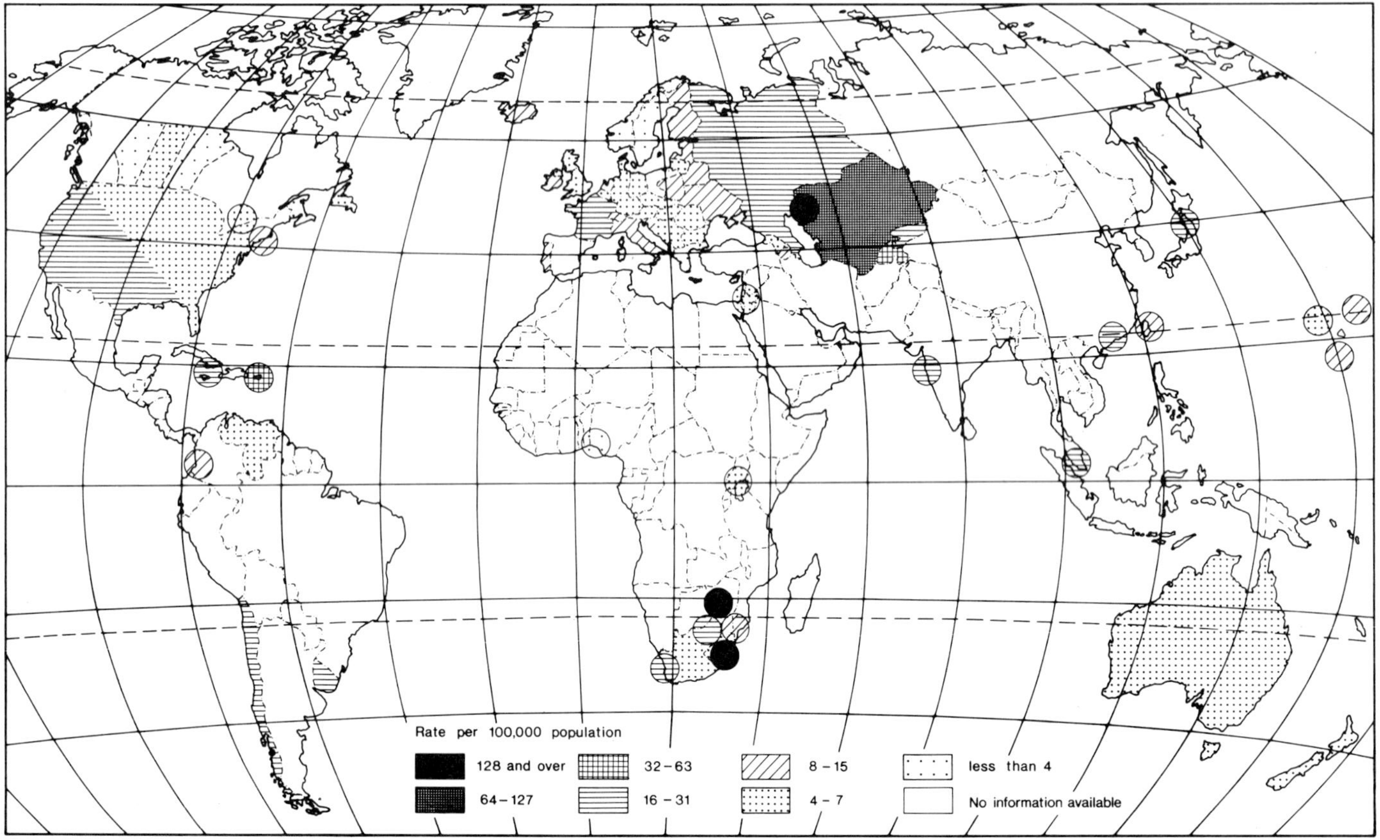

Fig. 19.6 Oesophageal cancer: incidence rates for males 35–64 years (adapted from Doll, 1967).

Equally important, the disease has only recently reached its present epidemic proportions there; this disease has occurred within the practising lifetime of doctors in this region. In Europe where the incidence is very much lower, France has comparatively high rates. Here again the high rates have been associated with the consumption of drinks containing alcohol. However, along the littoral of the Caspian Sea where there are areas of highest incidence, no alcoholic drinks are consumed. In France, some of the areas with the highest incidence of alcoholism show rates for oesophageal cancer similar to those for the country as a whole; in other areas where alcoholism is equally high, notably Brittany, rates for oesophageal cancer are higher than the average for the French population (Tuyns, 1970). Alcohol alone is not considered carcinogenic. A further intriguing factor is that, within the areas of very high incidence of oesophageal cancer, such as those found in Africa and the Caspian littoral, there are zones where comparatively high and low frequencies of oesophageal cancer can be demonstrated separated by as little as 100 miles. In the Caspian littoral area, the high incidence of oesophageal cancer has been associated with the ingestion of hot fluids. These fluids remain longest in the middle third of the oesophagus, the commonest site of this cancer. These associated factors are compounded by the practice of cigarette smoking. Cigarette smoking by itself and when combined with alcohol, has been shown to have a strong influence on the development of oesophageal cancer. It has been difficult to demonstrate the influence of alcohol on its own as those who drink heavily often smoke heavily as well. A further complicating factor is the presence of nitrosamines which are known to be powerful carcinogens in animals and which the human body can synthesize endogenously. Nitrosamines exist in many foods, fluids and soil types. However, it is a fact that substances which are carcinogenic in animals are not necessarily carcinogenic in man and vice versa. Thus while all of these factors may be associated with oesophageal cancer, the task facing medical geographers, environmentalists and epidemiologists is to find how each of these factors operates in the chain of causality (Gillis and Carter, 1976). If local environmental factors are to be adequately understood so that the geographical differences indicated may be accounted for, then much closer collaboration between medical geographers and others in the field of cancer studies must take place.

GASTRIC CANCER

Gastric cancer is considerably more common than oesophageal cancer. On the world scale, the most important feature is the gradient from Eastern Europe across to the western seaboard of the U.S.A. where this disease is apparently much less common than in Eastern Europe (Fig. 19.7). Of current importance is the fact that new techniques for early diagnosis have found extremely high rates of early gastric cancer in Japan. When similar techniques of diagnosis have been introduced in Europe, they have confirmed the suspicion that the comparative figures for Japan and European countries for early gastric cancer are likely to be correct. There is not the same decline in gastric cancer in males and females in Japan as noted for a similar time-period in Scotland (Figs 19.4 and 19.5).

Genetic factors are thought to play a part in the aetiology of this disease. Statistical evidence suggests that individuals with blood group A experience an incidence of gastric carcinoma as much as 20% greater than individuals having other blood groups. This applies whether the general incidence is high or low. It seems clear that genetic factors do not account for the considerable differences between geographical areas since these cross both ethnic and social boundaries.

The particular type of gastric cancer which relates to environmental characteristics shows a considerable decline in Japanese migrants to Hawaii where their experience of gastric cancer approximates to that of the general population. A correlation between incidence of gastric ulcer and the subsequent development of gastric cancer has been considered in many parts of the world but, in most Western countries, clinical observations infer that only in a very small proportion of cases do gastric ulcers lead to gastric cancer.

A variety of factors have been studied in the aetiology of stomach cancer and no clear understanding of the cause is apparent. Certainly there are no important epidemiological associations between gastric cancer and the intake of alcohol and spices, the extent to which food is chewed, the rapidity with which it is eaten, or the temperature at which it is consumed.

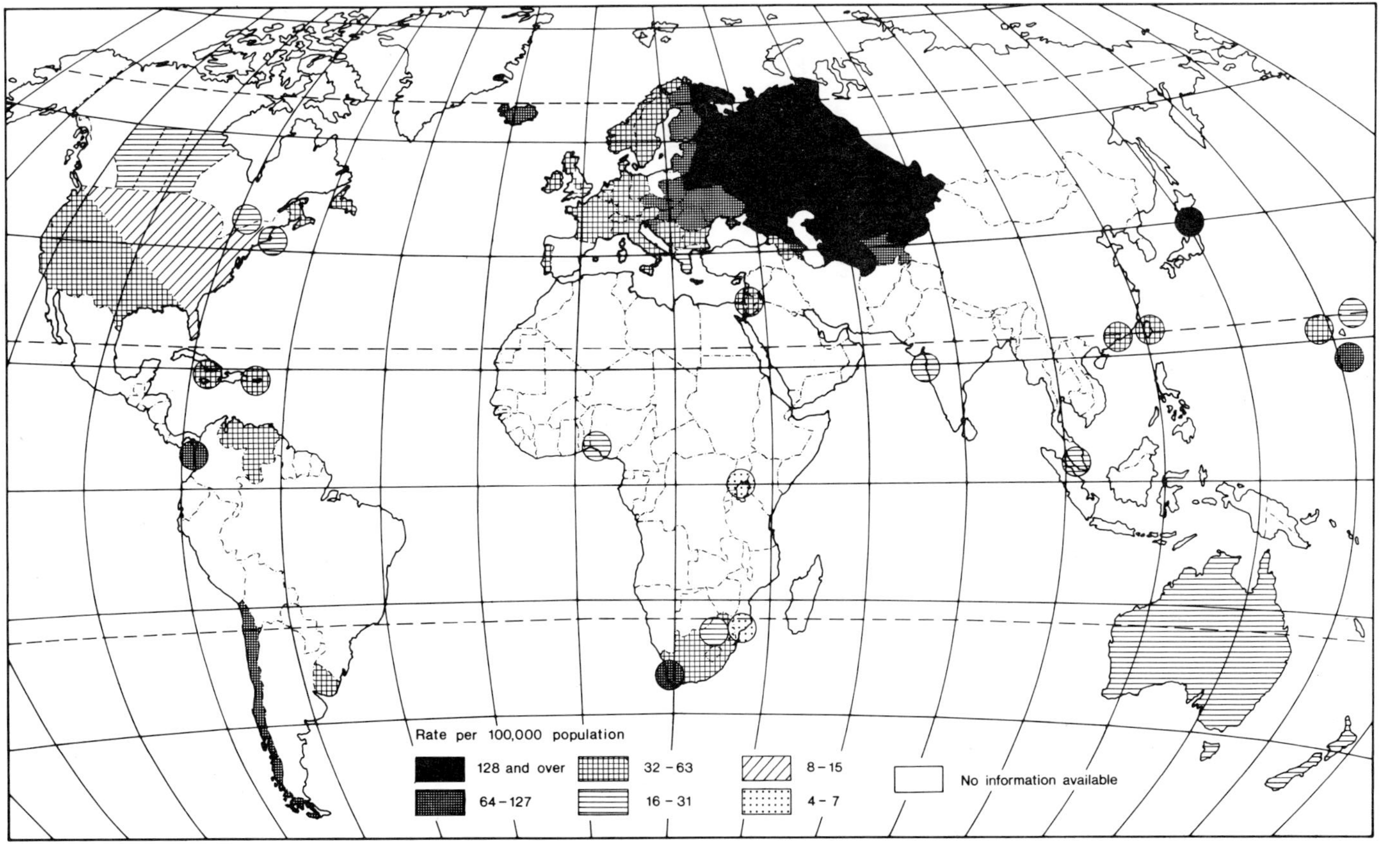

Fig. 19.7 Stomach cancer: incidence rates for males 35–64 years (adapted from Doll, 1967).

CANCER OF THE COLON

Cancer of the colon shows a world distribution which is almost the opposite of that for cancer of the stomach (Fig. 19.8). Highest rates are observed in Western America, lowest rates in Eastern Europe. This gradient must be environmental rather than genetic, added to which incidence studies in the U.S.A. suggest that changes in risk have occurred over too short a period for genetic factors to be implicated. This evidence is supported by rates for migrants to the U.S.A. from Norway and Poland (countries which have considerably lower incidence of colon cancer) which show a distinct tendency to rise to the level of the U.S.A. Though Japanese migrants, both in the U.S.A. and in Hawaii, have lower rates to those generally observed in the U.S.A., rates for Japanese in Japan itself approximate to the rates in the U.S.A. However, Japanese in Hawaii have rates comparable to whites in Hawaii. Rates for whites in the U.S.A. are only slightly higher than those for non-whites and there are no socio-economic differences which are strikingly obvious in either North America or Western Europe; there is however still some argument about this. There may be some hereditary predisposition to cancer of the colon. Various immune deficiencies and other diseases of low incidence which run in families, such as familial polyposis, have been implicated. Other diseases which may predispose to cancer of the colon include ulcerative colitis and possibly Chron's disease. However, environmental factors are clearly more important than hereditary factors. Diet is an obvious environmental variable and Burkitt (1971) has been responsible for drawing attention to the association between the amount of roughage in the food eaten which in its turn relates to the transit time of food through the intestine—an association which appears to be consistent on an international basis.

CANCER OF THE FEMALE BREAST

Cancer of the breast, like cancer of the colon, also shows a geographical distribution which is the inverse of that for stomach cancer (Fig. 19.9). There appears to be a tendency towards familial aggregation in breast cancer but again hereditary factors cannot account for the geographical variations illustrated. Cancer of the

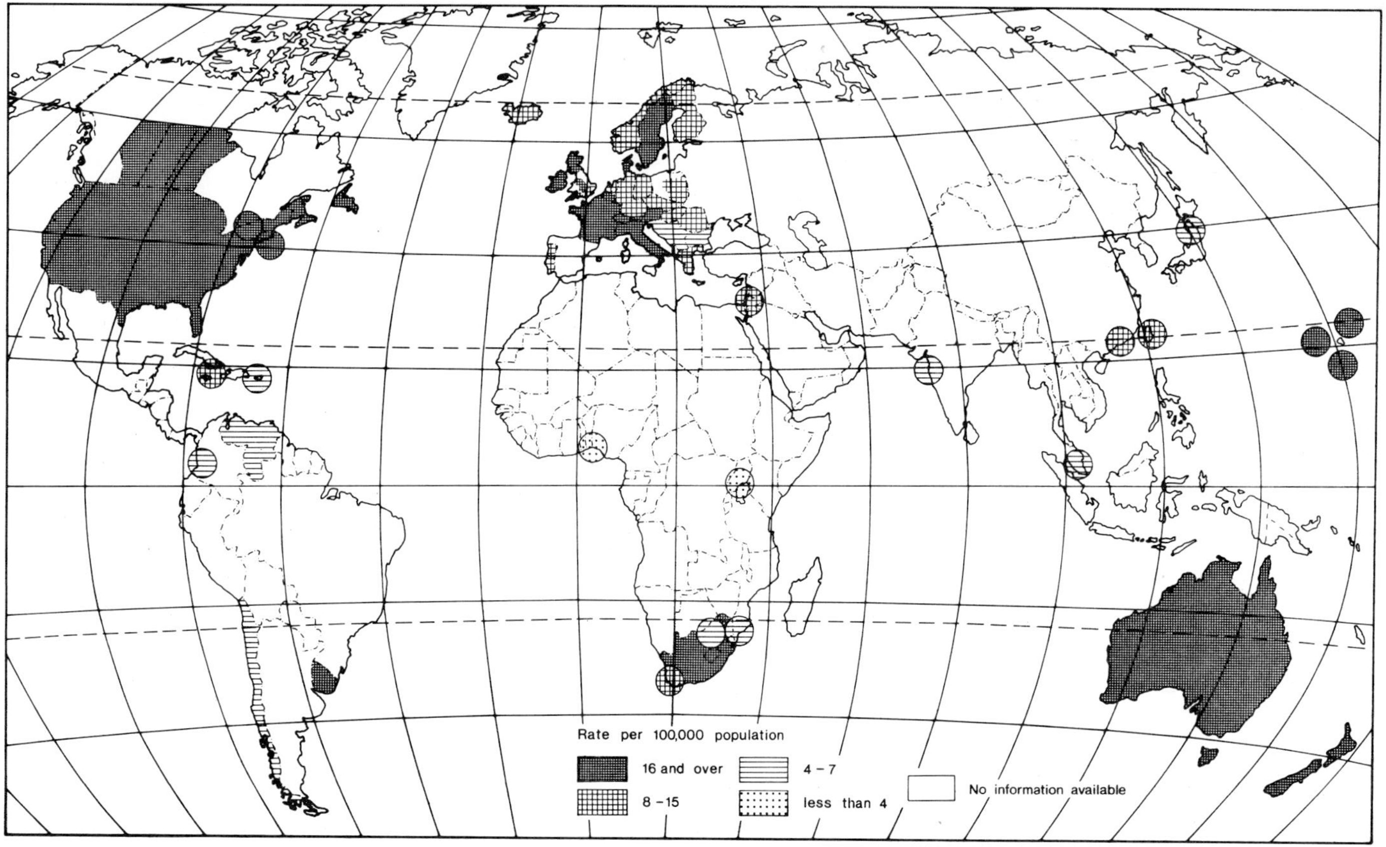

Fig. 19.8 Colon cancer: incidence rates for males 35–64 years (adapted from Doll, 1967).

breast is the commonest cancer in females and is only rarely seen in males. The incidence of breast cancer has increased in most Western countries though in the U.S.A. this increase has been more apparent for non-whites than whites. However, survival has also increased thus accounting for the fact that mortality rates for this disease have remained relatively unchanged over the past 30 years.

Polish migrants to the U.S.A. appear to have an increased risk of developing breast cancer, a risk which approximates that observed for native white Americans. To date, Japanese migrants have not displayed a tendency for their originally low rates of breast cancer to rise to the level of the U.S.A. Breast cancer is relatively unknown among Chinese living in the U.S.A., similarly among American Indians. While these data give some support to the importance of hereditary factors, the distribution shown in Fig. 19.9 emphasizes the influence of geographical factors. It is noteworthy that both colon and breast cancer show opposite geographical trends to gastric cancer.

In a study of cancer mortality for U.S.A. counties between 1950 and 1969 (Mason *et al.*, 1976), cancers of the colon and rectum showed a strikingly similar spatial pattern to that for breast cancer, suggesting that this disease may have an environmental factor or stimulus in common with cancer of the large intestine; Doll, on numerous occasions, has suggested that this factor may be related to diet. Other factors which have at one time or another been associated with a higher risk of female breast cancer are race (Caucasian), ethnic group (Jewish), marital status (single), age at first pregnancy (older), number of pregnancies (fewer), age at menarche (earlier), artificial menopause (absent), benign breast disease, socio-economic status (higher) and obesity.

CANCER OF THE LUNG

Cancer of the lung is perhaps the commonest cancer in most Western countries (Fig. 19.10) and is the only one of those cancers previously mentioned where the cause is now well defined, both in the general population and in specific occupational groups (see below). When available mortality and morbidity statistics are examined, the association between lung cancer and cigarette smoking appears to be consistent in all countries.

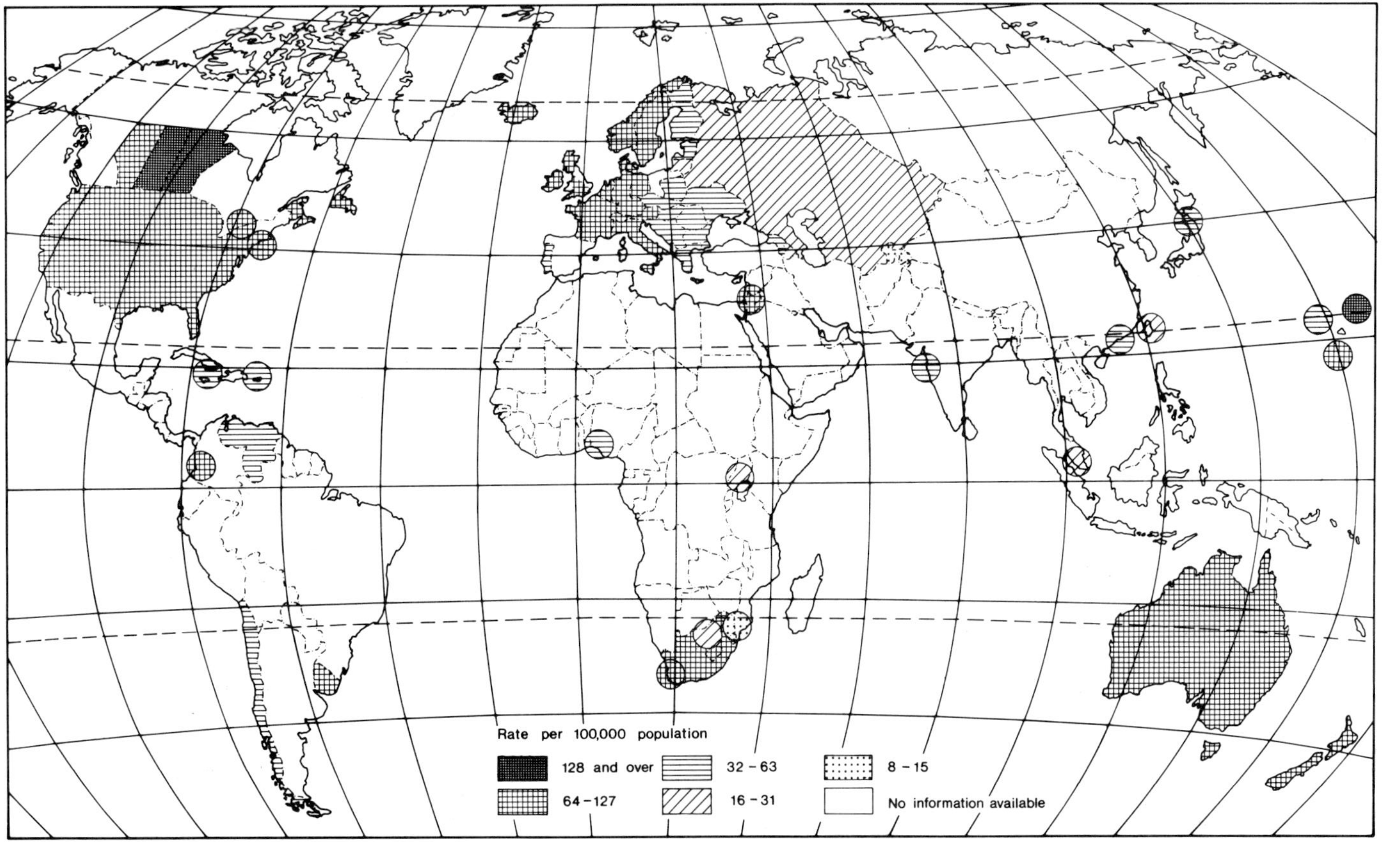

Fig. 19.9 Breast cancer: incidence rates for females 35–64 years (adapted from Doll, 1967).

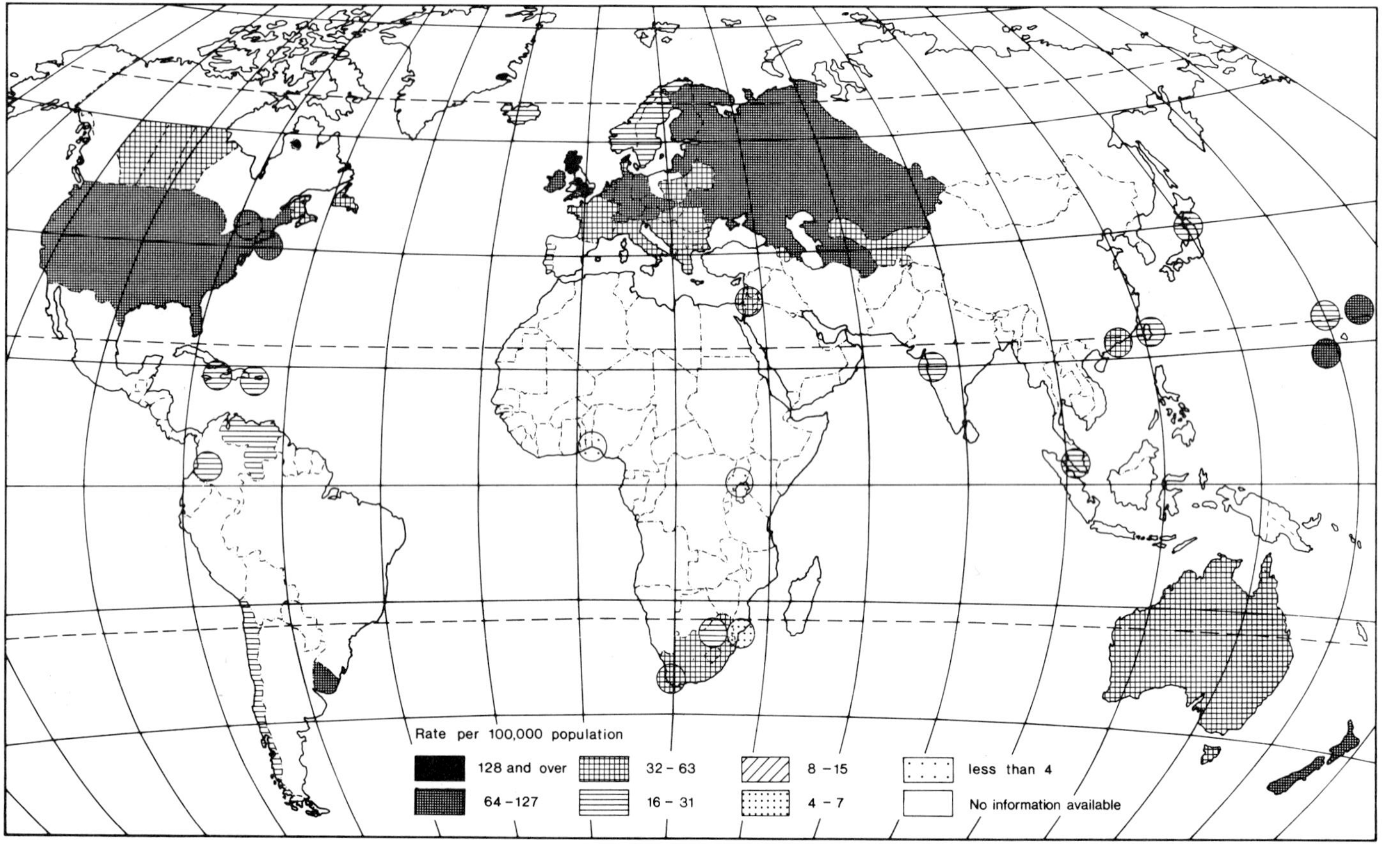

Fig. 19.10 Lung and bronchus cancer: incidence rates for males 35–64 years (adapted from Doll, 1967).

The incidence of the disease is considerably higher in Britain than in Australia or Canada and, although atmospheric pollution on its own has been considered as a causative factor, it is unlikely that this operates without the component of cigarette smoking. In Scotland, where the morbidity rate for lung cancer is amongst the highest recorded anywhere in the world, and where death rates are still increasing, morbidity rates for age-specific groups under 60 years of age fail to show a similar increase. It is not known whether the absence of any increase in the younger age group is due to (a) a fall in cigarette consumption, (b) the introduction of control measures for atmospheric pollution, or (c) the rapid rise in mortality in the younger age groups due to coronary heart disease preventing such individuals reaching an age where they might have otherwise contracted lung cancer. On the other hand, the disease itself may be changing in its nature over time. It may be that the "epidemic" of lung cancer being witnessed in Britain should be considered as a cohort phenomenon affecting those who had heaviest exposure to cigarette smoke during the First World War. Certainly, in Scotland, no subsequent age group appears to be experiencing a mortality rate which is quite as high. In other countries, the chewing of tobacco, either on its own or mixed with betel or lime, has been implicated in cancer of the mouth and pharynx; it is not simply the effect of heat on tobacco which makes it carcinogenic.

CANCER OF THE LIVER

The geographical variation in primary liver cancer, which is a rare cancer in most parts of the world, can vary very considerably between low and high incidence areas (Fig. 19.11). The incidence has sometimes been confused with differences in the distribution of carcinoma of the bile ducts. The latter appears to have a uniformly low distribution throughout the world, except in the Far East where the rate of bile duct cancer is associated with infestation with *Clonorchis sinensis* and other liver flukes (Gibson, 1971). Doll, in his map of liver cancer, has used the age group 15–44 years since this form of cancer appears early in adult life in those countries where it is common. Consideration of this younger age group also avoids confusion with secondary liver cancer which is common in all age

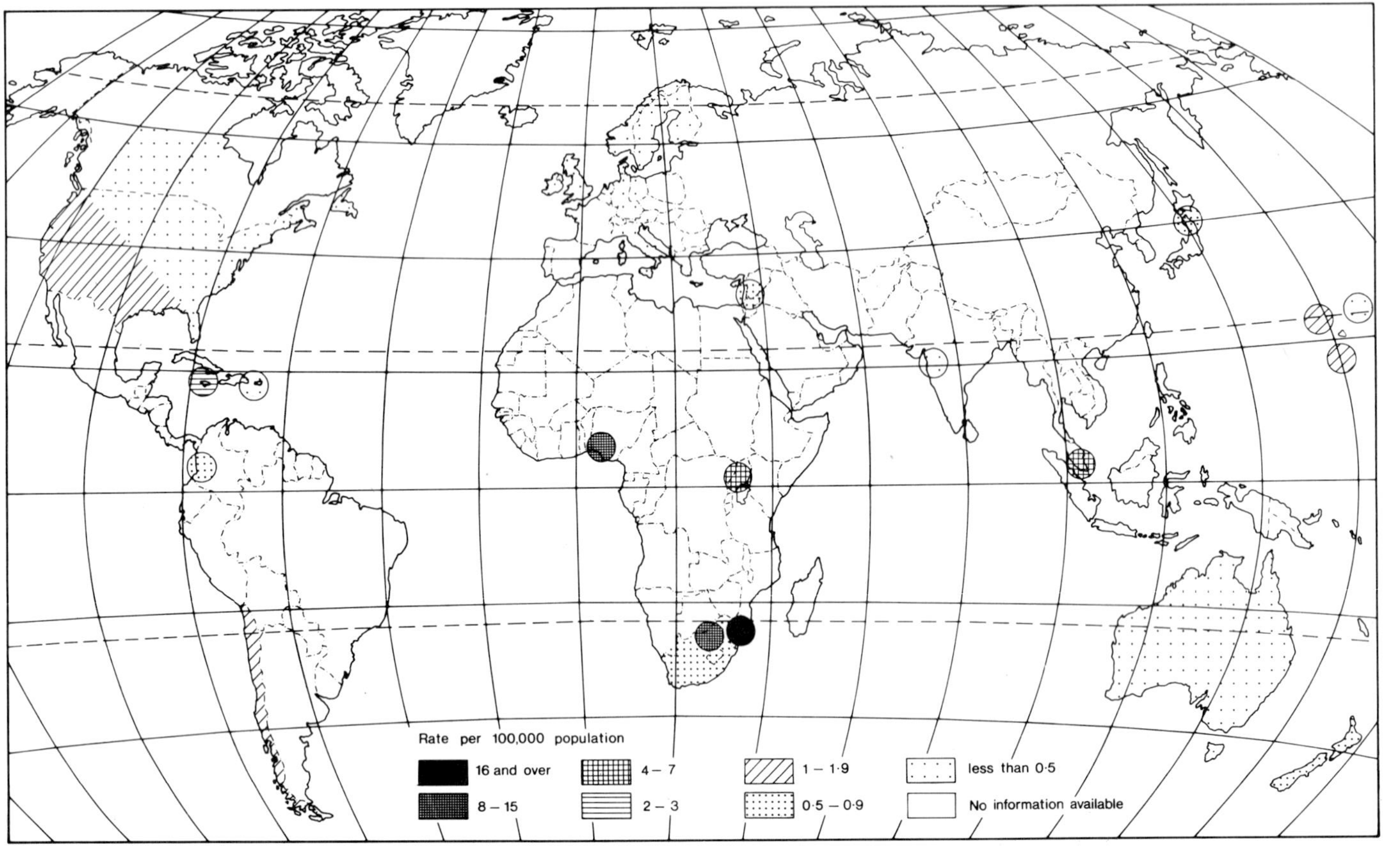

Fig. 19.11 Liver cancer: incidence rates for males 15–44 years (adapted from Doll, 1967).

groups and with many other cancers. In Europe and North America, 5–15% of patients with cirrhosis of the liver—a possible predisposing disease—develop liver cancer. Evidence suggests that this figure may be rising slowly in Western countries. In Africa and the Far East, the risk of developing liver cancer appears to be far greater. In South Africa, it was found that while the incidence of cirrhosis was approximately the same in European and African populations, the frequency of liver cell cancer in those with cirrhosis was 6% in Europeans and 44% in Africans (Becker and Chatgidakis, 1961). There was also a difference in the type of cirrhosis between the Europeans and the Africans. However, in Africa and in the Far East, alcohol does not appear to be a major factor in the aetiology of cancer of the liver. Aflatoxins, serum hepatitis and Australia antigen have recently been identified as having possible causal association in human liver cell cancer (Editorial, B.M.J., 1972).

Evidence is accumulating which suggests that distillery workers may be at higher risk than other occupational groups.

BURKITT'S LYMPHOMA

This tumour (Burkitt and Davies, 1961) is rare or almost unknown outside Africa and New Guinea and has the striking feature that it does not exist in areas where temperatures fall below 16°C (61°F) or where the annual rainfall is less than 76 cm (30 ins) (Haddow, 1964). The viruses responsible for yellow fever and O'nyong and nyong fever, at that time common in those parts of Africa, were known to be carried by mosquitoes and it was the maps showing the distribution of these insect vectors for these different diseases that first gave support to a viral hypothesis in the aetiology of this cancer since they had a remarkable similarity to those for Burkitt's lymphoma in Africa. The "EB" virus has since been implicated and further support for this tumour being regarded as having an infective aetiology is the demonstration of space/time clustering (see below) (Morrow *et al.*, 1971).

HODGKIN'S DISEASE

Hodgkin's disease is a form of cancer affecting the lymph glands in the body. On the global scale, there appear to be two major incidence peaks, one in childhood and young adult life, the other in the elderly. It has been suggested that Hodgkin's disease may be more than one disease entity, perhaps with an infective aetiology in young people and a different form of cancer in older age groups. Bimodal peaks in age-specific incidence rates in both males and females occur in almost all countries where adequate data are available. Detailed local studies have been made and an association with prior tonsillectomy found (Davies and Vianna, 1976). This adds some weight to the evidence for an infective aetiology in young people suffering from this disease. Other studies have yet to substantiate the hypothesis of infectivity.

LEUKAEMIA

Mortality rates for all forms of leukaemia differ from country to country but none of these differences are as prominent as those for other forms of cancer. Because of the recent improvement in the effectiveness of treatment for leukaemia it is difficult to know whether some of the differences which occur reflect variations in case finding or the influence of different environmental and/or genetic factors. Although genetic factors in leukaemia have been implicated, studies among immigrants to the U.S.A. suggest that rates for leukaemia among immigrants have more in common with U.S.A. rates than with rates in the country of origin of the individual immigrant. Many studies of geographical differences in leukaemia rates reflect largely the availability of medical care and correlate well with social class and income. However, there has probably been a real increase in the number of cases of leukaemia in the course of this century, particularly with the experience of the atomic explosions over Hiroshima and Nagasaki. It is also well known that different age distributions relate to different forms of leukaemia and, in general, children have different types of leukaemia from those seen in adults.

Leukaemia is a form of cancer which has some relation to ethnic group. For instance there is a striking lack of chronic lymphocytic leukaemia among the Japanese and other Oriental groups. Others would argue that the patterns of adult leukaemia reflect genetic constitution. Either way, the study of environmental factors makes both arguments uncertain. It may be that the genetic hypothesis has more weight since chronic lymphocytic leukaemia is rare in Japanese immigrants to the U.S.A. while leukaemia of all types is more common in Jews than in non-Jews. It has been suggested (Graham *et al.*, 1970) that the risk of leukaemia in Jews is confined to adults and in particular in Russian-born Jews; it is not related to variation in case finding, medical care, or exposure to X-rays or other forms of ionizing radiation.

Leukaemia appears to exhibit a seasonal variation in its incidence as summer peaks have been found (Lee and Gardner, 1965).

Lastly, the work of Jarrett (1974), wherein he has shown the ability of cats to transfer leukaemia to each other by a viral mechanism, may have important implications for mankind.

OTHER CANCER ASSOCIATIONS

It is a matter of speculation that if all cases of skin cancer were recorded this might be the second commonest form of cancer. One reason why it does not occupy this position in the morbidity tables for cancer is that potentially skin cancer is the most curable form of the disease. Many patients with skin cancer are cured without the necessity of an in-patient attendance. It follows that they are insufficiently documented to enter the statistical records.

On a global scale, evidence for the implication of *ultra-violet irradiation* in skin cancer includes the following. (a) coloured people have far less skin cancer than non-coloured; (b) skin cancer occurs most often on the exposed areas of the head, neck, arms and hands; (c) among white people, there is apparently more skin cancer in outdoor workers than those who work indoors; (d) the incidence of skin cancer in white people is highest (as in Scotland) in areas of greatest isolation and there is also a change with latitude, greater incidence being found towards the equator, an association related to latitude which is not found with other cancers.

Such evidence suggests the importance of ultra-violet irradiation in the aetiology of skin cancer, but the issue is rather more complicated in the case of malignant melanoma. Here the relationship of melanoma to exposure or history of sunburn is less marked. Indeed, the report of the Queensland Melanoma Project (Beardmore, 1972) suggests that sunlight has both a direct and an indirect effect in the causation of melanoma.

When cancer is studied in relation to *occupation* and to specific occupational groups, such as miners, it is frequently identified as an occupational hazard. Cancer of the lung is the commonest anatomical site and such minerals as silver, cobalt, uranium, chromate, ferrous ore, nickel and asbestos which reach the lungs by inhalation, have been held responsible. In the case of asbestos now used in the manufacture of many components of our daily life, exposure to particles can be dangerous since the amount of exposure required to produce cancer may be small. If individuals who have been exposed to asbestos particles also smoke cigarettes, then their risk of lung cancer is many times greater than that of cigarette smokers in the general population. Although soot is a common constituent of our atmospheric environment, it was known long before Percival Pott described cancer of the scrotum among chimney sweeps in Britain (1775) that these workers had a greater than expected experience of "sootwart" or scrotal cancer. This finding was not so well marked in Scotland or in Europe. It is an example of how such preventive measures as washing may be used in the protection of occupational groups from certain forms of cancer.

Factors of *soil* and *climate* have already been commented upon in relationship to specific cancers. Such relationships are clearly worthy of further study, and the stimulus given to researchers by Stocks and Davies (1964) when they found an association between the zinc and copper content of the soil and the incidence of various cancers has not elicited a sufficient response.

ASPECTS OF CANCER IN SCOTLAND—A CASE STUDY

It is perhaps appropriate to conclude this chapter with a brief note on aspects of cancer in Scotland. The author is able to qualify the statistical statements relating to this topic from his own epidemiological experience.

In Scotland, there is considerable geographical variation in the frequency of occurrence of some of the most common cancers (Fig. 19.12). Even more interesting geographical variations present themselves when the frequency of cancer in the Islands off the West coast of Scotland is examined in relation to Scotland as a whole (Fig. 19.13). While it is clear that cancer of the lung is an important

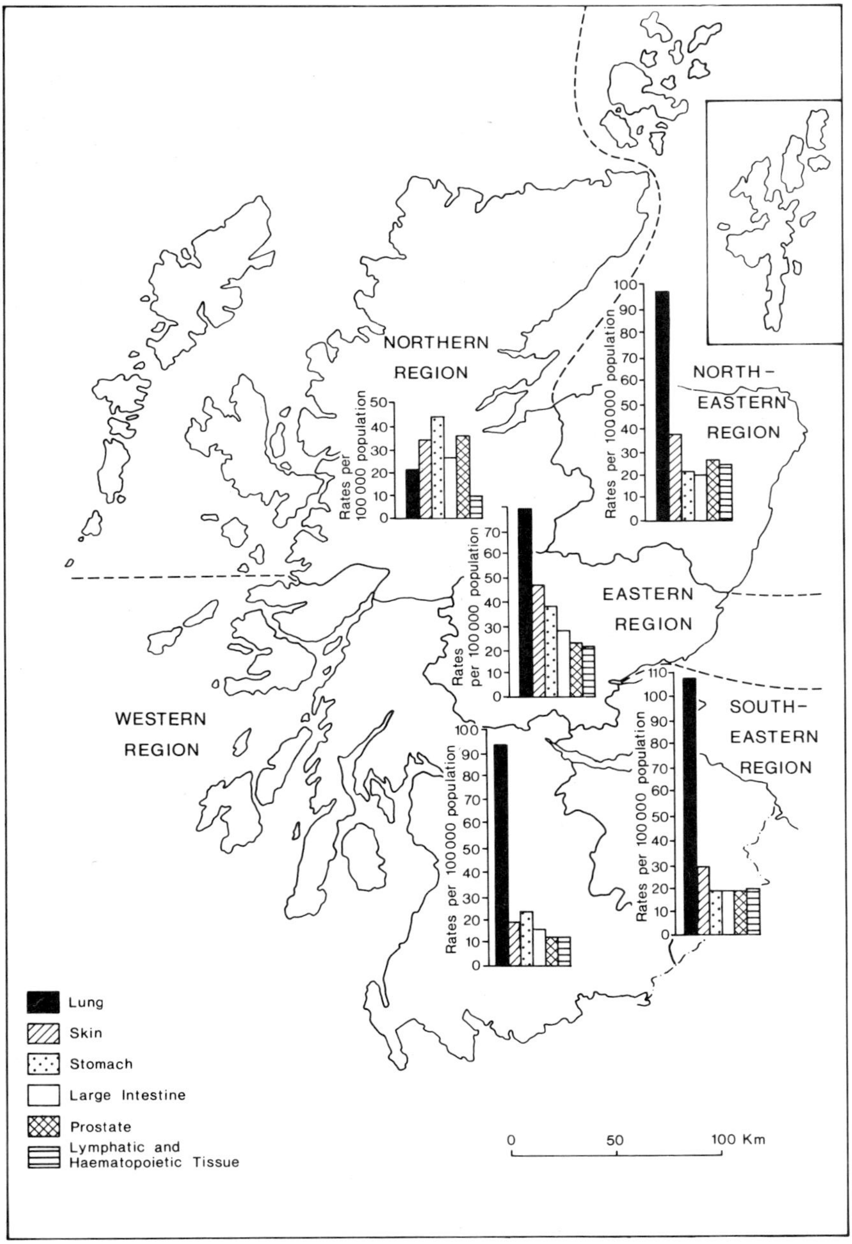

Fig. 19.12 Most common cancers in males in Scotland: registration in 1967.

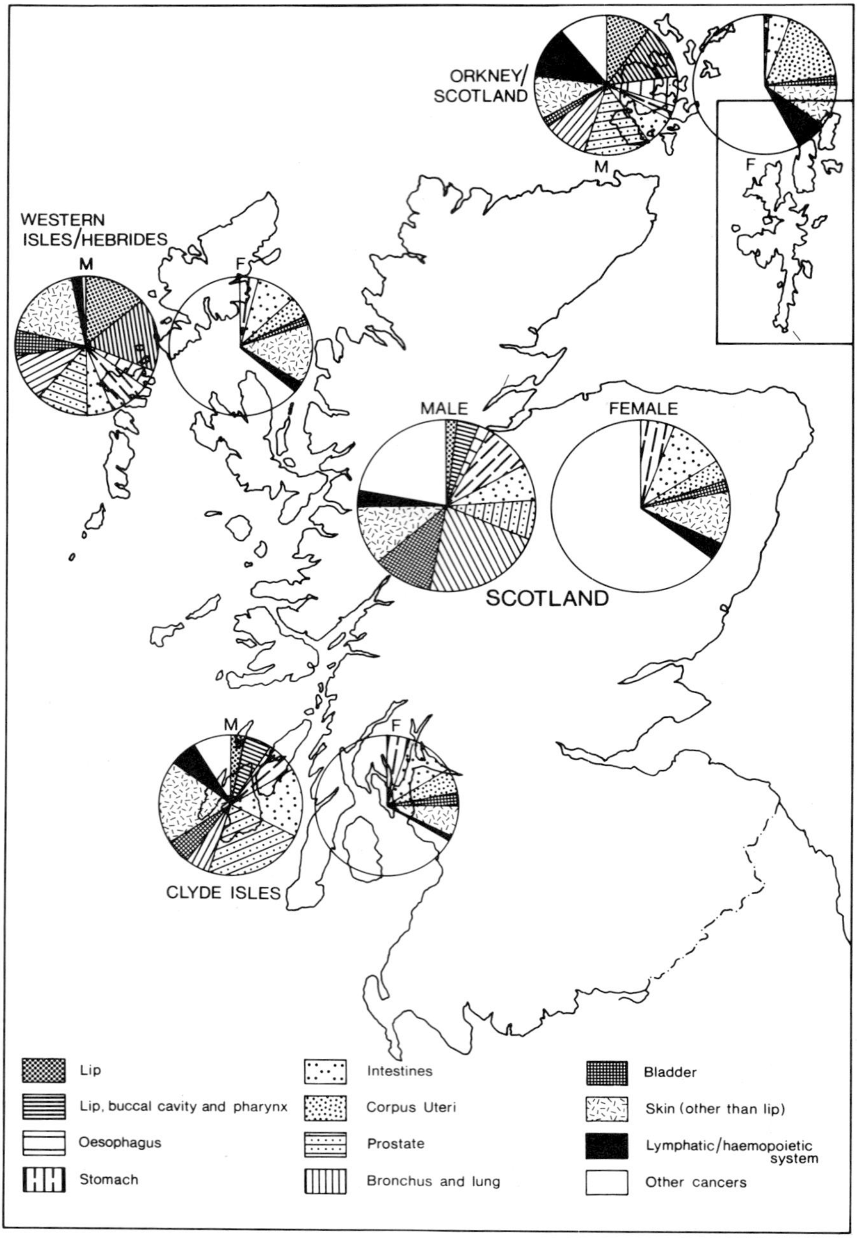

Fig. 19.13 Selected cancers: proportional incidence in Scotland.

problem not only for the industrial belt in Scotland,* the illustrations for the Highlands and Islands exemplify some of the associations between environmental factors and cancer. This applies particularly to cancer of the lip. Cancer of this site is many times more common in the islands than on the mainland. Sunlight may certainly be considered as a contributory factor but a further factor might be the fishermen sucking the tarry twine when mending their nets. This higher incidence of lip cancer does not appear in fishermen in the ports of the southern mainland of Scotland. Are the characteristics of these individuals different from their colleagues on the Islands? Such problems can be solved only by prospective epidemiological investigation using reliable population data. In addition to a reliable population denominator, accurate occupational numerators are also necessary. As in so many other occupational groups, such information is difficult to obtain. Observed differences in incidence on the Scottish mainland are very much in accord with the expected and relate to level of urbanization and social class.

At this more local level of investigation, the geographical approach can assist only where accurate data are available. One such area is the administrative county of Ayr in South-West Scotland. Here, during an examination of the bracken-fern hypothesis concerning the aetiology of alimentary cancer (Evans and Osman, 1974), it was necessary, in the absence of data relating population density and occupational numerators, to report to space/time clustering methods (Mantel, 1967). Anecdotal evidence was available which suggested that both humans and cattle who had been in close contact over a period of years had contracted alimentary cancer at approximately the same time. It was not possible to substantiate the bracken hypothesis, but during scrutiny of patients' addresses it was observed that there were also instances of oesophagus, stomach, large and small intestine and rectal cancers apparently living close to each other (Fig. 19.14). The spatial aspect of this phenomenon was intriguing especially as it appeared consistently in other geographical areas of the administrative county. The cases were analysed to find whether they clustered closely in both time and space. Statistically meaningful results were obtained.

* Morbidity from cancer of the lung appears lower in the West of Scotland than in the South East of Scotland. This is due to persistent under-registration of this form of cancer. Mortality statistics show a reverse picture.

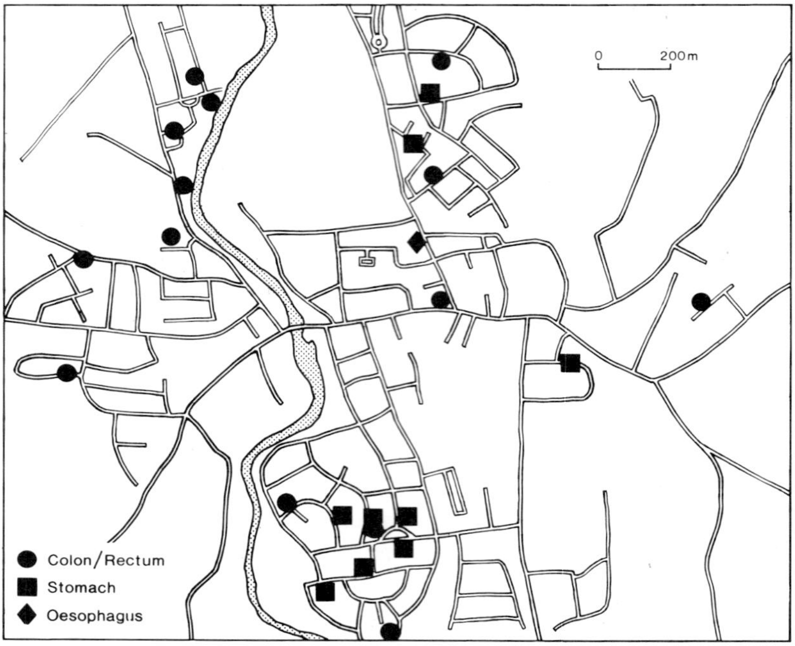

Fig. 19.14 Alimentary cancer: spatial aspects of clustering.

The demonstration of space/time clustering has been traditionally associated with communicable disease. As already noted, the phenomenon of micro-epidemicity has been demonstrated in childhood leukaemia as well as in Hodgkin's and Burkitt's lymphoma. Thus this finding in Ayrshire is of interest in that it could lead to the easier identification of a viral or chemical or other carcinogen in the aetiology of alimentary cancer. The use of space/time clustering techniques, relying on the use of map grid co-ordinates combined with good data, makes this a powerful research tool in the further identification of problems which can range from aetiology to the planning of social services for cancer patients in the future. Most of the major forms of cancer tend to cluster in space but none more so than alimentary cancer (Waterhouse, 1974). If all forms of alimentary cancer are taken together, then it becomes the second commonest cancer in both males and females in Scotland.

In conclusion it may be noted that the foregoing contribution illustrates some of the ways in which the study of geography and the total environment can assist in the identification of specific hazards.

For those engaged in cancer research, the geographical approach to problems affords pointers to those areas or localities where in depth research may be undertaken in order to validate hypotheses generated either in the laboratory, at the bedside or in the community. What matters most in research, however, is contact and collaboration between workers. With the emergence of organizations for the study and care of cancer, it is hoped that the multi-disciplinary approach will become more apparent—"the whole is greater than the sum of the parts".

ACKNOWLEDGEMENTS

Figures 19.6–19.11 have been adapted from "The Prevention of Cancer: Pointers from Epidemiology" by kind permission of Sir Richard Doll of The Nuffield Provincial Hospital Trust. Thanks are due also to Mr. D. S. MacLean, Statistician, West of Scotland Cancer Intelligence Unit for assistance in the preparation of Figs 19.1, 19.2 and 19.4–19.5.

REFERENCES

American Cancer Society (1965). The classification of cancer. *In* "Systematized Nomenclature of Pathology". College of American Pathologists, Chicago.

Beardmore, G. L. (1972). The epidemiology of malignant melanoma in Australia. *In* "Melanoma and Skin Cancer" (Ed. W. H. McCarthy). Government printer, Sydney, N.S.W., Australia.

Becker, B. J. and Chatgidakis, C. B. (1961). Primary carcinoma of the liver in Johannesburg. *Acta Un. Int. Cancer* **17**, 650.

Burkitt, D. and Davies, J. N. P. (1961). Lymphoma syndrome in Uganda and tropical Africa. *Med. Press* **245**, 367.

Burkitt, D. P. (1971). Epidemiology of cancer of the colon and rectum. *Cancer* **28**, 3–13.

Davies, J. N. P. and Vianna, N. J. (1976). Epidemiology of some human cancers: (5) Hodgkin's Disease. *In* "Scientific Foundations of Oncology" (Eds T. Symington and R. L. Carter). William Heinemann Medical, London.

Doll, R. (1967). "Prevention of Cancer: Pointers from Epidemiology". Nuffield Provincial Hospitals Trusts, London.

Doll, R., Muir, C. and Waterhouse, J. (1970). "Cancer Incidence in Five Continents", Vol. II. U.I.C.C., Geneva.

Editorial, 1972. Aetiology of liver cancer. *Brit. Med. J.* **I**, 261–262.

Evans, I. A. and Osman, M. A. (1974). Carcinogenicity of bracken and shikimic acid. *Nature*, 250.

Gibson, J. B. (1971). Parasites, liver disease and liver cancer. *In* "Liver Cancer", I.A.R.C. Scientific Publications No. 1. I.A.R.C., Lyon.

Gillis, C. R. and Carter, R. L. (1976). Epidemiology of some human tumours: (2) Oesophagus. *In* "Scientific Foundations of Oncology" (Eds T. Symington and R. L. Carter). William Heinemann Medical, London.

Graham, S., Gibson, R., Lilienfeld, A., Schuman, L. and Levin, M. (1970). Religion and ethnicity in leukaemia. *Amer. J. Publ. Hlth* **60**, 266–274.

Haddow, A. J. (1964). Age incidence in Burkitt's lymphoma syndrome. *E. Afr. Med. J.* **41**, 1.

Heasman, M. A. and Lipworth, L. (1966). "Accuracy of Certification of Cause of Death. Studies on Medical and Population Subjects". General Register Office, London.

Jarrett, W. F. H. (1974). Cat leukaemia and its viruses. *In* "Advances in Veterinary Science" (Eds C. A. Brandly and C. E. Cornelius), Vol. 19. Academic Press, New York and London.

Lee, J. A. H. and Gardner, M. J. (1965). Season and malignant disease. *In* "Current Research in Leukaemia" (Ed. F. G. J. Hayhoe). Cambridge Univ. Press, New York.

Mantel, N. (1967). The detection of disease clustering and a generalized regression approach. *Cancer Res.* **27**.

Mason, T. J., McKay, F. W., Hoover, R., Blot, W. J. and Fraumeni, J. F. (1976). Atlas of Cancer Mortality for U.S. Counties 1950–1969. U.S. Department of Health, Education and Welfare, DHEW Publication No. NIH. 75–780.

Morrow, R. H., Pike, M. C., Smith, P. G., Zeigler, J. L. and Kisuule, A. (1971). Burkitt's lymphoma—A time-space cluster of cases in Bwamba County of Uganda. *Brit. Med. J.* **2**, 491.

Pott, P. (1775). "Chirurgical Observations Relative to the Cataract, the Polypus of the Nose, the Cancer of the Scrotum, the Different Kinds of Ruptures and the Mortification of Toes and Feet". Hawes, Clarke and Collins, London.

Stocks, P. and Davies (1964). Zinc and copper content of soils associated with the incidence of cancer of the stomach and other organs. *Brit. J. Cancer* **18**, 14.

Tuyns, J. A. (1970). Cancer of the esophagus—further evidence of the relation to drinking habits in France. *Int. J. Cancer* **5**, 152.

Verhasselt, Yola (1975). "Maps on Cancer Distribution". Geografisch Instituut, Vrije Universiteit Brussel (circulated).

Waterhouse, J. A. H. (1974). Clustering in alimentary cancer. Leeds Colorectal Conference, Leeds (communicated).

Waterhouse, J., Muir, C. and Correa, P. (1976). "Cancer Incidence in Five Continents", Vol. III. U.I.C.C., Geneva.

W.H.O. (1967). "Manual of the International Statistical Classification of Diseases, Injuries and Causes of Death" (8th Revision). Geneva.

W.H.O. (1975). "Manual of the International Statistical Classification of Diseases, Injuries and Causes of Death" (9th Revision, to be implemented 1979). Geneva.

20. Deficiency Diseases

Jacques M. May

INTRODUCTION

The causes of deficiency diseases are multiple but three major factors can be identified: ignorance, poverty, and the presence of an irrational economic pattern. Ignorance is most probably the dominant cause of malnutrition. People do not know what their nutrition should be or, least of all, what foods to grow to meet their needs. While the feeling of general hunger is well-known and is a pleasant one at the beginning, the more subtle feeling of tissue hunger is not recognized. As a result, poor diets are maintained for centuries because they assuage general hunger while the damage they cause to the suffering tissues increases, resistance to infections or other diseases diminishes, and life expectancy is reduced.

Poverty is only second in importance among the many causes of deficiency diseases. Men do not buy the food their tissues need—they buy or grow the food they like, usually the food their parents preferred before them. If they become more affluent, they increase their intake of these traditional foods, or they buy prestige foods (soft drinks, spirits or manufactured foods made enticing by advertisements, regardless of their nutritional value).

Irrational economic patterns cover a considerable number of sins. The preference given by states and producers alike to cash crops over food crops may lead to hungry people sitting on bags of unsold coffee or fibres. Drilling for oil that none can drink, or mining for bauxite that none can eat, is also responsible for much malnutrition.

Experience proves that the money these enterprises earn does not find its way back to the masses of the population in significant enough amounts to improve their diets. Rather, the profits, if any, are funnelled toward the purchase of luxury products or war machines, or both. The cult of the gross national product (GNP) is also a profound reason for the dispersion of hunger over half the world's population. Evidence is available to show that the first decades of industrialization usually bring more hunger, more segregation of incomes, more class-conscious societies, more cluttering of unsanitary urban slums and more misery than there was before.

A deficiency disease is that alteration of the cells and tissues of a living thing that jeopardizes its survival. It is the result of a diet which fails to provide the nutrients needed to maintain the histological, and hence the functional, integrity of the tissues and cells. The geographic extent of the occurrence of these diseases is not accurately known. First, this is because the cases emerge only where there is a trained health worker to recognize them. Thus, whenever one or more new cases of deficiency disease are recognized, the logical assumption to make is that many more exist that never reach the physician's orbit. Second, the bottom of the bag of nutritionally-caused diseases has not yet been reached, i.e. many of the observed disease symptoms have not yet been related to their true origin.

Nutrition consists essentially of two operations: first, the food is broken down by the body into enzymes and the components used to rebuild the tissues as life erodes them; second, oxygen is consumed and heat generated as a result of the first operation. Hence foods provide man with two major needs: nutrients, measured in grams or fractions of grams; and fuel, measured in calories. The quantities of nutrients and the amount of calories required by each individual vary with age, size, physical exertion, physiological requirements, sex and climatic characteristics of the environment. Thus the demands of a given body may or may not be supplied by a given diet and deficiencies or surpluses of both nutrients and calories may exist, each with different consequences.

Deficiency can only be defined as an approximate value established by subtracting the nutrients supplied by the diet from the theoretical requirements of the individual body in the environment in which it functions. Since the intensity of the symptoms presented by the patient is usually related to the size of the inadequacy, minor deficiencies may very well remain hidden for long periods of time. This does not mean that they do not have a deleterious effect on the tissues of the host. This effect may remain below the threshold of clinical visibility, but it is assumed that it is cumulative in nature and over the years may be responsible for a multiplicity of consequences, such as short life expectancy, poor levels of functioning and a reduced resistance to infection.

It is entirely possible that compensatory mechanisms may be within the genetic power of some individuals who could conceivably, stimulated by an unmet need, synthesize in the body an essential item of nutrition. This is powerfully exemplified by the fact that several amino acids—breakdown products of proteins needed for survival—can be synthesized in the body while 10 or 11 of them cannot be synthesized and must be provided by the diet.

The geography of deficiency diseases is the geography of what is seen or detected by the clinical senses, aided by X-ray machines, microscopes, spectrofluorometers and other instruments; such a geography is by no means a true and exact representation of reality.

NUTRIENTS AND DEFICIENCY DISEASES

Nutrients may be classified into major groups on the basis of their role in human nutrition. Since deficiencies in any or all create specific problems of health and physiological development, a short resume of what these nutrients are and what they mean to man is essential to an understanding of the subject.

Carbohydrates

These are a combination of carbon, hydrogen and oxygen. Their list is long but the nutritionist is mainly interested in sugars and starches because they provide fuel. No normal diet should be entirely free of them because if they are not available, and if at the same time fat is not provided in adequate quantities, the proteins in the diet will be burned as fuel which, in most ordinary circumstances of human behaviour, is uneconomical.

Cellulose is also important among carbohydrates because it provides the bulk essential to stimulate the muscles of the bowels and insure its movements. Except for exclusively liquid diets, such as the milk diet consumed by some nomadic tribes (e.g. the Somalis of the Horn of East Africa), no diet is totally free from bulk-making fibres and cellulose. People on a liquid diet may remain months without having any bowel movement and yet experience no inconvenience.

Fats

These play many important roles in nutrition. Like carbohydrates, they provide calories, being the most concentrated source of energy there is. They take up iodine and are also needed as solvents for certain vitamins, such as A, D, E (Alpha-tocopherol) and K. No one knows exactly what the human fat requirements are. It has been calculated that fats should represent 15% of all calories consumed by infants. Some nutritionists estimate that 20% of the adult caloric intake should come from fats.

Proteins

These are probably the most important of body constituents, deriving their name from the Greek word *protos*, which means "first". All proteins include some nitrogen, carbon, hydrogen, oxygen and sulphur in different combinations. They are degraded by digestion into smaller molecules forming the protein-proteoses-peptones-peptides-amino acids chain. Some proteins are rich in amino acids, others are not. Gelatin, for example, is a protein that contains almost no amino acids and therefore has little nutritive value. Certain amino acids, such as glycine, can be synthesized in the body from other components of the diet; others, such as lysine and tryptophane, cannot be synthesized and must be consumed preformed. The latter are called "essential amino acids".

The amount of protein needed every day varies with age, sex, size, physiological condition, work performed, etc. One gram per kilogram of weight is an acceptable figure for rough evaluation of the optimum value of a protein ration. But in order to cover the body's need for high-quality protein, a fraction (25–30%) should come from animal sources, such as meat, fish, milk or eggs, in which the essential amino acids are sure to be found.

Adequate protein intake is especially important in infants and

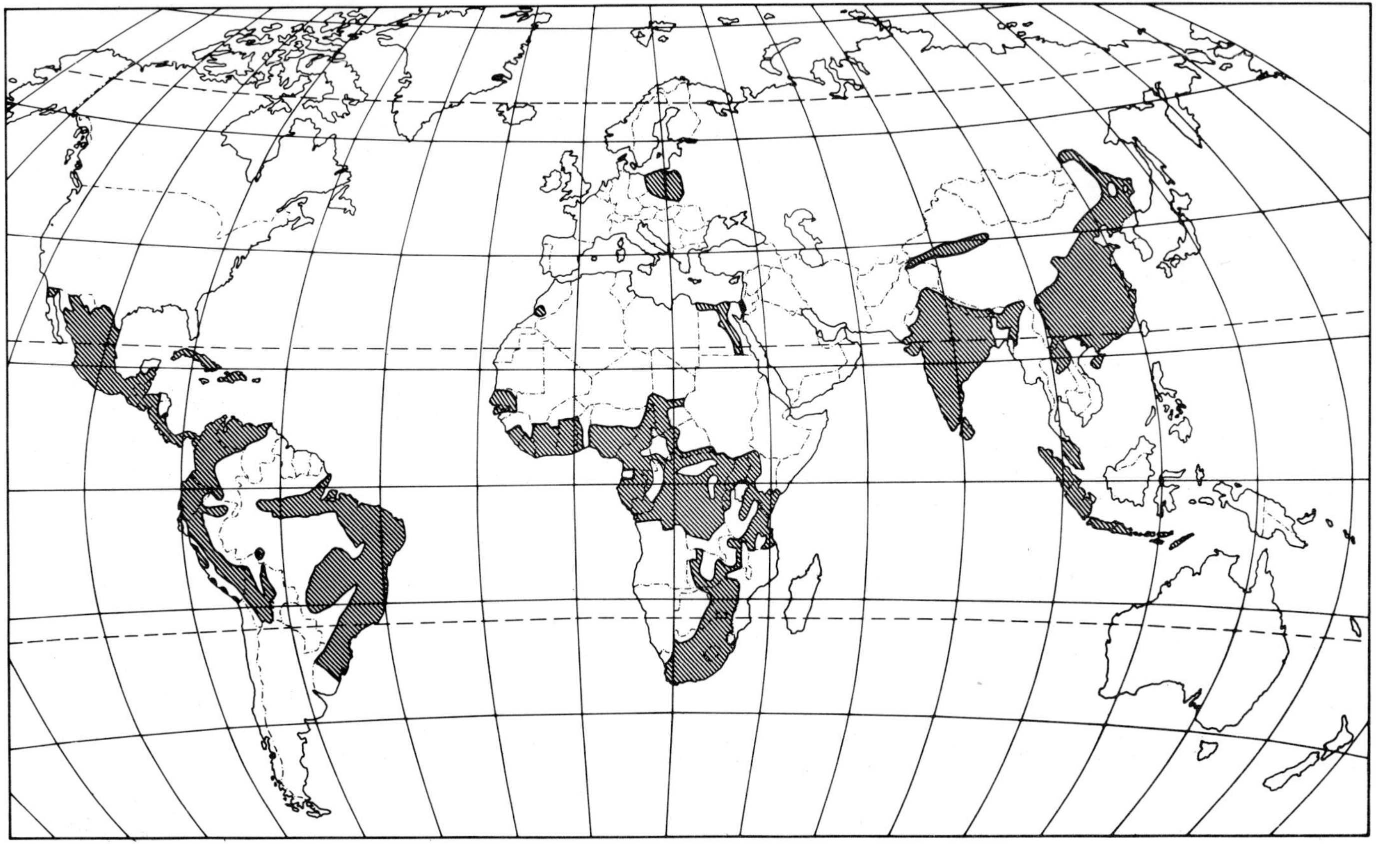

Fig. 20.1 Protein deficiencies.

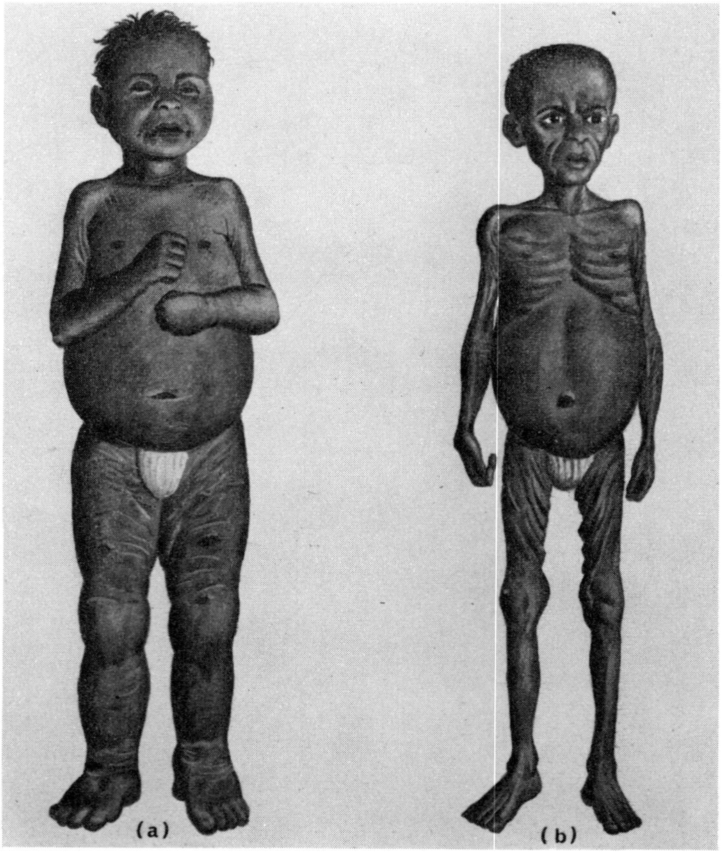

Fig. 20.2 Misshapen bodies tell the tragic story of malnutriton, a condition affecting perhaps as many as 1.5 billion people. Medical science identifies two major types, which usually occur in combination. (a) Kwashiorkor is typified by the bloated look so incongruous with starvation. Accumulated fluids pushing against wasted muscles account for the plumpness of hands, feet, belly and face. Emaciated shoulders reveal true thinness. Caused by an acute lack of protein, kwashiorkor (a West African word) can bring brain damage, anaemia, diarrhoea, irritability, apathy and loss of appetite. (b) Marasmus. Stick limbs, bloated belly, wide eyes, and the stretched-skin face of an old person mark victims of marasmus, a word taken from the Greek "to waste away". Lacking calories as well as protein, sufferers may weigh only half as much as normal. With fat gone, the skin hangs in wrinkles or draws tight over bones. With marasmus comes anaemia, diarrhoea, dehydration and a ravenous appetite. Children, whose growing bodies require large amounts of protein, are afflicted in greatest numbers, but perhaps only 3% of all child victims suffer the extreme stages illustrated. (National Geographic Society.)

young children because it is an essential factor in the growth of cells. In recent years, a number of studies have provided strong evidence that protein insufficiency in the first 5–6 years of life, when the brain attains 90% of its total cells, can lead to irreversible brain damage.

Protein malnutrition is known as kwashiorkor (Fig. 20.1). The combination of protein-calorie malnutrition is called marasmus and results in muscle wastage, dehydration, apathy and, in severe cases, even in death (Fig. 20.2).

Minerals

A variety of minerals is necessary for human survival. The quantities needed vary from a number of milligrams daily to minute traces. In terms of quantity, calcium is the most important mineral. It is essential to the growth, rigidity and resilience of bones and teeth and it plays an important role in blood coagulation, muscle contraction, myocardial function and neuromuscular irritability. It operates in conjunction with vitamin D, which is needed to "fix" calcium in the bones. The exact amount of calcium needed by man per day is not known with precision. An arbitrary figure of 500–800 mg per adult per day has been recommended by the U.S. National Academy of Science, but many populations manage to survive on a much lower level of intake. Milk, meat and eggs are the major sources of calcium but it is also present in cereals and other foods.

Phosphorous acts with calcium to promote bone growth and strength and it also acts independently in energy metabolism. A number of diseases have been attributed to calcium and phosphorous deficiency and to an inadequate ratio between the two, especially rickets and osteomalacia. However, since bone growth is also affected by vitamin D, rickets and osteomalacia are less prevalent where vitamin D is plentiful, either preformed in the diet, or synthesized as a result of the action of sunlight on the skin.

Sodium governs the volume of body fluids retaining water in proportion to its own amount while potassium is concerned with the enzymatic function of the cells. The growth of animals is retarded by deficiencies in either of these minerals. Potassium is abundant in diets predominantly based on plant foods.

Iron is also an essential mineral element in a balanced diet. About 3 g of iron are contained in an adult human body, 70% of which is in the blood. Iron plays an important role in the formation of haemoglobin, essential to respiration. Because iron is not destroyed or eliminated from the body, the nutritional requirements are small except when large haemorrhages occur. Iron-deficiency anaemia is a common result of insufficient iron intake or faulty iron metabolism. Populations living at high altitudes, as in Andean Latin America and in northern India, have higher iron requirements than those living at sea level. At high altitudes, where the atmospheric pressure is lower, the body produces more red cells. This, in turn, increases the requirement for haemoglobin to adequately oxygenate the tissues.

Iodine is an integral part of the thyroid hormones, which have important metabolic roles. Iodine deficiency leads to thyroid enlargement or goitre as a result of increases in the size and number of the cells in the gland. Some types of goitre lead to cretinism. Endemic goitre continues to be a problem of worldwide importance since about 200 million cases are believed to exist (see Chapter 18 and Fig. 18.6). The status of iodine nutrition may be assessed by use of iodine isotopes to study the avidity of the thyroid gland for iodine or by determination of the stable iodine content of urine samples. Good natural sources of iodine are seafoods and sea salt. Dairy products and eggs may be satisfactory sources when the animals themselves have had access to iodine-enriched rations. Most cereal grains, legumes, roots and vegetables are low in iodine content. Iodization of salt is one of the most common methods used by governments to prevent iodine deficiency.

Vitamins

Are substances which are essential to support life. Their name was coined by Casimir Funk in 1912: "vita" because they are so necessary to life and "mine" because they were at that time thought to be made of a chemical compound classified as "amine". Vitamins are protein molecules to which one or more groups of non-protein substances are attached. These nutrients are usually required in varying small amounts and their usefulness is based on their catalytical rather than metabolic properties. The medical ecologist is hard put to condense a geographical study of vitamin deficiencies to manageable size because the field is so extensive and because most of it is still unexplored. Hence the discussion has to be limited to those vitamins which, given the state of contemporary knowledge, seem to be the most important and result in the most serious clinical syndromes when deficient in the diet. Only vitamin A, thiamine (vitamin B_1), niacin (vitamin P.F.), riboflavin (vitamin B_2), ascorbic acid (vitamin C) and calciferol (vitamin D) will be considered in this discussion (Figs 20.3–20.8).

Vitamin A deficiency may lead to impairment of vision and even to total blindness. A specific amount of this vitamin is essential for the formation of rhodopsin, a substance which permits the normal functioning of the retina. A person suffering from vitamin A deficiency has an impaired adaptation to darkness and fails to see at low levels of illumination. Another function of vitamin A is to contribute to the integrity of epithelial membranes and the skin. When vitamin A is lacking, a dryness of the cornea occurs which is known as xerophthalmia. This soon leads to keratinization of the eye epithelia, which is called keratomalacia and causes blindness. Other functions of vitamin A include the defence against infection. The main sources of vitamin A are carrots, sweet potatoes, amaranth leaves, lettuce, spinach, pumpkins, peppers, chillies, apricots, peaches, mangoes, papayas, egg yolks, liver and butter. Vitamin A is a fat-soluble substance, hence avitaminosis A can occur in spite of a high level of vitamin A intake if the diet is fat-free or low in fat.

Thiamine is a water-soluble vitamin discovered by R. R. Williams in the early 1930s and synthesized in 1936. It is important in carbohydrate metabolism and as a result its requirements are related to the number of carbohydrate calories ingested. Only small amounts of thiamine are stored in the body. Symptoms of deficiency appear shortly after the intake becomes inadequate and include polyneuritis, oedema and eventually heart failure. The syndrome is known as beriberi. Thiamine is found in yeast, rice millings, peanuts, wheat, barley, millet, pork and liver. It is also found in lesser quantities in many legumes and in small amounts in milk, eggs, corn, fish and other meats. Its water solubility may result in its being lost during the cooking or washing of foods.

Riboflavin was identified and separated from thiamine around 1920. It regulates the utilization of foods and plays a role in the growth and building of tissues since it is closely related to protein metabolism and utilization. It is also essential to maintain the skin, the tongue and lips in good condition. Like thiamine, riboflavin requirements are linked to caloric intake. Riboflavin deficiency is

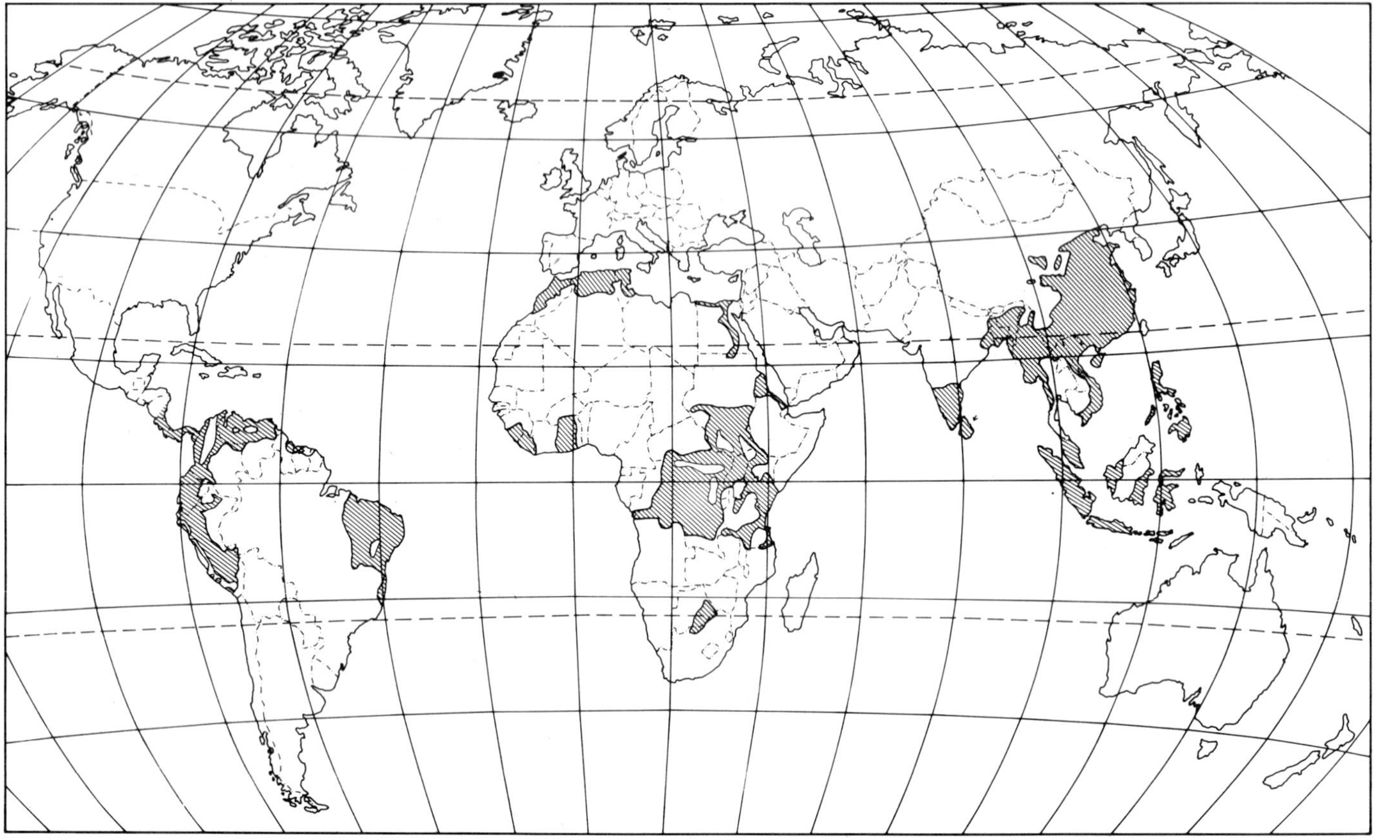

Fig. 20.3 Vitamin A deficiency (night blindness, keratomalacia, etc.).

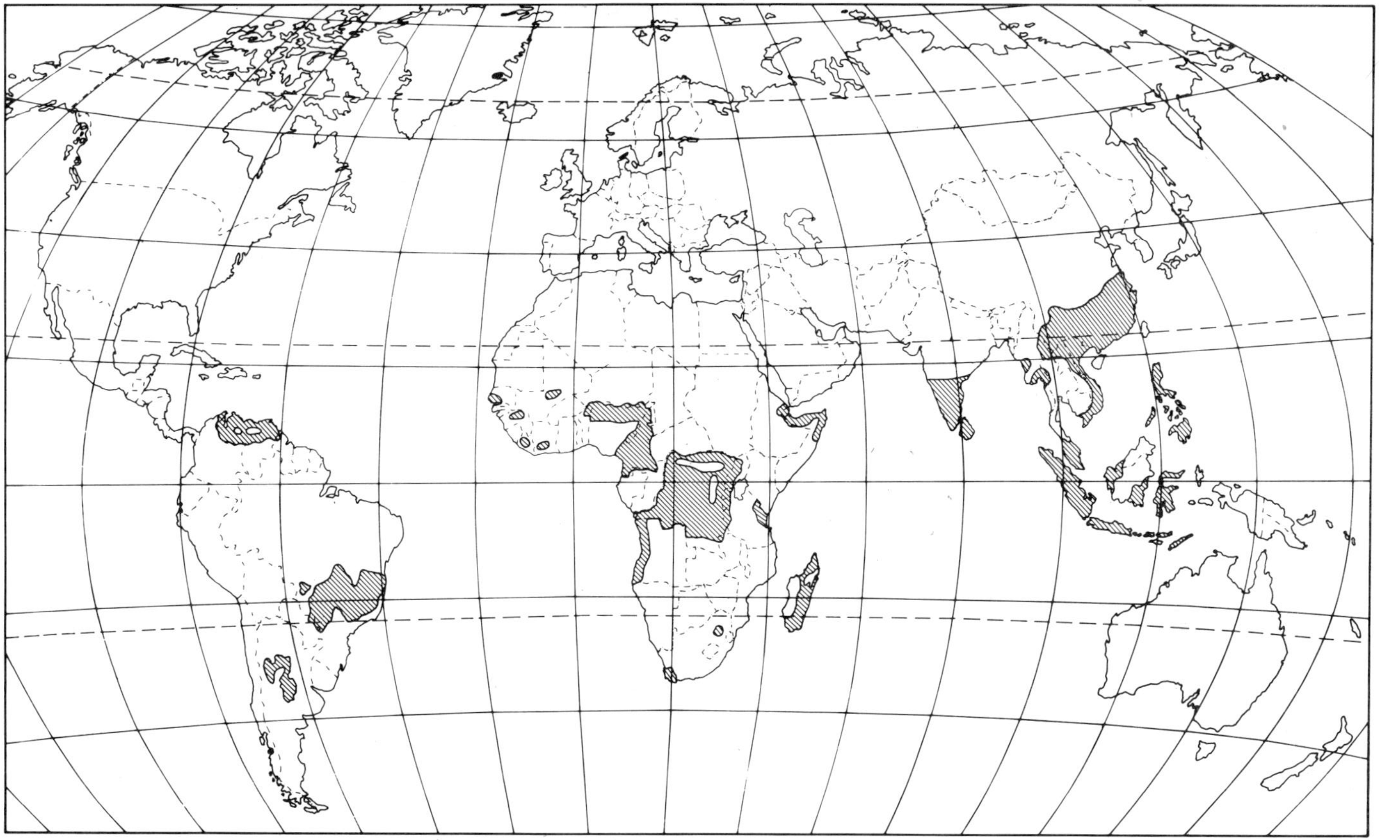

Fig. 20.4 Vitamin B_1 deficiency (beriberi).

T

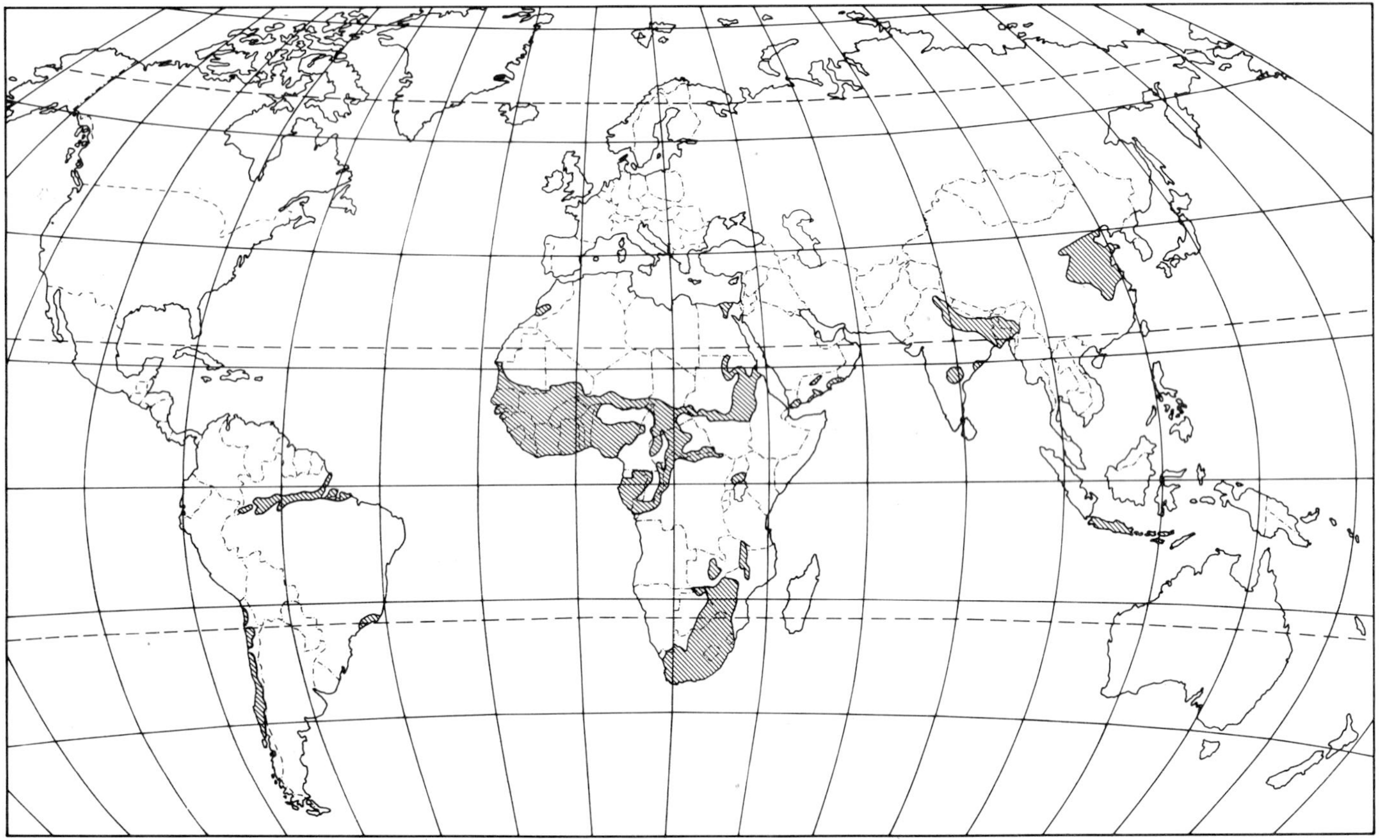

Fig. 20.5 Niacin deficiency (pellagra).

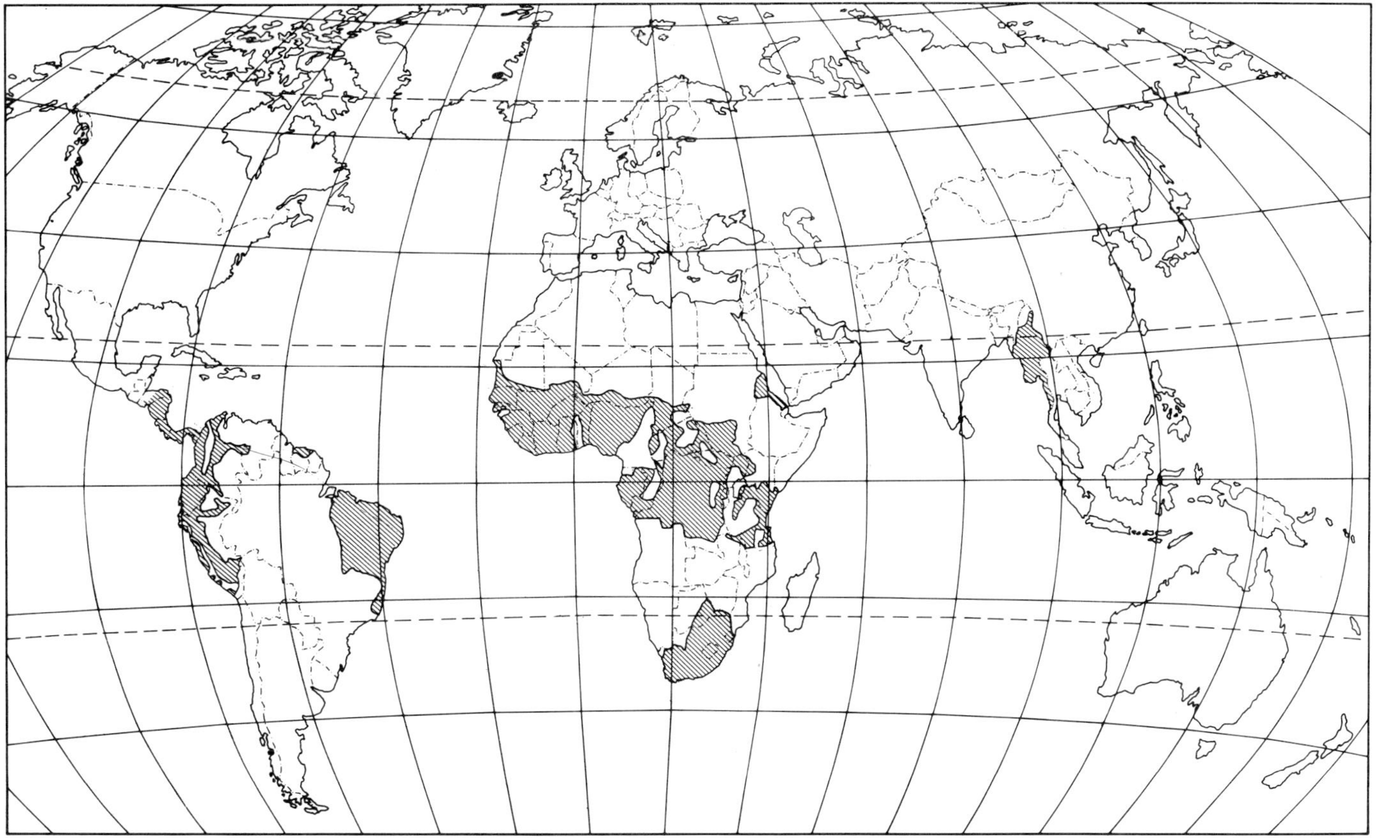

Fig. 20.6 Vitamin B_2 deficiency (ariboflavinosis).

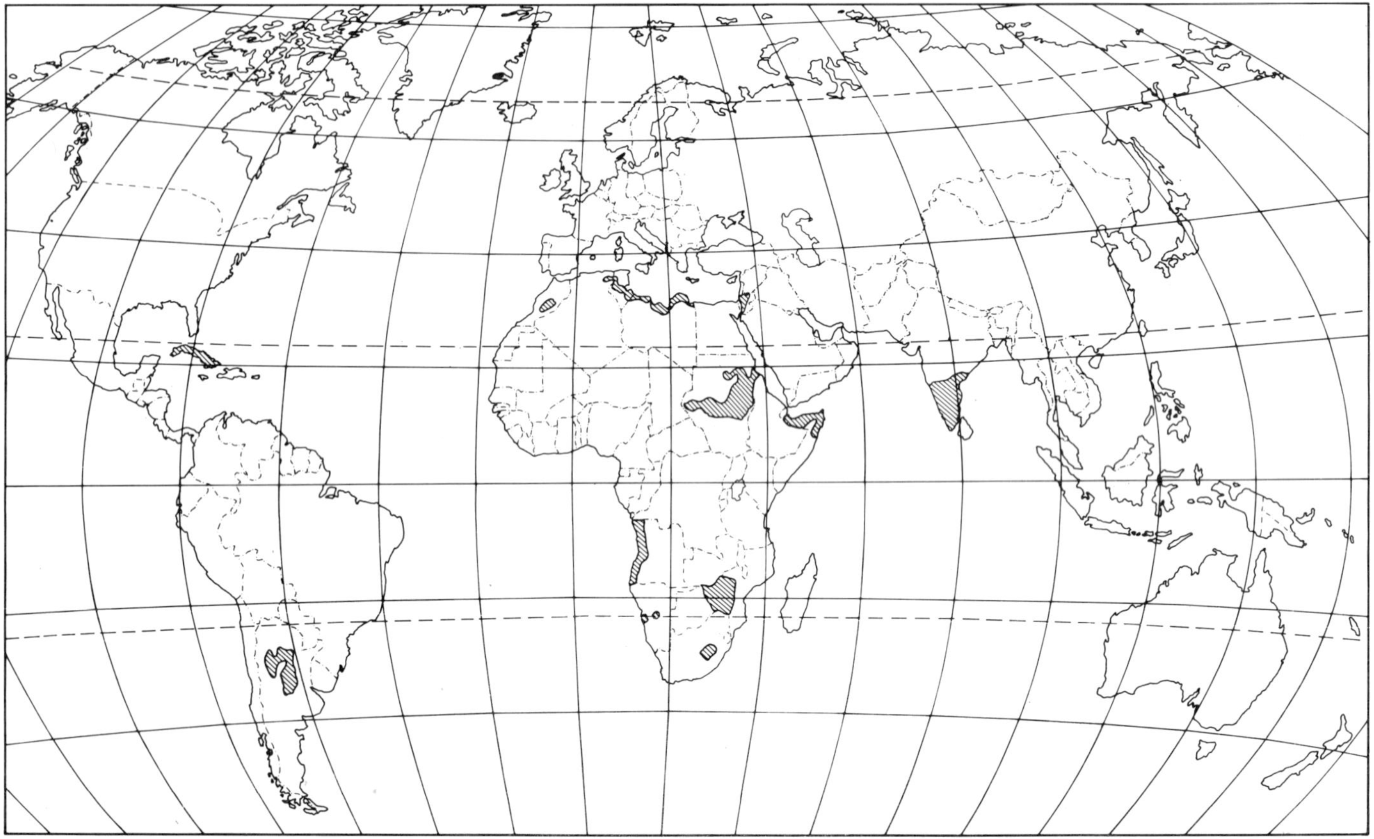

Fig. 20.7 Vitamin C deficiency (scurvy).

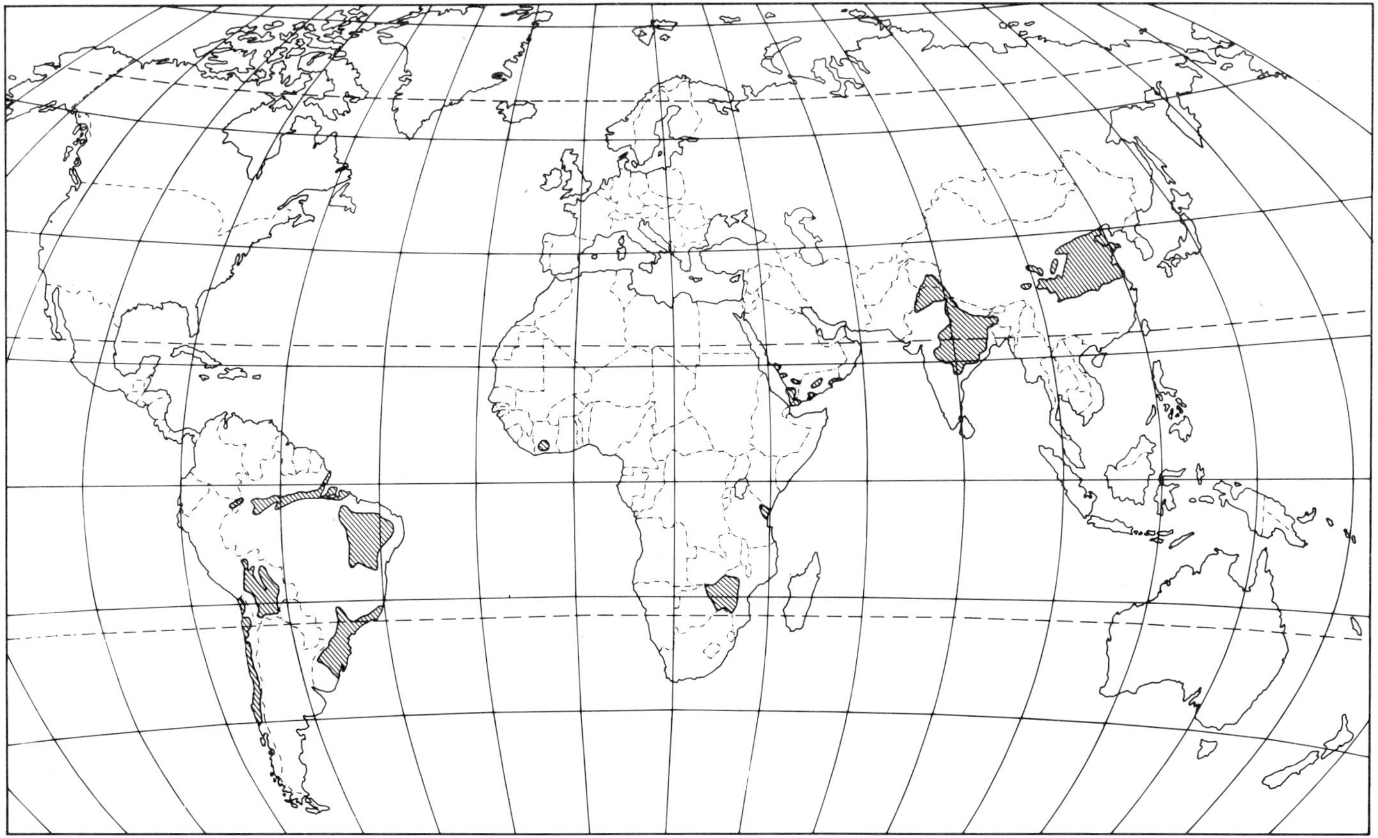

Fig. 20.8 Vitamin D deficiency (rickets, osteomalacia).

called ariboflavinosis and results in fissuration of the tongue, lesions of the lips and commissures of the mouth. Foods rich in riboflavin include corn (maize), oatmeal, wheat and legumes, which even synthesize riboflavin during germination. Various leaves, especially those of certain almonds such as *Prunus amygdalus*, are especially rich. Kidneys offer a good source of riboflavin, as do fish and eggs.

In 1926, Goldberger found that niacin, an acidic substance extracted from yeast, could be effective against a disease called pellagra. At first it was considered to contain a "pellagra-preventive" factor, hence the name vitamin P.P. was given to it by many scientists, especially in Europe. Others attached this substance to the B group of vitamins which has created a great deal of confusion. Niacin includes both nicotinic acid and nicotinamide. It is incorporated in certain enzymes playing an important role in the metabolism of carbohydrates, and it is dependent upon its association with other vitamins. The amino acid tryptophane is a precursor of niacin and can be transformed into niacin in the body. Niacin deficiency, or pellagra, is characterized by an alteration of the skin that leads to a scaly dermatitis. In fact, the name of the disease comes from two Spanish words meaning "rough skin". The syndrome includes lesions of the gastro-intestinal mucosa which result in diarrhoea, while pathology of the nervous system eventually leads to psychosis. Like the other water-soluble vitamins, thiamine and riboflavin, niacin requirements vary with the caloric intake. Niacin is present in yeast, wheat, rice, lean meat, liver and fish.

Although vitamin C (ascorbic acid) was identified only in 1933, scurvy, the disease which occurs when vitamin C is deficient in the diet, has at least a 400 year-old history. More than 100 years ago, the British Navy understood that lime juice was useful in protecting sailors from the bleeding gums and gradual weakening of the body that are typical symptoms of scurvy. Ascorbic acid has many functions and it cannot be synthesized in the human body but has to be ingested preformed. It is, of course, effective against scurvy once the disease is established but, better still, it prevents scurvy if present in the diet in adequate amounts. Vitamin C is found in a large number of fruits and vegetables, especially citrus fruits. Unfortunately, it is easily destroyed by oxidation and by temperatures in excess of 56°C.

Vitamin D (calciferol) is a fat-soluble vitamin charged mainly with fixing calcium at adequate levels in the skeleton and in the teeth. The lack of vitamin D in the diet results in rickets in children and in osteomalacia in adults. Large sources of vitamin D exist in the skin of men and can be mobilized by sunlight and irradiation with ultra-violet rays. Thus, the presence of rickets, in North Africa and in countries such as Pakistan where the sun is abundant, can only be explained by the customs of the people who protect their children from the sun or keep them indoors unnecessarily. Purdah in Moslem countries has been rightfully incriminated as a cause of osteomalacia in adult women.

THE GEOGRAPHY OF FOOD CULTURES

A geography of disease makes sense only if related to culture and if studied as evidence of maladjustment between society and the environment in which that society lives. A brief description of the food cultures is thus a necessary introduction to a listing of the ills they generate.

Food cultures are a consequence of the soil and climate of the environment and the traditions and economic potential of the human society involved. There are, of course, overlaps between food culture areas. Some of the overlaps result in a corrective dietary effect (as when rice and legumes or wheat and dairy products co-exist), other overlaps are detrimental (as when maize (corn) and manioc combine their deficient compositions). Examples of almost all deficiencies can be found everywhere. What the following discussion will show is a generalized picture of area-related combinations of deficiencies centred around one most conspicuous ill.

While diets may be varied *ad infinitum*, in any given cultural tradition, there is always a basic food which man feels he must eat in larger quantities than others in order to be satisfied, both psychologically and organically. An Asian from South India, South China or Japan does not feel fed if he has not eaten rice, regardless of the other components of the meal. Many black Africans consider cornmeal to be essential, while those living along the southern margins of the Sahara have a strong attachment to millet, sorghum and groundnuts. The following discussion will focus on the deficiency diseases usually found among people living in regions of rice culture, corn culture, wheat culture, millet–sorghum culture and manioc–tuber culture.

The rice culture

Rice is the basic food of more than half of the world's population. The time when it was first introduced as a human food is not known, but there is some indication that rice was cultivated in Thailand in 3500 B.C. and in the the Yangtze valley around 1650 B.C. The rice culture region includes countries of the South-East Asian peninsula (Cambodia, North and South Vietnam, Laos and Thailand), South China, Korea, Indonesia, Japan, South India, Nepal, Bangladesh, the Philippines and Burma. Rice is also basic in such other places as Madagascar and some of the countries of West Africa (Sierra Leone, Liberia). It is becoming the preferred luxury food in several areas such as Senegal where millet was until recently dominant and has taken hold in Latin America.

The main disease of the rice culture is beriberi. This is the consequence of three concurrent factors: a high percentage of caloric intake based on rice; excessive milling of the rice, resulting in a greater portion of the thiamine-rich scutellum of the grain being removed; and a lack of diversification of the diet, preventing the replacement of the missing thiamine from other sources. Hard physical labour predisposes rice eaters to beriberi in virtue of the heavy caloric intake their work requires. Pregnant women develop beriberi more frequently than non-pregnant females because of their increased biological activity (Fig. 20.4).

In its full form, beriberi often begins with an acute onset during which swelling, abdominal pain, vomiting and very early paralysis are not uncommon. In other cases, the paralysis installs itself gradually and the swelling is limited. There is also a dry form in which the swelling is at a minimum but paralysis of the lower limbs with atrophy and pain of the muscles dominate. The dry and chronic form is more difficult to recognize unless the acumen of the physician is on the alert. Infantile beriberi is present in areas where the diet is inadequate and results from poor amounts of thiamine in the mother's milk. Cardiac beriberi is not uncommon, resulting in heart enlargement and early heart failure. This form was often seen in the concentration camps of Asia during the Second World War. Given proper treatment and time, recovery is the rule. Large doses of thiamine (50–100 mg per day) or good food containing proper amounts of the substance usually restore health.

The prevalence and incidence of beriberi are very much influenced by the type of milling practised. When the rice crop was universally milled by pestle and mortar, enough or nearly enough thiamine was left sticking to the grain to minimize the adverse effect of milling. With mechanical milling, the dehulling is more thorough and beriberi more probable.

In Thailand, the rice is increasingly polished and milled mechanically, and a considerable amount of its nutritive value is thereby removed; in only a few areas is the rice still milled at home by wooden pestle in a wooden mortar. Since the densely-populated Menam Delta area is where most farmers use the commercial rice mills, it is not surprising that Delta farmers have the highest incidence of beriberi in Thailand. The Thai government has made a considerable investment in enriching rice by adding a small amount of specially-treated rice grains to a large bulk of milled rice. The grains are impregnated with thiamine and other nutrient supplements according to the needs of the particular area and they are then made comparatively resistant to washing and cooking losses by applying a final waterproof coating.

Thiamine deficiency may be compensated by including protective elements in the diet. Most rural areas in Thailand have large supplies of fresh vegetables and fish but, in the northeast, these additional foodstuffs are lacking. Fish is available but it is consumed usually after some degree of decomposition has occurred. It has been reported that an enzyme called thiaminase may develop in decomposed fish which allegedly destroys the thiamine in the fish and whatever thiamine may have survived in the rice.

The practice of parboiling rice decreases the incidence of beriberi since, even when highly polished, parboiled rice retains a significant amount of thiamine. In certain parts of India, e.g. Madras and the east coast, parboiled rice is preferred. It is prepared by soaking the paddy in cold or lukewarm water for varying lengths of time then steaming it until the grain becomes soft and partly or wholly cooked. The excess water is drained off and the paddy is spread out to dry. The parboiled paddy is then hulled, giving the rice its special appearance and flavour. The treated grain appears slightly coloured and is more resistant to the tooth than the original rice grain.

A detrimental practice commonly found in other parts of India is the washing of rice in plenty of water before cooking. The first washing is responsible for the loss of 40–50% of the thiamine and the draining of the water after cooking is responsible for additional losses. Fortunately, however, this practice is not general and some families know how to prepare good rice without throwing away the water. In some parts of India, rice water is used for breakfast and/or to cook vegetables so the thiamine is not lost.

In Sri Lanka, the main food is boiled rice, especially eaten at the midday meal. Along with the rice go curries made from meat (beef, mutton, pork, fowl), eggs, fish or vegetables, with fruits or jams to which many spices and condiments are added. Although there is no gross malnutrition in Sri Lanka, signs of undernutrition are seasonally prevalent and beriberi as well as other vitamin deficiencies occur annually.

Beriberi has been reported from eastern Afghanistan on a relatively large scale. In Malaya, beriberi is still found in subclinical forms, showing isolated symptoms.

The corn (maize) culture

Corn is reputed to have originated in the Americas. There is evidence that corn was eaten after 7000 B.C. in the Tamaulipas area of Mexico. It is still the most important food crop and the basic staple of nutrition in Mexico. There is also some evidence that corn was brought under cultivation in Peru between 6000 and 5000 B.C. Columbus is said to have brought corn to Europe from the Americas and Magellan is supposed to have had some corn with him on his final ill-fated voyage. Eventually, this cereal was transplanted to Africa and now corn cultivation is dispersed all over the world. Yet, what can truly be called the corn culture is confined to some regions of the Americas, particularly Mexico and Central America, and some areas of Africa, especially Kenya, Swaziland, Lesotho and Rhodesia, although millet and sorghum are close seconds in most of these African countries. Corn is also grown and well-liked in northern India, Pakistan and China.

The main deficiency disease of the corn culture is pellagra which was identified by Gaspar Casal in 1735. The seasonal aspect of pellagra has been noted by many investigators who observe that, in Southern Africa, mental hospitals fill up during the hungry season when practically nothing is available to eat except cornmeal, salt pork and molasses. The hospitals empty rapidly when other cereals, fresh vegetables, fruits and tryptophane-rich foods become available again (Fig. 20.5).

The wheat culture

Leaving aside the so-called developed countries of North America and Western Europe where wheat is the preferred cereal but not the basic food, the wheat culture extends mainly along the northern coast of Africa eastwards into the Middle East and beyond to the northern half of both India and China. Wheat is known to have been cultivated in the Mediterranean area several millenia before the birth of Christ. In countries where wheat is not the staple, it is considered a luxury food, and it is being grown more and more abundantly even in areas where corn or rice were hitherto the basic crops. Durum wheat, the coarse type with which unleavened bread is made, is gradually being replaced by the soft wheat with which Europeans and North Americans make their bread. In North Africa, for example, the demand is such that quite often soft wheat has to be imported. Wheat is also the main cereal of most of the larger cities of the world. Without placing the following countries in the wheat culture area, it must be said that this cereal is becoming more and more popular in South America where its cultivation is increasing in Brazil, Argentina, Uruguay, Chile, Bolivia and Peru.

There are no specific deficiency diseases connected with wheat as there are with rice and corn. This is probably in part because the countries of the wheat culture have a far more varied diet than the countries where corn or rice are significantly predominant. The wheat grain is a good cereal with one exception: its protein is deficient in the essential amino-acid lysine. Hence a diet limited to wheat products may be deficient in protein. Experiments are being undertaken in some parts of the world, especially in Tunisia, to enrich wheat flour with lysine as well as with a number of vitamins and minerals.

The millet–sorghum culture

Millet is an ancient cereal which was consumed several millenia before Christ in the various areas where it is still consumed today. It is the main staple mostly in Africa, especially in the Sahel—the intermediate region between the Sahara and the forests—where it is eaten from the valley of the Senegal river in the west to the coast of the Indian Ocean in the east. With or without sorghum, it is the basis of the diet in those countries strung along Middle Africa: Senegal, northern Togo, northern Dahomey, northern Nigeria, northern Cameroon, Niger, Mali, the Upper Volta, Sudan, Somalia, parts of Uganda and Tanzania. It is a supportive crop in Kenya and Ethiopia and it vies with corn for importance in Uganda. It is also eaten in northern China. The food-producing areas of China can be divided into two major regions: a northern wheat region and a southern rice region. The north is subdivided into spring wheat, winter wheat and millet, and winter wheat and kaoling areas; there is no millet consumed in the south. Prosomillet (*Panicum miliare*) is grown at high altitudes because this variety is the only one that can grow to maturity in a short crop season. Two crops may be grown in some particularly favourable areas. In India, where two generalized rice and wheat zones exist, millet is an important part of the diet in certain states of the wheat zone: Andhra Pradesh, Bombay, Madras, Mysore, Madhia-Pradesh. Millet is a good cereal, richer in protein than corn and rice. It is not associated with a specific deficiency disease. Yet, like rice, corn or any other cereal, it needs to be accompanied by other foods to provide a balanced diet.

The manioc and other tuber culture

The tuber food culture is associated with the rain forests of Equatorial Africa and South America. The major problem with this type of diet is that manioc and tropical tubers, such as yams, taros, and sweet potatoes, are poor in protein. This deficiency must be compensated by other foods rich in protein which are usually not available, or only at prices that the less-privileged members of the population cannot afford. By comparing maps showing the manioc culture and the main sources of protein, it is easy to see that the two do not coincide. The areas of manioc culture are, therefore, understandably linked with such major deficiency diseases as kwashiorkor and marasmus (Figs 20.1–20.2).

THE GEOGRAPHY OF DEFICIENCY DISEASES

Having related certain deficiency diseases to the diet cultures within which they occur, it is desirable to sketch out briefly the problems by region and country.

North America

A record of the nutritional status of the population of the U.S.A. is to be part of a major nationwide health and nutrition examination survey which will reflect the findings of a 2-year field study (1971–1973). Final results are not yet available, but some preliminary reports have been made. It was found, for instance, that socio-economic condition, sex and race do not affect the height and weight of U.S. children. It was also found that the differences between the sizes of U.S. children from socio-economic extremes, though real, were extremely small, and that even the children from the lowest economic stratum in the U.S.A. were larger than most of the children from all countries of the world except those most culturally and technologically similar to the U.S.

In Canada the report of a recent (1970–1972) nutrition survey provides a description of the nutritional status of the Canadian population. In summary, it was found that about 5% of the children under 6 years of age had moderate degrees of weight deficit which was usually higher among the Indian and Eskimo populations than among the general population. A protein and calorie deficiency was found among a significant proportion of children under 6 years of age, and again this finding was more severe among Indian and Eskimo children. Widespread deficiency of iron was also found among these children. Intakes of calcium and vitamin D were below desirable levels for children, but no clinical signs of rickets were obvious. While there was no clinical evidence of vitamin A deficiency among the samples examined, levels of vitamin A in the blood implied a moderate risk to health for about 25% of the children and toddlers, 15% of the school-age children and 5% of the adolescents. The findings for vitamin C were similar. There was no evidence of shortage of thiamine, riboflavin or niacin. Adequate amounts of iodine were consumed by all three major population groups, general, Eskimo and Indian. Some degree of thyroid enlargement was observed among adolescent girls in the general population but not among the Indians and Eskimos. This finding was prevalent among the people living in the prairie regions.

Among adults, 50% of the sample population seemed to be overweight. Dietary protein intakes were found to be deficient in 25% of the men and 50% of the women of the older age group. This tendency was most marked among Indians while Eskimo men had adequate intakes but women fared no better than those of the same age group in the general population. There was a high prevalence of iron deficiency among men and women in all three populations.

Calcium intake was deficient among 25% of females of the general population and more so among the older Indian and Eskimo males and females. There was no evidence of vitamin A deficiency in spite of conspicuous shortages in the dietary intake. This suggests good storage capabilities in the body. There was no clear clinical evidence of vitamin deficiency in the general population, but there was some such evidence concerning a small percentage of Indian young men. Eskimos showed some prevalence of symptoms of vitamin C deficiency.

A substantial proportion of the adults in the general and Indian population (more frequently women and older people) presented signs suggesting thiamine deficiency, but none was found among the Eskimos. This was confirmed by the excretion levels of thiamine in the urine which were in the normal range among Eskimos but below normal for Indians and the general population.

While many adults consumed less than adequate amounts of riboflavin, urinary excretion seemed normal. Urinary excretion of iodine indicated adequate intakes, except among 10% of the Eskimos observed. Nevertheless, these Eskimos showed no signs of clinical enlargement. Moderate goitres were found in a significant percentage of the women in the general population.

In Mexico a number of serious deficiencies are continuously reported. Cravioto *et al.* (1960) have seen kwashiorkor at the Children's Hospital in Mexico City. Pellagra, together with many other deficiency diseases, is endemic in the Yucatan and Campeche departments. It is more frequent during the months of April, May and June. A rate of 2.5 cases per 1000 inhabitants has been observed by Chavez and Rosado (1967) in a rural community of Campeche. The annual incidence is 4% of the adults.

Goitre in Mexico was known by the Aztecs and the Mayas. In the mountainous regions of Mexico, there are still areas of endemic goitre due to the low iodine content of the water. In the area of Tpetlixua, thyroid enlargement was found in 92% of 866 children aged 6–14 years surveyed in 1962. Following the introduction of an iodine supplement, in 1965 the prevalence in the same area was 68%, in 1967 the rate had diminished to 50% and in 1968 the prevalence was only 38%.

Central America

In Guatemala, kwashiorkor or marasmus has been diagnosed in 1.9% of the children under 5 years who were surveyed. The protein-calorie shortages in the diets of children appear to be the most important cause of their slow development. Corn is the staple cereal in Guatemala, followed by sorghum and rice. Despite the high level of corn consumption, no cases of pellagra were found by investigators from the Institute for Nutrition in Central America and Panama (I.N.C.A.P.) in 1969 when a national nutrition survey was conducted. It is highly possible that other elements of the Guatemalan diet compensate for the lack of niacin in the corn.

In Belize, corn, together with beans and rice, is the staple of the diet—corn and beans among the Indians and *mestizos*, rice and beans among the Creoles. Yet, as in Guatemala, few cases of pellagra have been reported, most probably because of the compensatory effects of the beans and rice. Kwashiorkor is reported to be a serious problem in the rural Stamm Creek area, where local physicians blame early weaning practices and the use of cassava lab, a weaning food which is nothing more than a combination of manioc, water and sugar. In Belize City, where sophistication of the urbanite prevails, children are bottle-fed very early and the milk used is usually imported condensed milk diluted with unsterile water. The mixture rapidly deteriorates and causes a large number of infantile diarrhoeas, some of them fatal, often associated with the syndrome known as marasmus.

In a survey of the Republic of Honduras, 21.4% of all children under 5 years of age revealed hair changes usually indicative of kwashiorkor. Protein-calorie malnutrition exists in Nicaragua where minor changes in the hair and pretibial eodema have been seen in a small percentage of the children under 5 years of age.

In El Salvador, where corn is the staple, there is no evidence of pellagra, which leads to the belief that enough tryptophane is included in most diets to add its own niacin-generating potential to the niacin actually consumed, and that the habit of soaking cornmeal in lime water liberates the niacin in sufficient quantities to protect the consumer from niacin deficiency. Although low levels of nutrition have been recorded by investigators, they are not reflected in a widespread picture of nutritional diseases.

In Panama, the consumption of corn is second only to that of rice and the problem of pellagra does not exist. Goitre is found throughout Central America, especially in the mountainous areas.

South America

In a country as extensive as Brazil, diets are different in each region and so are the nutritional deficiency disease patterns. The worst off of all is the north-east where there is an endemic deficiency of protein. Malnutrition is serious among children up to 5 years of age in this region and constitutes the main cause of mortality during this period of life. Vitamin A deficiency is observed, as well as delayed physical growth. Early weaning is very common in the region and is the result of the general insufficiency of maternal milk. Gum and tongue abnormalities among a significant percentage of children examined are suggestive of pre-scurvy or scurvy conditions. Signs of riboflavin deficiency are noticeable on the face, particularly among males over 45 years of age and females in the 15–45 age range. Liver enlargements have been observed in 28.2% of the males of all ages examined and in 43.3% of the females. More important, perhaps, is the high prevalence of goitre, which is very common in Latin America, although recent vigorous prophylaxis has considerably reduced the endemicity. Kwashiorkor and marasmus have been reported frequently from North-East Brazil and remain a serious problem there. Quite recently, preliminary data gathered for an inter-American investigation on mortality in childhood indicated that 64% of all children under 5 years of age in Recife had first-degree malnutrition.

In the state of Maranhão, protein malnutrition and signs of deficiencies of the vitamin B complex and vitamins A and D are common. Anaemia is frequent among the population and is reportedly due to lack of iron in the diet. In Bahia, it is believed that about one-third of the total infant deaths in the capital city of Salvador are caused by malnutrition or hunger rather than by the obvious gastro-intestinal disorders reported. Babies are breast-fed as long as possible but seldom beyond the third month, after which they receive manioc flour or corn pap. Milk given to these children is well-diluted with water. Among the lower income groups, meat consumption is minimal and consumption of sweet potatoes, manioc. and yams is very high. Even in the rich state of São Paulo, pockets of malnutrition exist and signs of vitamin A, B complex and C deficiencies can be found. Protein deficiency in children is common in public hospitals and undoubtedly is the largest nutritional problem in the state. Iron deficiency, and consequently hypochromic microcytic anaemia, is also a nutritional problem of considerable importance.

According to Neto, nearly 11 million Brazilians are afflicted with endemic goitre. There are three distinct areas of endemicity: (a) the east meridianal south and west regions where the incidence is high; (b) the north and north-east occidental regions where the endemicity is moderate; and (c) the north-east oriental and east septentrional areas which are free of significant prevalence. The state of Mato Grosso seems to have the highest rate of prevalence at 58.9%. A 1953 law requires that iodine be added to salt in Brazil in the proportion of 10 mg per kg of refined salt.

Although deficiency diseases are found in the Gran Chaco region of Uruguay and in the poorest provinces of Argentina, they exist only in pockets of little national significance. These two cattle countries have a privileged situation in the map of nutritional deficiencies, thanks to their meat and milk diets. Goitre, however, is found in Argentina, especially among closed Indian groups such as the Mapuche of Neuquen.

Even though other deficiencies exist, goitre is one of the most important nutritional diseases in Colombia. Gaitan and Wahner (1968) report that the high incidence of endemic goitre in the Cauca valley of Colombia has been known for many years. Prevalence rates as high as 80% have been reported in the past but have decreased since iodized salt was introduced in 1955. Nevertheless, endemic goitre persists among the child population of the Cauca valley in spite of ample iodine intake and the possibility of positive goitrogenic factors has been considered. Recent studies suggest that volatile components in some of the drinking water may have a goitrogenic effect.

In Ecuador, signs of possible riboflavin deficiencies, such as nasolabial seborrhea, angular lesions of the lips and filiform papillary atrophy of the tongue, have been found at low altitudes; follicular hyperkeratosis is common at high altitudes. This suggests vitamin A deficiency, although it has been difficult to associate this symptom with real shortages of vitamin A. Endemic goitre is found in the Andean region, with prevalences running as high as 67% in certain villages compared with less than 9% in the coastal areas. Experiments are being conducted in Ecuador in the use of iodized oil injections to prevent goitre.

In Bolivia, few data are available on the prevalence of nutritional deficiency diseases. In addition to goitre, whose prevalence is high, especially in the departments of Cochabamba, Santa Cruz, Beni, Chuquisaca and Tarija, few marked symptoms of malnutriton have been found in the rest of the population. Nutrition survey investigators have seen follicular hyperkeratosis in 4.1% of the children examined in Cochabamba and in the same percentage of adults in Oruro. The symptom was thought to be related to the low level of vitamin A consumption observed in these areas. Very few signs of protein-calorie malnutrition have been reported, yet the condition is said to be commonly seen at hospitals in Cochabamba, Riberalta and La Paz.

In Peru, the roots and tubers that form the base of the diet in certain areas include white potatoes, sweet potatoes and manioc. No obvious cases of kwashiorkor or marasmus have been identified during surveys made by investigators. The only well-established nutritional deficiency observed in high- and medium-altitude Peru was the enlargement of the thyroid gland so commonly seen in South America. The existence of goitre in the Inca empire is well-established and it was clearly discussed during the colonial period. A survey made by the Peruvian National Institute of Nutrition in 1963 proved that goitre prevalence is higher in the sierra and jungle areas of Peru than along the coast where, nevertheless, 10% prevalence persists. The Government is well-aware of the problem and started a salt iodization programme in 1969.

In Chile, the main nutritional problem is the deficiency in caloric intake. The marginal character of the diet results in growth deficiencies in infants, children and even adolescents. Babies are born with the same weight as U.S. children but, soon after birth and until the diet has been suitably broadened, they show increasing signs of growth retardation and mental apathy, to which Dr. Monckeberg of Santiago has drawn attention. In addition to growth retardation, which is perhaps one of the most important signs of nutritional deficiency in Chile, clinical findings of other deficiencies seem to be widespread. Most significant is follicular hyperkeratosis, which is usually described as a symptom of vitamin A deficiency. It is practically ubiquitous in Chile and, in view of the large diversity in climate that characterizes this country, this is an argument in favour of a nutritional cause rather than a climatic one. Riboflavin deficiency can be suspected when angular lesions of the lip appear at fairly high rates of prevalence. Such is the case in Valdivia, Antofagasta and on the island of Chiloe. Filliform papillary atrophy of the tongue also suggests some vitamin B complex deficiencies. This symptom is particularly in evidence at Osorno, Santiago, Quillota and La Serena. Rickets has been commonly reported and protein-calorie malnutrition is frequently seen in Chilean hospitals, leading to the suspicion that many undiagnosed and untreated cases exist in the towns and villages. A series of systematic studies conducted since 1954 has demonstrated the existence of endemic goitre in Coquimbo, Santiago, Linares, Nuble, Malleco and Cautin and Aisén.

Africa

North Africa

The northern coast of Africa from Morocco to Egypt is an area with many ethnic and geographical similarities. Cultures are comparable and so are the deficiency disease patterns. The area includes, from west to east, Morocco, Algeria, Tunisia, Libya and Egypt. All these countries belong to the wheat culture.

Signs of nutritional deficiencies are widespread in Morocco. Approximately 2 million people are estimated to suffer from malnutrition in one form or another. Rickets is common in all the North African countries and Morocco is no exception. It is caused by living in the sunless hovels of the casbahs rather than by a calcium deficient diet. Kwashiorkor is also common, reaching a peak among

2-year-old children. Not infrequently, the signs of kwashiorkor have occurred in breast-fed children. This has led to an exploration of the composition of mother's milk, revealing that it contains an average of 8.36 g of protein per litre against a normal 12–15 g. In the Rabat area, there is a significant correlation between the incidence of new cases of kwashiorkor and the driest months of July and August. It is hypothesized that the need for water results in an over-consumption of fluids on the part of nursing women which prevents intakes of other foods, thus lowering considerably the protein content of the breast milk.

Signs of vitamin A deficiency are frequently observed. Cutaneous symptoms can be detected in 16% of the population. Night blindness is present among the inhabitants of the Riff Mountains. Goitre, caused mainly by iodine deficiency, is common in the area of Ouarzazate and particularly in the village of Skoura where prevalence reaches 59% of the boys and 56% of the girls. Riboflavin deficiency, however, is seldom observed and vitamin C deficiency is not seen.

In Algeria, where the dietary culture is very similar to that of Morocco, the general picture of dietary deficiency is much the same. Kwashiorkor, goitre and iron deficiency anaemia are common. Night blindness afflicts some of the sedentary people of the northern Sahara. The pastoral nomads, although surrounded by livestock, are deprived of sufficient amounts of animal protein because of their cultural attitude concerning their herds, which provide prestige rather than meat. Rickets among very young children is not rare; the efforts to protect children from sunlight are all too successful.

In Tunisia, a national nutrition survey is now being conducted and it would be premature to anticipate the conclusions, but earlier small-scale surveys have indicated that the most important deficiencies are protein, vitamin A and vitamin D. According to Tunisian estimates, 80% of the lower classes present signs of malnutrition in varying degrees. As in Morocco, investigators insist that kwashiorkor is closely related to the poor quality of mother's milk which does not give adequate nutrients to the child in his first year. The diet of the mother herself is often composed of carbohydrates, little fat of animal origin and inadequate protein.

In Libya, evidence of malnutrition in the samples examined in the early 1960s was found to be general. Anaemia was common among women, especially pregnant women. Males and females were commonly found to be underweight in rural areas, indicating caloric undernutrition. Clinical symptoms pointed to riboflavin deficiency, pellagra and goitre. Now that the country has entered an era of oil affluence, it will be interesting to discover whether the new wealth will result in modifying the general picture of nutritional deficiencies.

An analysis of the prevalence of deficiency diseases in Egypt is difficult because information on the occurrence and incidence of nutritional diseases there is meagre. The picture is complicated by the widespread existence of parasitic infestation which aggravates the effects of poor diets. Although the caloric intake and total protein consumption equals or exceeds recommended levels, most of the proteins consumed are of vegetable origin and the total consumption of animal products is at an extremely low level. Pellagra occurs in areas where corn is the principal cereal. Rickets and osteomalacia are more commonly seen for the same cultural and dietary reasons that cause these diseases to be prevalent in Morocco and Algeria. Iron deficiency anaemia is also present.

Sahel

The semi-arid southern margins of the Sahara Desert have always been zones of undernutrition and malnutrition where climate and culture combine to give rise to unwanted results. Some tribes, who combine cattle-raising and farming, produce millet in quantities that do not meet their needs and groundnuts sold for cash. Cattle are a symbol of wealth and prestige and are not slaughtered for food. In consequence, diets are high in carbohydrates with little intake of animal protein. The introduction of Western culture has added new material criteria of prestige. It seems to have contributed to more malnutrition by increasing non-food expenditures.

Investigators in Senegal report that 38.8% of the children between 8 months and weaning age exhibit some sign of nutritional deficiency. Pre-kwashiorkor conditions, riboflavin and vitamin A deficiencies are commonly seen. After weaning the situation becomes worse. Kwashiorkor is not common among the milk-drinking Peuls but is found among the fish-eating Lebous. It is strange that the fish found in the Cap Vert waters do not protect against kwashiorkor as well and uniformly as does milk. In the middle Senegal valley, mild forms of kwashiorkor have been observed in spite of a relatively balanced diet. Signs of vitamin A deficiency, such as some degree of xerophthalmia, are encountered from time to time. Signs of ariboflavinosis are seen in children after the age of 9 years but indications of scurvy are rare. Goitre is present in Senegal at an average rate of only 3.6% but isolated islands of the disease occur. In Ziguinchor, 59% of the inhabitants are afflicted. Beriberi has been observed among the rice-eating people from lower Casamance who have migrated into the city of Dakar.

In Upper Volta, where a number of different tribes exist side by side, poor diets prevail. Vitamin A deficiency and mild forms of kwashiorkor have been seen in about 3% of the children examined by investigators. As a result of the drought of 1973, the prevalence of many deficiency diseases is likely to have reached high levels. One may assume that the tradition of eating almost anything may have saved many, albeit at a near starvation level. Rats, various kinds of birds, frogs, snails, winged termites, locusts and cockroaches are all probably consumed in greater amounts than is realized and make a contribution to the animal protein share of the diet. Yet, such resources are also likely to disappear when widespread drought makes most life virtually impossible.

In normal times, Mali produces 1 million tons of millet per year, but in 1973 the prolonged drought resulted in true famine, the consequences of which are still being felt. In certain villages, 70% of the people have a daily intake of less than 1000 calories, 50% of which comes from carbohydrates. Seasonal fluctuations are considerable and nutritional diseases are common.

The Sudan and the Horn

In the Sudan, the most important and widely consumed cereal is sorghum or millet of which there are a variety of species. Subnutrition has always existed in most parts of the country with marked shortages in proteins. Kwashiorkor and marasmus are common, perhaps due in part to the widespread custom in Africa of allowing fathers and older boys to eat first, leaving women and children to fend for themselves as best they can. In many parts of the Sudan and the rest of Africa, the milk of a pregnant woman is deemed bad for a child and is supposed to be the cause of the frequent cases of diarrhoea observed in infants. The cure, however, is believed to be to stop nursing the child, rather than to avoid pregnancy; hence three people suffer instead of two thriving. Ariboflavinosis is observed in a high percentage of kwashiorkor cases. Swelling of the gums, which responds to ascorbic acid deficiency, is common, as is anaemia. Beriberi and pellagra are frequent. Xerophthalmia occurs in the Nuba mountains. All these nutritional diseases peak during the pre-harvest "hungry season". Goitre has been reported among the Azande tribe in southern Sudan.

In Ethiopia, the staple food is a cereal called teff (*Eragrostis abyssinica*). It is a grass which produces tiny grains weighing only about 0.0023 mg each. It comes in white, red and mixed varieties. The calcium, phosphorus and iron contents of teff are high, but the niacin value is as low as that of corn. Malnutrition in its various forms is manifest in Ethiopia. Protein-deficiency syndromes, scurvy, vitamin A deficiency and ariboflavinosis are found in relatively high percentages of the population. Rickets is widespread despite the fact that Ethiopia is a country with 12 months of sunshine. Again, overprotection of the child by the mother is responsible for this condition. It appears to be the fear of an evil eye that leads Ethiopian mothers to seclude their children in sunless areas. Endemic goitre is very common in some regions and also affects pre-school children, but a programme of salt iodization is under way. Anaemia is widespread and could be the consequence of the iron in teff being made unabsorbable by binding with phytic acid.

In Somalia, the major cereal crop is sorghum, distantly followed by corn. This grain, cooked into a porridge or baked into a cake and eventually eaten with butter, is one of the basic foods of the Somali diet. Unfortunately, no adequate nutrition survey has been made in Somalia, so little is known about the prevalence and incidence of deficiency diseases there.

The intertropical area—West Africa

Sierra Leone belongs to the rice culture but also partakes of the manioc and tuber culture. While the deficiencies associated with the latter are present, beriberi linked with the consumption of rice is not. It would seem that in 1923 Indian rice began to be imported into the country and with it the parboiling technique. Malnutrition is a major cause of infant mortality, either directly or indirectly. Kwashiorkor, marasmus, anaemia, ariboflavinosis, especially during pregnancy all have been reported from several districts, but especially from Kono and Koinoduga.

Togo and Dahomey owe the dual character of their diets to their long north-south axes. In the north, the Mobas and Cabrais eat millet and sorghum whereas, in the south, the tribes use manioc, corn, yams, groundnuts, beans and palm oil. Several deficiency problems are related to these cultures. In the sorghum- and millet-eating areas the conversion of grain into beer is detrimental to nutrition because of the nutrient loss it causes. It has been computed that the equivalent of 30 meals per capita per year are lost as a result of brewing beer. In the south, kwashiorkor and anaemia are common. Deficiencies of vitamin A, riboflavin and niacin in various degrees have been found among all tribes living in the Togo-Dahomey area.

In Portuguese Guinea, kwashiorkor is a major problem. Signs of anaemia as well as vitamin A, riboflavin and vitamin C deficiencies affect over 37% of the child population, especially among the Bijago tribe.

In Ghana, where infant mortality is still above 100 per 1000 live births, kwashiorkor is common, especially in the manioc-eating area. Anaemia due to iron deficiency is frequent.

In Nigeria, an immense territory that includes various cultures and ways of life, kwashiorkor is frequently seen in city hospitals. Mothers do not connect this with nutrition. Vitamin deficiencies are widespread, depending upon the various types of diet and the season.

In Cameroon, the dietary pattern and attendant deficiencies can be likened to Togo and Dahomey and divided into north and south. In the north, a diet of millet and sorghum, legumes and milk prevents a heavy deficiency disease load; in the south, where manioc, yams and bananas are the mainstays, kwashiorkor is common and illustrates the poor balance of the post-weaning and early infancy diet.

In Zaire, kwashiorkor used to be common, especially in the Kivu and Kassai areas, when nutrition surveys were made. None has been carried out in recent years but there is no reason to believe that the picture has improved much. Pellagra and scurvy have been found and goitre is common in the Upper Ouele region. Ariboflavinosis seems to be an important problem. Anaemia is very common due to a combination of iron deficiency, malaria and intestinal parasitism. It is interesting to compare the plight of such tribes as the Twa and Bushong. The Twa have gradually abandoned their original hunting way of life in favour of sedentary agriculture while the Bushong have not. Kwashiorkor has appeared among the Twa but not among the Bushong.

In the mountain areas of Rwanda and Burundi, endemic goitre is common, especially around Kitabi where 28% of the general population is reported to be affected.

East Africa

The three major countries of East Africa—Uganda, Kenya and Tanzania—suffer from a wide spectrum of deficiency diseases connected mostly with the corn diet, the lack of animal protein, iron deficiency and with the rapid urbanization. In Uganda, corn is second to millet but still expanding. White corn is preferred, in spite of its poorer value. The most common type of deficiency seen at the Mulago Hospital near Kampala is kwashiorkor and marasmus. Even in areas like Karamoja and Ankole where cattle and their milk are available, the development of children is impaired due to the lack of caloric intake which results in the protein diet being consumed for energy. Anaemia is common because of iron deficiency and is often associated with protein deficiency. Pellagra is occasionally reported in Uganda, Kenya and Tanzania. The rapid urbanization of these societies is resulting in considerable increases in mass feeding through factory canteens. Corn replaces millet as a staple food in such places with the loss in protein level this cereal implies. The preparation of legumes also leaves something to be desired in mass feeding kitchens. While on the East African farm, the pulses are usually left to simmer in water long enough for the envelope to be peeled away and only the substantial grain to remain; in canteens everything is boiled together, loading the dish with non-digestible cellulose at the expense of the protein-rich inner substance.

In Angola where diets based on corn and manioc are dominant, deficiency syndromes are common. These are alleviated somewhat in certain areas like the north where legumes provide proteins, the coastal areas where fish are abundant and the south where cattle are raised. But in the central part of the country, kwashiorkor is observed among the Ovimbundu population. Rickets, ariboflavinosis and scurvy are also reported. Pellagra is seen in areas where corn is the staple of the diet.

In Malawi, kwashiorkor is found and, in Zambia, protein deficiencies are also common. This is often ascribed to a shift in the way of life of rural families who have emigrated to the cities where the diet must be procured with money that is not generally available. The Zambian government is sponsoring a national nutrition programme which may improve the situation.

In Mozambique, a country that belongs to the corn culture, pellagra is now slowly disappearing. The main area of remaining endemicity is the Zambezia district but the disease is seasonal. Beriberi is still observed and kwashiorkor is common. Signs of vitamin A deficiency are frequently observed but usually disappear during the mango and papaya season. Signs of riboflavin deficiency are very common.

In Rhodesia, corn is planted almost everywhere in the African sectors since it is the staple food of the black population. There is even a surplus which brings an income to the grower. Pellagra, although not rampant, is still occasionally observed.

In South Africa, pellagra is still a serious problem and affects particularly the young children; it can also involve working adults. Other deficiency diseases, including rickets and scurvy, are also present.

Asia

The Middle East

In Lebanon, frank deficiency diseases are relatively rare, although subclinical vitamin A, C and D deficiencies are common among the poorer inhabitants. It is almost impossible at this stage to give a picture of the state of nutrition in Israel. The conditions of life there at present do not allow the drawing of valid conclusions.

In Syria, according to rather old data, frank clinical deficiency diseases do not appear to be frequent, but subclinical signs and symptoms are commonly found. Thirty-three percent of the children in the 5–16 year age group studied in one survey were found to show clinical signs of vitamin A deficiency. The high consumption of whole wheat and other cereal products is probably responsible for the comparative absence of vitamin B-complex deficiences. Scurvy is rare but subclinical vitamin C deficiencies were found in 58% of the children investigated. These signs of subclinical vitamin C deficiency appear to be more common in the grain-producing areas where little fruit is grown. Ariboflavinosis is reportedly rare. Cases of rickets are common, especially in urban areas. In Damascus, 14% of young children at maternal and child health centres or admitted to hospitals have been shown to exhibit frank signs of rickets. Iron deficiency anaemia, associated with poor nutrition and aggravated by hookworm infestation, is a common cause of admission to hospitals of young children.

Malnutrition is considered to be one of the major health problems of Iraq. Actual starvation is rare, but the majority of the inhabitants subsist on a diet grossly deficient in caloric content and nutritional balance. Under-nutrition, anaemia and avitaminosis are prevalent, especially among low-income town dwellers and farmers. As a result of the deficiency of good quality proteins, some kwashiorkor has been occasionally reported. Clinical manifestations of vitamin A deficiency are widespread but pellagra is absent and beriberi is rare. However, clinical signs of vitamin C deficiency are commonly observed and cases of scurvy are reportedly numerous. Vitamin C is absent from the diet for as much as 3 months a year. As in North Africa and the remainder of the Middle East, deficiencies in intake of calcium and especially in the consumption and production of vitamin D result in numerous cases of osteomalacia and rickets. Minor symptoms of ariboflavinosis are frequently observed.

Saudi Arabia is a country originally included in the wheat culture which is now drifting towards the rice culture. Yet, the conversion is not complete and wheat, millet and sorghum are still the most important cereals. In spite of the enormous petroleum wealth of the country, the majority of the inhabitants of the Arabian peninsula suffer from undernourishment and malnutrition. Night blindness is reportedly prevalent in Saudi Arabia as well as vitamin C deficiency, scurvy, rickets, ariboflavinosis and nutritional anaemia. Beriberi is rare and pellagra is said to be sporadic.

In Turkey, wheat consumption is high and is increasing steadily. One half of the total caloric intake is supplied by wheat, prepared in a variety of ways in addition to its use in bread. Frank deficiency diseases are generally not a serious problem but they do occur in certain areas and at certain seasons. The most common are rickets and osteomalacia. Scurvy has been a problem, especially in the north-east. Pellagra has been reported among the inhabitants of the Black Sea region where the diet is largely based on corn. The intake of vitamin A and carotene is low and follicular keratosis, often associated with low vitamin A intake, has been observed.

Three major cereals are grown in Iran, viz. wheat, barley and rice. Wheat, however, is the most important crop. The few nutritional surveys that have been carried out in Iran indicate that a considerable proportion of the population shows clinical signs and symptoms of nutritional deficiencies ranging from mild to severe. Vitamin deficiencies are reportedly widespread. Obvious signs of vitamin A and vitamin C deficiencies as well as ariboflavinosis are found, especially in children from Bushire, Abadan, Shiraz, Ishfahan, Teheran, Tabriz and Risht. Rickets is reportedly common, especially in urban areas, and osteomalacia is common in the south-east. Night blindness is prevalent in the adult population of the cities. Pellagra is said to occur in corn-eating areas. Recent investigations have shown that consumption of large amounts of phytate in the form of unleavened whole wheat bread by the rural population interferes extensively with the utilization of mineral nutrients including calcium, iron, zinc, magnesium and phosphorus. Preliminary experiments indicate that the phytate of village bread is more potent in its effects upon calcium and zinc metabolism than is pure sodium phytate. The prevalence of rickets and osteomalacia, retardation of growth and sexual development, and iron deficiency anaemia are direct effects of these high phytate intakes.

A large proportion of the rice consumed in India is of the parboiled type. In certain regions and in a few communities, raw milled rice is preferred and eaten. This practice can be traced to social or religious prejudices against parboiled rice, although certain groups sometimes resented the offensive odour. As elsewhere in areas where kwashiorkor has been described, it occurs in children receiving a faulty diet after weaning, essentially based on starchy foods among families which cannot afford the purchase of proteins. Vitamin A deficiency is common, manifested by a thickening and folding of the scleral conjunctiva, by Bitot spots and by keratomalacia. The latter symptom is said to be common in Calcutta where it has been observed by certain researchers in 10.5 per 10 000 persons. Night blindness is also often found in children of the poorer classes of India although the point is made that not all cases of night blindness are the result of vitamin A deficiency. Dry and rough skin is frequently encountered among children, often associated with dryness of the eye. Indian investigators believe that vitamin A deficiencies are not the only cause of this symptom, but hypothesize that it may also be correlated with fatty acid deficiencies. Angular stomatitis and scrotal eczema also occur, indicating probable important deficiencies in nicotinic acid and riboflavin.

Thiamine deficiencies are prevalent among the rice-eating population. The most important centres of occurrence are the districts of Ganjan, Vizagapatan, Guadivari, Krishna, Guntur and Vellore. In addition, a few circumscribed areas of beriberi occur in West Bengal and Assam. Pellagra occurs sporadically throughout India, although it is more common in the parts of the state of Madras where beriberi is endemic. Patwardan remarks that pellagra does not affect large numbers of the population at any one time but causes cases to occur continuously in small numbers. Vitamin C deficiency is not one of the current manifestations of malnutrition although the usual intake of vitamin C in poor Indian diets is low. Rickets and osteomalacia are found, especially in the state of Bombay. In Orissa, the incidence of rickets has been reported at 0.2–1.6% of the children, while 3.2% of the children of Uttar Pradesh are estimated to be afflicted. Osteomalacia is particularly common in the Punjab. Simple goitre is endemic in the Himalayas and the South Himalayan region. Urinary calculi, especially in the bladders of young children, are common. This is believed by some to be the result of the precipitation of minerals, especially calcium, in urines low in nitrogen. This is the case in vegetarian diets and in areas where the consumption of protein is low.

In the South-East Asian peninsula, the deficiency disease situation has much improved over the past 10 years. While there is no information on Burma, it is known that Thailand has practically controlled beriberi. In South Vietnam, with the exception of areas in the previous war zones or in the congested suburbs of Saigon, deficiency diseases are only rarely seen. Beriberi and signs of vitamin A deficiency are becoming rare.

Little is known about nutrition in modern China. As for the Asian part of the U.S.S.R., all that is known is that general malnutrition existed in the 1950s in what has now come to be known as "the Gulag Archipelago" (Solzhenitsyn).

CONCLUSIONS

Given the multiplicity of causes of deficiency diseases, no single panacea can be accepted as a cure. The only general recommendation that can be made to planners is to consider the spectrum of causes that create the problem, evaluate priorities and conceive plans which reflect the local circumstances. Certainly co-operation between governmental authorities, international agencies and foreign-aid donors should be intensified. Nutrition education is probably the most important tool available to correct deficient diets since the missing nutrients are often available in unused or misused local resources.

ACKNOWLEDGEMENTS

Figures 20.1, and 20.3–20.8 have been adapted from the American Geographical Society's "Atlas of Diseases". Figure 20.2 and caption are reproduced with permission from the National Geographic Society.

REFERENCES

Baker, H. and Frank, O. (1968). "Clinical Vitaminology". Wiley Interscience, New York.

Chávez, A. and Rosado, A. P. (1967). *Bol. Of. Sanit. Panamer.* **55**, 398–404.

Cravioto, J., Gómez, F., Ramos-Galvan, R., Frenk, S., Montano, E. L. and Garcμa, N. (1960). *Bol. Of. Sanit. Panamer.* **48**, 383–391.

Gaitán, E. and Wahner, H. W. (1968). *In* "Endemic Goiter" (Ed. J. B. Stabury), pp. 267–290. Pan American Health Organization, Washington, D.C.

Institute of Nutrition of Central America and Panama (1969). "Evaluación Nutricional de la Población de Centro América y Panamá". I.N.C.A.P., Guatemala City.

Madeiros-Neto, G. A., Lobo, L. C. G. and Nicolau, W. (1968). *In* "Endemic Goiter" (Ed. J. B. Stanbury), pp. 179–182. Pan American Health Organization, Washington, D.C.

May, J. M. (1961). "The Ecology of Malnutrition in the Far and Near East". Hafner, New York.

May, J. M. (1963). "The Ecology of Malnutrition in Five Countries of Eastern and Central Europe". Hafner, New York.

May, J. M. (1965). "The Ecology of Malnutrition in Middle Africa". Hafner, New York.

May, J. M. (1966). "The Ecology of Malnutrition in Central and South-Eastern Europe". Hafner, New York.

May, J. M. (1967). "The Ecology of Malnutrition in Northern Africa". Hafner, New York.

May, J. M. (1968). "The Ecology of Malnutrition in French-Speaking Countries of West Africa and Madagascar". Hafner, New York.

May, J. M. and McLellan, D. L. (1970). "The Ecology of Malnutrition in Eastern Africa and Four Countries of Western Africa". Hafner, New York.

May, J. M. and McLellan, D. L. (1971). "The Ecology of Malnutrition in Seven Countries of Southern Africa and in Portuguese Guinea". Hafner, New York.

May, J. M. and McLellan, D. L. (1972). "The Ecology of Malnutrition in Mexico and Central America". Hafner, New York.

May, J. M. and McLellan, D. L. (1973). "The Ecology of Malnutrition in the Caribbean". Hafner, New York.

May, J. M. and McLellan, D. L. (1974). "The Ecology of Malnutrition in Eastern South America". Hafner, New York.

May, J. M. and McLellan, D. L. (1974). "The Ecology of Malnutrition in Western South America". Hafner, New York.

Monckeberg, F. *et al.* (1967). *Rev. Chil. Ped.* **38**, 491–522.

National Academy of Sciences (National Research Council) (1968). "Recommended Dietary Allowances". National Academy of Sciences, Washington, D.C.

Nutrition Canada (1973). "Nutrition: A National Priority". Information Canada, Ottawa.

Tannahill, R. (1973). "Food in History." Stein and Day, New York.

Glossary of Selected Terms

(to be used in conjunction with the Index)

Some of the terms are not, or only partially, explained in the text

---

Acanthocheilonema (perstans, streptocerca)—filarial worms. Their offspring (microfilaria) circulate in the blood stream. They are transmitted by blood-sucking *Culicoides* (midges).

Aëdes—a genus of mosquitoes which carry the virus that causes yellow fever.

Aestivate—adaptions to permit survival or to become dormant during summer (cf. to hibernate in winter).

Amoebocytes—wandering cells.

Anaphylactic—having an increased susceptibility to foreign protein.

Anoxia—deficiency of oxygen in the tissues.

Antibody—a natural substance that protects the body against a disease or infection.

Antigenic structure—the structure of that fraction (usually a protein) of an invading organism which elicits an antibody response.

Anthropophilic—preferring human beings to other animals; usually applied to blood sucking insects, esp. mosquitoes.

Arbovirus—virus transmitted by arthropods.

Arteriosclerosis—thickening, hardening and loss of elasticity of the arterial wall, usually due to atherosclerotic changes. The arteries may become narrower and cause impairment of the flow of blood.

Atherosclerosis—lesions on the inside of the arteries with fibrous and fat deposits that lead to thickening, hardening, narrowing or even occlusion of the arteries and thus impede the flow of blood through the arteries.

Aucthonous—found in places of formation or development; not removed to a new situation.

Bancroftian filariasis—a tropical disease caused by thread-like parasitic worms called filaria (*Wuchereria bancrofti*), often resulting in large swellings.

Cancer—any one of several diseases that result when the process of cell division, by which tissues normally grow and renew themselves, gets out of control and leads to the development of malignant cells. These cancer cells multiply in an unco-ordinated way, independently of normal growth-control mechanisms, to form a tumour.

Carcinogen—any substance or irritant that contributes to the development of cancer.

Cardiac arrest—cessation of the heart's contractions.

Ceiling temperature—temperature beyond which a germ will not grow.

Cercaria—the free-swimming larval stage of a trematode (fluke) which emerges after development in a snail.

Cerebrovascular diseases—any brain disease caused by impaired blood flow. The main forms are cerebral haemorrhage, cerebral thrombosis and cerebral embolism.

Chemotactic—attraction of living cells to (positive) or repulsion from (negative) other organisms by chemical stimulation.

Chorio-allantois of developing chick embryo—membrane around a fertilized hen's egg; virus can be grown on it.

Chrysops—a blood sucking fly.

Cohort (study in epidemiology)—the study over a prolonged period of time of a group of individuals with a common characteristic, e.g. the year of birth.

Commensal—a parasitic micro-organism that co-exists with its host. The commensal derives benefit but the host is neither harmed nor benefitted.

Communicable disease—a disease that is transmitted from one person to another, or from an animal to a person. It may or may not be contagious; an infectious disease.

Conjunctiva—the transparent mucous membrane or fine lining of the inner surfaces of the eyelids; it also covers part of the front of the eyeball.

Contagious—spread of disease by direct contact with the body of the infected individual.

Contractile vacuoles—a pulsating fluid-filled cavity in protozoa which discharges its contents periodically to the exterior; it controls the water content of the cell.

Coronary arteries—arteries that supply blood to the tissues of the heart.

Coronary or ischaemic heart disease—cardiac disability from insufficient supply of blood to the heart muscles: in most cases caused by advanced atherosclerosis in the coronary arteries.

Cross-section (study in epidemiology)—the study of individuals of different ages and sexes at one specified point in time.

Culicine mosquitoes—mosquitoes of the genera *Culex mansonia* (including vectors of some filarial infections) and *Aedes* (including vectors of dengue and urban yellow fever).

Dextral—(of snail shell) coiled to the right.

Digenetic—having two stages of multiplication, a sexual one in the mature forms, an asexual one in the larvae forms.

Dilation—expansion, e.g. of pupil of the eye, or of blood-vessels.

Dioecious—having two sexes in separate individuals.

Discoid—flat and circular in shape.

Disseminated—scattered over a wide area.

Embolism—occlusion or blockage of a blood vessel by a detached clot or by some other particles, including bubbles of air or other gas, or particles of fat.

Endogenous—originating within the organism, reactivation.

Endotoxin—toxin within the bacterial cell.

Enzymatic structure—the molecular structure of an enzyme.

Eosinophils—type of white blood cell containing granules, so-called because they take up acidic dyes such as eosin. The cells are formed in the tissues and in the blood in the reaction to parasites. In such a reaction the cells occur in large quantities in the blood (oesinophilia).

Epithelial cells—surface cells of skin or mucous membrane.

Epizootic—descriptive of a disease (a) of high morbidity that is *temporarily* prevalent among animals; (b) attacking many animals in any region simultaneously, the disease spreading rapidly.

Erythrocytic phase—the phase of the life-cycle of *Plasmodium* spent in human red blood cells; so-called exoerythrocytic phase is now known to be spent in the human liver.

Exogenous—reinfection, developing or originating from outside.

Exotoxin—toxin produced and liberated by bacteria into their environment.

Faculative parasite—an organism that can survive independently but which may be parasitic, i.e. co-exist with another.

Feral—wild, untamed; resembling a wild animal; sometimes applied to domestic animals which have broken off their associations with humans and are living an independent existence.

Fibrin—a protein precipitate, a precursor of which occurs in the blood. This precipitate occurs at an early stage in the reaction against certain parasites.

Fibrinogen—the soluble protein in the blood that is the precursor of fibrin.

Fulminating—overwhelmingly severe, cf lightning.

Geotropic—a tendency to move towards (positive) or away from (negative) the earth.

Glycogen—an energy-rich carbohydrate.

Haemorrhagic (hypertoxic)—highly toxic form of disease in which haemorrhage occurs into skin or from body openings, e.g. rectum, urethra.

Haematuria—the passage of blood in the urine.

Haemocete—the body cavity of an insect.

Heart attack—a sudden disturbance of heart function that occurs in coronary and certain other heart diseases.

Hermaphroditic—an organism having both male and female sexual organs.

Herxheimer reaction—an anaphylactic reaction usually produced by a drug in which all the symptoms of infection are rapidly increased due to the release of breakdown products of the parasite.

Holoendemic areas—areas in which effectively the whole population is affected by a disease.

Hypertension—high blood pressure, abnormal elevation of arterial blood pressure as a result of narrowing of the small arteries. Essential hypertension is hypertension of unknown origin, the most common form of consistently elevated blood pressure.

Iliac crests—flared bones above the hip.

Imagocidal—killing the imago or adult insect.

Immunology—the study of immunity and the immune processes.

Infectious disease—*see* communicable disease.

Intradermal inoculation—injection into the layers of the skin.

Ischaemic—*see* coronary.

Labile—unstable, changeable.

Loa loa—parasitic African threadworm.

Lyse—to break up, to cause lysis, or dissolution.

Macrophages—large cells derived from a type of white blood cell (monocytes) with the property of engulfing and destroying foreign particles (such as micro-organisms and parasites).

Maculo-papulus—spot of skin midway between a flat spot (macule) and a raised spot (papule).

Metronidazole—a chemotherapeutic agent used in the therapy of certain infections by protozoa such as amoebiasis, trichomoniasis and giardiasis, and of infections by gram-negative bacteria.

Miracidium—free swimming larva of the trematode which emerges from the egg.

Morphology—shape of germ; its structure as seen under microscope.

Mucous membrane—lining of body channels, e.g. nose, mouth, respiratory and intestinal tract are covered with mucous.

Myocardial infarct or infarction—a manifestation of acute ischaemic heart disease.

Necrosis—the death of cells, tissues or a portion of an organ in the living body.

Nematode—a long, cylindrical parasitic worm with protective outer coating covering a muscular body, with a simple nervous system and an intestine.

Neoplasm—a new and abnormal growth in the body; a tumour.

Obligatory parasite—an organism that depends for its survival on co-existing with a host organism.

Operculate—having a lid or cover.

Osmotic action—action whereby fluid moves into the egg, raising the pressure and causing the egg shell to rupture.

Overt—open.

Parenchyma—the functional elements of an organ, as opposed to its structural elements.

Phage—accepted abbreviation of the term "bacteriophage"—which is not unlike a virus. Specific types of phage affect certain bacteria and cause their dissolution. In some cases the bacterium becomes resistant to the phage which may remain associated and lead to a change in the function of the bacterium.

Phototropic—a tendency of an organism to turn to (positive) or away from (negative) light.

Piperazines—a group of chemical substances which are effective against nematodes.

Plexus—network of veins. Vesical: of the bladder; mesenteric: of the fold of tissue which attaches the bowel to the posterior abdominal wall.

Pre-eruptive state—stage of a disease before the typical rash appears.

Prodromal stage—stage of a disease just before typical symptoms appear.

Prospective incidence (study in epidemiology)—the follow-up of large groups containing individuals of varied age and sex.

Pustules—blisters containing pus.

Quadrinucleate cyst—a cyst containing four nuclei; usually applied to the infective stage of the dysentery amoeba.

Reticulo-endothelial cells—special cells, mostly in the liver and spleen, which are concerned with the control of infection.

Rheumatic fever—a sequel to infection by group A streptococci characterized by heart disease and/or acute pain and inflamation of the joints.

Rheumatic heart disease—damage to the heart valves and heart muscle resulting from rheumatic fever.

Scintigraphy—radioactive scanning.

Serological tests—tests for presence of antibodies against germs in blood of infected person.

Serology—the study of serum, with particular reference to immunity reactions.

Single antigenic virus—a virus which remains constant in composition, e.g. smallpox; a vaccine prepared against one strain of smallpox virus protects against all strains. Influenza virus, in contrast, is constantly changing, and vaccines against influenza must be altered when a change in virus strain takes place.

Sinistral—(of snail shell) coiled to the left.

Skin epithelium—the surface cells of the skin.

Sporocyst—the sac within the snail containing the reproductive cells.

Stroke—any cerebrovascular disease having an abrupt onset. The leading symptom is paralysis of the body.

Thermolabile—sensitive to external heat.

Thrombin—an enzyme which can clot many hundred times its own weight of fibrinogen.

Thrombosis—occlusion or blockage of a blood vessel by clotting within the vessel itself at the site of occlusion.

Trematode—a fluke.

Trimester—a term of three months.

Trochanter—the hip bone.

Tumour—a swelling on or in part of the body, resulting from either abnormal growth of tissue or, as in a cyst, from a collection of fluid. Tumours may be *benign* (non-cancerous) or *malignant* (cancerous).

Variola—smallpox.

Vector—a carrier.

Vesicles—blisters.

Viraemia—the presence of virus in the bloodstream.

Zoonosis—an animal disease that may affect man.

Zoophilic—preferring animals.

Subject Index

J

O

Q

R

U